Practical Guide to Interpret Visual Fields

Practical Guide to Interpret Visual Fields

Fourth Edition

GR Reddy MS (PGI Chandigarh)
Managing Director
GR Reddy Eye Care Center
Tadepalligudem, Andhra Pradesh, India
grreddy_ophthal@hotmail.com

Co-Author
G Jayamadhury DNB (Oph)

Foreword
R Ramakrishnan

JAYPEE

JAYPEE BROTHERS MEDICAL PUBLISHERS
The Health Sciences Publisher
New Delhi | London

Jaypee Brothers Medical Publishers (P) Ltd

Headquarters
Jaypee Brothers Medical Publishers (P) Ltd
4838/24, Ansari Road, Daryaganj
New Delhi 110 002, India
Phone: +91-11-43574357
Fax: +91-11-43574314
Email: jaypee@jaypeebrothers.com

Overseas Office
J.P. Medical Ltd
83 Victoria Street, London
SW1H 0HW (UK)
Phone: +44 20 3170 8910
Fax: +44 (0)20 3008 6180
Email: info@jpmedpub.com

Website: www.jaypeebrothers.com
Website: www.jaypeedigital.com

Practical Guide to Interpret Visual Fields

First Edition: 2003
Second Edition: 2006
Third Edition: 2010
Fourth Edition: 2020, Reprint: 2023

ISBN 978-93-89587-01-2

Printed in India

Dedicated to

My brother Dr Satya G Reddy
(Professor of Pediatrics, Women and Infants Hospital,
Brown University, Providence RI, USA and An Eminent
World-renowned Vitamin D Scientist)
Who inspired me to think rationally and conclude logically

Foreword

It is always a pleasure to write the foreword for GR Reddy's *Practical Guide to Interpret Visual Fields.* Humphrey visual field plays an important role not only in the diagnosis of glaucoma, but also monitoring the visual field progression. I appreciate GR Reddy for his wonderful work on his fourth edition of the book. After thoroughly understanding the basics of Humphrey, he has analyzed his own cases of glaucoma and written the book. He is bringing something new in every edition. This 4th edition is an updated version of the earlier edition with lots of illustrations and case scenario. The book will be really useful for the postgraduates, fellows and practicing ophthalmologists. He has simplified the complex subject and has given in a way that is easy-to-understand by all. It is nice that he has given new concept of perimetry-based classification for primary open-angle glaucoma (POAG) which is based on the location and direction of progression of field defect. This will definitely help to know the severity of glaucoma and to set a target intraocular pressure (IOP). In this book, a new chapter has been added regarding a new point pattern 24-2C SITA Faster which will help to pick up field defect starting in the bare area between 3° and 9° circle points in 24-2. He has made this book more comprehensive, readable and easily understandable. Definitely, it will be a useful guide for all.

R Ramakrishnan
Head of Glaucoma Services
Aravind Eye Hospital
Tirunelveli, Tamil Nadu, India

Preface to the Fourth Edition

This book has journeyed through three editions since its inception in 2003. Ever since its first publication, there has been a significant change in my understanding of visual fields. The first few pages of this edition dealing with the fundamentals of automated static perimetry and understanding of single field analysis (SFA) remain the same as in the previous editions. The interpretation of single field analysis printout has been stressed in this edition.

All these years, fields were interpreted depending on the stage of glaucoma being early, established or advanced and recommended the 10-2 point pattern only for advanced cases of glaucoma. I have based this book on my clinical experience. My concepts and understanding of the disease has been changed when I happened to see a case with a prominent retinal nerve fiber layer (RNFL) defect in the macular area (10° field) which became evident only in 10-2 but not in 24-2 owing to large bare area. Since then I started to give more importance to the location of field defect. In this edition, I have emphasized on the indications to repeat the test with 10-2 point pattern.

By definition, glaucoma is a progressive neuronal loss and its management depends on location, extent, depth and the direction of progression of the field defect. Of the above parameters, the location of the field defect and its relation to fixation is of utmost importance. This book intends to throw light on the development of 2 new classification systems of glaucoma based on the location of the field defect (perimetry-based classification) and step by step analysis of SFA correlating with the fundus pictures and the optical coherence tomography (OCT) images. I propose to highlight the importance of location and the direction of progression of field defect in setting the target IOP and reemphasize that the older ideology of reserving 10-2 point pattern for advanced glaucoma is no longer tenable.

A chapter has been added on a new point pattern 24-2C SITA faster; which was introduced by Zeiss, where 10 additional points are created in the bare area between 3° and 9° circle of 24-2 point pattern. This can aid in picking up early glaucoma and may warrant the need of 10-2.

Visual field index (VFI) which forms the basis in glaucoma progression analysis (GPA) is not calculated in 10-2 point pattern. As this book highlights the importance of 10-2 even in early cases of glaucoma, GPA has not been discussed in this book.

I am grateful to Dr R Ramakrishnan, Head, Glaucoma Services, Aravind Eye Hospital, Tirunelveli, Tamil Nadu, India, for his foreword to this edition. My sincere thanks to Professor Tanuj Dada, Glaucoma Department, AIIMS, New Delhi; Dr SR Krishna Das, Director-HRD, Aravind Eye Care System and Medical Consultant, Glaucoma Services, Aravind Eye Hospital, Madurai, for their comments about this book. My heartful thanks to my children Dr G Jayamadhury and Dr Sandeep Reddy for their help in preparing this final copy. Most importantly I can never forget the loving cooperation of my wife Mrs Laxmi in supporting me as

I wrote this book. I thank my parents for inculcating in me the idea that any subject can be understood with a rational approach.

I would like to thank Shri Jitendar P Vij (Group Chairman), Mr Ankit Vij (Managing Director), Ms Chetna Malhotra Vohra (Associate Director—Content Strategy) of M/s Jaypee Brothers Medical Publishers (P) Ltd, New Delhi, India, for their untiring support.

GR Reddy

Preface to the First Edition

The primary intention of this book is to present automated perimetry in a simple and illustrated manner devoid of all technical details and theoretical abstractions which abound in standard perimetry textbooks. It is designed to serve as a handbook for practicing ophthalmologist by providing information to supplement what is available in currently prescribed textbooks. Its contents have been so organized to facilitate easy use by all practicing ophthalmologists and postgraduate students and to serve as a guide in the interpretation of visual field printouts of automated perimetry.

Emphasis is laid on the fundamentals of automated perimetry; especially the units used to express light intensity and retinal threshold value, selection of the test and interpretation of single field analysis printouts. Change analysis printouts of selected cases gleaned from my personal experience, have been included for a broader perspective.

This book owes its existence to an update lecture I delivered at Kakinada to the appreciative gathering of colleagues and friends. I convey my special thanks to Dr R Sriram, Nayana Eye Care Center, Kakinada, for inviting me to the above conference on behalf of Kakinada Ophthalmic Association. I am deeply indebted to a large number of talented and thoughtful colleague ophthalmologists who helped me in many ways during the preparation of this book. To each of these my dearest friends, I wish to express my most sincere gratitude.

I am grateful to Dr Amod Gupta, Professor and Head of the Department of Ophthalmology, PGI, Chandigarh, for giving his Foreword. My sincere thanks to my father Sri G Subbi Reddy, Retd. Principal, Bobbili College, mother Smt Jayalakshmi, wife Lakshmi and children Dr Jaya Madhury and Dr Sandeep Reddy for their support in completing this book.

I hope the readers of this book will find it useful in their day-to-day practice. I am conscious that my first endeavor may have shortcomings and hope discerning readers will help me to improve it in the future.

I am thankful to Dr K Vengala Rao, Former Professor and Head of the Department of Ophthalmology, Guntur Medical College (AP), Dr G Chandra Sekhar, Director, VST Center for Glaucoma Care, LV Prasad Eye Institute, Hyderabad and Dr K Viswanath, Professor and Head of the Department of Ophthalmology, Osmania Medical College, Hyderabad for their comments in this book.

GR Reddy

Contents

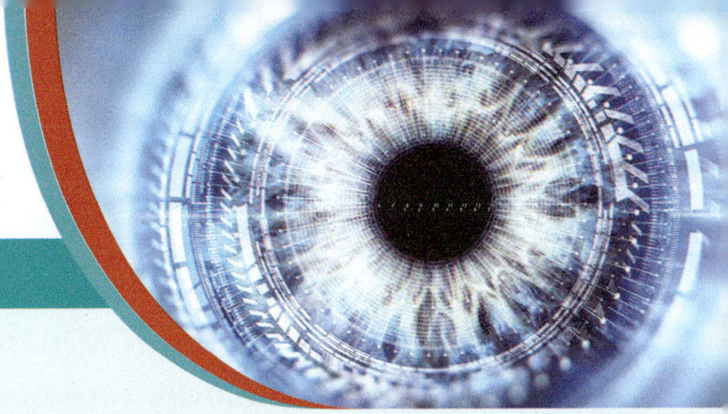

CHAPTER

1

Introduction to Automated Static Perimetry

Automated perimetry is the current gold standard to diagnose and manage glaucoma. The main aim of this book is to help the ophthalmologist to understand the basic fundamentals of automated static perimetry, to select the most appropriate test to the clinical condition one is dealing with, to understand the visual field printouts and to interpret the printouts without much difficulty so that one should be able:

1. To identify a field defect.
2. To decide whether the field defect is due to glaucoma.
3. To set target intraocular pressure (IOP).
4. To make a reasonable decision whether the defect is progressive or not.

REASONS FOR COMPUTERIZED PERIMETRY

1. Reproducible testing conditions.
2. *Data-storage capability*: Results can be compared overtime and analyzed using expert system software.
3. More sensitive testing. Many researchers claim static perimetry to be superior to kinetic perimetry to identify defects.
4. Easy operation and menu-driven software make automated perimetry easy to learn and to use.
5. Requires little technician training for reliable results.

HISTORY

1970: The original octopus perimeter was first introduced. It never gained popularity due to its very large room size and high expense.

1982: Humphrey field analyzer was first displayed at American Academy of Ophthalmology.

1983: August-Michael Patella showed its first clinical trial.

1984: February-started production and became very popular because of its small size and affordable price.

ROLE OF VISUAL FIELDS IN THE FIELD OF OPHTHALMOLOGY

Every ophthalmologist in his/her daily practice requires visual fields mainly for two purposes:

1. To diagnose various clinical conditions:
    a. Ocular conditions—glaucoma and optic nerve disorders
    b. Central nervous system (CNS) conditions—optic nerve pathway disorders, CNS tumors and occipital lobe disorders)
2. To manage glaucoma.

Role of Visual Fields in Making a Diagnosis

The loss of retinal sensitivity will present in three forms: Localized form, uniform generalized form and irregular generalized form with a definite pattern of the field defect, from which we diagnose various conditions. So, we must know the pattern of the field defect even when it is masked by generalized depression due to cataract, media opacities, uncorrected refractive error, optic atrophy, etc. to diagnose various conditions.

The pattern of field defect in glaucoma: It depends on the stage of glaucoma. Visual fields are required to diagnose glaucoma at an early stage. In early stage it can present as nasal step, Seidel scotoma, irregular loss of sensitivity on either side of horizontal axis and isolated scotomas either in the arcuate nerve fiber zone or within 10° circle area around fixation.

The pattern of the field defect due to cataract: Mostly it is a uniform generalized field defect. Occasionally, it may present with irregular generalized field defect with more loss of sensitivity at the center. This type of field defect is usually seen in dense central lenticular opacities.

The pattern of the field defect due to optic nerve disorders:

1. Optic neuritis—generalized depression, central scotomas.
2. Anterior ischemic optic neuropathy—altitudinal field defects.

The pattern of the field defect due to tumor pressing the central binasal fibers of optic chiasma: Bitemporal hemianopia.

The pattern of the field defect due to occipital lobe infarcts: Homonymous hemianopia. The most important role of visual field is to tell us the pattern of the field defect through which we can diagnose various conditions.

Role of Visual Fields in the Management of Glaucoma

In established cases of glaucoma we need to know the details of the field defect regarding its location, extent, depth, direction of progression of the field defect and the foveal status. The target IOP will be decided on these factors. In advanced cases of glaucoma, we need to know the details of sensitivity around fixation point to explain the prognosis to the patient. Our aim in the management of glaucoma is to arrest progression of the field defect due to glaucoma. Hence we require a base line visual field and the follow-up fields preferably on a single sheet so that the comparison of the fields becomes easy. With this background the single field analysis printout and the overview printout have been developed.

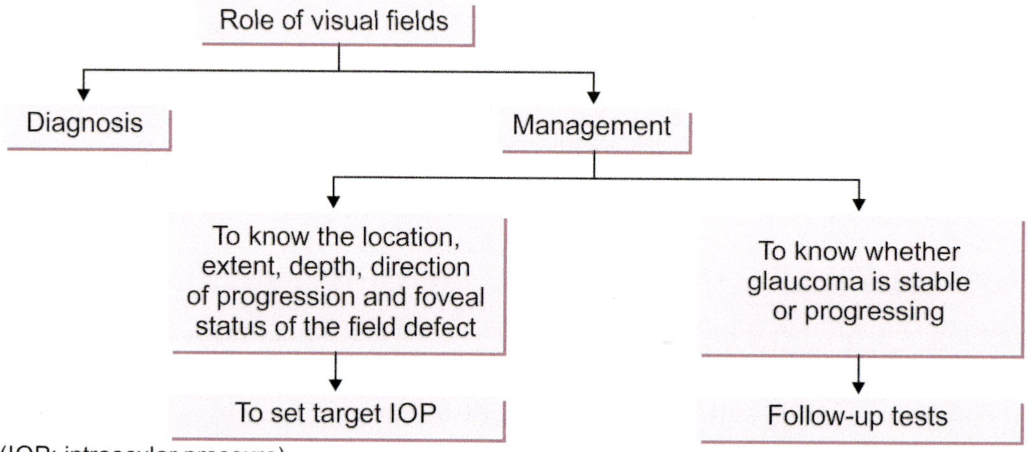

(IOP: intraocular pressure)

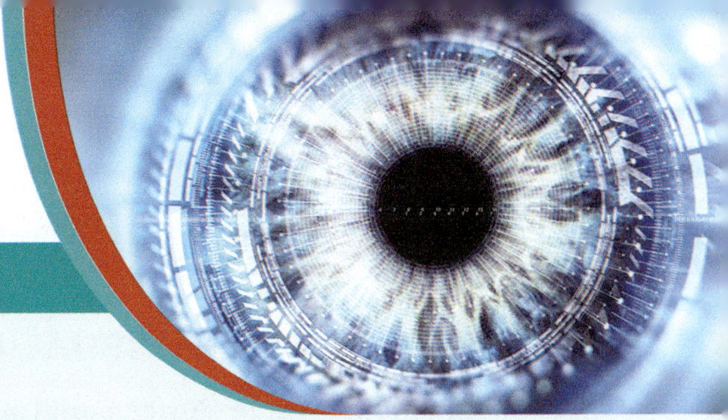

CHAPTER

2

Fundamentals of Automated Perimetry

DEFINITION OF VISUAL FIELD

The visual field is defined as that part of the environment that is visible to the steadily fixing eye. The extension of visual field is as follows:

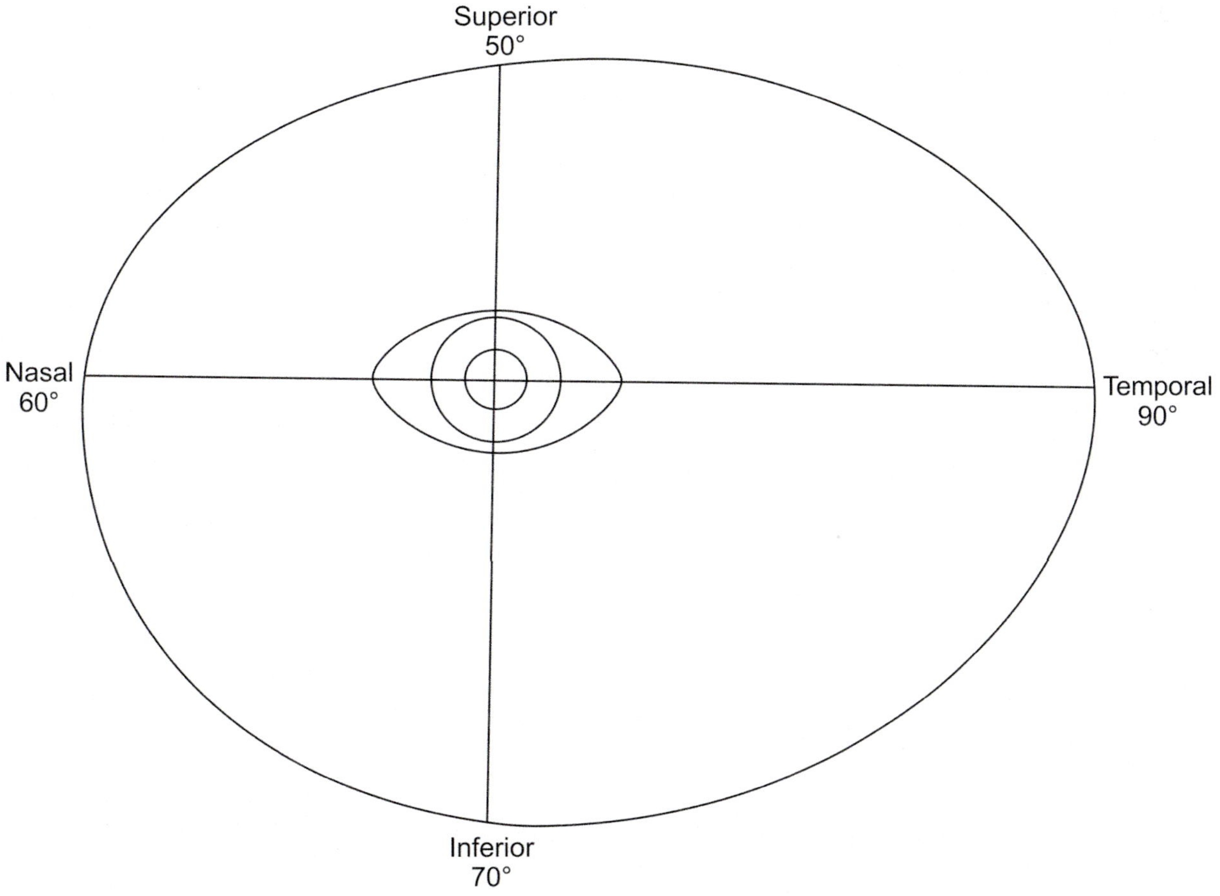

The functional boundaries of normal visual field approximate a spiral; 50° above, 60° nasally, 70° below and 90° temporal.

MEASUREMENT OF VISUAL FIELDS

The visual field is three-dimensional and is measured in two ways:

1. **Kinetic perimetry**
2. **Static perimetry**

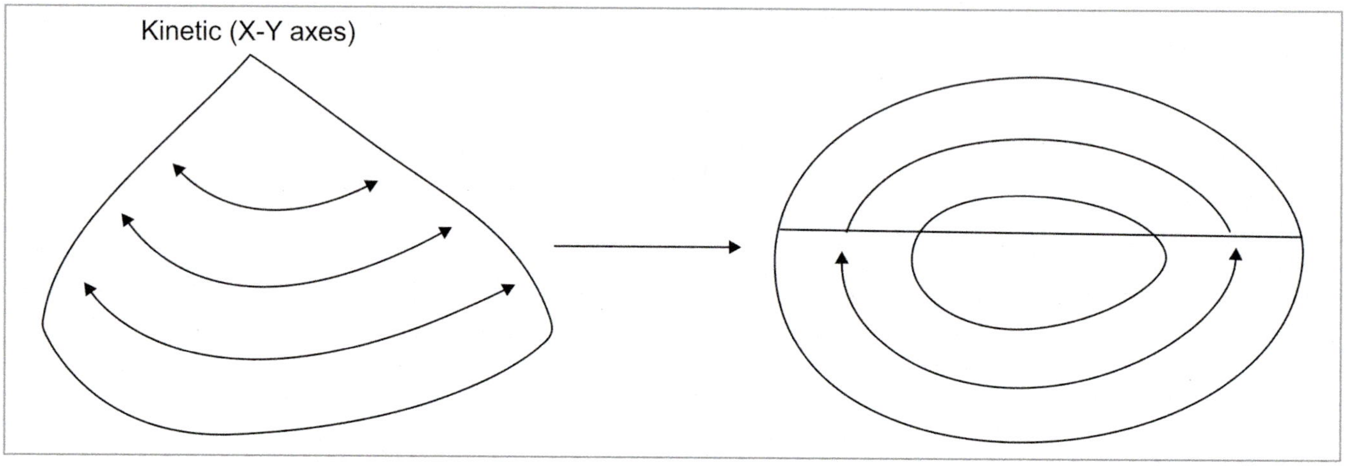

When the island hill of vision is kinetically explored along the X-Y axis (i.e. a plane parallel to the surface of the sea), the locations of points with the same threshold are identified; these are isopters.

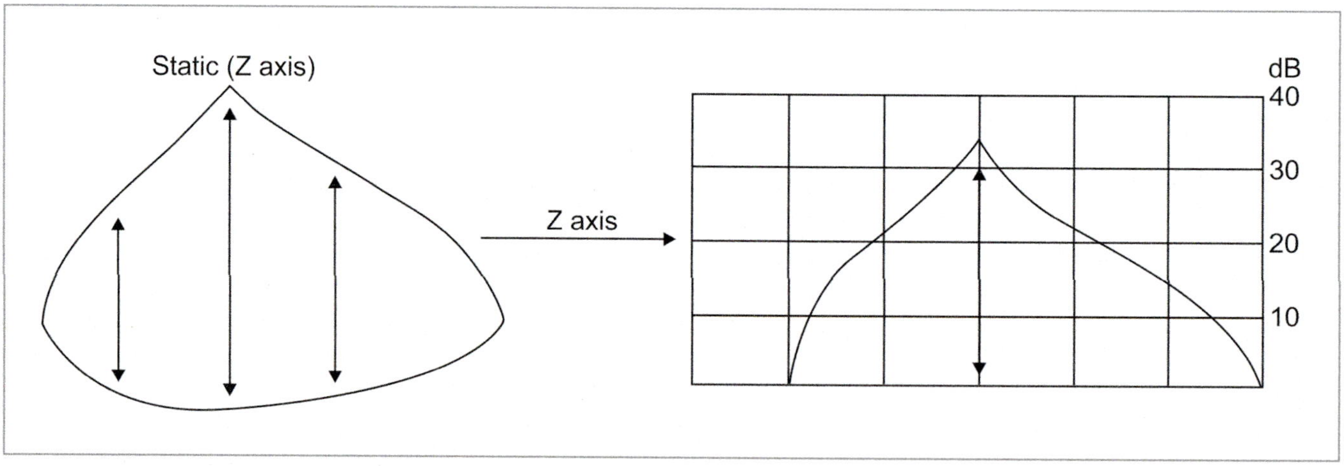

When the island hill of vision is statically explored along the Z axis (i.e. in a plane perpendicular to the surface of the sea) the varying points of sensitivity are identified; these are the thresholds displayed as meridional cut.

KINETIC PERIMETRY

Measuring along X-Y axis, the border of the visual field is outlined when the object is moved from a non-seeing area to seeing area.

Disadvantages

Kinetic tests are suprathreshold and are not always reproducible and are highly dependent on skill of the technician. Early or subtle changes may be overlooked.

STATIC PERIMETRY

The main aim of static perimetry is to find out the threshold of retina at various fixed points. Static perimetry is a technique where the patient looks at a small fixation point, located at the center of a white hemispherical bowl and the light stimuli are briefly presented at fixed stationary locations usually for about 200 milliseconds duration. The patient presses a response button when the stimulus is detected. Usually the factors affecting the stimulus visibility are stimulus size, background illumination and brightness of the stimulus. In static perimetry the size of the stimulus and the background illumination remain constant, the light intensity is varied according to a staircase (bracketing) procedure to define the minimum intensity necessary for the detection of stimulus.

Size of the stimulus: The standard stimulus size for all perimeters is Goldmann size III. The size of the stimulus can be changed depending on the clinical conditions. The size III can be changed to size V in case of macular disorders and advanced glaucoma. Please note that during the entire test period, the size of the stimulus whether it is size III or size V will remain constant along with the background illumination while, the intensity of light stimulus varies.

Background illumination: The background illumination is not the same for all perimeters. The background illumination for different field analyzers are shown **below.**

Octopus 101	Octopus 1-2-3	Humphrey 700	Dicon
4 asb (1.27 cd/m^2)	31.4 asb (10 cd/m^2)	31.5 asb (~10 cd/m^2)	31.5 asb (~10 cd/m^2)

The stimulus intensity is varied by the use of attenuation filters. The attenuation of light is expressed in logarithmic unit and is more commonly in tenths of log units which are known as decibel (dB). 1 decibel = 1/10 log unit of attenuation of maximum available stimulus. (10000 asb units for the current Humphrey perimeters). The maximum and minimum intensities of light projected by each perimeter vary. The maximum intensity of light projected by Humphrey field analyzer is 10,000 asb units and 4000 asb units for octopus 1-2-3. The minimum intensity of light projected by Humphrey field analyzer is 0.1 asb unit and 0.4 asb unit is for octopus 1-2-3 model. The change in the stimulus intensity will be discussed in detail when we talk about the units used to express light intensity and retinal sensitivity later in this chapter.

Automated static perimetry uses a standardized test procedure which ensures that testing is performed in a unified manner from one time to another and one location to another. Because a standard test procedure is used, databases of normal values for individuals of all ages have been established for automated static perimetry. This allows the examiner to compare an individual's test results to age adjusted normal population characteristics, to identify whether various locations are within normal sensitivity limits or whether they are outside normal limits by a specific amount. However, the normative database does not include all ethnic groups.

THRESHOLD

Definition

Threshold for a given point is defined as that stimulus intensity which has a 50% probability of being seen. If light of a particular intensity is shown 100 times and if it is appreciated 50 times, that particular intensity of light is termed as threshold for that given point. If the stimulus intensity is seen >50% of times it is termed as suprathreshold and if it is seen < 50% of times, it is termed as infrathreshold. This is clearly shown in this below figure of frequency of seeing curve, the X axis represents the intensity of light in dB values and the Y axis represents the percentage of frequency of seeing.

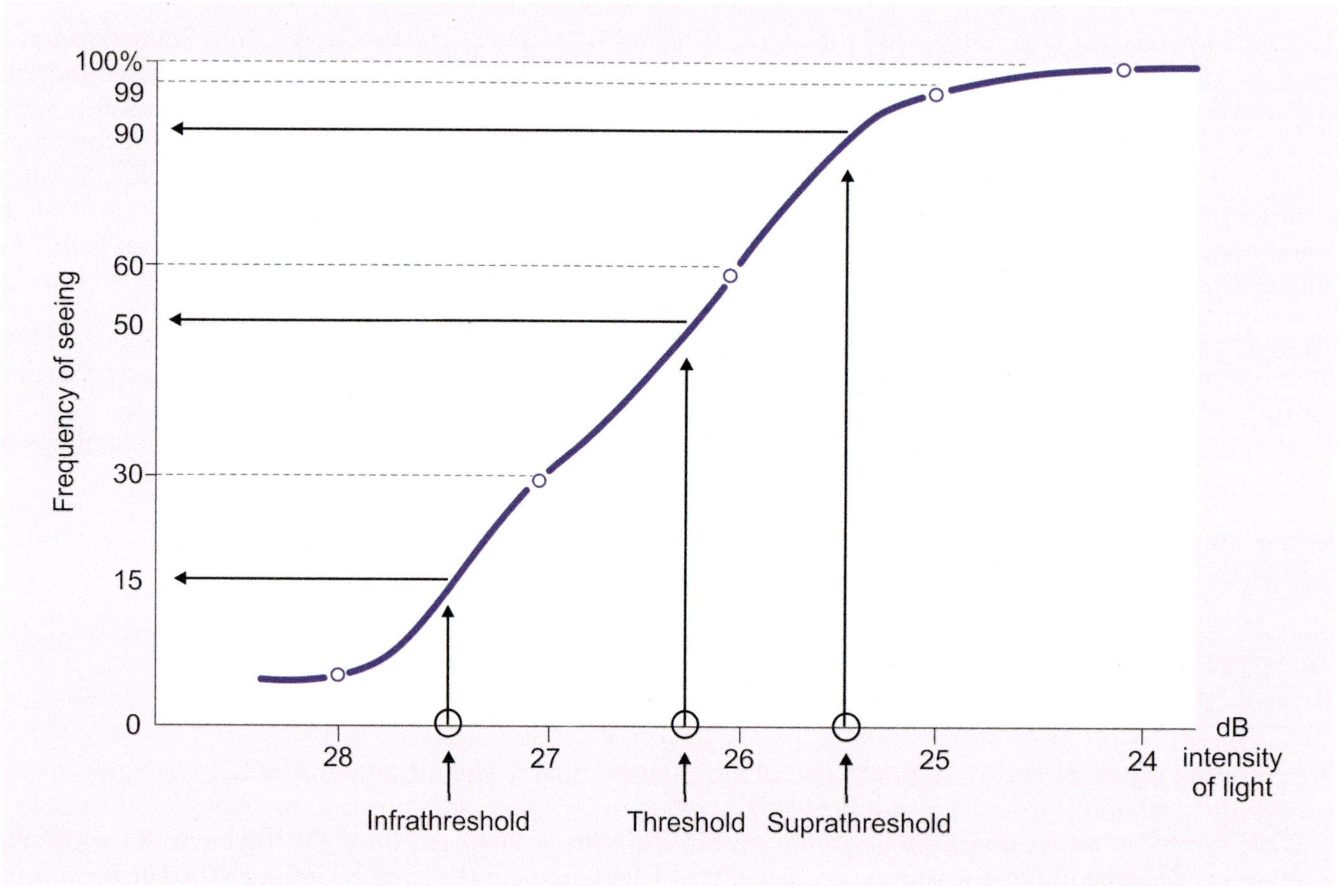

The most important point to be noted in this figure is as the dB value decreases, the light intensity increases.

From the frequency of seeing curve it is very clear that if a light intensity of around 27 dB is projected 100 times, it is appreciated 15% of the time indicating that the light intensity of around 27 dB is infrathreshold value of that point. If the light intensity of around 26 dB is projected 100 times, it is appreciated 50% of the times indicating that the light intensity of around 26 dB is the threshold value of that point. If the light intensity of around 25 dB is projected 100 times, it is appreciated 95% of the times indicating that light intensity of around 25 dB is the suprathreshold value of that point.

Units are Used to Express Light Intensity and Retinal Sensitivity

Apostilbs (asb units) are the fundamental units used to express light intensity. Apostilbs are converted to decibel (dB) units to express light intensity and retinal sensitivity. The brightness of the stimulus is attenuated by the use of filters in field analyzer. If there is no attenuation of light intensity, it is labeled as 0 decibel. So by convention the maximum intensity of stimulus is assigned a value of 0 decibel (which means there is no attenuation of light). The maximum intensity of light projected by Humphrey field analyzer is 10,000 Asb units. So in Humphrey field analyzer '0' dB value = 10,000 Asb units. The minimum intensity of light projected by Humphrey field analyzer is 0.1 Asb units. So in Humphrey field analyzer '50'dB value = 0.1 Asb units.

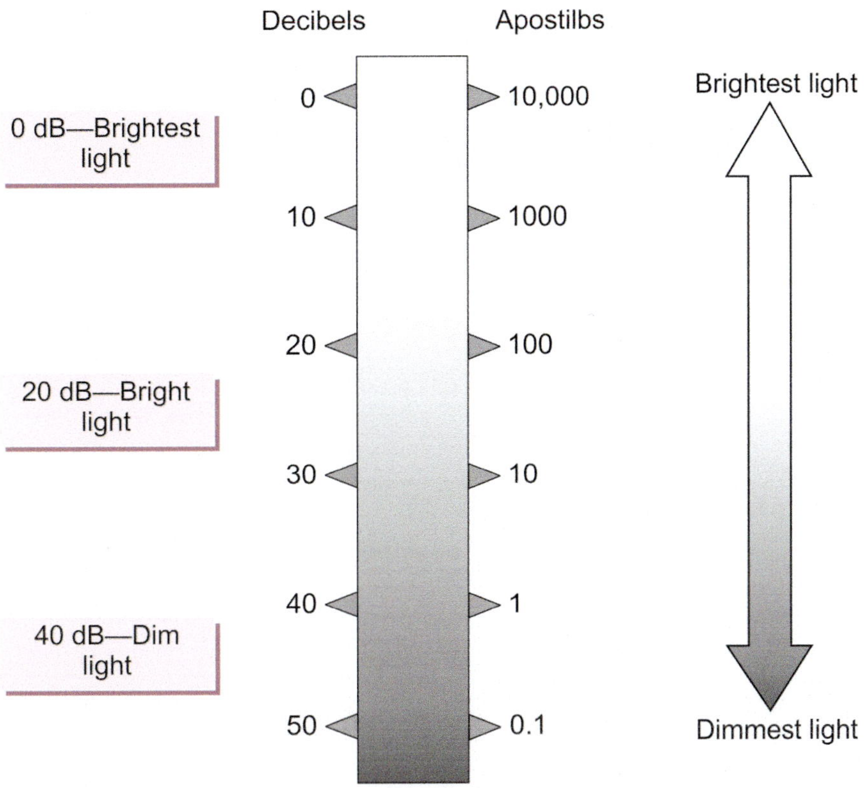

Apostilbs are absolute units of light intensity (100 asb intensity on one instrument is same as 100 asb intensity on another instrument). In contrast, the decibels are relative units. That means the decibel value depends on the maximum intensity projected by each perimeter.

As the brightest light projected by each perimeter varies, the dB value also varies. So decibel units are not absolute units but are relative units to express light intensity. For example, on Goldmann perimeter, the maximum light intensity is 1000 asb and 10 dB attenuation results in 100 asb light intensity. On Humphrey perimeter, the maximum intensity of light is 10,000 asb and 10 dB attenuation results in 1000 asb light intensity. Thus the 10 dB stimulus on Goldmann perimeter which is equal to 100 asb units is not the same intensity as a 10 dB stimulus on Humphrey field analyzer, which is equal to 1000 asb units. But 10 dB does represent the same percentage reduction from maximum intensity in both the instruments. The conversion from asb units to decibels is logarithmic and not a simple multiplication factor.

Decibel (dB) units are used to express both the light intensity and retinal threshold value.

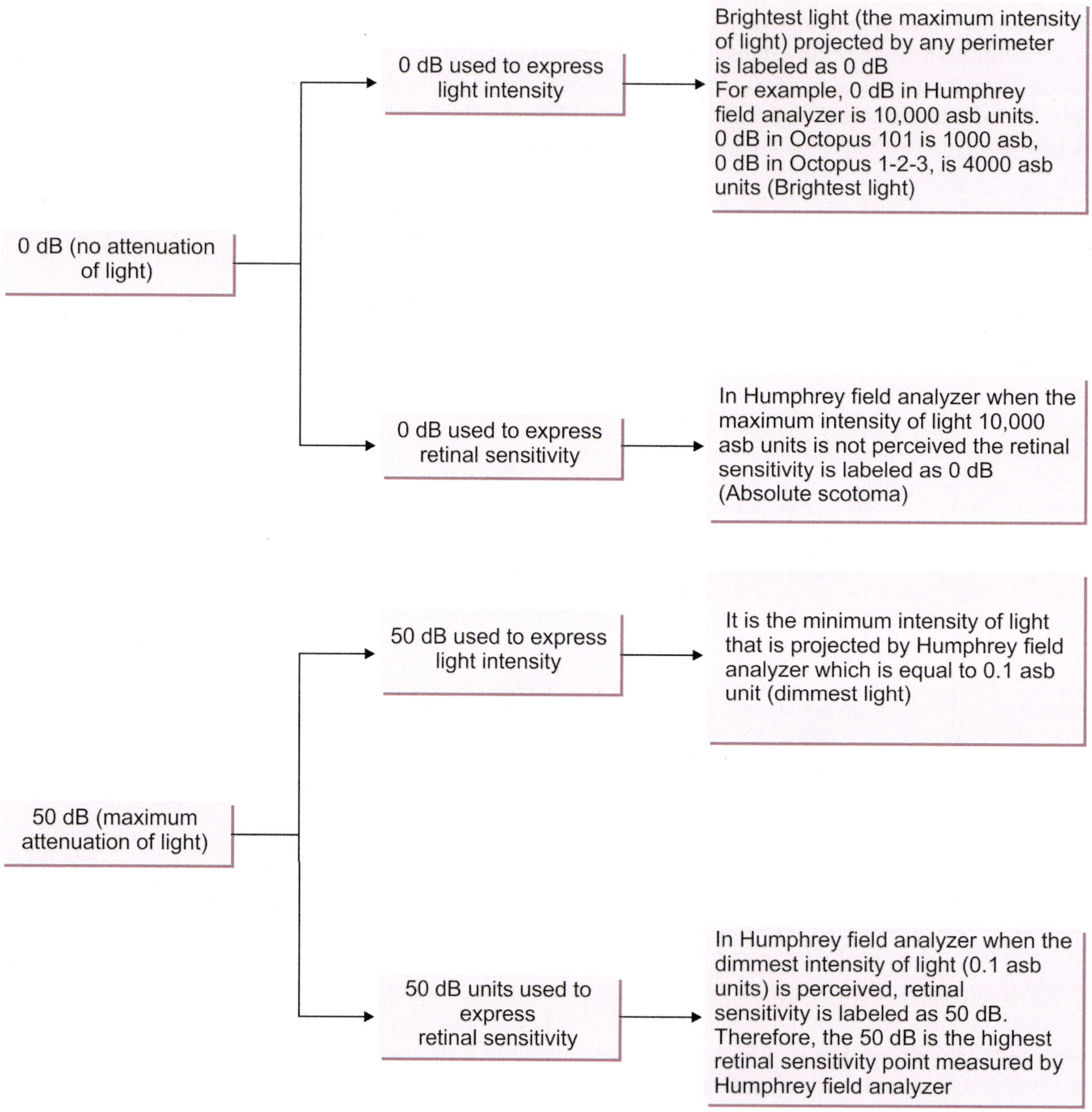

The asb units when used to express light intensity

High asb value denotes bright light and low asb value denotes dim light. Thus light intensity is directly proportional to asb value.

The asb units when used to express retinal sensitivity

If higher light intensity is required to get the response, it indicates the retinal sensitivity is low. As described above higher asb units represent bright light. Thus higher the asb units indicates that the retinal sensitivity is low. Thus retinal sensitivity is inversely proportional to asb units. The main disadvantage of expressing the retinal sensitivity in asb units is it's inversely proportional relation. When the maximum light intensity of 10000 asb units in Humphrey field analyzer is not perceived then the retinal sensitivity should be labeled >10000 asb; which denotes an absolute scotoma. Similarly the retinal sensitivity with a positive response to minimum light intensity of 0.1 asb unit should be labeled 0.1 Asb. Absolute scotoma is represented by 10,000 asb units and best sensitivity point is represented by 0.1 asb unit.

If we say the retinal sensitivity is >10,000 asb units, it gives impression as if the sensitivity is the best. But in real sense, it is an absolute scotoma. This is one of the reasons why asb units are not used for retinal sensitivity and they are converted to dB units. The main advantage of expressing retinal sensitivity in dB units is that the retinal sensitivity is directly proportional to dB value.

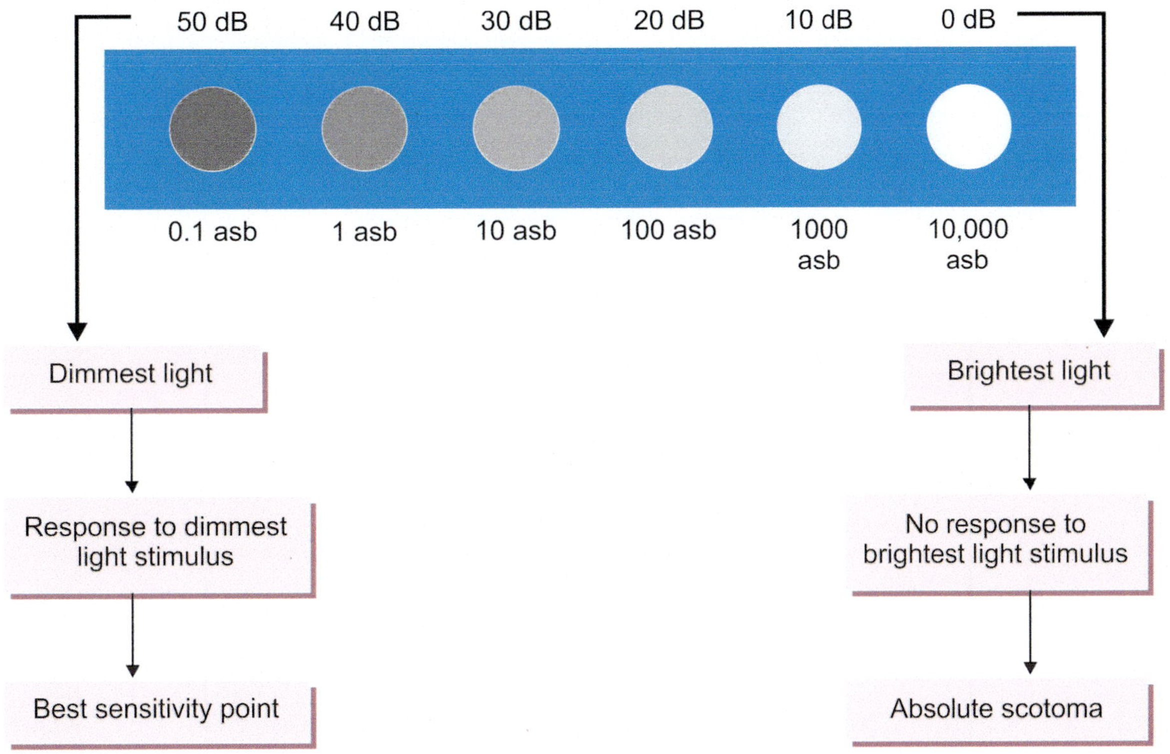

The most important point to be noted is that the dB units represent both the light intensity and the retinal threshold value.

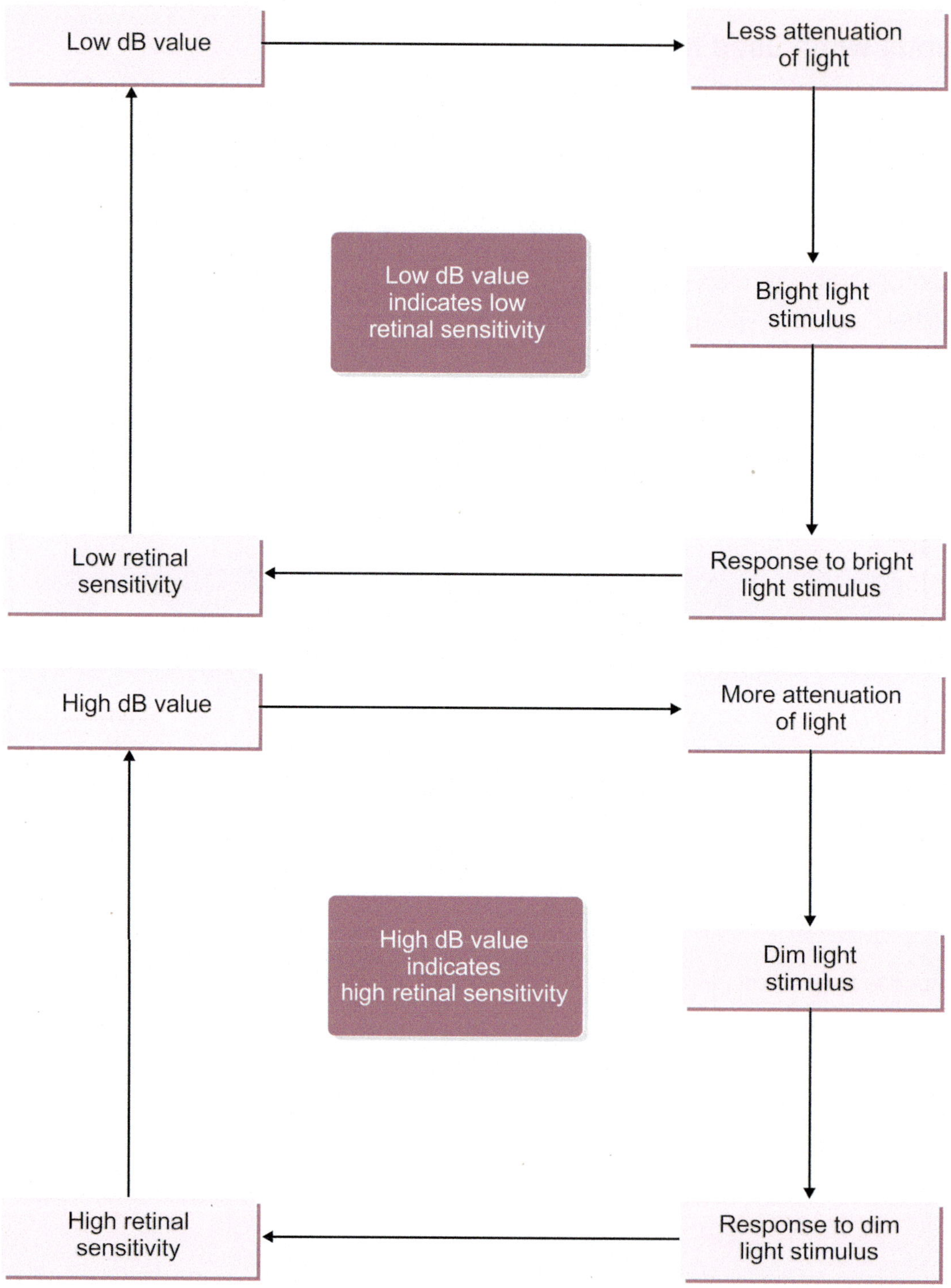

The retinal threshold value and its derivatives are expressed in dB units in all the visual field printouts.

Raw data:

The retinal sensitivity is expressed in dB units instead of asb units. To express retinal threshold values in asb units more space is needed. For example, a point with threshold value of 10 dB units has to be represented 1000 asb units. In order to avoid large numbers, retinal threshold value is expressed in dB units instead of asb units. Another advantage of expressing retinal sensitivity in dB units is that the retinal sensitivity is directly proportional to dB value.

Total and pattern deviation numerical plots:

The deviation values from normative data are expressed in dB units with no sign or (–) sign in front of each number.

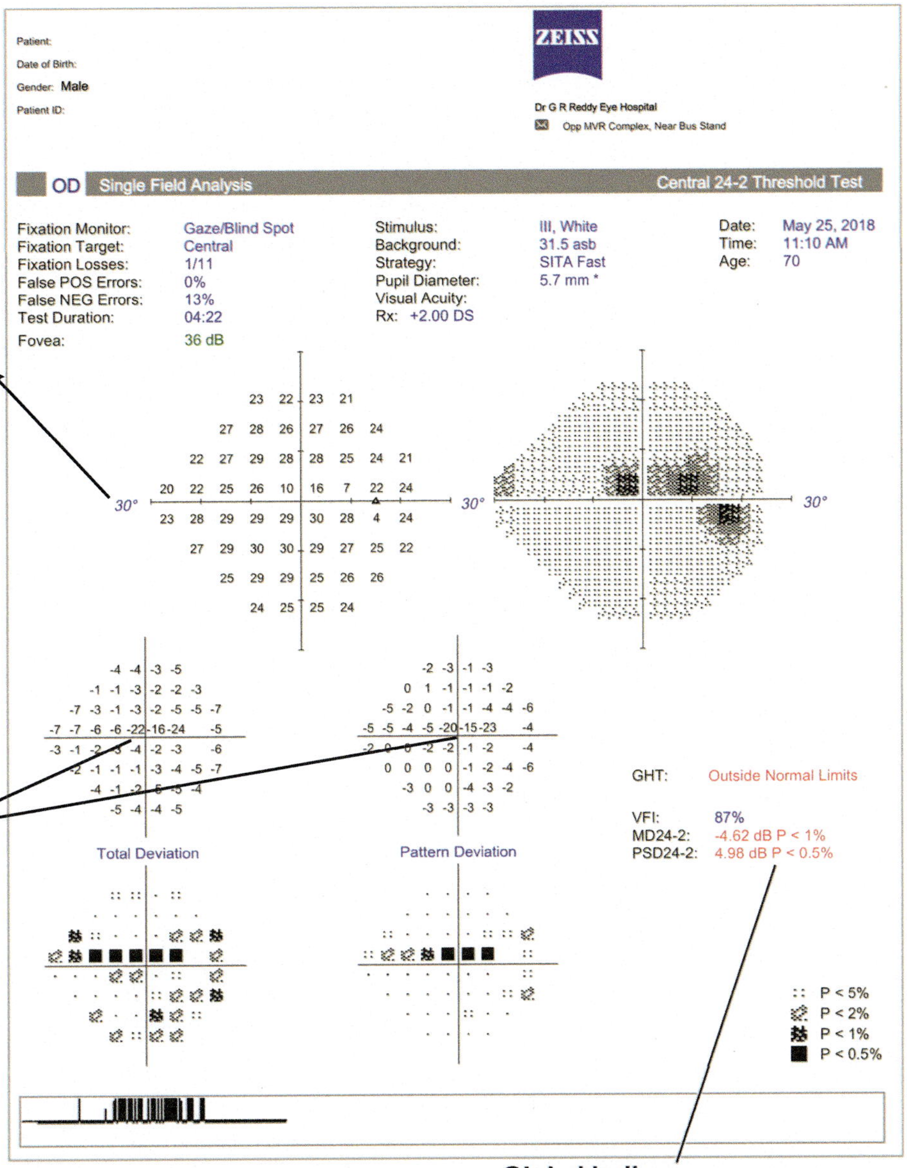

Global indices
Mean deviation index
Pattern standard deviation (PSD)
Visual field index (VFI)

To understand visual field printouts, one should have a very good concept on dB units. dB units are used to measure both retinal sensitivity and light intensity.

Classification of Humphrey Visual Field Tests

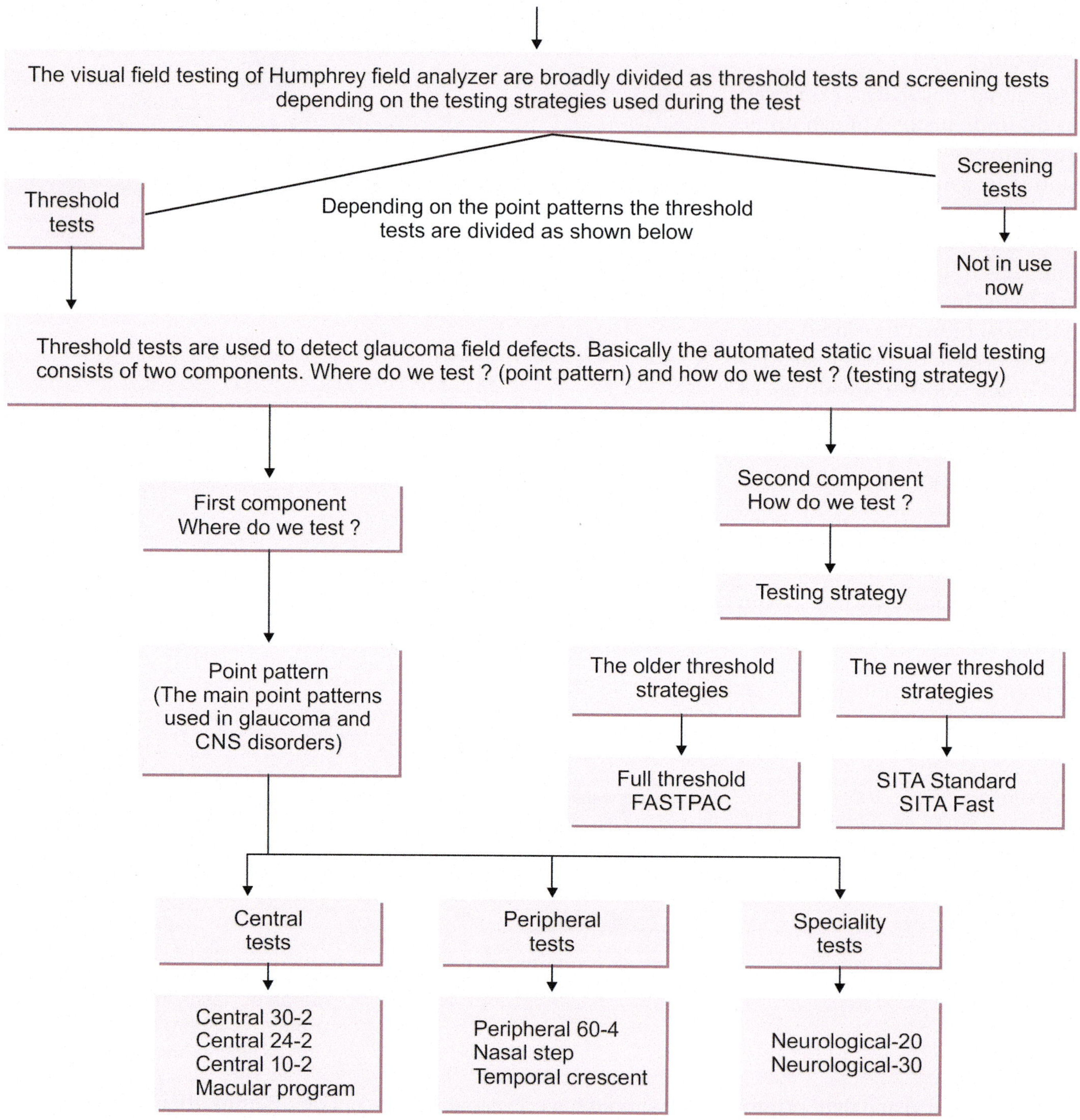

For example, the selected test is central 30-2 Swedish Interactive Threshold Algorithm (SITA) Standard. In this test the first component (point pattern) is central 30-2 and the second component (testing strategy) is SITA Standard. Now the point patterns and the testing strategies are discussed in detail.

POINT PATTERNS

Point patterns used for glaucoma are 30-2, 24-2, 10-2 and macular program. It was thought that 30-2 and 24-2 are for early and established glaucomas and 10-2 is for advanced glaucoma. Currently this concept has been changed as we are seeing good number of primary open-angle glaucoma (POAG) cases which start within the 10° circle area. The concept of 10-2 point pattern being reserved for advanced glaucoma no longer holds good. However 30-2 and 24-2 are selected in a suspected or established case of glaucoma. Selecting 10-2 point pattern depends on the sensitivities of the 16 points in the 10° circle area of 30-2 or 24-2 single field analysis (SFA) printouts and the direction of the retinal nerve fiber layer (RNFL) defect. If RNFL defect directs towards macula, 10-2 point pattern is selected even if 30-2 or 24-2 single field analysis printout shows early or no glaucomatous field defect.

30-2 Point Pattern

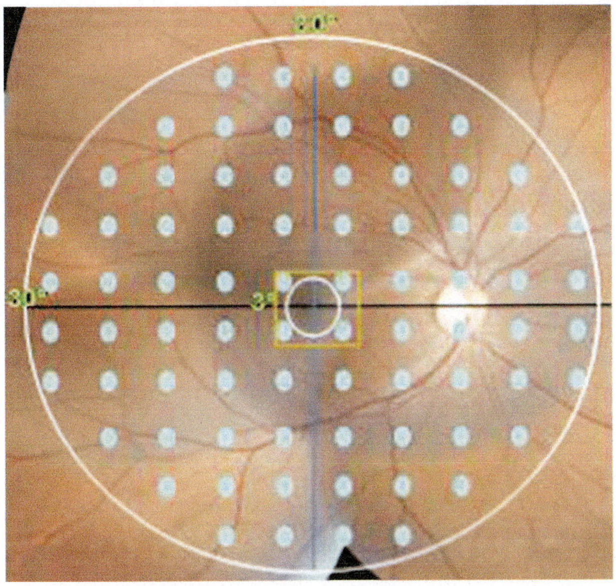

30-2 point pattern

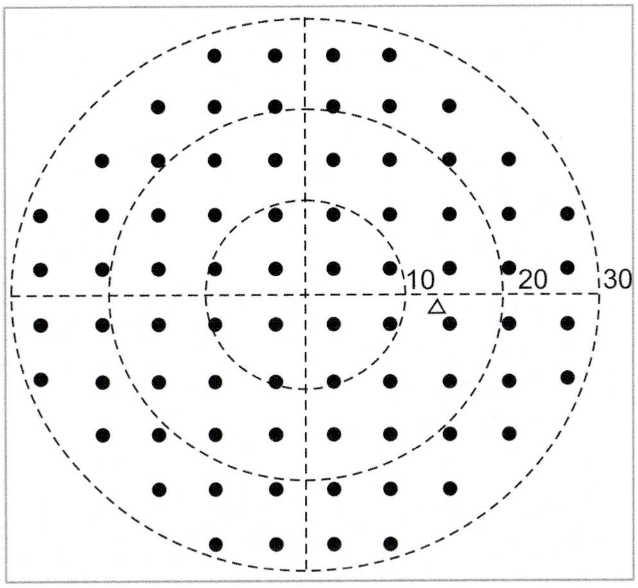

30-2 central field

- 30° represents the extent of the field being tested with fovea as center.
- 2 represents that no points are present on vertical and horizontal axis.
- The distance between each point is 6° and the distance between point and the center of fixation is 3°.
- 76 points are distributed in this entire area including the two points on the blind spot.
- The 3° circle around the center of fixation; which does not have any points is the bare area of 30–2 or 24-2 point pattern.

24-2 Point Pattern

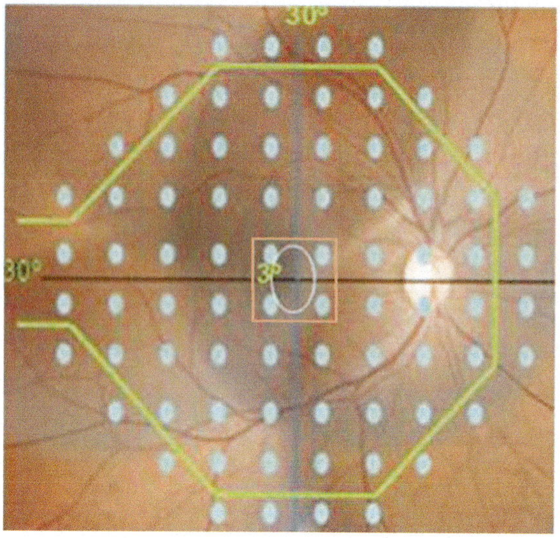

30-2 point pattern

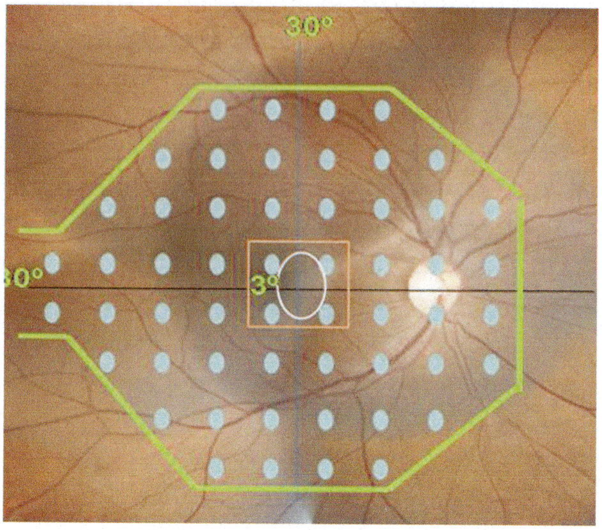

24-2 point pattern

The outer set of points except the two nasal points on either side of horizontal axis are eliminated from the 30-2 point pattern to form 24-2 point pattern. So the total points of 24-2 point pattern (76–22 = 54) will be 54 points. 24-2 pattern is nothing but the 54 points of 30-2 which are present within 24° circle area from the fixation point. Because of this reason, the results from 30-2 and 24-2 may be presented on one sheet in the overview printouts. But note that the two outer most points on the nasal side are 27° from the fixation point. So strictly speaking it is actually not 24-2 point pattern because the two nasal points on either side of horizontal axis are at 27° from fixation point (the two points on the outer circle 30-2).

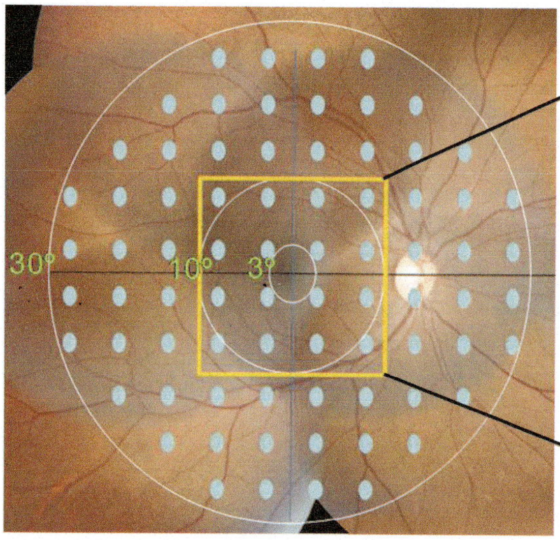

30-2 point pattern

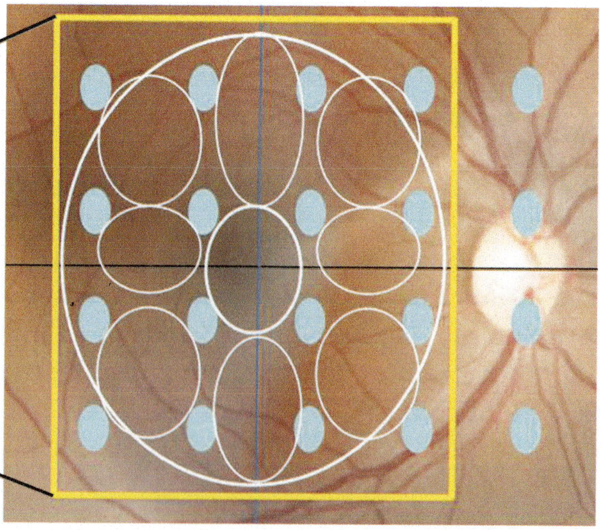

10° circle area of 30-2 or 24-2

10° Circle Area of 30-2 or 24-2

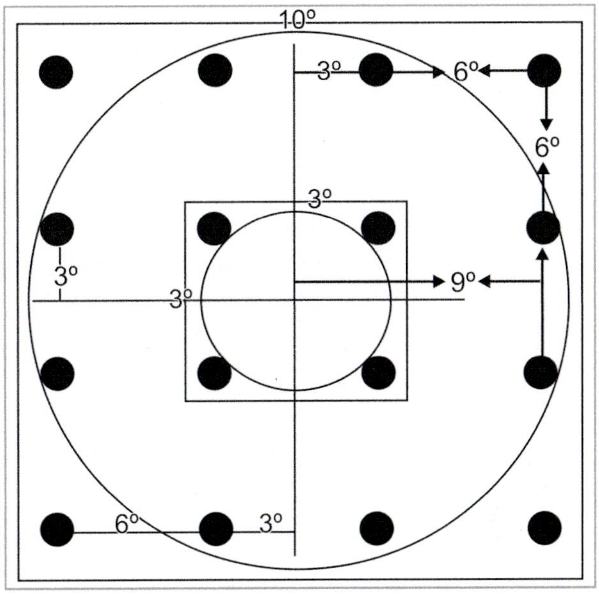

The 10° circle area of 30-2 or 24-2 contains two set of points. The outer set of points are related to 9° circle. They are 12 in number. The inner set of points are related to 3° circle. They are 4 in number. The total number of points in the 10° circle area of 30-2 or 24-2 are 16 points. The distance between each point is 6° and the distance between point and the axis is 3°. Concentrate on the sensitivities of these 16 points within the 10° circle area of 30-2 or 24-2. There are no points within 3° circle around the fixation point. Hence 30-2 and 24-2 point patterns are not suitable to assess foveal split. We always talk about the bare area of 3° circle around the fixation point in 30-2 and 24-2 point patterns.

But there is a huge bare area between the 3° circle points and 9° circle points of 30-2 or 24-2 point pattern. If glaucomatous damage occurs in this bare area, it will be missed in 24-2 or 30-2 point patterns. Significant loss of retinal sensitivity at any of these 16 points in 10° circle area of 30-2 or 24-2 point patterns is an indication to repeat the test with 10-2 point pattern and this aids in detecting glaucomatous damage at an earlier stage.

10-2 Point Pattern

1. **In 10-2 Point pattern-10** represents extent of testing area (10° radius circle with fovea as center) and 2 represents that there are no points on both the horizontal and vertical axis. (In 10-1 point pattern points are present on both the horizontal and vertical axis. The 10-1 point pattern is not in use now).
2. The distance between point to point is 2°.
3. The total number of points are 68 points in 10-2 Point pattern (The 10° circle area of 30-2 or 24-2 contains 16 test points).
4. In this point pattern the bare area around the fixation target is 1° radius of a circle because the distance between the point to the center of fixation is 1°.

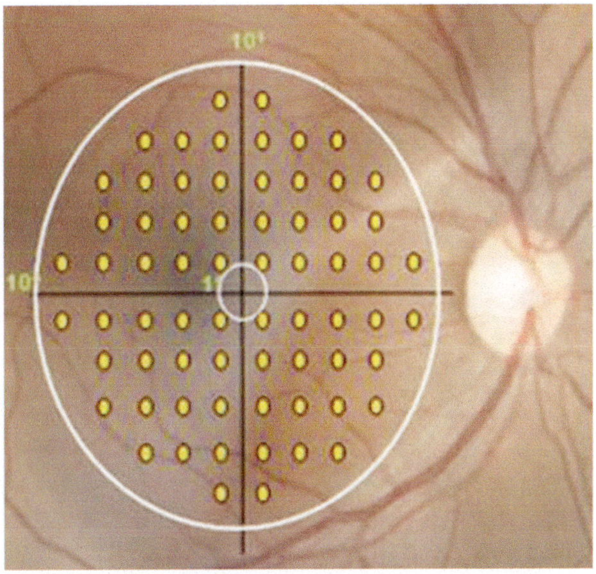

10-2 point pattern

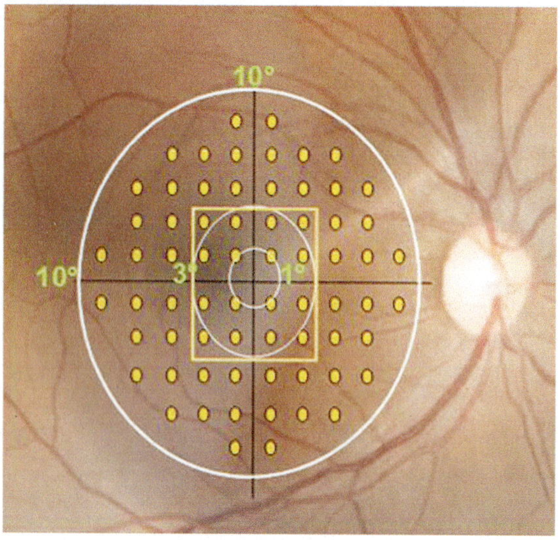

10-2 point pattern

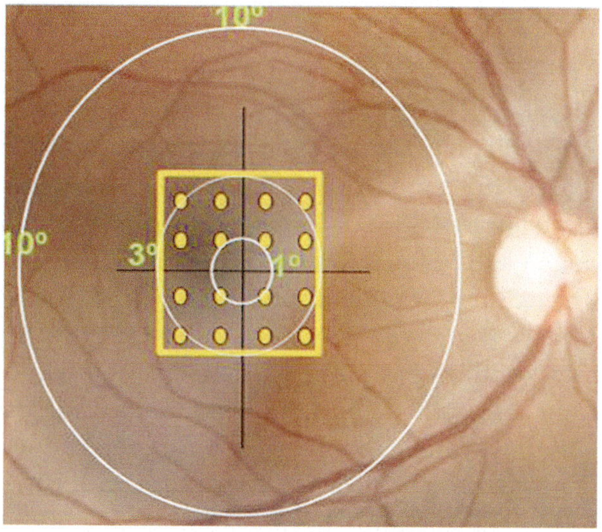

Macular program

The outer 3 sets of points of the 10-2 point pattern are eliminated to form the macular point pattern. Macular program has 16 central points of 10-2 which are present within 3° radius of a circle from fixation point. In this point pattern the bare area around the fixation spot is 1°. In advanced cases of glaucoma to assess the foveal status and to comment on macular split, macular program with stimulus size 111 or V can be ordered.

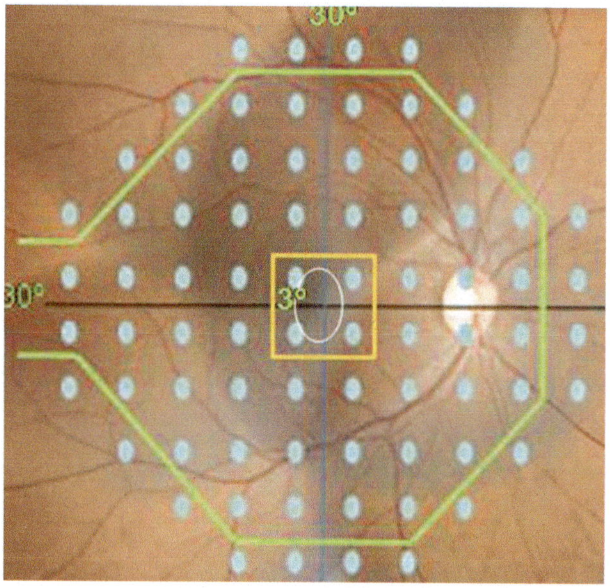

30-2 point pattern

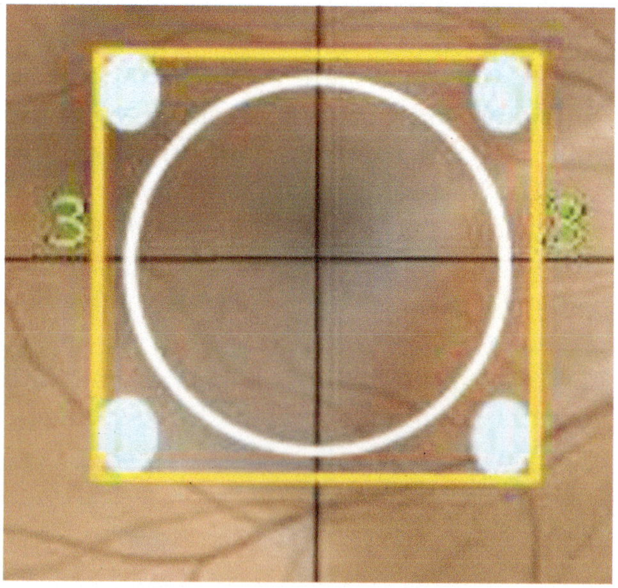

Bare area of 30-2 or 24-2 point pattern

The 3° circle around the center of fixation; which does not have any points in the bare area of 30-2 or 24-2 point pattern. As there is 3° circle bare area around the center of fixation; in the 30-2 or 24-2 point patterns, the foveal status should not be commented. Depending on the sensitivities of the 16 points in the 10° circle area, we should repeat the test with 10-2 point pattern to know the foveal status.

What are the indications to repeat the test with 10-2 point pattern?

The sensitivities of all the 16 points in the 10° circle area of 30-2 or 24-2 point pattern will decide whether the test should be repeated with 10-2 point pattern or not.

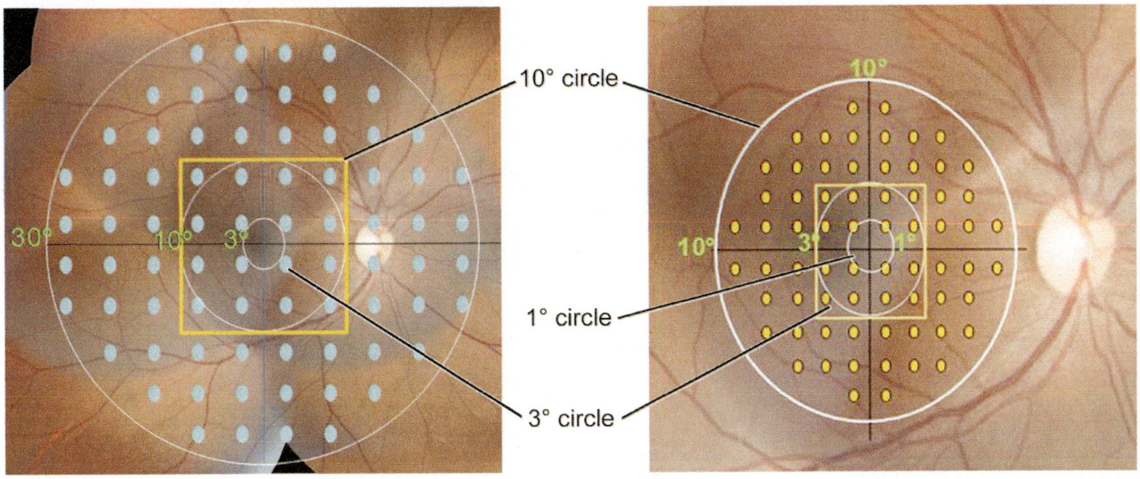

30-2 point pattern **10-2 point pattern**

There are 16 points in the 10° circle area of 30-2 or 24-2 point pattern. They can be divided as outer set of points (points placed at 9 degrees from the vertical and horizontal axis) and inner-set of points (points placed at 3° from the vertical and horizontal axis). The outer set of points are 12 in number and the inner set of points are 4 in number. The outer set of points are not included in the 10-2 point pattern. The 4 inner most set of points lie just outside the 3° circle are included in the 10-2 point pattern.

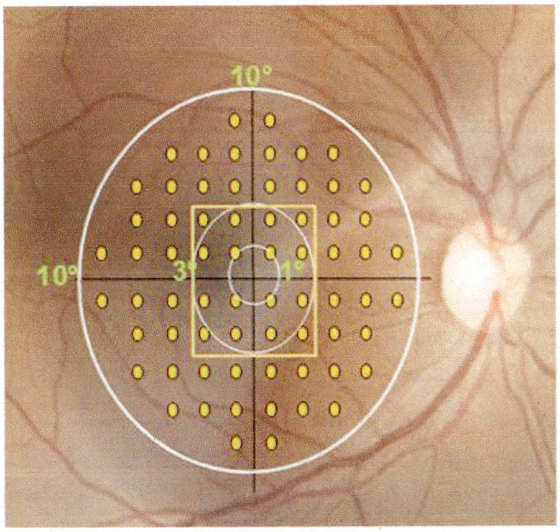

10-2 point pattern

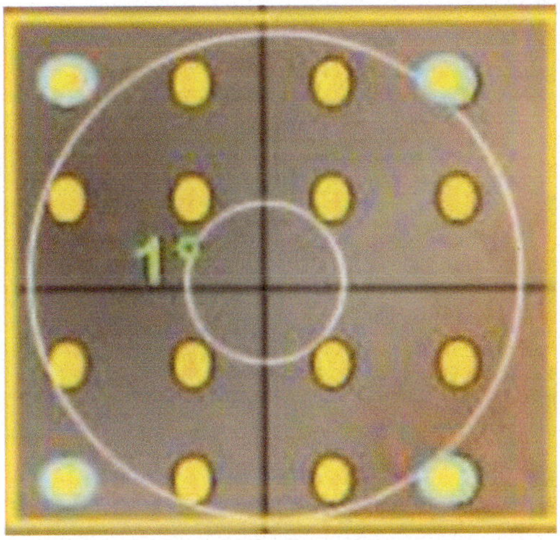

Macular program

In 10-2 point pattern, there are 16 points in the 3° circle area around the center of fixation (the bare area of 30-2 or 24-2 point pattern). Out of the 16 points, 12 points lie within the 3° circle and 4 points just outside the 3° circle. There is only 1° bare area in the 10-2 point pattern. So we almost test up to fixation in 10-2 point patterns. Now it is very clear that the foveal status should not be commented from the 30-2 and 24-2 point pattern.

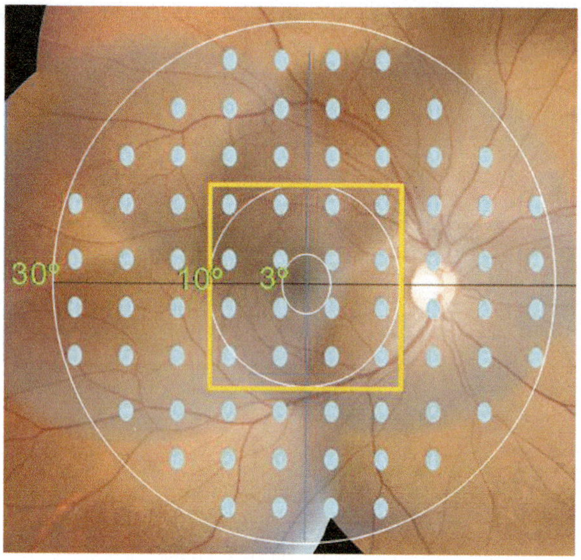

30-2 point pattern

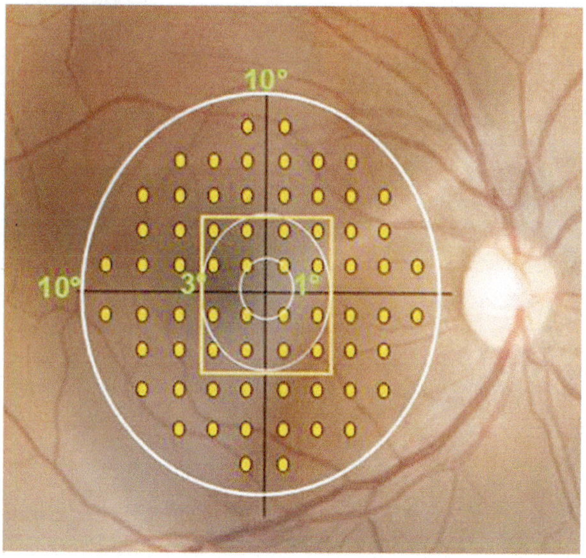

10-2 point pattern

10° Circle Area of 30-2 and 10-2 Point Pattern

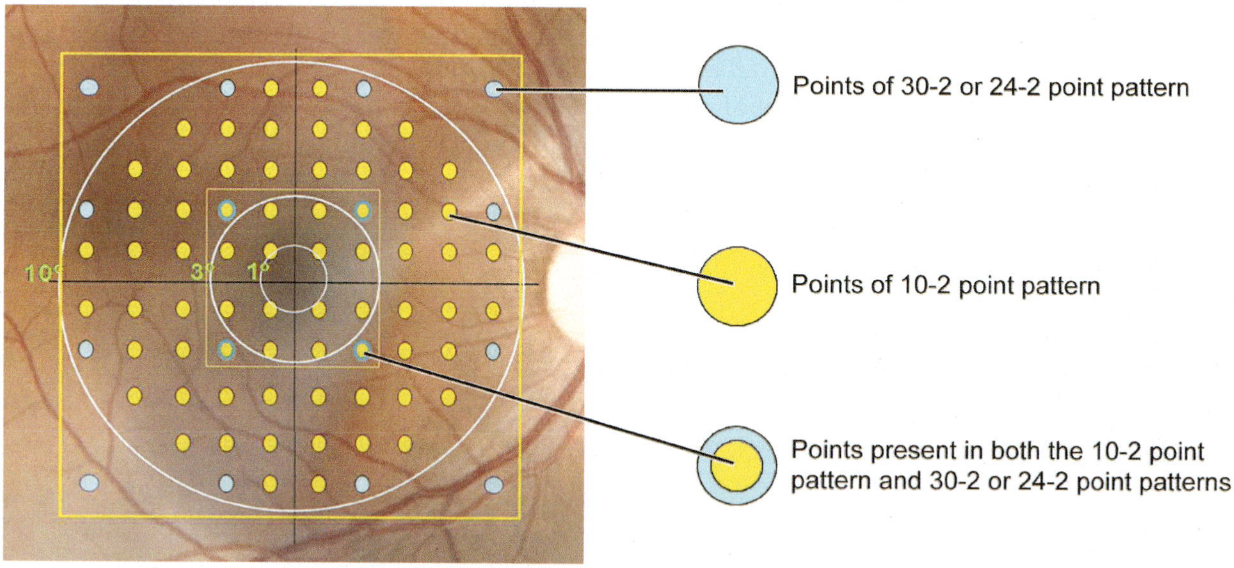

If we do the tests with both 30-2 and 10-2 point patterns, the total number of points tested in both 30-2 (24-2) and 10-2 in the 10° square area are 80.

Out of these 80 points, 12 points belong to 30-2 or 24-2 point pattern, 64 points belong to 10-2, and 4 points are present in both 30-2 or 24-2 and 10-2 point patterns.

Total number of points in 10-2 point pattern are 68 in number. But the 4 innermost set of points lie just outside the 3° circle are present in 30-2 point patterns also. The 4 innermost set of points lie just outside the 3° circle are present in 30-2 or 24-2 and 10-2 point patterns.

Selection of the Point Pattern

Point patterns used for glaucoma are 30-2, 24-2,10-2 and macular program. As discussed earlier it was thought that 30-2 and 24-2 are for early and established glaucomas and 10-2 and macular program tests are for advanced glaucoma. Originally primary open angle glaucomas are classified as POAG and normal tension glaucoma (NTG) on the basis of IOP. Later the concept has been changed. The most important factor in the management of glaucoma is the location of the field defect, i.e the exact location where the glaucomatous damage has begun. Now, the better way of classifying primary open-angle glaucoma is on the basis of location of the field defect. So the concept that 10-2 point pattern being reserved only for advanced glaucoma no longer holds good.

Classification of Primary Open-angle Glaucomas

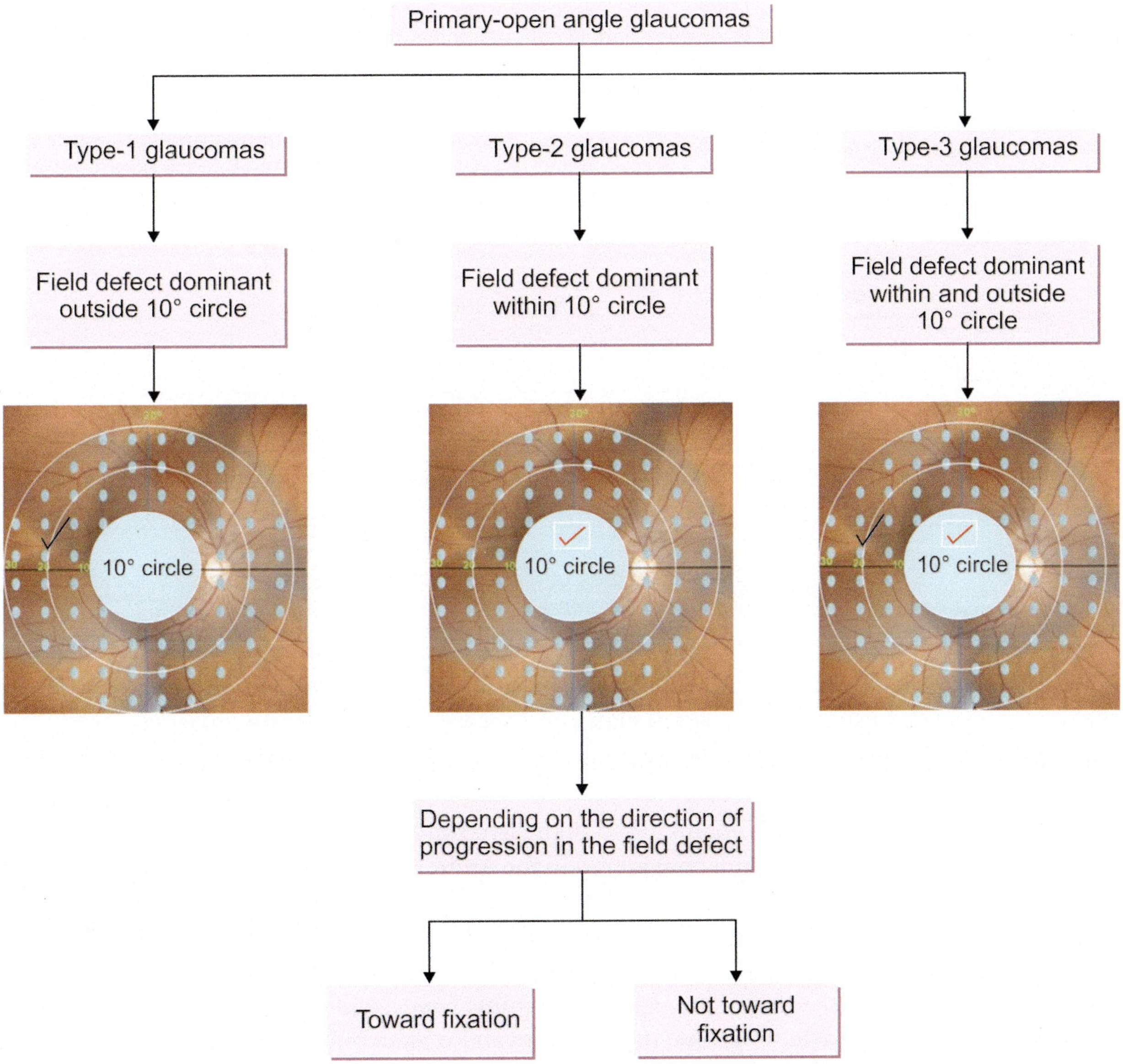

Summary of Selection of Point Pattern

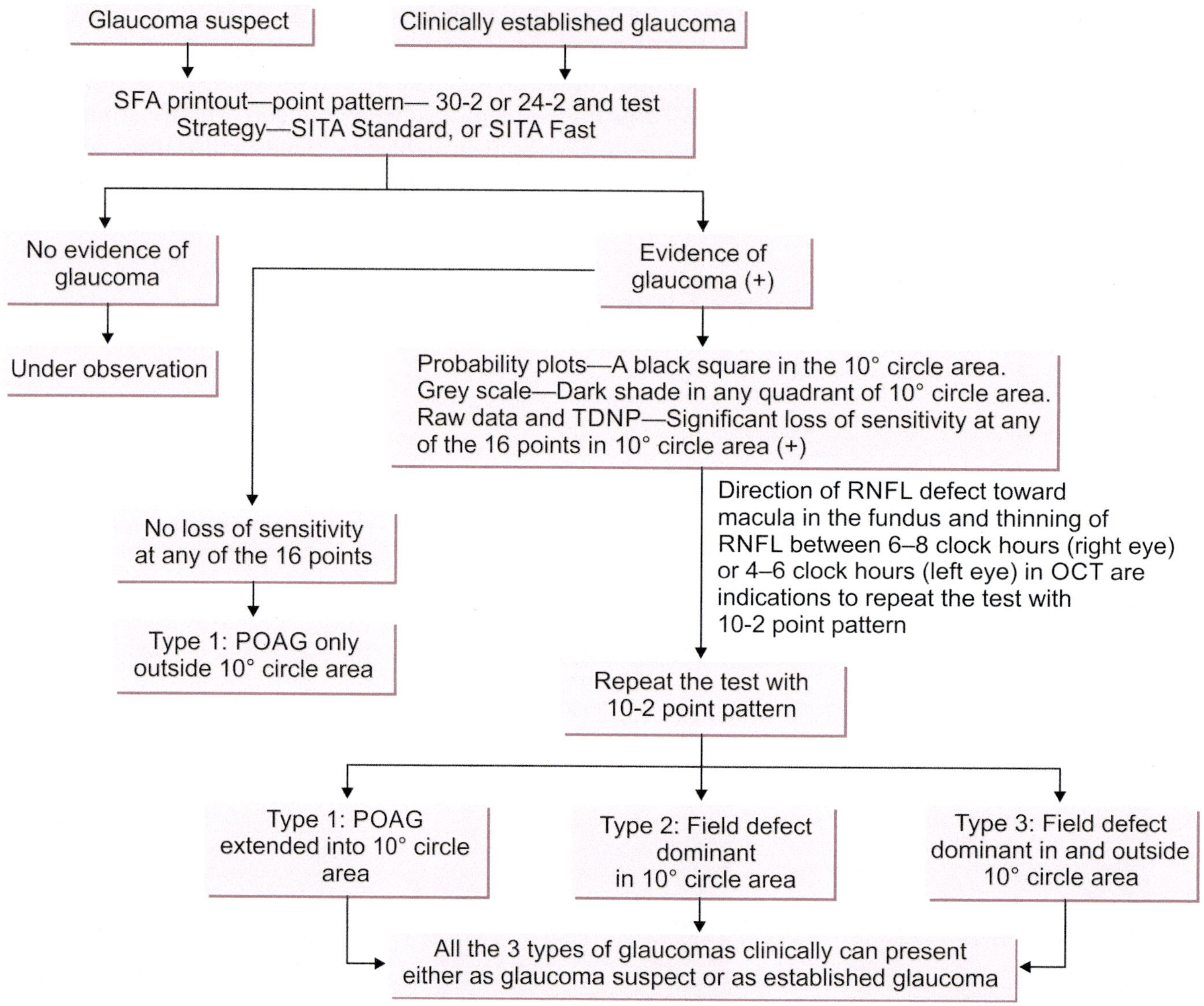

It is a general concept that we should select 30-2 point pattern in a glaucoma suspect. But 24-2 point pattern is the test of choice even in suspicious cases of glaucoma because of the following reasons.

1. The outer set of points of 30-2 are not considered while selecting the 7th best deviation point of total deviation numerical plot (TDNP)
2. The outer set of points of 30-2 are not included in the five zones of GHT (Glaucoma hemifield test).
3. The outer set of points of 30-2 are not considered in the Anderson's criteria to name the field defect due to glaucoma.
4. The outer set of points of 30-2 are tested last. The patient may be fatigued by that time and chances are more to get high fixation losses and false (–) ve errors.
5. The average normative data value of the peripheral points have a wide range. Taking all the points into consideration 24-2 point pattern became the choice even for glaucoma suspects.

   The details of the above said five points are dealt in the forthcoming chapters

THRESHOLD TESTING STRATEGIES

The test "strategy" refers to the method of presenting stimuli to the patient to attain the desired information. There are two types of strategies: screening or suprathreshold testing strategies and threshold testing strategies. In suprathreshold testing strategies (screening test), each stimulus is intense enough to be seen by nearly all normal patients. This strategy provides only general, qualitative information about the visual field and consumes less time. While threshold strategies consume more time, they provide detailed, quantitative information to find out the threshold at each selected point of retina. There are different threshold strategies available to the Humphrey field analyzer.

The testing threshold strategies are of 2 types

1. Old standard threshold strategies - 1. Full Threshold Strategy; 2. FASTPAC
2. Newer threshold strategies - 1. SITA Standard; - 2. SITA Fast

(SITA stands for Swedish Interactive Threshold Algorithm)

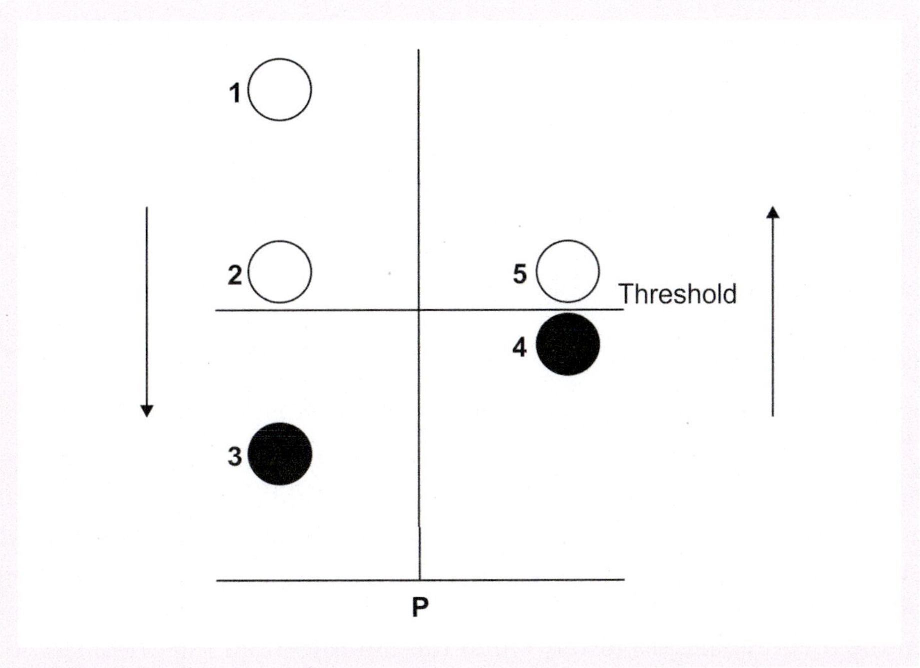

Threshold determination at a visual field point P, open circle indicates patient response to stimulus. Filled circle indicates no response to stimulus. Down arrow indicates stimuli decreasing in 4 dB steps. Up arrow indicates stimuli increasing in 2 dB steps. Numbers indicate order of stimulus presentation.

Staircase Method (Bracketing Method) of detecting threshold.

This method is used in full threshold strategy.

DETERMINATION OF THRESHOLD

To determine threshold at each point in the test grid, stimulus intensity varies in such a way that some stimuli will be suprathreshold (brighter than necessary to elicit a response most of the time) and some will be infrathreshold (too dim to elicit a response most of the time). Threshold is thus bracketed by the stimuli as the examination proceeds. This method of bracketing is also known as staircase method for determining threshold.

Explanation of Method (Bracketing) for Determining Threshold

First stimulus: The first stimulus presented at the point P is seen and hence it is labeled as open circle 1 (See the figure in the page no. 21).

Second stimulus: Because the first stimulus is seen the intensity of light is dimmed by 4 dB. In this example, the second stimulus is also seen and labeled as open circle 2.

Third stimulus: As the second stimulus is also seen, the third stimulus is dimmed further by 4 dB. The third stimulus is too dim to elicit a response and hence indicated by closed circle 3. This is the first crossing from seeing zone to nonseeing zone.

Fourth stimulus: Now the machine makes the stimulus brighter but in 2 dB steps. The fourth stimulus is also too dim to elicit a response and hence indicated by closed circle 4.

Fifth stimulus: The fifth stimulus is further brightened by 2 dB and this time, the patient responds by pressing the button and hence labeled as open circle 5. This is the second crossing of the threshold from nonseeing zone to seeing zone. Since the step size was 2 dB, threshold is the value that lies between the intensity values of the last 2 stimuli. Obviously if the first stimulus presented to the point was not seen, the machine will make the stimuli brighter in 4 dB steps until the threshold is crossed and then dimmer in 2 dB steps until the second crossing. This standard method is adapted in determining threshold in the full threshold strategy. Thus the theoretical best threshold resolution is 2 dB.

The Newer Threshold Strategies

The newer threshold strategies reduce the test time of the threshold tests by more than 40% by measuring threshold with an alternative strategy to the standard staircase method. The newer strategies change the stimulus in 3 dB steps and cross the threshold only once. The threshold assigned to each tested point lies between the two stimulus intensities where the threshold is crossed. The theoretical best threshold resolution is 3 dB rather than the theoretical 2 dB resolution of the full threshold (algorithm) The threshold values determined by the newer fast methods were found to be similar to those found on the standard testing strategies (full threshold strategy and FASTPAC).

It is very important to note that the Full Threshold strategy is a confusing terminology because there are no half threshold strategies. Because the standard staircase method is adapted in detecting the threshold in full threshold strategy it should have been named as standard threshold strategy rather than full threshold strategy.

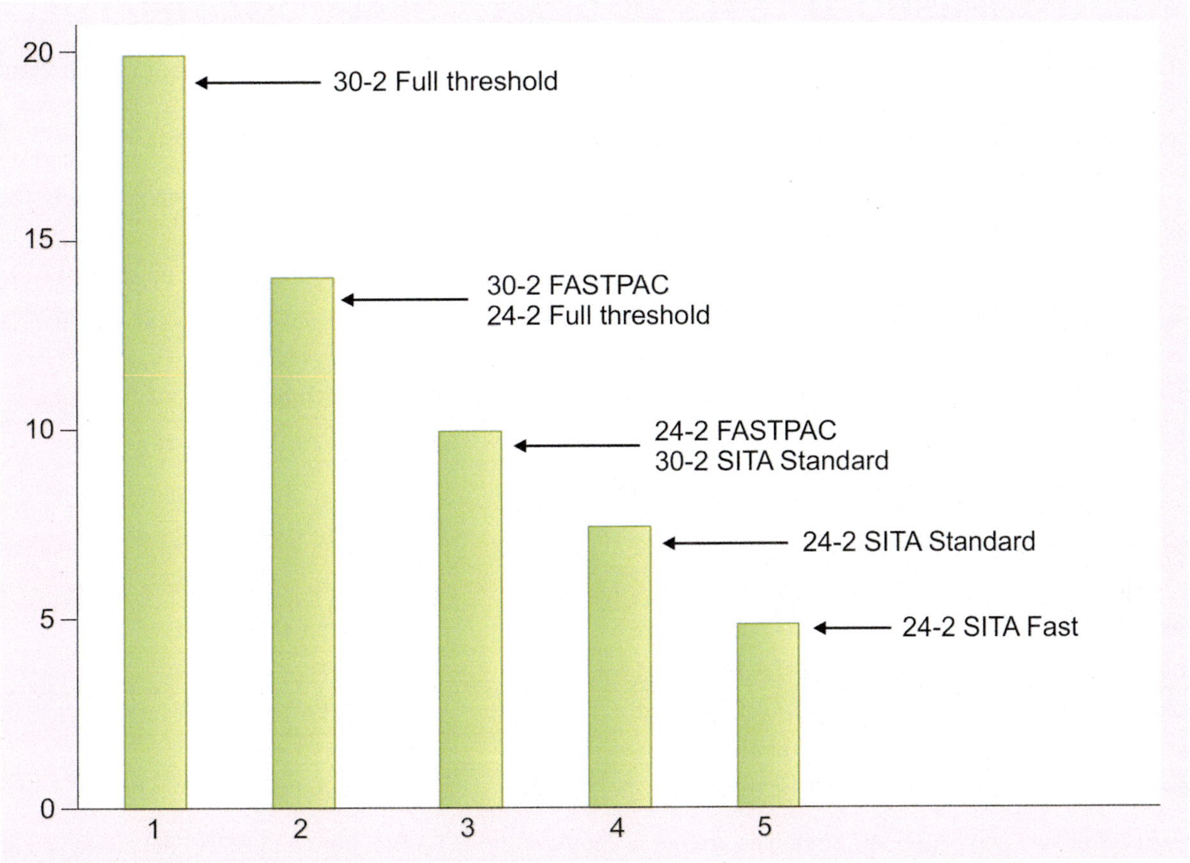

Typical test time ranges (minutes) comparative test times for four main threshold test algorithms. **Percentages are relative to typical test time for full threshold 30-2 testing.**

From the above figure, you understand the test time for each selection of the test is as follows:

1. 30-2 Full threshold—20 minutes.
2. 30-2 FASTPAC,
   24-2 Full threshold—14 minutes.
3. 24-2 FASTPAC,
   30-2 SITA Standard—10 minutes
4. 24-2 SITA Standard—7 minutes
5. 24-2 SITA Fast—5 minutes

IMPORTANT THRESHOLD TESTS TO DETECT GLAUCOMA FIELD DEFECTS

Now, we know the available point patterns and the testing strategies. Whenever we order for a visual field test always specify the point pattern and the testing strategy.

The usual available point patterns are as follows:

- 30-2 point pattern, 24-2 point pattern, 10-2 point pattern, macular program point pattern, and custom tests.
- Available threshold testing strategies: SITA Standard, SITA Fast.

Each of the above point pattern can be tested with any of the above threshold strategy as shown below:

1. 30-2 point pattern with SITA Standard.
2. 30-2 point pattern with SITA Fast.

   Similarly, the 24-2 point pattern and 10-2 point pattern can be done with all these strategies.

   Note that

   We can tabulate the above information as follows:

	Testing Strategy	
Point pattern	***SITA Standard***	***SITA Fast***
30-2 point pattern	SITA Standard	SITA Fast
24-2 point pattern	SITA Standard	SITA Fast
10-2 point pattern	SITA Standard	SITA Fast
Macular program	Full threshold	FASTPAC
Custom test	Full threshold	FASTPAC

In general full threshold and FASTPAC strategies are not in use now and SITA Standard and SITA Fast strategies are being used in most of the cases.

If the normative data is not available to the tests, Full threshold and FASTPAC strategies are being used.

PROFORMA OF ORDER FORM FOR VISUAL FIELD TESTING

Whenever we subject the patient for visual field testing we have to feed the field analyzer the details of the patient data and the test data accurately. For this purpose a proforma order form for visual field testing is designed. This proforma must be properly filled before subjecting the patient for visual field testing.

Patient Data	:	
Name of the patient	:	
Age/Sex	:	
VA/Refractive error correction for far and near	:	Both eyes
Pupil size	:	
Test Data	:	
Selection of the test	:	
Test point pattern	:	30-2/24-2/10-2 point pattern/Macular program.
Specify any special test	:	
Test strategy	:	SITA Standard/SITA Fast.
Fixation target	:	Central/Small diamond/Big diamond
Size of the stimulus	:	Size III/Size V
Indication for field testing	:	

Regarding fixation target, if nothing is mentioned it is understood that, it is the central fixation. In situations like macular degenerations, the fixation target has to be changed to small diamond or large diamond. Regarding the size of the stimulus, if nothing is mentioned it is understood that the stimulus size is size III. In situations like advanced glaucoma, to know macular status, size V stimulus can be used. To reduce high fixation losses sometimes we need to change the central fixation target to either small diamond or big diamond. The change of the size of the stimulus from size III to size V will also help to reduce the high fixation losses to make the test more reliable. The data in the proforma must be fed to the field analyzer accurately.

The patient should be carefully and fully educated about the performance of the test before beginning the test. Then the printout of Humphrey field analyzer will be available for interpretation.

Verify whether the test data and the patient data that are present in the visual field printouts are exactly similar or not to the data given in the proforma.

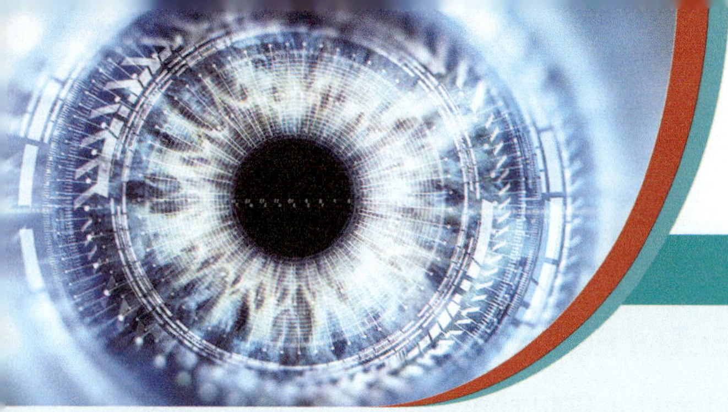

CHAPTER 3

Classification and Understanding of Visual Field Printouts

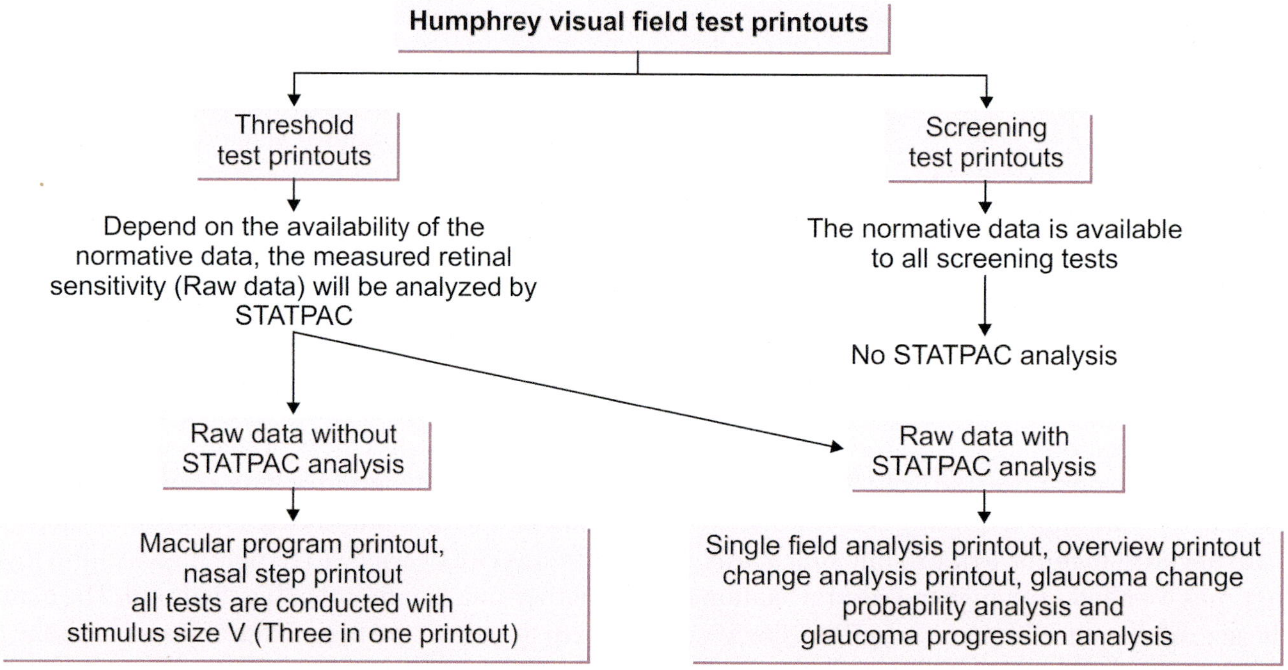

The normative data is available to the tests that are conducted with the following parameters. The STATPAC (The Humphrey field analyzer's statistical package) will analyze tests that fall within the parameters listed below.

Test pattern	:	Central 30-2, 24-2, 10-2
Test strategy	:	Swedish Interactive Threshold Algorithm (SITA) Standard, SITA Fast
Stimulus size	:	III
Fixation target	:	Central, small diamond, big diamond
Foveal threshold	:	On or off
Fluctuation	:	On or off

SINGLE FIELD ANALYSIS (SFA) PRINTOUT

In our daily practice we usually deal with Humphrey field analyzer's printouts. The Humphrey field analyzer's statistical package (STATPAC) can be used to produce an in-depth statistical analysis of visual field test results. The field analyzer determines the retinal sensitivity threshold at all predetermined points and plots them as raw data. From the raw data we have to find out the change in the retinal sensitivity from the normative data at each point. The retinal sensitivity is highest at the fovea and low at the periphery. The raw data has different retinal sensitivity values at each point even in normal field. So, it is difficult to identify early field defects just by seeing the raw data.

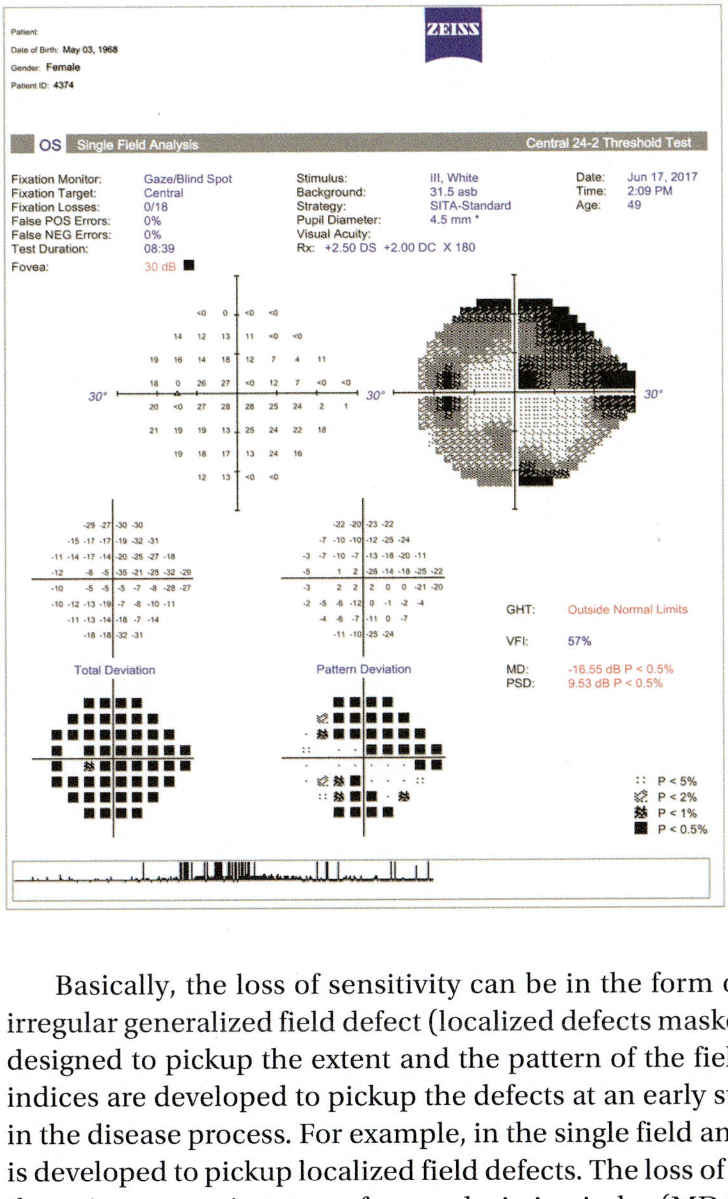

To know whether the sensitivity at any predetermined point is normal or not, the normal retinal sensitivity value at each point should be known, which is impossible to remember. To overcome this problem, the computer stores the mean normal threshold values at each point for all age groups. To establish the mean threshold values for different age groups, large number of normal population were tested keeping in mind the age of the patient, size of the pupil, refractive error correction, selection of the point pattern, selection of testing strategy, size of the stimulus, fixation center and reliability indices, etc. The raw data of the patient is now compared with mean normal threshold values of the same age group and the difference between the measured retinal sensitivity and the mean normal retinal sensitivity at all points is calculated and plotted as total deviation numerical plot (TDNP). TDNP is nothing but raw data expressed in terms of deviation values from normal values. The most important function of field analyzers is to establish the total deviation numerical plot. It becomes easy to know loss of sensitivity from TDNP.

Basically, the loss of sensitivity can be in the form of a localized defect/uniform generalized defect/ irregular generalized field defect (localized defects masked by generalized field defect). The field charts are designed to pickup the extent and the pattern of the field defects even in generalized field defects. Some indices are developed to pickup the defects at an early stage and also to pickup even the mild progression in the disease process. For example, in the single field analysis printouts, pattern standard deviation (PSD) is developed to pickup localized field defects. The loss of sensitivity is expressed as mean of all the points of the point pattern in terms of mean deviation index (MD index).

The STATPAC expresses the severity of PSD value and MD index in terms of statistical significance (P value). STATPAC calculates P value of each decibel deviation in the total deviation numerical plot and a symbol is allotted to each P value. Thus, each deviation value in the total deviation numerical plot is converted to symbolic form according to its P value and plotted as total deviation probability plot. One should never try to estimate the depth of the field defect from the probability plots. The STATPAC developed a new software-Glaucoma Hemifield Test (GHT) to pickup glaucoma at a very early stage. The software calculates the difference of retinal sensitivity values between the corresponding points on either side of the horizontal axis. In glaucoma, there will be a difference in the sensitivity between the corresponding points on either side of the horizontal axis. The localized field defects can be identified by similar total deviation probability plot and the pattern deviation probability plots (TDPP and PDPP show similar field defects), with a corresponding localized dark area in the grey scale and PSD with significant P value. The uniform generalized field defect can be identified by generalized field defect in the total deviation probability plot with a normal pattern deviation probability plot, uniform shade in the grey scale, high MD index and PSD without significant P value. The irregular generalized field defect can be identified by generalized field defect in the total deviation probability plot with a localized field defect in the pattern deviation probability plot, with different shades in the grey scale, high MD index and PSD value with significant P value.

From the above information one can know whether the field defect is generalized, localized or irregular generalized. If it is a generalized field defect, pattern deviation probability plot tells whether it is uniform generalized field defect or irregular generalized field defect. Now it is up to us to decide whether the field defect is corresponding to our clinical condition or not. Usually in early cases of glaucoma, a localized field defect is seen. In advanced cases of glaucoma and in cases of cataract with coexisting glaucoma, there will be irregular generalized field defect. When we suspect glaucoma in a case of cataract, the suspicion of glaucoma can be eliminated if the field shows generalized field defect in the total deviation probability plot without any localized field defect in the pattern deviation probability plot (i.e. cataract produces an uniform generalized field defect). The aim of creating the probability plots is to know the extent and pattern of the field defect. Once the field defect becomes generalized, the pattern of the field defect is not known in the total deviation probability plot. The next step is the conversion of total deviation plots to pattern deviation plots to know the pattern of the field defect in generalized depression. By the pattern of the field defect various conditions other than glaucoma like anterior ischemic optic neuropathy (AION), optic tract disorders, occipital lobe infarcts can be diagnosed even when these conditions are associated with diseases which can cause generalized depression.

UNDERSTANDING OF SINGLE FIELD ANALYSIS PRINTOUT

For better understanding and to interpret the visual fields systematically, the single field analysis printout is divided into 11 zones. Broadly, these 11 zones can be classified into 2 groups:

- Group 1 consists of zones independent of normative data and STATPAC analysis
- Group 2 consists of zones dependent on normative data and STATPAC analysis

ZONES OF SINGLE FIELD ANALYSIS PRINTOUT

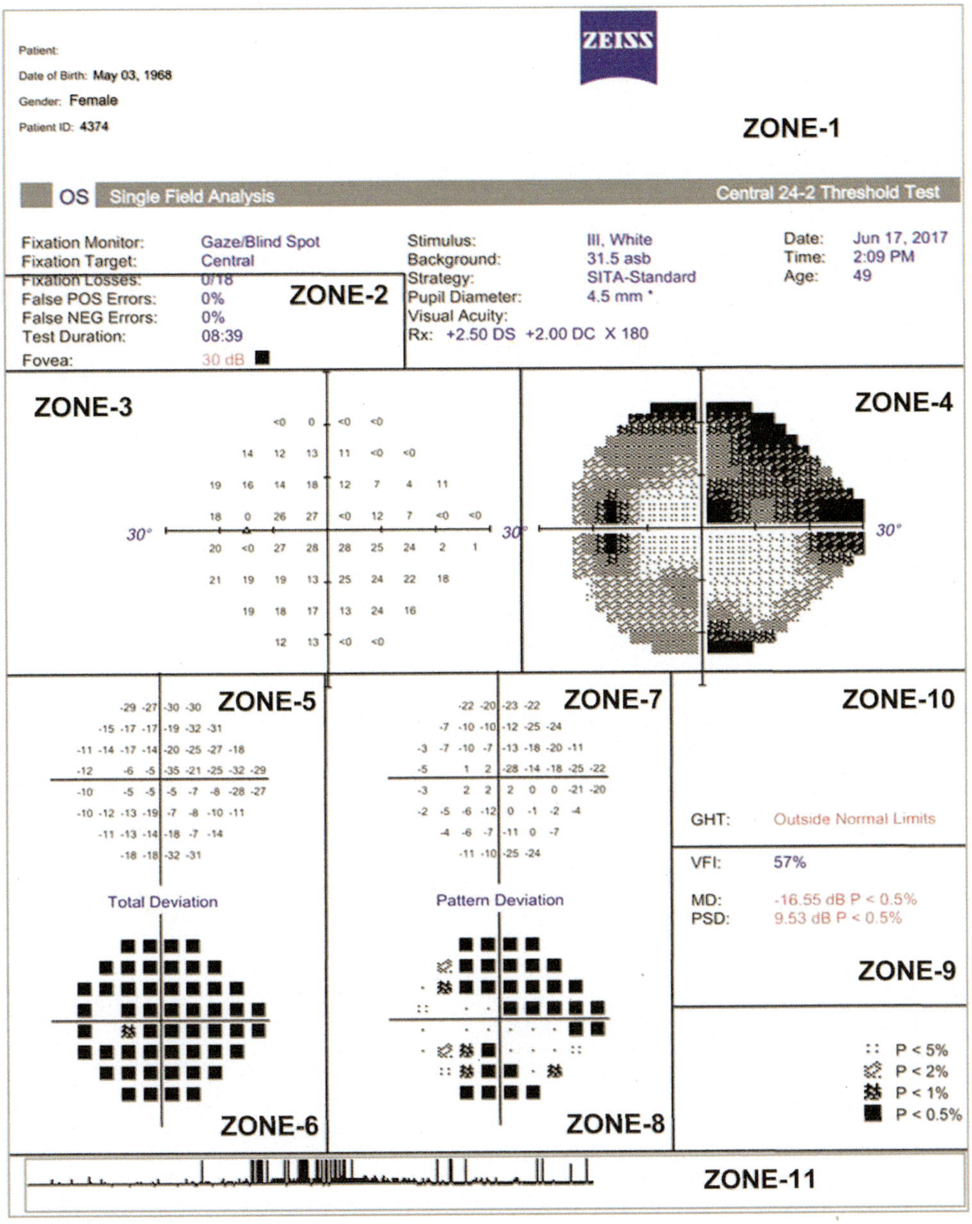

GROUP 1

Zones—Independent of normative data and STATPAC analysis.

Zone 1: Patient data/test data.

Zone 2: Reliability indices/foveal threshold.

Zone 3: Raw data.

Zone 4: Grey scale.

GROUP 2

Zones—dependent on normative data and STATPAC analysis.

Zone 5: Total deviation numerical plot (TDNP).

Zone 6: Total deviation probability plot (TDPP).

Zone 7: Pattern deviation numerical plot (PDNP).

Zone 8: Pattern deviation probability plot (PDPP).

Zone 9: Global indices.

Zone 10: Glaucoma hemifield test.

Zone 11: Gaze tracking.

From the above classification, it is understood that if normative data is not available, the zones dependent on normative data—STATPAC analysis will not be seen in the visual field printout charts.

ZONES OF SINGLE FIELD ANALYSIS PRINTOUT

ZONE 1 PATIENT DATA AND TEST DATA

ZONE 2 RELIABILITY INDICES
FOVEAL THRESHOLD

ZONE 3 RAW DATA

Measured retinal sensitivity of the selected point pattern

ZONE 4 GREY SCALE

Measured retinal sensitivity (Raw data) is shown in shades

ZONE 5 TOTAL DEVIATION NUMERICAL PLOT (TDNP)

To know the depth of the field defect

ZONE 6 TOTAL DEVIATION PROBABILITY PLOT (TDPP)

To know the extent and pattern of the field defect

ZONE 7 PATTERN DEVIATION NUMERICAL PLOT (PDNP)

General height of hill of vision is adjusted to bring out the pattern of the field defect in a generalized depression.

ZONE 8 PATTERN DEVIATION PROBABILITY PLOT (PDPP)

To know the pattern of the field defect in a generalized depression

ZONE 10

GLAUCOMA HEMIFIELD TEST

ZONE 9

GLOBAL INDICES, MD INDEX, VFI AND PSD

Probability symbols

ZONE 11 GAZE TRACKING

ZONE 1

Patient Data

Zone 1 is patient's data and the test data fed to the field analyzer. Patient's data includes name, date of birth, visual acuity, refractive error correction for near, pupil size.

Name of the patient—Name and age of the patient should be entered correctly. The name of the patient should be entered similarly in the follow-up tests to get the follow-up field reports on the same sheet (overview printout).

Date of birth—Date of birth of the patient should be entered correctly. Otherwise the patient's raw data will be compared to normative data of a wrong age group and thus the derived deviation values from normative data will be totally inaccurate. Thus, we will get an inaccurate total deviation numerical plot. All the zones except the first four zones (independent of normative data) will be inaccurate.

Visual acuity and refractive error correction—If visual acuity and foveal sensitivity correlate with each other, it indicates that the refractive error correction for near was correct. The patient's near vision refractive error must be accurate. The lens must be properly placed in the trial frame of the automated perimeter and the correcting lens should be very close to the testing eye. Otherwise it can produce artifacts.

Effect of the size of the pupil—Normally the size of the pupil should be between 3 mm to 4 mm (The normative data was obtained with the pupil size 3–4 mm). Constricted pupil is thought to give rise to diffuse visual field depression or edge scotomas. Pupil less than 2 mm is more likely to exert a significant effect on the overall level of the visual field particularly if media opacity is present in the visual axis.

Test Data (Selection of the test)

The test data includes three constant parameters. They are: (1) fixation monitor (Blind spot), (2) color of the stimulus (white), background illumination (31.5) asb. The fixation target, size of the stimulus, point pattern and testing strategy vary according to the clinical conditions but remain constant during the test.

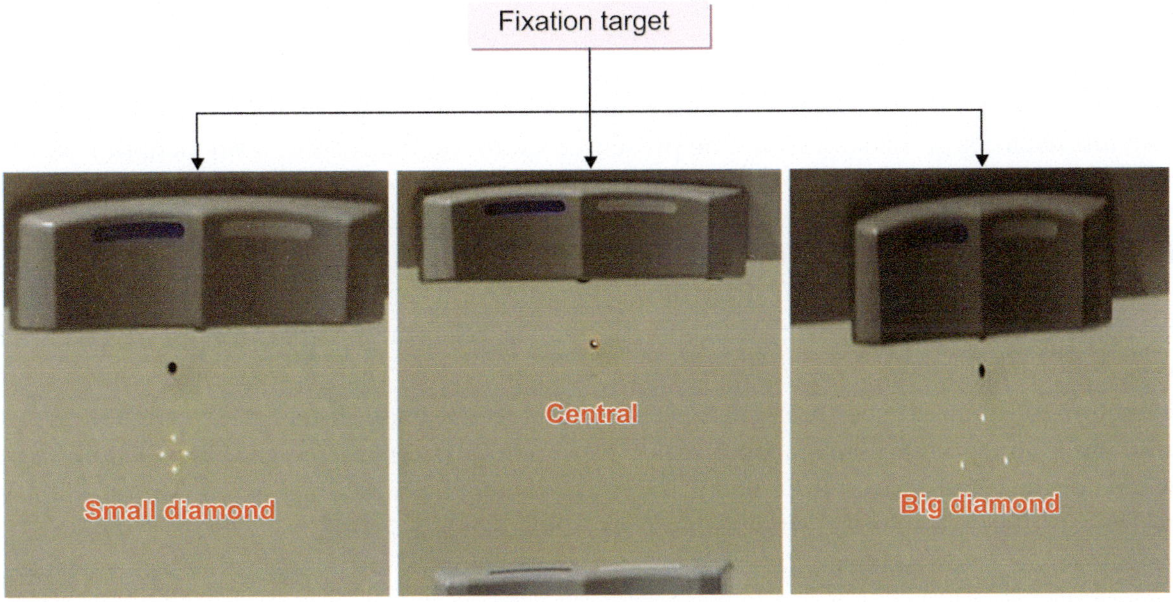

The fixation targets are of four types:

1. Central—Yellow light in the center of the bowl.
2. Small diamond—It is located below the central target and should be used if the patient cannot see the central fixation light, e.g. macular degeneration. The patient should look in the center of the diamond formed by the four lights.
3. Large diamond—It is located below the central target and is used for patient with central scotoma who cannot see either central fixation light or small diamond.
4. Bottom LED—Some tests have points in the superior visual field that require a lower fixation light than the central target. The target used is the bottom LED of the large diamond.

When testing with the superior 64 or superior 36 screening speciality tests, the bottom LED is the default fixation target. It is automatically illuminated at the beginning of a test. If no information is available regarding the fixation target the machine always adjusts the fixation target as central fixation. In special situations like macular disorders, the fixation target can be changed either to small or big diamond.

Size of the stimulus: The standard size of the stimulus is size III for all routine tests. But in situations like advanced glaucoma, the test may be conducted with size V to assess the status of macular split.

ZONE 2—FOVEAL THRESHOLD AND RELIABILITY INDICES

It is very important to measure foveal threshold at the very beginning of the test. If the patient has good visual acuity and significant reduction in the foveal sensitivity then the technician should become alert and check if the refractive error correction for near is correct or not.

Reliability Indices

The reliability indices include the fixation losses, false positive errors, false negative errors. Even if the test has very low reliability criteria this does not necessarily imply that the field will provide no useful information. It is just that such fields are not included in the data base and such fields should be interpreted with more caution.

Fixation Losses

During the test itself 5% of the stimuli will be presented on to the blind spot. If the patient fixes at central fixation target, the patient should not respond to the stimulus presenting on the blind spot area. If the patient responds to such a stimulus, he or she is not fixing at the fixation target. The patient's response to this stimulus presentation is due to shift of fixation. The fixation losses > 20% are considered to be unreliable. Always instruct the patient to look at fixation target what is fed to the machine because the location of the blind spot in the field chart depends on the fixation target. The machine locates the blind spot area according to the fixation target selected.

The location of the blind spot area changes according to the fixation target. The patient must look at the fixation target that is fed to the machine. If the fixation target was entered as central fixation target, the machine locates the blind spot by the small triangle just below the horizontal axis 15° temporal to fixation (fixation is at the intersection of the vertical and horizontal axes).

Fixation monitoring

Blind spot (Heijl-Krakau) monitoring
Most common perimetric method for fixation monitoring

Gaze tracking (Zone 11)
A patented, high precision system which uses real-time image analysis to verify if the patient is looking at the fixation target or not

Blind spot (Heijl-Krakau) monitoring

Moderately bright stimuli are presented periodically in the presumed location of the patient's blind spot.

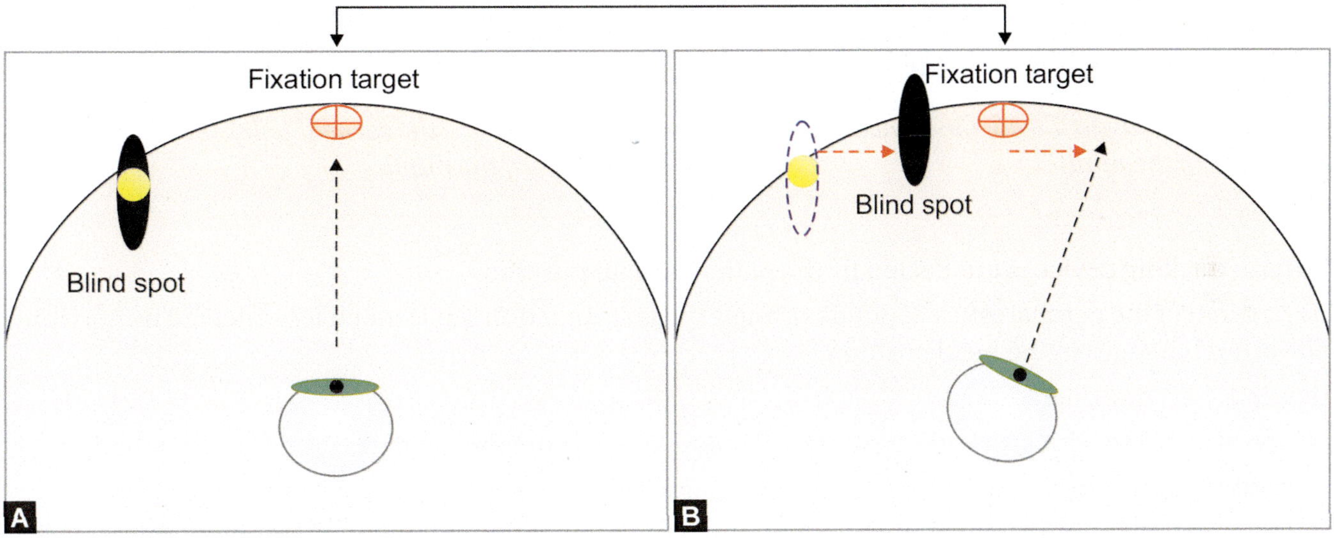

If the patient is fixating centrally, a stimulus presented within the blind spot should not be seen (See A).

If the blind spot check stimulus presented is seen, it must be because the patient is no longer fixating the central target (See B).

Sources of error

Depends on the accuracy of the blind spot location.

It does not constantly assess fixation.

Affected by patient's head tilt.

Humphrey Field Analyzer Fixation Monitoring: Gaze Tracking

Patented, high precision system which uses real-time image analysis to verify if the patient is looking at the fixation target. It measures the distance between the pupil center and the corneal reflex.

It is a two-variable gaze tracking system. Note that the measurement made is the distance between two features of the eye and is, therefore, independent of head movement.

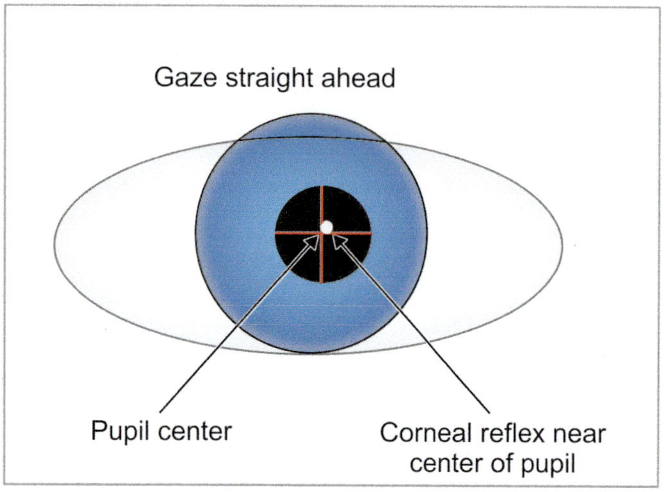

When gaze is straight ahead, the corneal reflex is near the center of the pupil.

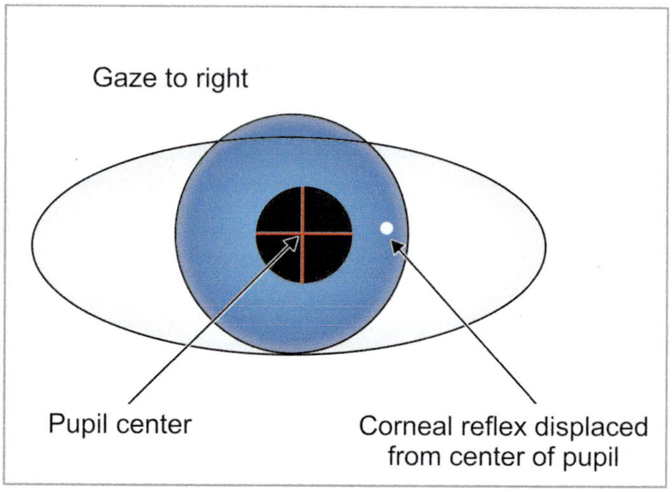

When gaze shifts, the corneal reflex is displaced from the center of the pupil.

The gaze tracking device is unaffected by the patient's head position.

The position of the corneal reflex depends strongly on gaze direction but is much less affected by horizontal and vertical changes in the head position.

Precision ~ +/- one degree.

Fixation is checked with every stimulus presentation (vs 5% of the time with the blind spot method).

No testing time is devoted to fixation check presentations.

The gaze tracking shown on the screen helps the technician monitor the test. The technician may decide to restart the test if gaze tracking shows that the patient is not cooperating or has not understood the test. In case of new patients, we recommend the technicians closely monitor gaze tracking to make sure that the patient has fully understood the instructions.

HFA GAZE TRACKER (ZONE 11)

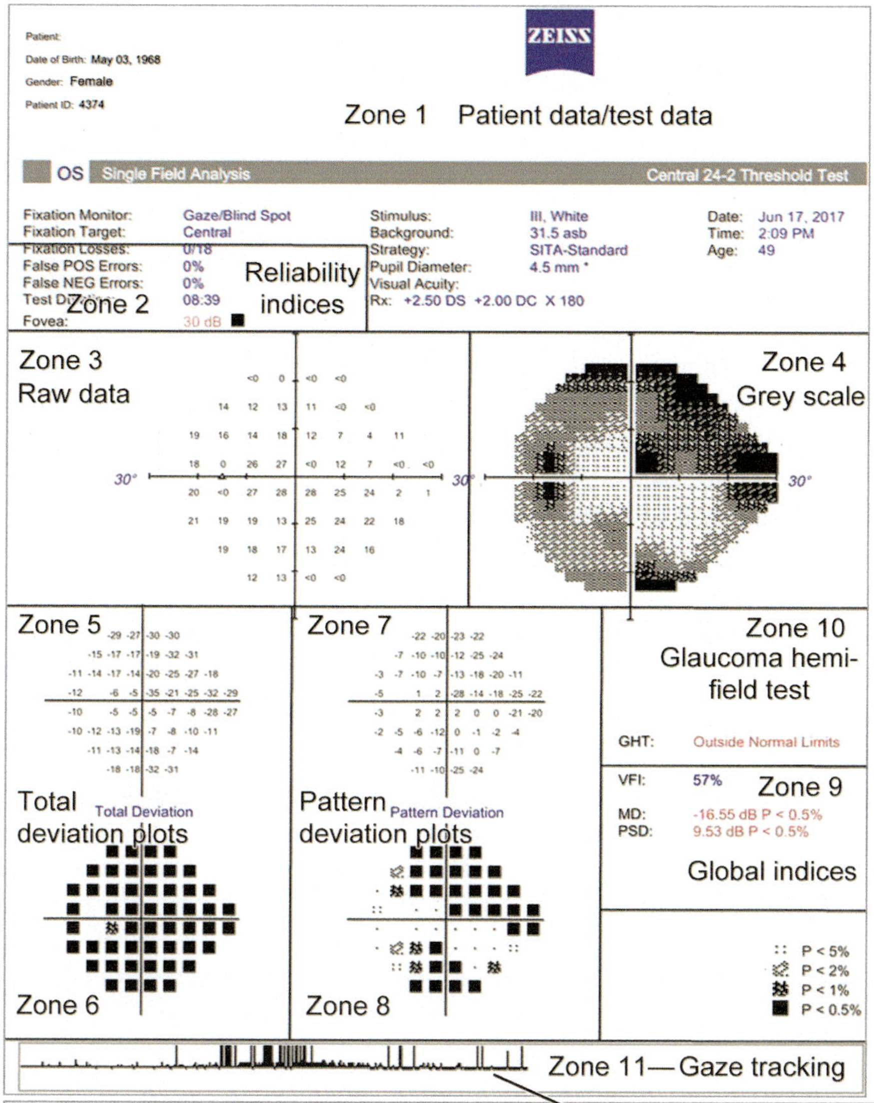

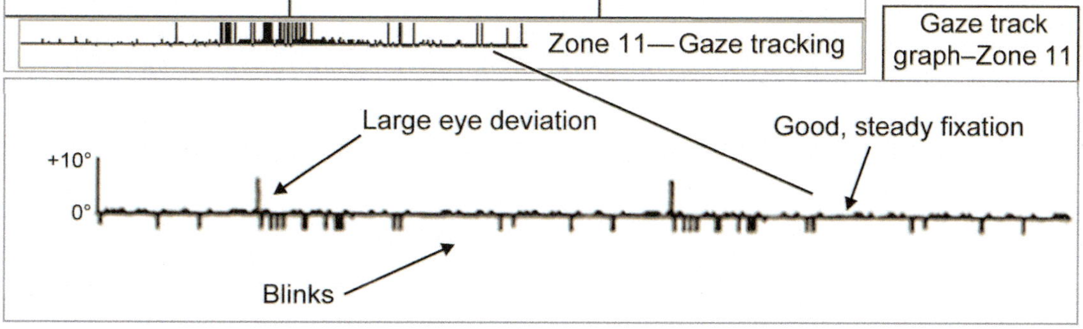

A continuous record of fixation is available on the test screen for monitoring during the test.

The Gaze Track graph is included on the printout to provide a permanent record of the patient's fixation.

A general estimate of the usefulness of the test results can be made.

Gaze stability history can help clinicians interpret certain findings. For example, if fixation deteriorates towards the end of testing, points tested last (on the periphery) would be most affected.

Upward deflections indicate gaze error.

Downward deflections indicate absent pupil images or corneal reflexes, usually due to blink. On the gaze tracking record, lines extending upward indicate the amount of gaze error during each stimulus presentation, with full scale indicating gaze errors of 10° or more. Lines extending downward indicate the unsuccessful measurement of gaze direction, for instance, because of a blink.

Even highly experienced perimetry patients show occasional gaze errors, and such fixation patterns are generally associated with reliable test results.

False Positive Errors

If the patient pushes the response button to the nonprojected stimulus or responding to a dimmer light stimulus for which he or she should not respond will be recorded as false positive response. Most patients will have some false positive responses during the test. If the false positive rate exceeds 33% the printout will indicate so by printing "XX" next to rate. "XX" next to any of the indices is considered to be unacceptable by the machine and indicative of unreliability. With high rate of false positive responses the grey tone printouts show multiple white scotomas corresponding to areas of abnormally high sensitivity.

False Negative Response

Failure to respond to the brightest stimulus in an area previously determined to have some sensitivity is a false negative response. High false negatives may indicate lack of attentiveness, fatigue or hypnosis. In general greater than 20% rate of false negative response is considered to be abnormal though the machine defaults to 33%. Fields should not be considered unreliable solely upon a false negative response rate, particularly if there is a great deal of pathology. In patients with advanced glaucomatous optic nerve damage we may get more than 50% false response which can be attributed to small shifts in fixation.

Always try to get the false positives, false negatives and fixation losses to zero, and zero respectively in suspicious case of glaucoma. Even 1% FL, FP and FN will have an impact in the interpretation of the single field analysis printout. In established and advanced cases of glaucoma up to 20% of false positives, false negatives and fixation losses are considered to be acceptable.

Importance of locating blind spot before interpreting the visual field analysis

100% fixation losses are seen in figure (next page) resulting from proper localization of the blind spot followed by performance of the test while fixating on the lower fixation target instead of the center. An unusual cause of high fixation losses is shown in the single field analysis printout. The selected fixation target is central and is fed to the machine. The machine locates blind spot area for central fixation (below the horizontal meridian 15° temporal to fixation). Due to lack of proper understanding of the test, patient performed the test while fixing on the lower fixation target (small diamond or big diamond) in the bowl instead of fixing on the central fixation target.

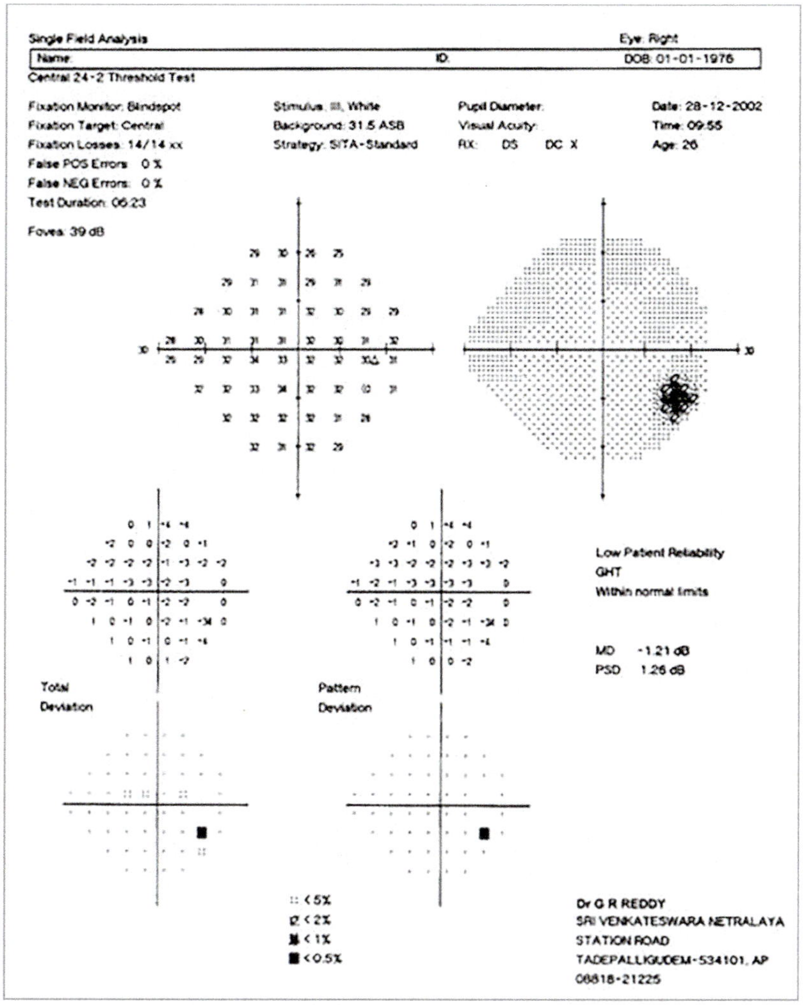

If the patient performs the test while fixing on the small diamond or big diamond (lower fixation target in the bowl instead of fixing on the central fixation target) the eye rotates down and actual blind spot area moves down in the field and the located blind spot area for the central fixation becomes seeing area. During the test 5% of the stimuli will be presented on to the blind spot area located for central fixation by the machine which is no longer a blind spot area. Each fixation loss catch trial was in actuality projected on to seeing retina and elicited a response, resulting in the 100% fixation loss rate recorded. Care must be taken in all aspects of test performance to avoid such problems. This point's measured retinal sensitivity 0 dB appears as a black spot below the horizontal axis on the grey scale representing the shifted blind spot.

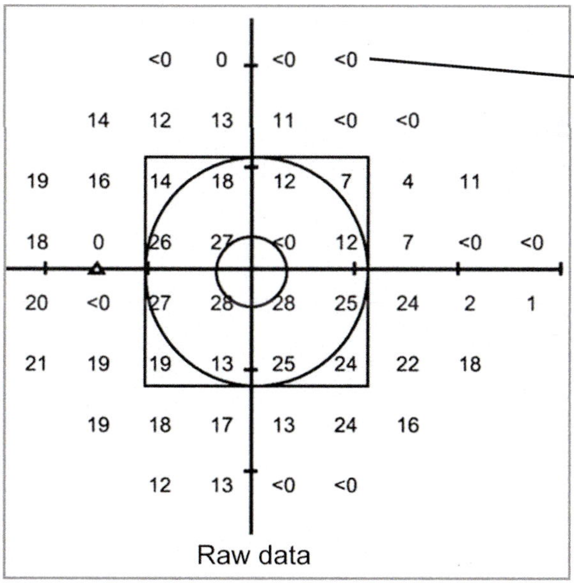

ZONE 3—RAW DATA

(<0) indicates no response to the maximum intensity of light projected by the field analyzer it means that the point is an absolute scotoma.

Point pattern 24-2

Testing strategy—SITA standard

Raw data is the exact retinal sensitivity in dB units of the selected points calculated by field analyzer. Only the numerical value is displayed and the dB unit is omitted. '0' indicates absolute scotoma (no response to the maximum intensity of light intensity—10,000 asb units in Humphrey field analyzer). The number 50 indicates response to (0.1) asb unit. The number 50 is the highest retinal sensitivity that can be recorded by the Humphrey field analyzer (HFA) because 0.1 asb unit of light intensity is the dimmest light that can be projected by Humphrey field analyzer. In the same patient, the raw data calculated by different strategies is not exactly similar. So raw data is strategy specific. Hence, for follow-up tests, one should select the same strategy which was used for the previous test. Only the result of the latest test will be compared with the previous test to assess progression.

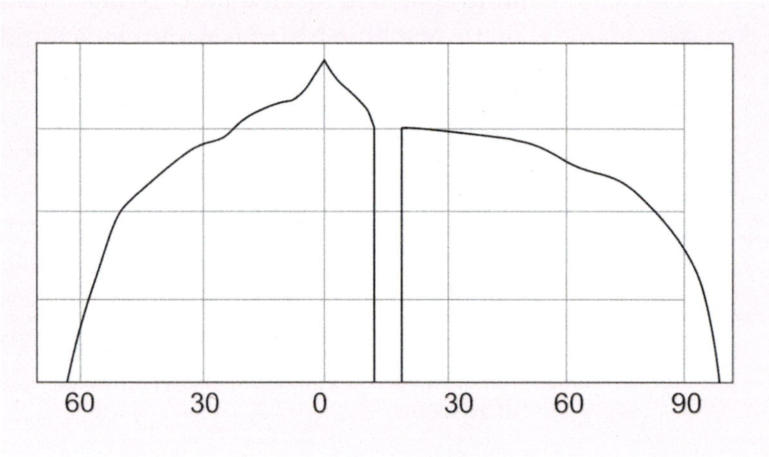

The hill of vision

Even though the measured retinal sensitivity is normal at all the points, the raw data contains different sensitivity values at each point because the retinal sensitivity is not the same at all points. It is highest at the fovea and as we go towards periphery the retinal sensitivity decreases. The retinal sensitivity at 5° from the fovea is always higher than the retinal sensitivity at 10° from the fovea. So the normal slope (contour) of the hill of vision is smooth. Depending on the type of field defect, changes will occur in the average height of hill of vision, with or without change in the contour of hill of vision.

Normally (<) sign is seen only in front of (0). But in this raw data there is (<) in front of (1). That means the maximum intensity of light projected by field analyzer is not 10,000 asb units but it is less than 10,000 asb units. If there is no response to this maximum intensity of light (less than 10,000 asb units), an (<) sign infront of any digit other than 0. This indicates that the light is dim and it is time to replace the bulb or it requires recalibration.

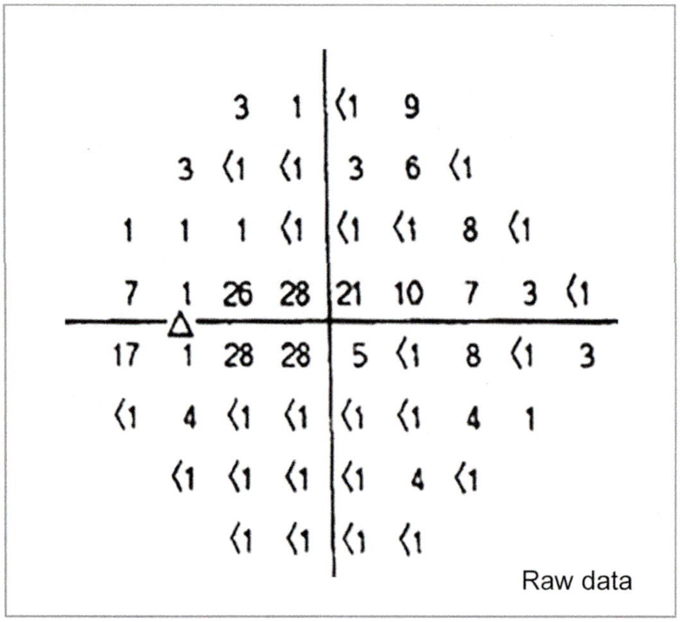

Point pattern 24-2
Testing strategy—SITA Standard.

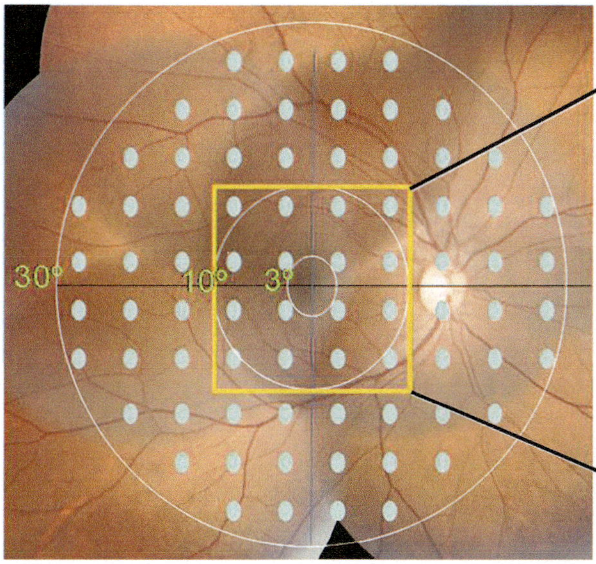

30-2 point pattern

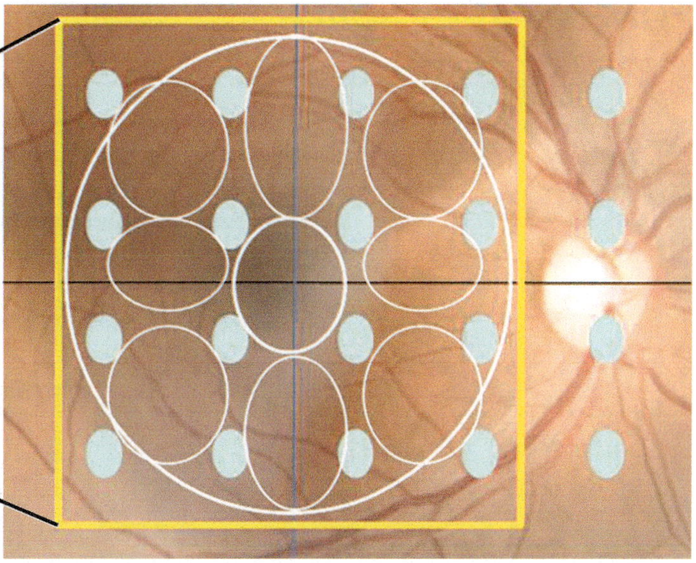

10° circle area of 30-2 or 24-2 point pattern

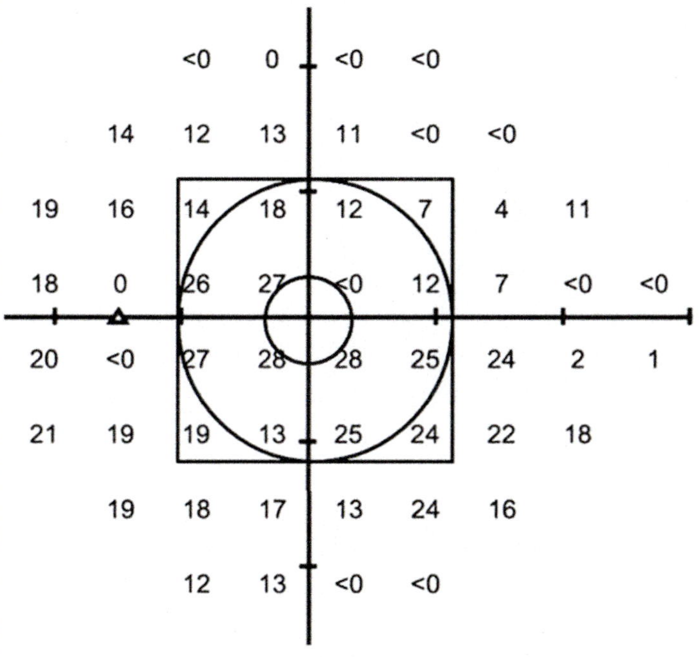

Raw data

In 30-2 or 24-2 point pattern the central 3° radius circle area is not having points. Hence, these point patterns are not suitable to know foveal split. The sensitivities of all the 16 points present in the 10° circle area play an important role to decide if the test has to be repeated with 10-2 point pattern or not.

Concentrate on the sensitivities of the 16 points in the 10° circle area. If there is severe loss of sensitivity even at one point among the 16 points, we should repeat the test with 10-2 point pattern. If the probability plot shows a black square at any point, do not come to any conclusion whether the black square is an absolute scotoma or a relative scotoma till you see the raw data. A 0 dB in the raw data indicates absolute scotoma.

Macular split—Never come to a conclusion regarding the foveal status from the probability plots (even from 10-2 point pattern). Never say that there is foveal split, unless you see the 0 dB sensitivity at any of the four points on 1° circle around fixation in 10-2 point pattern.

ZONE 4—GREY SCALE

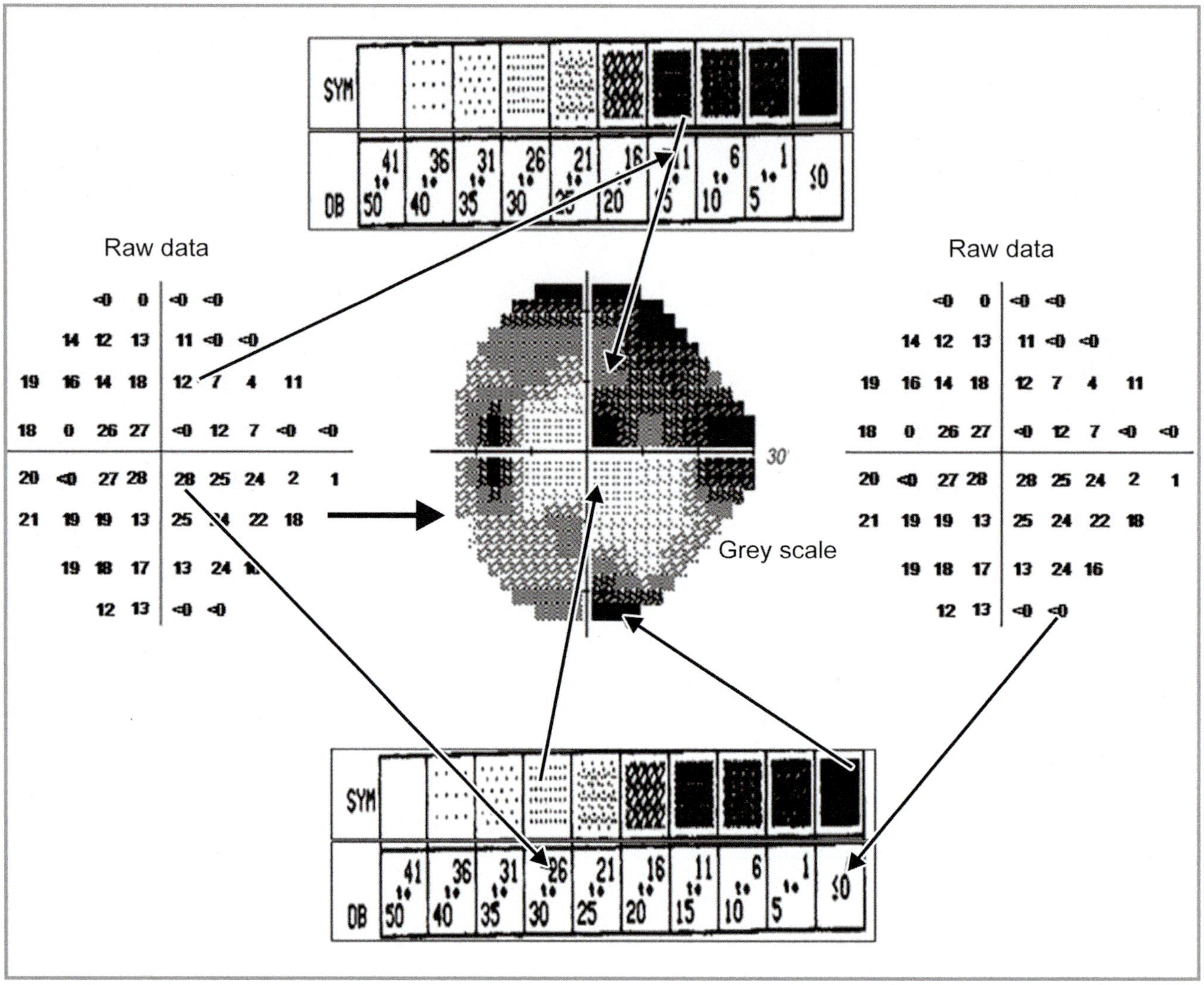

The sensitivity values from the best (50 dB) to absolute scotoma (0 dB) are divided into 10 groups. Each step of the pattern corresponds to a change of 5 dB intensity, except the first column represented by 50 dB to 41 dB. Now, the numerical values of the raw data in (dB) units are presented graphically according to a grey scale form in which, areas of high sensitivity are denoted by lighter shades and areas of low sensitivity are denoted by darker shades. The conversion of the raw data to grey scale does not involve any statistical calculations or normative analysis.

Do not make any definitive diagnosis on the basis of grey scale. It only gives an idea about the pattern and the depth of the field defect. In high false positives, areas of white zones will be appreciated. When there are high false negatives the grey scale gives a clover leaf appearance. The grey scale is also useful to explain the seriousness of the condition to the patient. The grey scale can also give a rough idea of the pattern of visual field loss. Now, I will be discussing the advantages and disadvantages of grey scale.

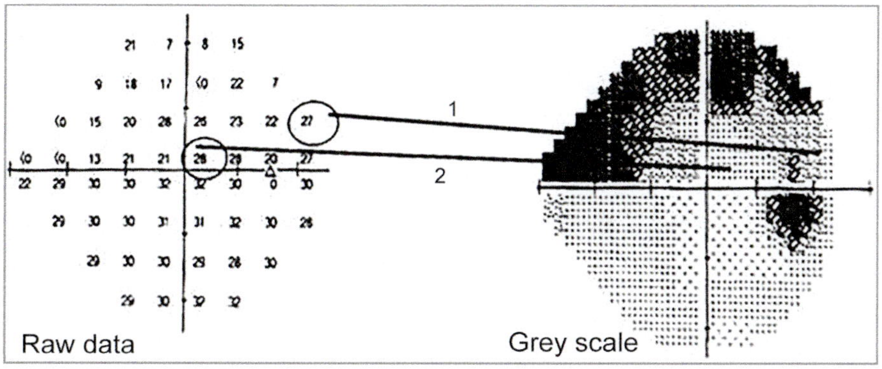

The two main drawbacks in the conversion of raw data to grey scale are as follows:

The retinal sensitivity is highest at the fovea and lowest at periphery. In this raw data two points are selected. One point is on 3° circle and the second one is from the outer most set of points (The other name commonly used for the outer most set of points is edge points).

In the example-1, the retinal sensitivity of the point on 3° circle is 28 dB, and the retinal sensitivity of the point from the outer most set of points is 27 dB. So both the points are given the same shade. If you carefully observe the retinal sensitivity 28 dB on 3° is not normal (the expected normal value at that location is around 35 dB. So there is a loss of sensitivity by 7 dB), whereas the retinal sensitivity of edge point is 27 dB which is almost normal (the expected normal value at that location is around 29 dB. So there is a loss of sensitivity by 2 dB). So points of 2 dB loss and 7dB loss are represented by the same shade.

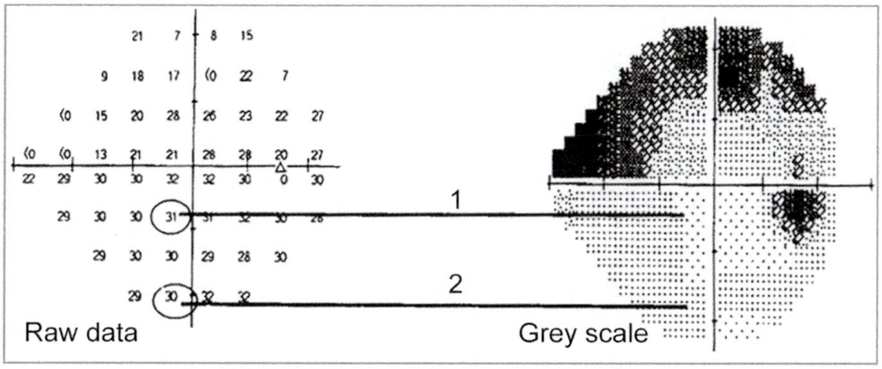

In the example-2 two locations are selected. At the location 1 the sensitivity is 31 dB and the location 2 the sensitivity is 30 dB. Though there is only 1 dB difference between the two locations, the shades given to them differ grossly. If you observe carefully at location 1, the sensitivity is 31 dB (the expected normal value at that location being 34 dB. So there is a loss of sensitivity by 3 dB).

The sensitivity at location 2 is 30 dB. The expected normal value at that location is around 29 dB. So there is no loss of sensitivity at this location. Between these two points, the normal location 2 is given a worse shade when compared to location 1, which is expected to be abnormal. Observe the sudden shift of the shade by 1dB difference (here from 30 dB to 31 dB). These are some more limitations of grey scale. But still it has got its own importance in picking up early localized field defects, pattern of the field defects, false (+) white areas and is very useful in glaucoma progression analysis (overview printouts). The depth of the field defect is better appreciated in grey scale than the probability plots. A thick black shade in grey scale indicates absolute scotoma. But a black square in the probability plot need not be an absolute scotoma.

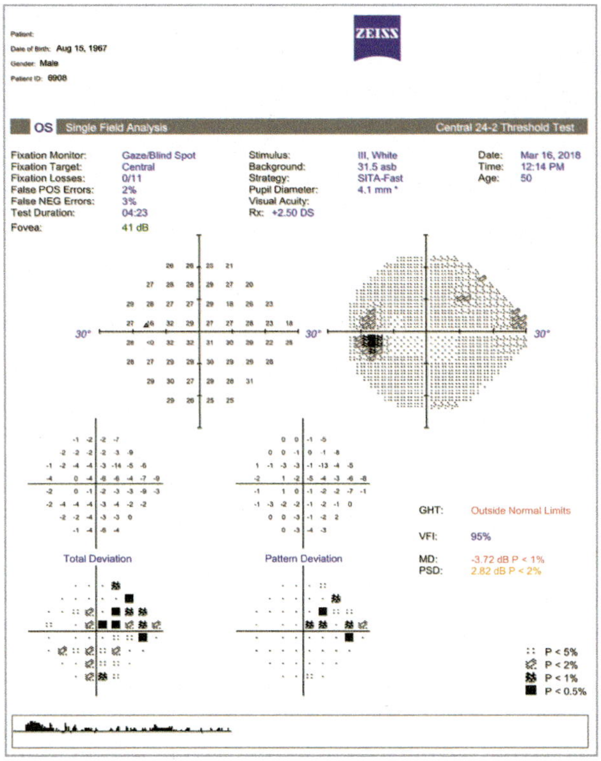

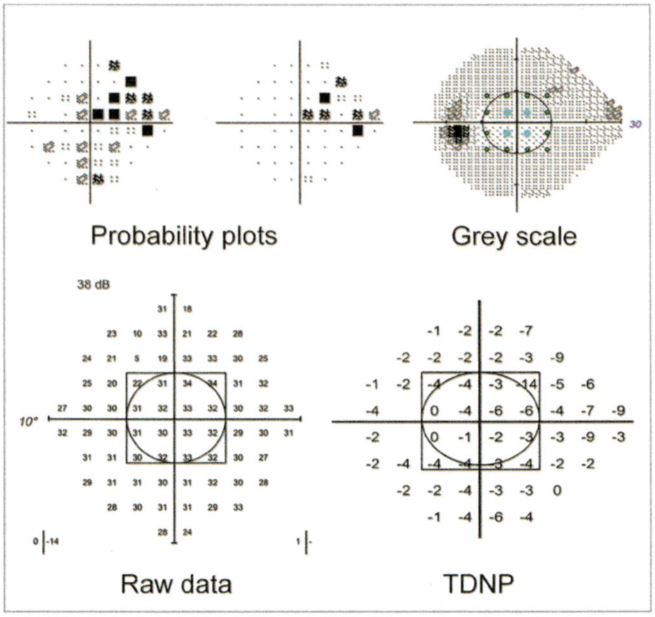

The most important disadvantage of the grey scale—Though TDNP is showing the loss of sensitivity at some of the points in 10° circle area as 4 dB and 5 dB, the sensitivity of these points is 28 dB or 29 dB because the sensitivity of the points in the macular area is high. Still 28 dB or 29 dB will have good shade in the grey scale. So minimal loss of sensitivity of the points of 10° circle area will not be appreciated in the grey scale. But minimal loss of sensitivity will be appreciated in the probability plots as shown here.

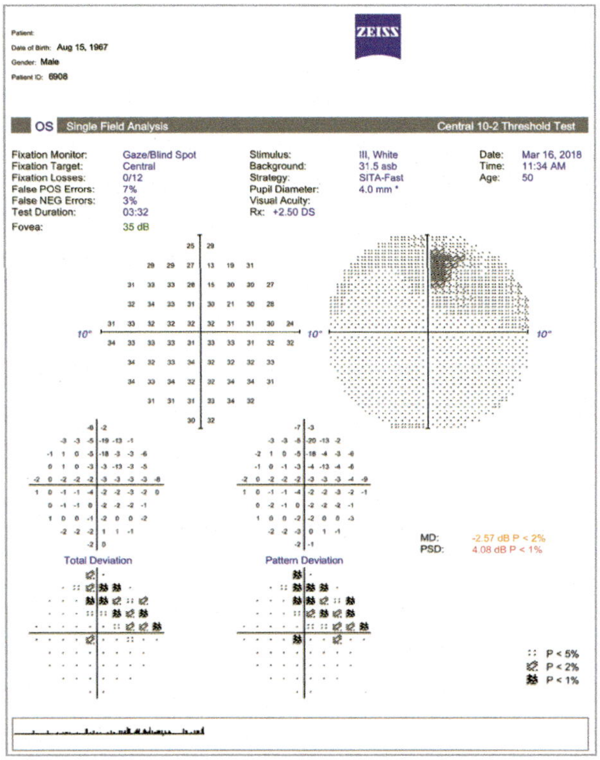

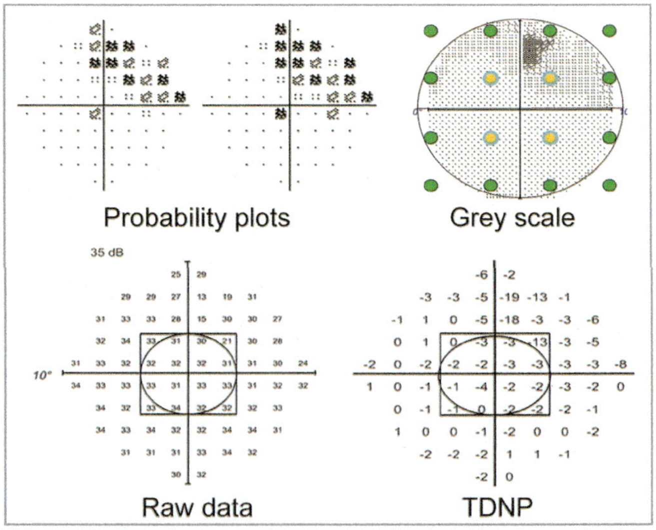

From these two examples, it is very clear that the early field defects in the 10° circle area will not be picked up the grey scale, but will be appreciated in the probability plots as shown here.

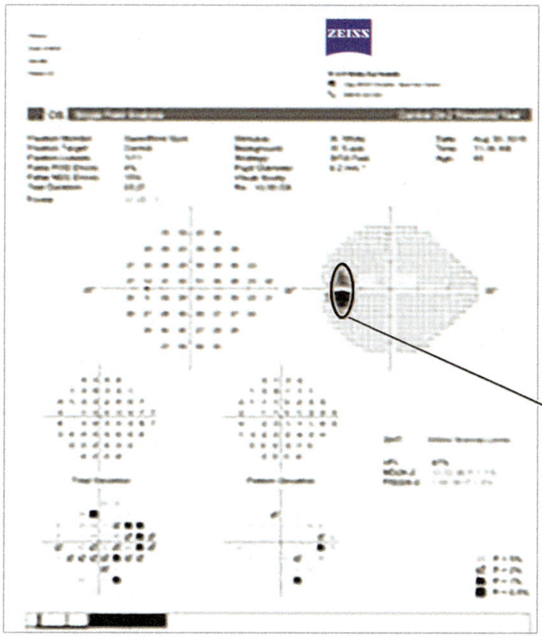

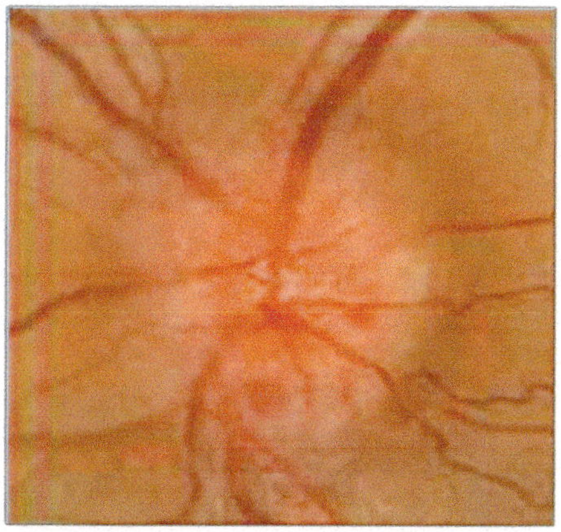

Enlargement of the blind spot is well appreciated in the grey scale than in the probability plot.

Normal size and location of the blind spot

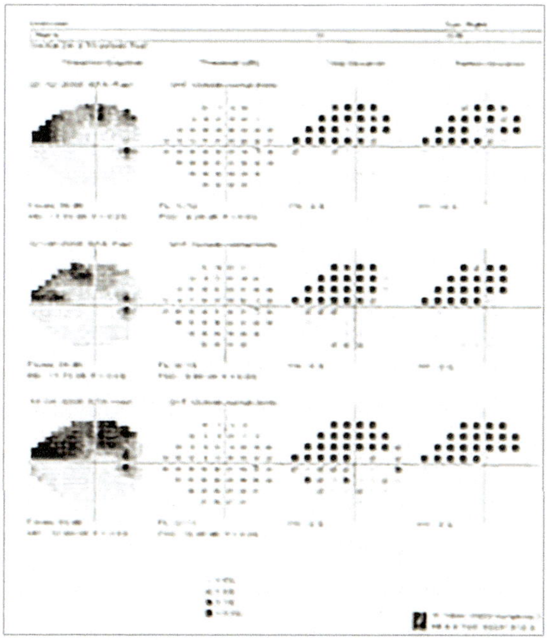

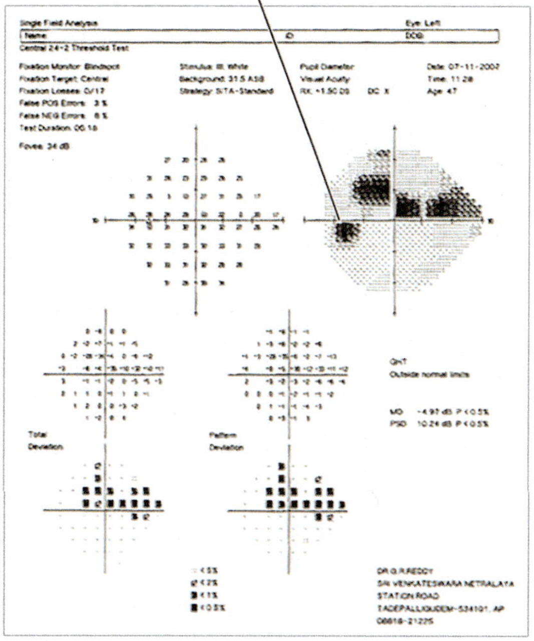

In this example, probability plots are similar and there is increased darker shade in the grey scale from the 1st to last test. The darker shade reflects a deeper scotoma. So the change in depth of the scotoma is better appreciated in the grey scale than in the probability plots.

In this example, grey scale is showing multiple areas of dark shades which suggests multicentric origin of glaucoma. Multicentric origin of glaucoma is better appreciated in the grey scale than the probability plots.

ZONE 5—TOTAL DEVIATION NUMERICAL PLOT (TDNP)

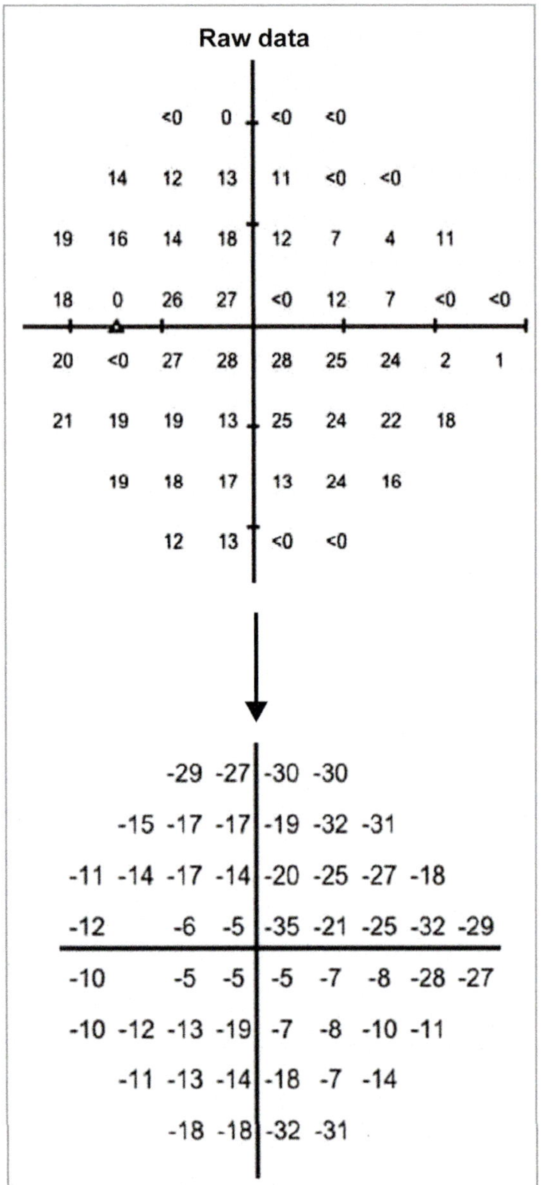

Total deviation numerical plot

In this example of TDNP, there is not zero (0) deviation point and deviation point without sign. All the deviational values are having (-) sign infront of them.

The measured retinal sensitivity of each point (raw data) is now compared with the normative data of same age group and the difference between them at each point is plotted as TDNP. TDNP is nothing but raw data expressed in terms of deviation values from normal values. TDNP contains values deviated from the normative data.

In this example of TDNP, there is no zero (0) deviation point and deviation point without sign. All the deviational values are having (-) sign in front of them. Zero (0) deviation in the total deviation numerical plot means the measured retinal sensitivity and the normal value are same. So zero in TDNP means that there is no loss of sensitivity at that point. The deviation value without sign means that the measured sensitivity value is better than the normal value. The deviation value with (-) ve sign indicates loss of sensitivity at that point. The loss of sensitivity is directly proportional to the numerical value. The high deviation values with (-) in front of them indicate that the loss of sensitivity at that point is heavy (deep scotomas) and lower deviation values with (-) sign in front of them indicate superficial scotomas. For all practical purposes, we can label the total deviation numerical plot as loss of sensitivity plot. The loss or change of retinal sensitivity will be well appreciated by the deviation values of the TDNP.

If there is no significant field loss, TDNP contains the deviation values in the range of zero (0) deviation. If there is a localized field defect, we can identify it by locating high (-) deviation values at those particular areas. If there is a uniform field loss, TDNP contains almost similar (-) deviation values at all points and the difference between the highest (-) deviation point and lowest (-) deviation point of TDNP will be minimal. If there is irregular loss of sensitivity, TDNP contains dissimilar deviation values and the difference between the highest (-) deviation point and lowest (-) deviation point will be very high. The total deviation numerical plot becomes the platform for the calculations of global indices [mean deviation index/visual field index (VFI) and pattern standard deviation].

Concentrate on the deviation points with (-) sign in front of them. The exact loss of sensitivity at each point is known from the TDNP. Please get into the habit of seeing TDNP to know the depth of the field defect. It gives the exact change of sensitivity at each point from the normative data of the same age group. For all practical purposes the TDNP can be considered as loss of retinal sensitivity plot.

Understanding of total deviation numerical plot: Example 1

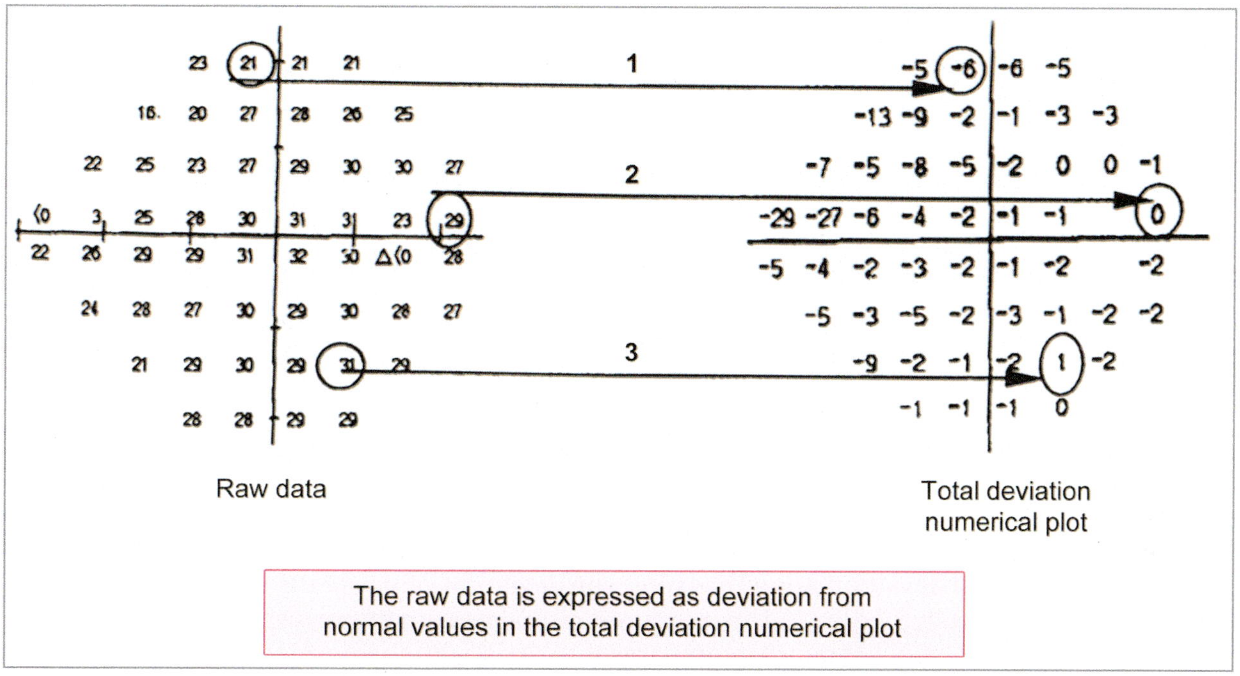

The existing retinal sensitivity (measured retinal sensitivity) of the patient is named as raw data. The raw data is expressed in terms of deviation values from normal values in the total deviation numerical plot. The most important point one should know is "why total deviation numerical plot is created?". The motto behind ordering for field is to know whether there is loss of sensitivity or not. We have to express the measured sensitivity in terms of deviation values from the normative data. Note that even 1 dB loss from normative data can be appreciated in the TDNP and the same cannot be appreciated in the raw data because, we do not know the normal value at that particular point.

1. The measured retinal sensitivity corresponding to arrow number 1 in the raw data is 21 dB and this 21 dB is expressed as -6 dB in the total deviation numerical plot. The field analyzer compares the 21dB with its age normal value which was stored in the field analyzer and expresses 21 dB as -6 dB deviation in the total deviation numerical plot. That means the normal sensitive value at this point is 27 dB which was stored in the field analyzer as normative data. -6 dB in the TDNP means that there is loss of sensitivity by 6 dB at this point. In TDNP, if any number carries (-) sign in front of it, it indicates that there is loss of sensitivity at this point.
2. The measured retinal sensitivity corresponding to arrow number 2 in the raw data is 29 dB and this 29 dB is expressed as zero (0) in the total deviation numerical plot. The field analyzer compares the 29 dB with its normative data which was stored in the field analyzer and expresses 29 dB as zero (0) deviation in the total deviation numerical plot. A (0) in the TDNP means that there is no loss of sensitivity at this point. That means the normal sensitivity value is 29 dB which was stored in the field analyzer as normative data. If there is 0 in TDNP, it indicates that there is no loss of sensitivity at this point.
3. The measured retinal sensitivity corresponding to arrow number 3 in the raw data is 31 dB and this 31 dB is expressed as 1 dB in the total deviation numerical plot. The field analyzer compares the 31 dB with its age normal value and expresses 31 dB as 1 dB deviation in the total deviation numerical plot. The deviation value 1dB in the TDNP means that at this point the sensitivity is better than normal by 1 dB. That means the normal value is 30 dB. Number without sign in TDNP indicates that the measured retinal sensitivity is better than its normal value.

Understanding of total deviation numerical plot: Example 2

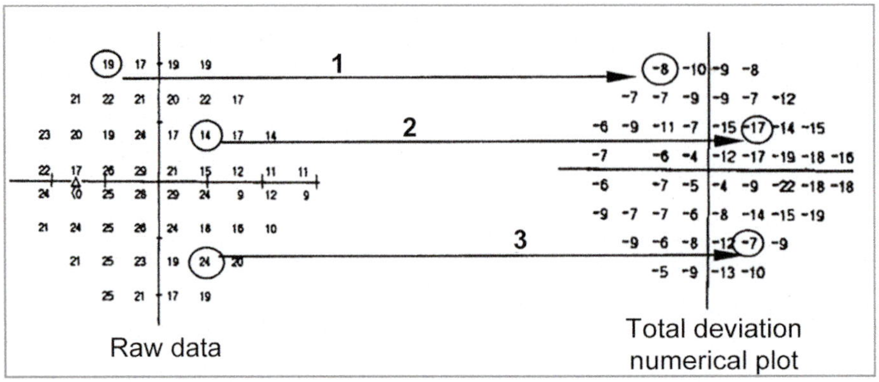

(1) The measured retinal sensitivity corresponding to arrow number 1 in the raw data is 19 dB. The field analyzer compares this 19 dB with its normative data and expresses 19 dB sensitivity as -8 dB deviation in the total deviation numerical plot. The deviation value -8 dB in the TDNP indicates loss of sensitivity at this point is by 8 dB. (2) The measured retinal sensitivity corresponding to arrow number 2 in the raw data is 14 dB. The field analyzer compares this 14 dB with its the normative data and expresses 14 dB sensitivity as -17 dB deviation in the total deviation numerical plot. The deviation value -17 dB in the TDNP indicates loss of sensitivity at this point is by 17 dB. (3) The measured retinal sensitivity corresponding to arrow number 3 in the raw data is 24 dB. The field analyzer compares this 24 dB with the normative data and expresses 24 dB sensitivity as -7 dB deviation in the total deviation numerical plot. The deviation value -7 dB in the TDNP indicates loss of sensitivity at this point is by 7 dB.

Understanding of total deviation numerical plot: Example 3

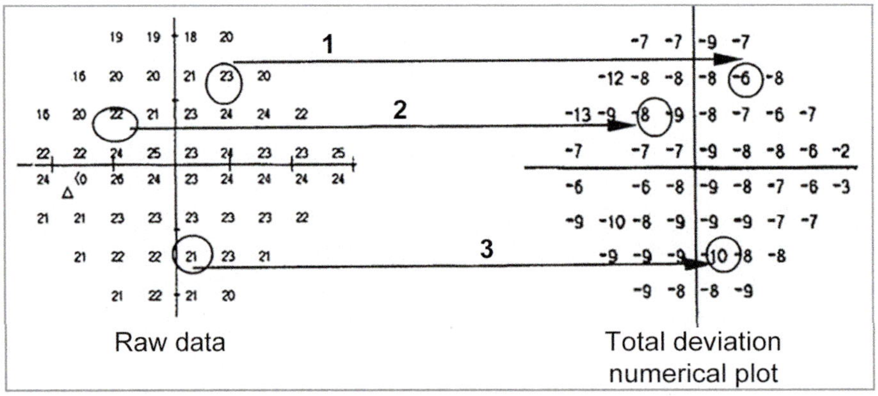

(1) The measured retinal sensitivity (raw data) corresponding to arrow 1 is 23 dB which is expressed as -6 dB in the TDNP. -6 dB in the TDNP indicates that there is loss of retinal sensitivity by 6 dB at that point. (2) The measured retinal sensitivity (raw data) corresponding to arrow 2 is 22 dB. The retinal sensitivity is 22 dB in the raw data is expressed as -8 dB in the TDNP indicating that the loss of sensitivity at that point is by 8 dB. (3) The measured retinal sensitivity (raw data) corresponding to arrow 3 is 21 dB. The sensitivity 21dB in the raw data is expressed as -10 dB in the TDNP. The deviation value -10 dB in the TDNP means that there is loss of retinal sensitivity by 10 dB at that point.

> The exact depth of the field defect is known in the TDNP. For all practical purposes the TDNP is loss of retinal sensitivity plot. A point with (0) deviation in TDNP means the measured sensitivity is normal. But (0) in raw data is an absolute scotoma.

ZONE 6—TOTAL DEVIATION PROBABILITY PLOTS (TDPP)

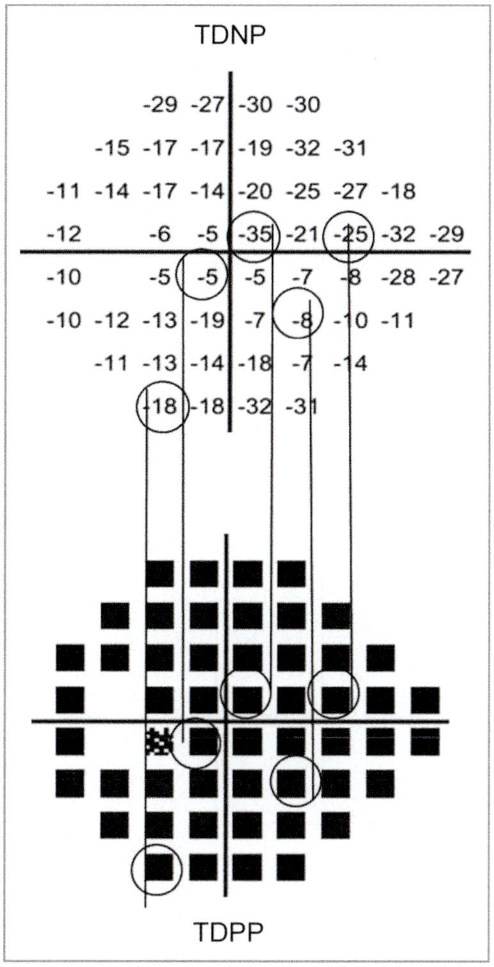

The main aim of total deviation probability plot is to give the extent and pattern of the field defect but not the depth of the field defect. STATPAC calculates the P value of the points with loss of sensitivity in total deviation numerical plot. Each deviation value of the total deviation numerical plot is given a symbol on the basis of its P value and is plotted as total deviation probability plot. Thus, loss of sensitivity value in the total deviation numerical plot is converted to scotomatous form in total deviation probability plot according to its P value. If you carefully observe the total deviation numerical plot, the loss of sensitivity more than 8 dB has the P < 0.5% which is represented by black square in the total deviation probability plot. A black square in this total deviation probability plot represents a wide range of deviation values from -8 dB to > (-40) dB. Just by seeing a black square in the total deviation probability plot, we cannot tell the loss of sensitivity at that point whether its value is -8 dB or -12 dB or -30 dB, etc. The numerical values of TDNP are converted into their symbolic form of P value to show the loss of sensitivity in scotomatous form in probability plots. Because the loss of sensitivity is converted to symbolic forms the extent and the pattern of the field defect is well appreciated as the scotomatous form in the probability plots. The STATPAC calculates the P value for the points where there is loss of sensitivity. P value is not calculated for those points whose sensitivities are better than normal. This is a very important point to be remembered.

P VALUE

P < 5% indicates that this degree of loss of sensitivity at that point is seen in <5% of normal population. The P < 5% is represented by:

P < 2% indicates that this degree of loss of sensitivity at that point is seen in <2% of normal population. The P < 2% is represented by:

P < 1% indicates that this degree of loss of sensitivity at that point is seen in <1% of normal population. The P < 1% is represented by:

P < 0.5% indicates that this degree of loss of sensitivity at that point is seen in <0.5% of normal population. The P < 0.5% is represented by:

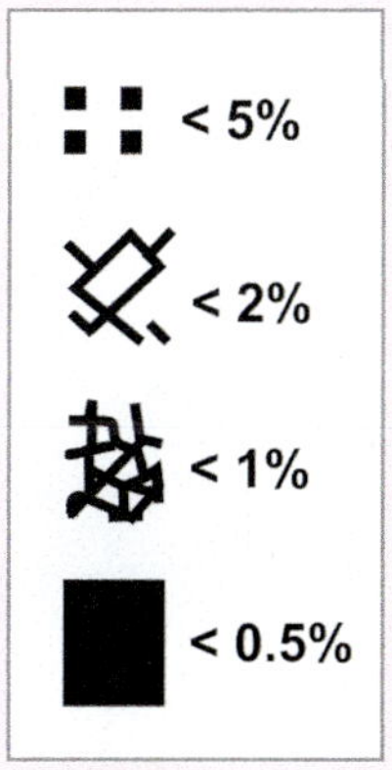

ZONE 7 AND 8—PATTERN DEVIATION PLOTS

Among the 11 zones of the single field analysis (SFA) printout, pattern deviation plots are the most important and difficult zones to understand. But if you know why they are created? and, how they are created?, it becomes very easy to understand these zones.

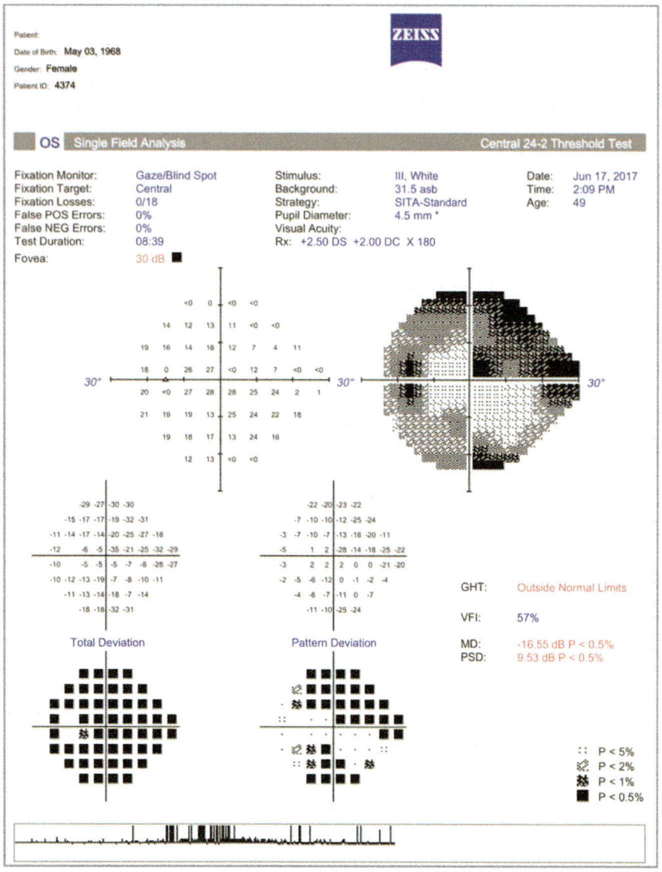

In SFA printout, the basic zone is the measured retinal sensitivity (raw data) and all the remaining zones represent raw data in different formats with a purpose. Now we study the raw data of this SFA printout.

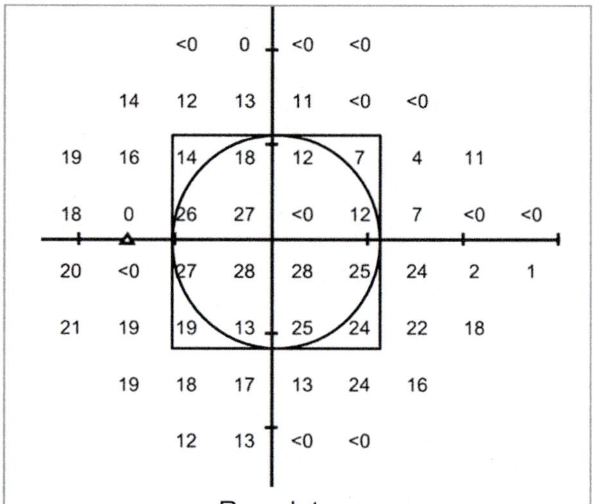

Raw data

The raw data shows a decreased sensitivity predominantly in the upper nasal quadrant. Some points became absolute scotomas. The central 10° area is less affected, as a whole raw data is showing irregular generalized loss with deep scotomas predominantly in the upper nasal quadrant. The information seen in raw data should reflect in grey scale, total deviation numerical plot and total deviation probability plot.

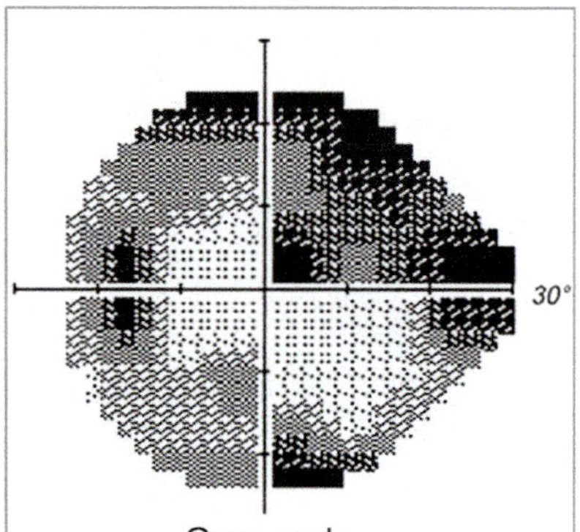

Grey scale

Zone 4—Grey Scale

Measured retinal sensitivity (raw data) is expressed in terms of shades in grey scale. From the grey scale it is clearly evident that there is generalized loss of sensitivity, more in the upper nasal quadrant and the less affected area is the central 10° area except the upper nasal quadrant.

By seeing the grey scale we can come to an idea regarding the type of field defect, pattern of the field defect and depth of the field defect. So raw data is reflected in grey scale.

Zone 5—Total Deviation Numerical Plot

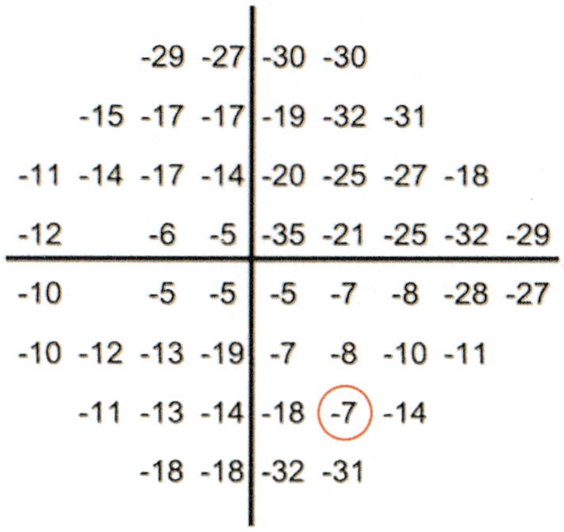

TDNP

Measured retinal sensitivity (raw data) is expressed in terms of deviations from normal values. The main aim of TDNP is to know the depth of the field defect. All the points in the TDNP are represented by numerical values with (-) sign in front of them. It is a generalized field defect with more loss of sensitivity in the upper nasal quadrant. The loss of sensitivity is less in central 10° area. So raw data is reflected in TDNP.

By seeing TDNP we can come to an idea regarding the type of field defect and depth of the field defect.

Zone 6—Total Deviation Probability Plot

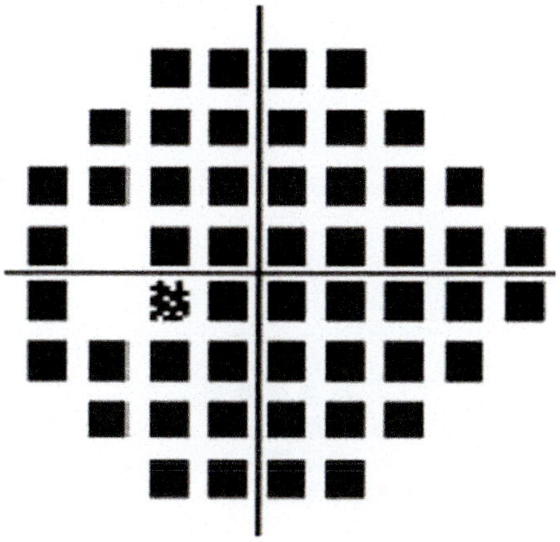
Total deviation probability plot

The aim of probability plot is to know extent and pattern of the field defect. In this probability plot, all points have the $P < 0.5\%$, and hence all the points are represented by black squares. In this printout the raw data is having generalized depression with localized field defects. This information of raw data is not reflected in TDPP. So we require another plot (PDPP) to tell whether this TDPP is representing a uniform generalized field defect (PDPP plot without field defect) or irregular generalized field defect (localized field defect in PDPP).

When raw data has generalized depression with localized field defects, TDPP shows generalized depression and PDPP highlights the localized field defects in the generalized depression.

When raw data has uniform generalized field depression, TDPP shows generalized depression and PDPP will be without a field defect.

When raw data has localized field defect, TDPP shows localized field defect. Raw data is reflected in TDPP itself and PDPP is not required. In localized field defects TDPP and PDPP look similar.

The pattern deviation plots are created to identify the localized field defects (deep scotomas) in the generalized field defect.

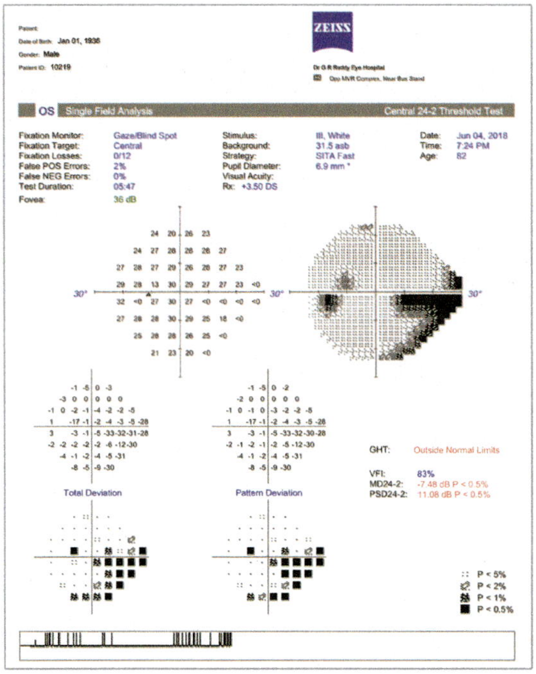

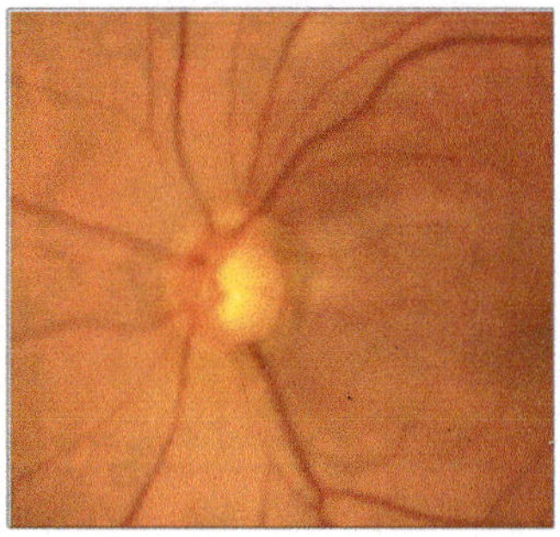

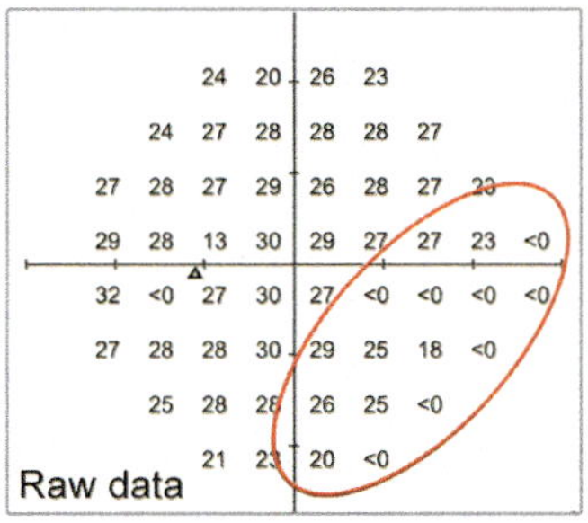

This is a known case of primary open-angle glaucoma (POAG) under follow-up since 2006. The raw data is showing decreased sensitivity points in the lower nasal quadrant. This loss of sensitivity area in the raw data is well-appreciated in grey scale, TDNP and TDPP.

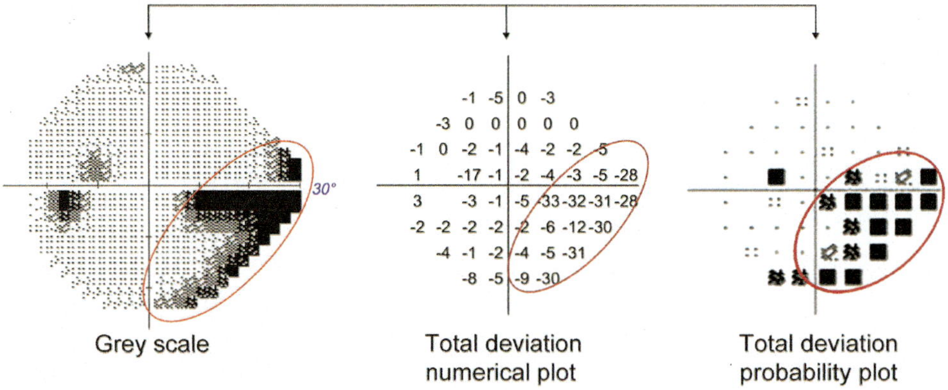

When it is a localized field defect, the pattern and extent of the localized field defect is well appreciated in the total deviation probability plot it self. There is no need to have another plot. But the software converts the TDNP to PDNP immaterial whether it is required or not.

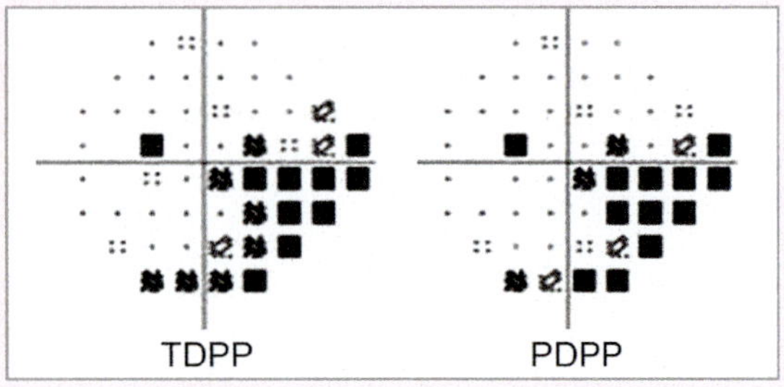

The most important observation is that TDPP and PDPP look similar in localized field defects. Why do they look similar will be explained later in this chapter.

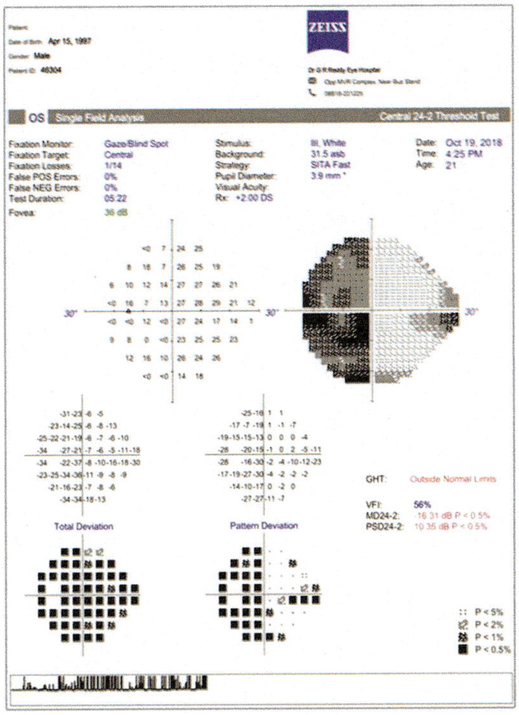

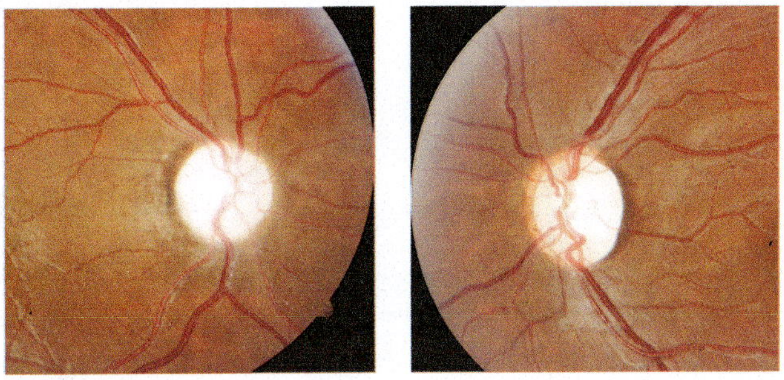

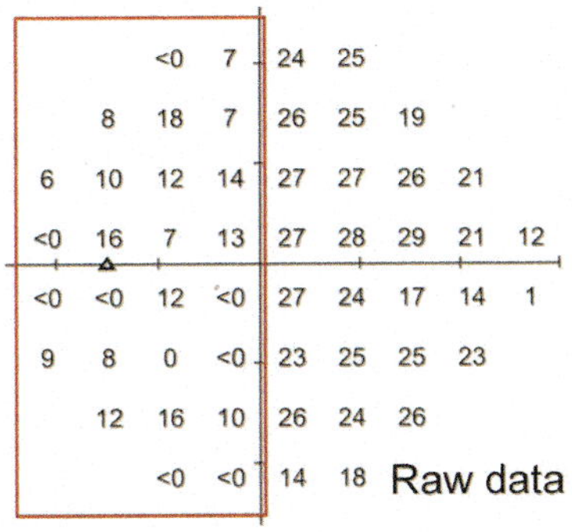

This is a case of pituitary adenoma causing right eye optic atrophy and left eye field is showing temporal hemianopia in generalized depression

The deep vertical half of the field defect what we are seeing in the raw data is well appreciated in grey scale and total deviation numerical plot and is not appreciated in the total deviation probability plot.

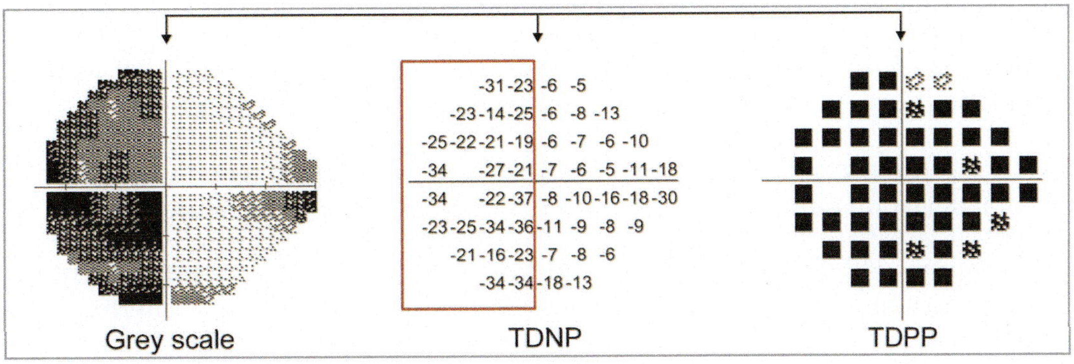

We are appreciating the temporal hemianopic field defect in the grey scale and total deviation numerical plot. As all the points are represented by black squares in this total deviation probability plot we require another plot to appreciate the temporal hemianopic field in a generalized depression.

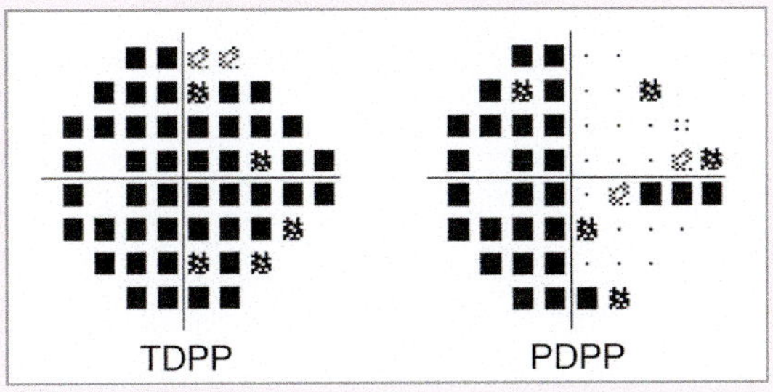

The pattern deviation plots are created to identify the localized field defects which are already appreciated in the raw data, grey scale and total deviation numerical plot, but masked in the generalized depression of TDPP.

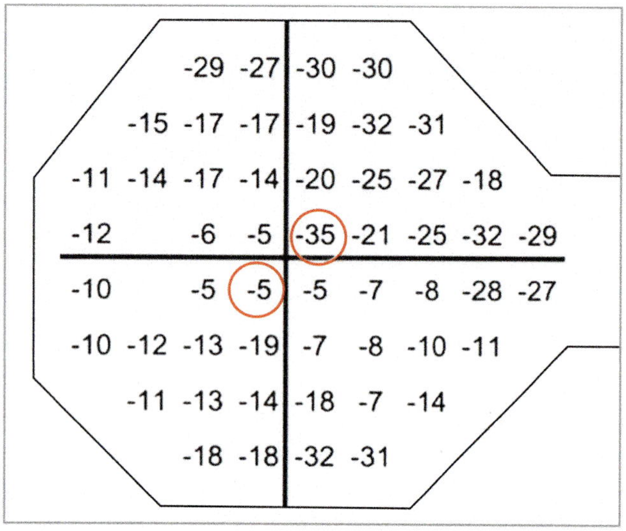

Total deviation numerical plot

Conversion of total deviation numerical plot to pattern deviation numerical plot can be explained in three steps:

Step 1: Selection of 7th best deviation point of TDNP

The most important key point for the conversion of total deviation numerical plot to pattern deviation numerical plot is the selection of 7th best deviation point of the total deviation numerical plot (TDNP). Before selecting 7th best deviation point in TDNP the following points are to be noted.

1. In 30-2 point pattern only points of 24-2 point pattern are considered
2. In 30-2 and 24-2 point patterns, the three points in the area of blind spot are ignored.
3. In 10-2 point pattern all points are considered. Since there is no blind spot in 10° field (Total number of points—68)

Selection of 7th best deviation point of TDNP

On the basis of deviation values from the normative data, numerical values of the total deviation numerical plot are divided into three groups to select the 7th best deviation point of TDNP

First group: The deviation values without sign. (Deviation value without sign indicates measured retinal sensitivity is better than its normative data). In this total deviation numerical plot there is no point without sign.

Second group: Zero (0) deviation points (0) in TDNP indicates that there is no loss of sensitivity at those points) In this total deviation numerical plot there are no zero (0) deviation points.

Third group: The points with (-) ve sign in front of the deviation value. These points represent loss of sensitivity. Higher the numerical value higher the loss of sensitivity. Lower the numerical value, lower the loss of sensitivity. All 52 points are with (-) ve sign in this TDNP.

-5 dB deviation point is the best deviation point of this TDNP.

-35 dB deviation is the worst deviation point of this TDNP.

Total deviation numerical plot

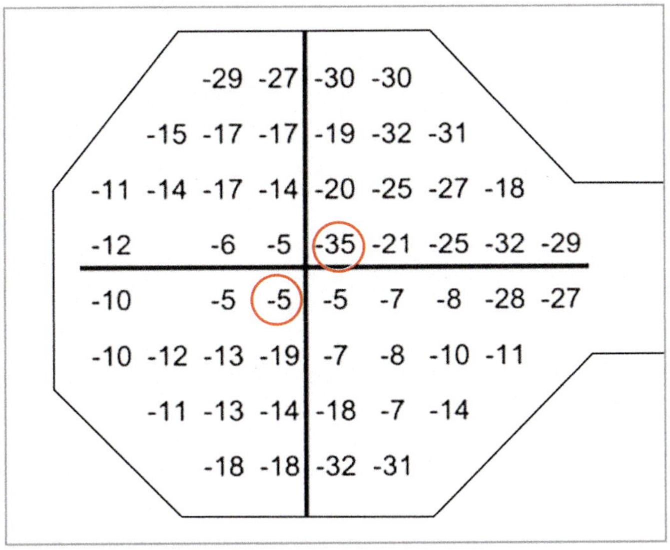

Step 1: Selection of 7th best deviation point of TDNP

Now the computer arranges the deviation points of the total deviation numerical plot in a chronological order on the basis of deviation values from the normative data. The first point being the best deviation point and the last point being the worst deviation point and selects the 7th best deviation point after ignoring the mentioned points while arranging the deviation values in a chronological order. All these calculations will be done by the software in the field analyzer.

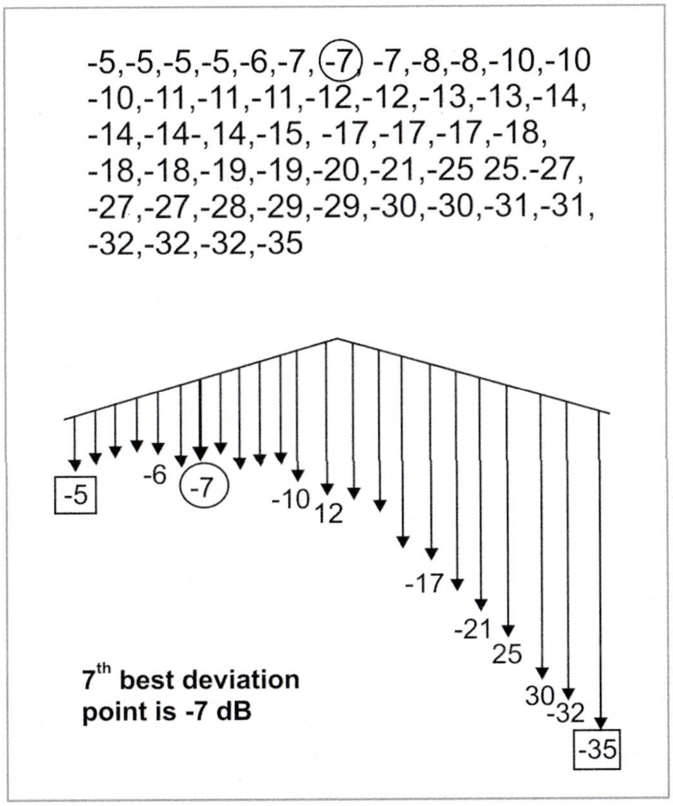

Total deviation numerical plot

7th best deviation point is -7 dB

Step 2: Establishing the dB value that converts 7th best deviation point of TDNP to zero (0) deviation.

Since -7 dB is the 7th best deviation point of TDNP, (+) 7 is the dB value to convert the 7th best deviation point to zero (0) deviation

Step 3: The dB value that converts the 7th best deviation point of TDNP to zero (0) deviation is added to all points of TDNP to convert it to PDNP

Since -7 dB is the 7th best deviation point of TDNP, (+) 7 dB is added to all the points of total deviation numerical plot to convert it to pattern deviation numerical plot. Thus by eliminating generalized depression, the localized scotoma if present, will be highlighted in the pattern deviation plots without affecting the contour of hill of vision.

Why 7th best deviation point was taken into consideration during the conversion of TDNP to PDNP?

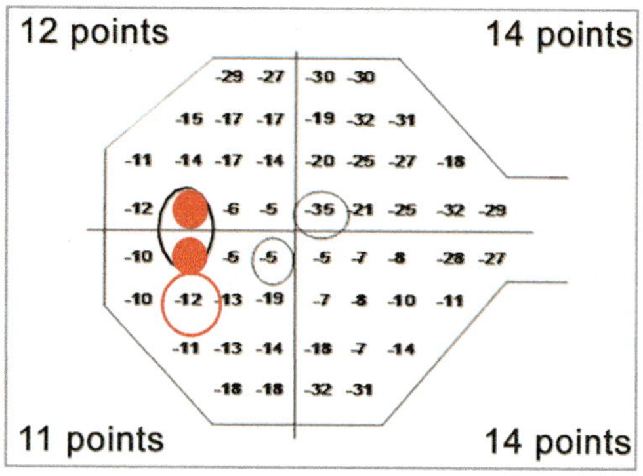

Total deviation numerical plot

-5,-5,-5,-5,-6,-7 ,-7,-7,-8,-8,-10,-10-,-10,-11,-11,-11,-12,-12,-13,-13,-14,-14,-14,-14,-15,-17,-17,-17,-18,-18,-18,-19,-19,-20,-21,-25,-25,-27,-27,-27,-28,-29,-29,-30,-30,-31,-31,-32,-32,-32,-35

Total number of points are 51

5th best deviation point is –6 dB
7th best deviation point is –7 dB
25th best deviation point is –15 dB

The most important key point for the conversion of total deviation numerical plot to pattern deviation numerical plot is converting certain percentage of point of TDNP with no significant P value without affecting the contour of hill of vision of TDNP. So, the dB value of each point in TDNP should be elevated by certain dB value till certain percentage of point will not be represented by any significant P value symbol in PDNP. From this, it is very clear that pattern plot is never a generalized depression and it always contains minimum certain percentage of points without a symbol and pattern of the field defect will be appreciated in pattern deviation plot when TDPP shows generalized depression.

Before knowing why 7th best deviation point is taken into consideration to convert TDNP to PDNP, we will see how PDNP looks if we select 5th, 25th and 7th best deviation point into consideration to convert TDNP to PDNP?

TDNP		PDNP
-5,-5,-5,-5 ,-6 ,-7,-7,-7,-8,-8,-10,-10 ,-10,-11,-11,-11,-12,-12,-13,-13,-14 ,-14,-14,-14,-15,-17,-17,-17,-18,-18 ,-18,-19,-19,-20,-21,-25,-25,-27,-27 ,-27,-28,-29,-29,-30,-30,-31,-31,-32, -32,-32,-35	5th best deviation point is -6 dB → (+) 6 dB is added to all points of TDNP to convert TDNP to PDNP	1,1,1,1,0,-1,-1,-1,-2,-2.-4,-4,-4,0,-5,-5,-5,-6,-6,-7,-7,-8,-8,-8,-8,-9,-17,-17,-17,-12,-12,-12,-12,-13,-13,-14,-15,-19,-19,-21,-21,-21,-22,-23,-23,-24,-24,-25,-25,-26,-26,-26,-29.

In PDNP, there will be minimum 5 points out of 51 points (around 10% of the points) will not be represented by any significant P value symbol in PDNP and 5th best deviation point becomes normal (0) deviation point in PDNP.

We see how PDNP looks like if 25th best deviation point is selected.

TDNP		PDNP
-5,-5,-5,-5,-6,-7,-7,-7,-8,-8,-10,-10 ,-10,-11,-11,-11,-12,-12,-13,-13,-14 ,-14,-14,-14,-15,-17,-17,-17,-18,-18 ,-18,-19,-19,-20,-21,-25,-25,-27,-27 ,-27,-28,-29,-29,-30,-30,-31,-31,-32, -32,-32,-35	25th best deviation point of TDNP (–) 15 dB → (+)15 dB is added to all points of TDNP to convert it to PDNP	10, 10, 10, 10, 9, 8, 8, 8, 7, 7, 5, 5, 5, 4, 4, 4, 3, 3, 2, 2, 1, 1, 1 ,1, 0,-2,-2,-2, -3 ,-3, -3, -4, -4, -5, -6, -10, -10, -12, -12, -12, -13, -14,-14,-15,-15,-16,-16,-17, -17,-17,-20.

There will be minimum 25 points out of 51 points (around 50% of the points) will not be represented by any significant P value symbol in PDNP and 25th best deviation point becomes 0 deviation point in PDNP. If more percentage of points become normal, some of the superficial scotomas (recent onset scotomas) of the localized scotoma in generalized depression of TDNP may become nonsignificant in PDNP and hence the direction of progression may not be appreciated.

We see how PDNP looks like if 7th best deviation point is selected.

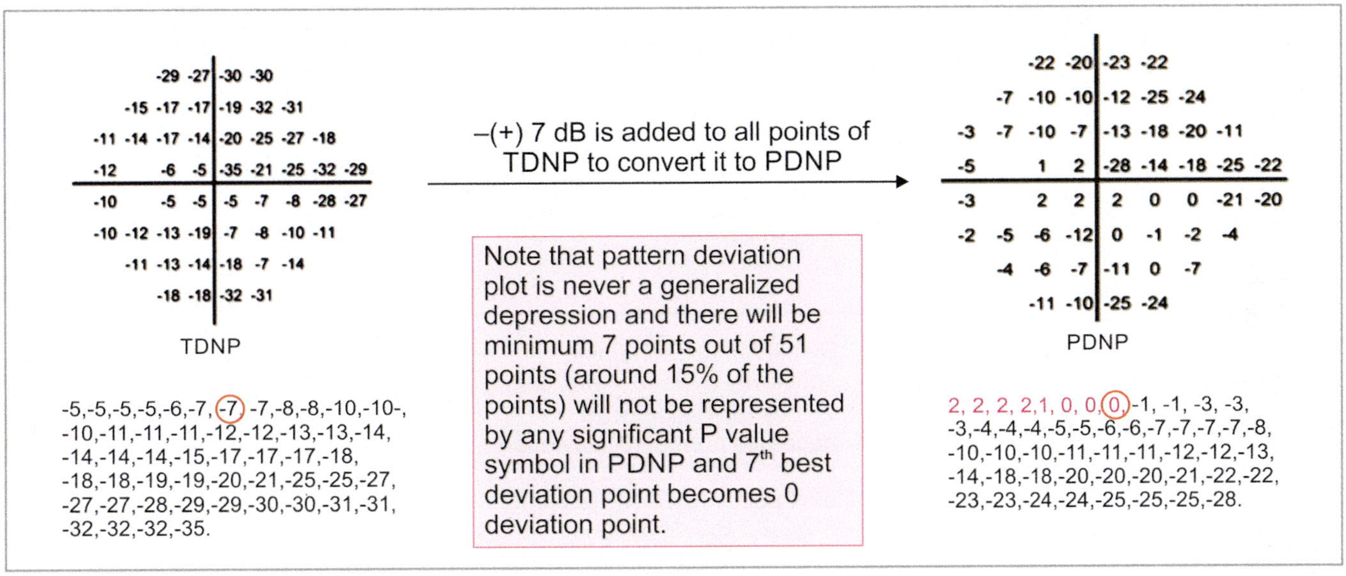

When we select 7th best deviation point is taken into consideration to convert TDNP to PDNP, 15% of the points (shown in red color) will not be represented by any significant P value symbol in PDNP. These 15% of normal points are enough to highlight the pattern and the direction of progression of the localized scotoma in a generalized depression. That is why 7th best deviation point was selected to convert TDNP to PDNP.

In a localized scotoma the loss of sensitivity is confined to few points out of 51 points and the 7th best deviation point will be either normal (0) deviation or minimal deviation and no or minimal dB value will be added to TDNP to convert it to PDNP. Hence both TDNP and PDNP will be almost similar. This is the reason why both the probability plots look similar in localized scotomas.

In a uniform generalized depression the dB value of 7th best deviation point and the dB value of all the remaining deviation points will be almost same. The dB value that converts 7th best deviation point of TDNP to 0 deviation, will also converts all the remaining points to around (0) deviation points in PDNP. This is the reason why PDNP looks normal in uniform generalized depression.

Conversion of total deviation numerical plot to pattern deviation numerical plot

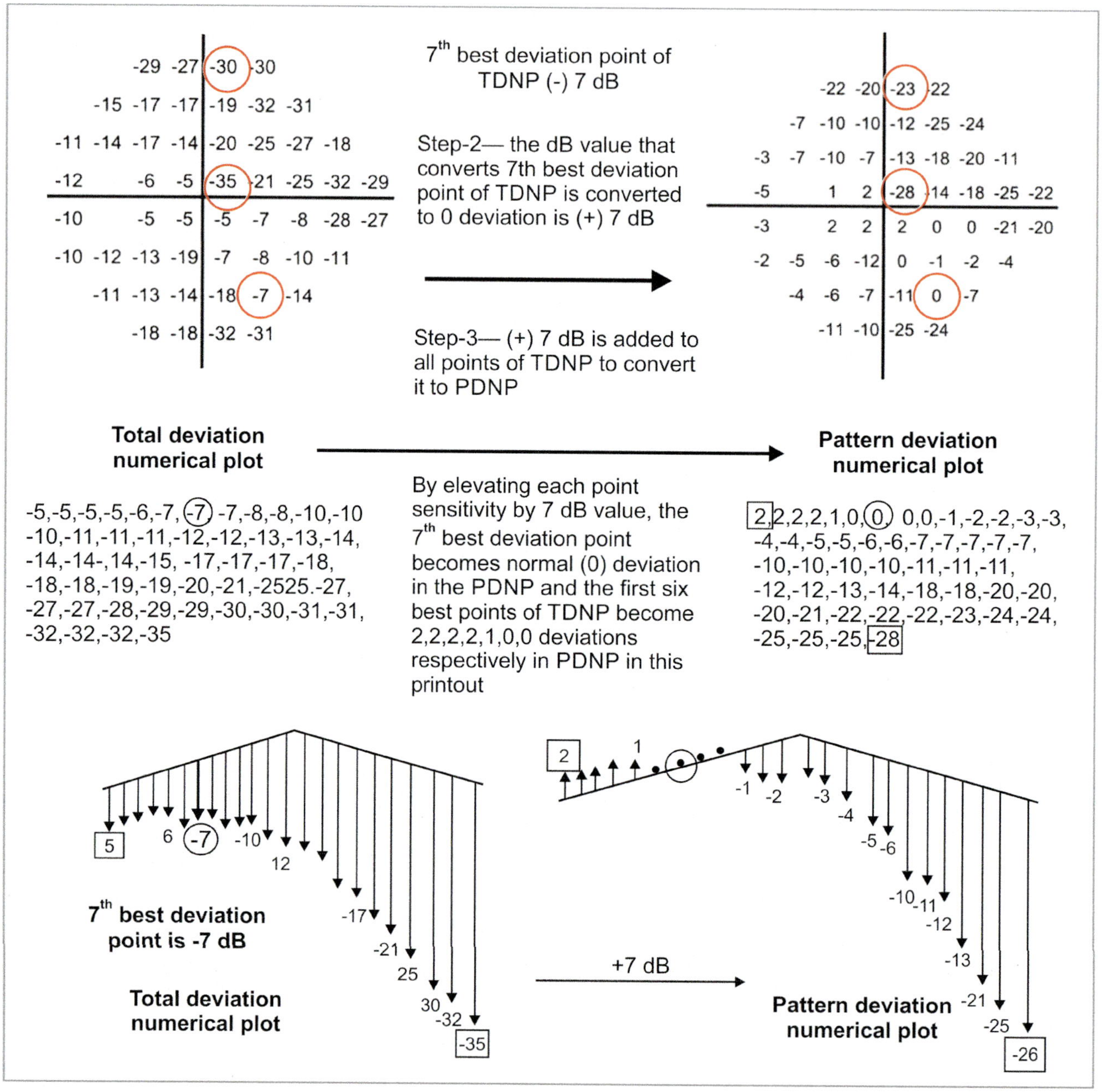

From this, it is very clear that the pattern deviation probability plot will never show generalized depression and always will have at least seven points without loss of sensitivity and so these minimum seven points will not be represented by any symbol in the pattern deviation probability plot. Each deviation value of the pattern deviation numerical plot is given a symbol on the basis of its P value and plotted as pattern deviation probability plot. Since pattern deviation plot will never show generalized depression, the pattern and extent of the field defect will be appreciated in any situation in PDPP.

Conversion of total deviation plots to pattern deviation plots: Example 1

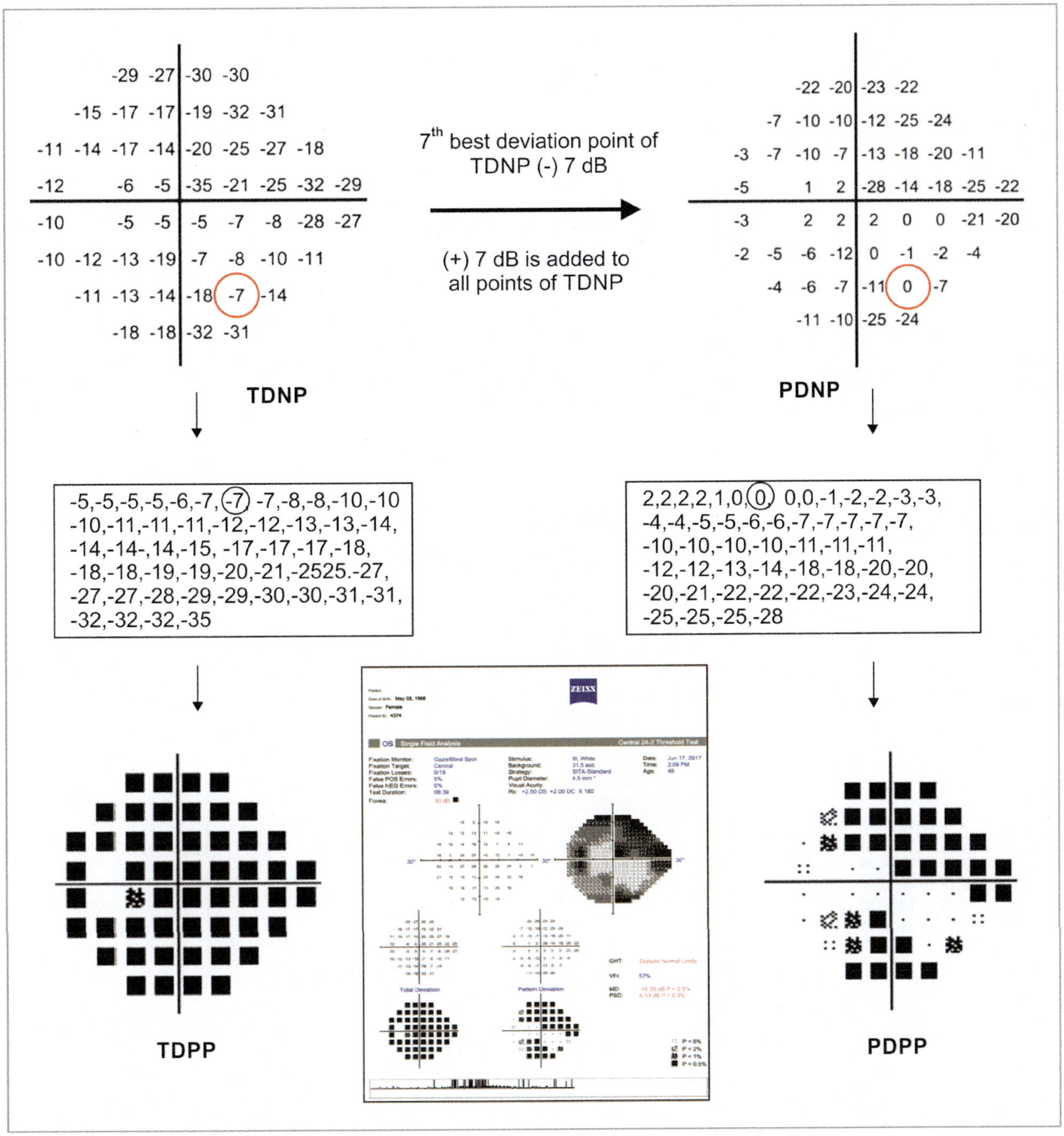

Each deviation value of the pattern deviation numerical plot is given a symbol on the basis of its P value and plotted as pattern deviation probability plot. The pattern deviation probability plot is nothing but the symbolic representation of P value of each deviation value of TDNP after eliminating the generalized depression worth of the dB value that converts the 7th best deviation point of TDNP to 0 deviation

Conversion of total deviation plot to pattern deviation plot: Example 2

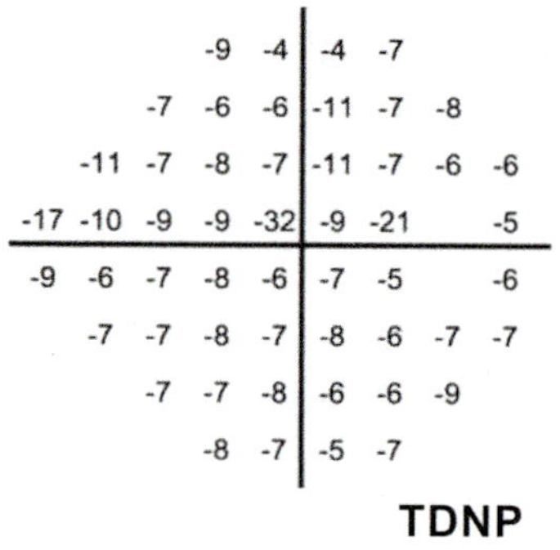

-(+) 6 dB is added to all points of TDNP to convert it to PDNP

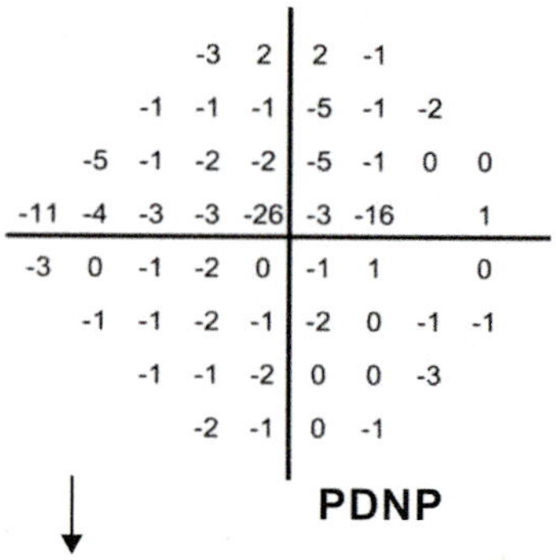

-4,-4,-5,-5,-5,-6, -6(-6)-6,-6,-6, -6,-6,-6,-6,-7,-7,-7,-7,-7,-7,-7,-7,-7,-7,-7,-7,-7,-7,-7,-7,-7,-7,-7,-8,-8,-8,-8,-8,-8,-8,-9,-9,-9,-9,-9,-10,11,-11,-11,-17,-21,-32

Each deviation value of the pattern deviation numerical plot is given a symbol on the basis of its P value and plotted as pattern deviation probability plot

2,2,1,1,0,0(0)0,0,0,0,0,0,-1,-1,-1,-1,-1,-1,-1,-1,-1,-1,-1,-1,-1,-1,-1,-1,-1,-1,-1,-2,-2,-2,-2,-2,-2,-2,-2,-3-,3,-3,-3,-3,-4,-5,-5,-5,-11,-16,-26

7th best deviation point of TDNP (-) 6 dB

Suspected glaucoma in a case of cataract

7th best deviation point of of PDNP is (0 dB) deviation

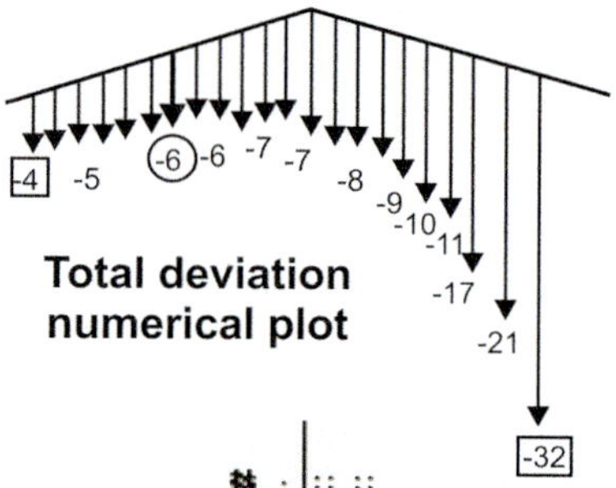

Total deviation numerical plot

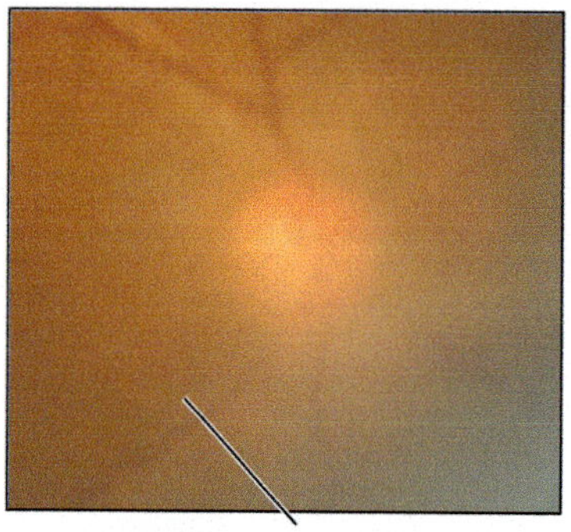

RNFL Defect

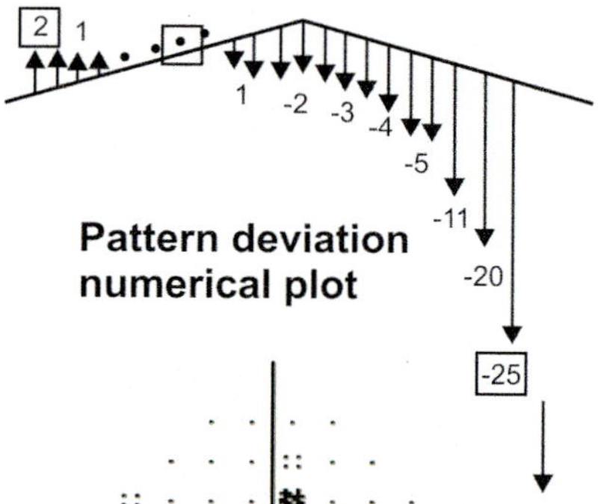

Pattern deviation numerical plot

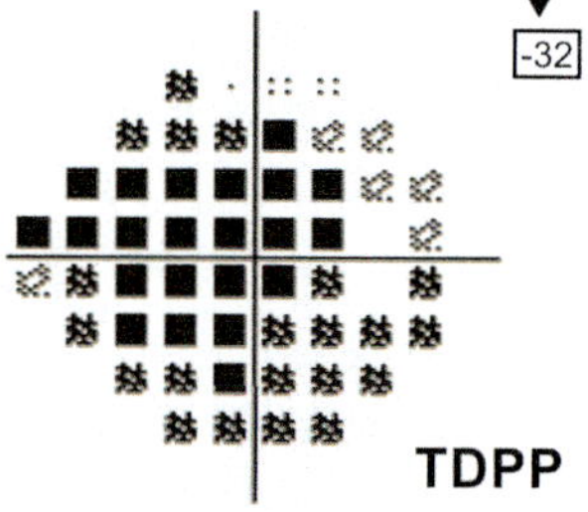

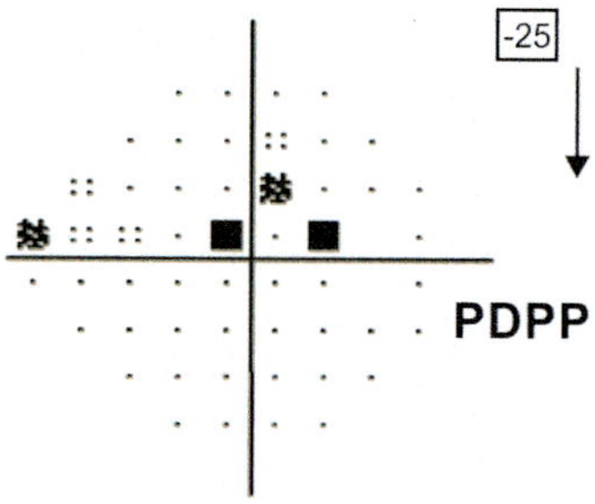

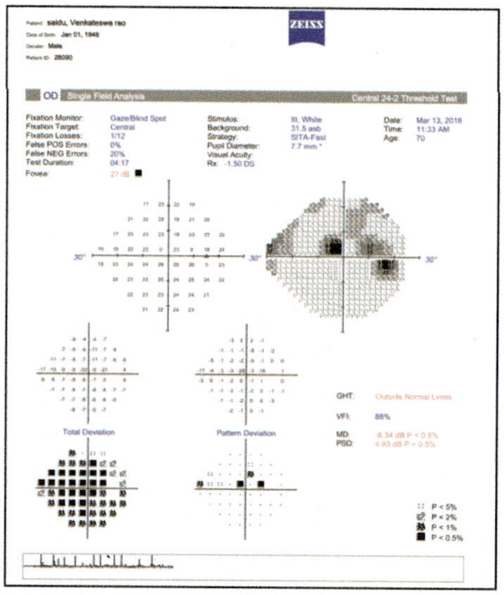

In a case of cataract, loss of sensitivity at most of the point will be >8 dB. Hence all the points will be represented by black squares. If this patient develops glaucoma, how to appreciate the localized field defect in this generalized field defect

The field defect of glaucoma masked in generalized depression is highlighted in the pattern deviation probability plot. To appreciate the localized field defect in generalized field defect, the pattern deviation plots are created. If glaucoma is not present the PDPP will be normal

Conversion of total deviation plots to pattern deviation plots: Example 3

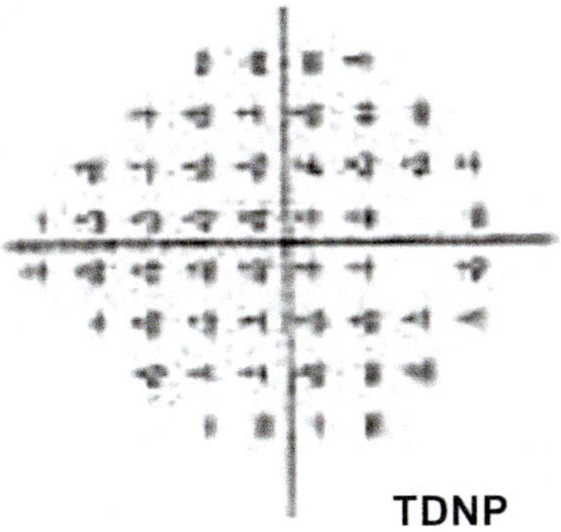

TDNP

(+)7 dB is added to all points of TDNP

7th best deviation point is -7 dB

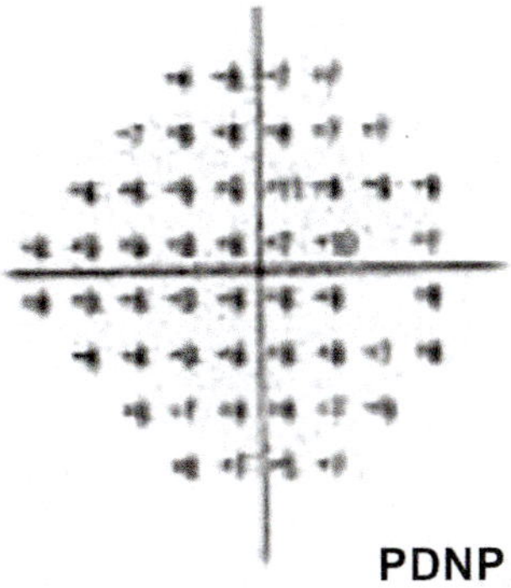

PDNP

-4,-5,-6,-6,-6,-6,-7,-7,-7,-7,-7,-7,-7,-7,-7,-7,-7,-7,-8,-8,-8,-8,-8,-8,-8,-8,-8,-8,-8,-8,-8,-8,-8,-8,-8,-8,-8,-8,-9,-9,-9,-9 -9,-9,-9,-9,-9,-9,-9,-10,-11,

2,1,1,1,1,0,0,0,0,0,0,0,0-1, -1,-1,-1,-1,-1,-1,-1,-1,-1,-1,-1,-1,-1, -2,-2,-2,-2,-2,-2,-2,-2,-2,-2, -2,-2,-2,-2,-2,-2,-2,-2,-3,-3, -3,-3,-3,-4,-4,

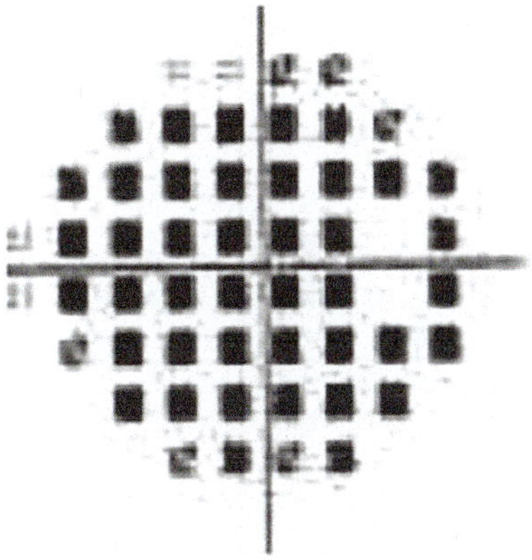

TDPP

By elevating each point's sensitivity by 7 dB, the 7th best sensitivity point of total deviation numerical plot became normal (0 deviation) and the first six best points of TDNP became 2,1,1,1,1,0,0, deviations respectively. The deviation values in PDNP are varying mostly from -2 dB deviation to -4 dB deviation. So the sensitivity of most of the points of PDNP are in the normal range and hence are not represented by any significant P value symbol and thus a normal pattern deviation probability plot.

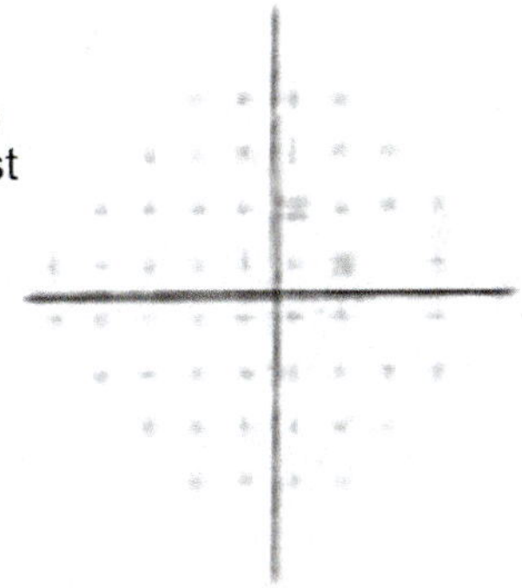

PDPP

Total deviation probability plot with generalized depression and a normal pattern deviation probability plot indicate that it is a case of uniform generalized field defect. In such a situation always think of the conditions like cataract, media opacities, small pupil, and check if the fields were done with proper refractive error correction or not. Apart from glaucoma, some neurological conditions like AION, occipital lobe infarcts, etc can be diagnosed on the basis of the pattern of the field defect. When these conditions are suspected in the presence of cataract, the pattern deviation probability plot plays a major role in picking up these diseases. If the pattern deviation probability plot does not show any field defect (Uniform generalized field defect) as in this case, we can eliminate the above said conditions. If the pattern deviation probability plot shows a localized field defect (irregular generalized field defect) the diagnosis can be made depending on the pattern of the field defect.

Conversion of total deviation plots to pattern deviation plots: Example 4

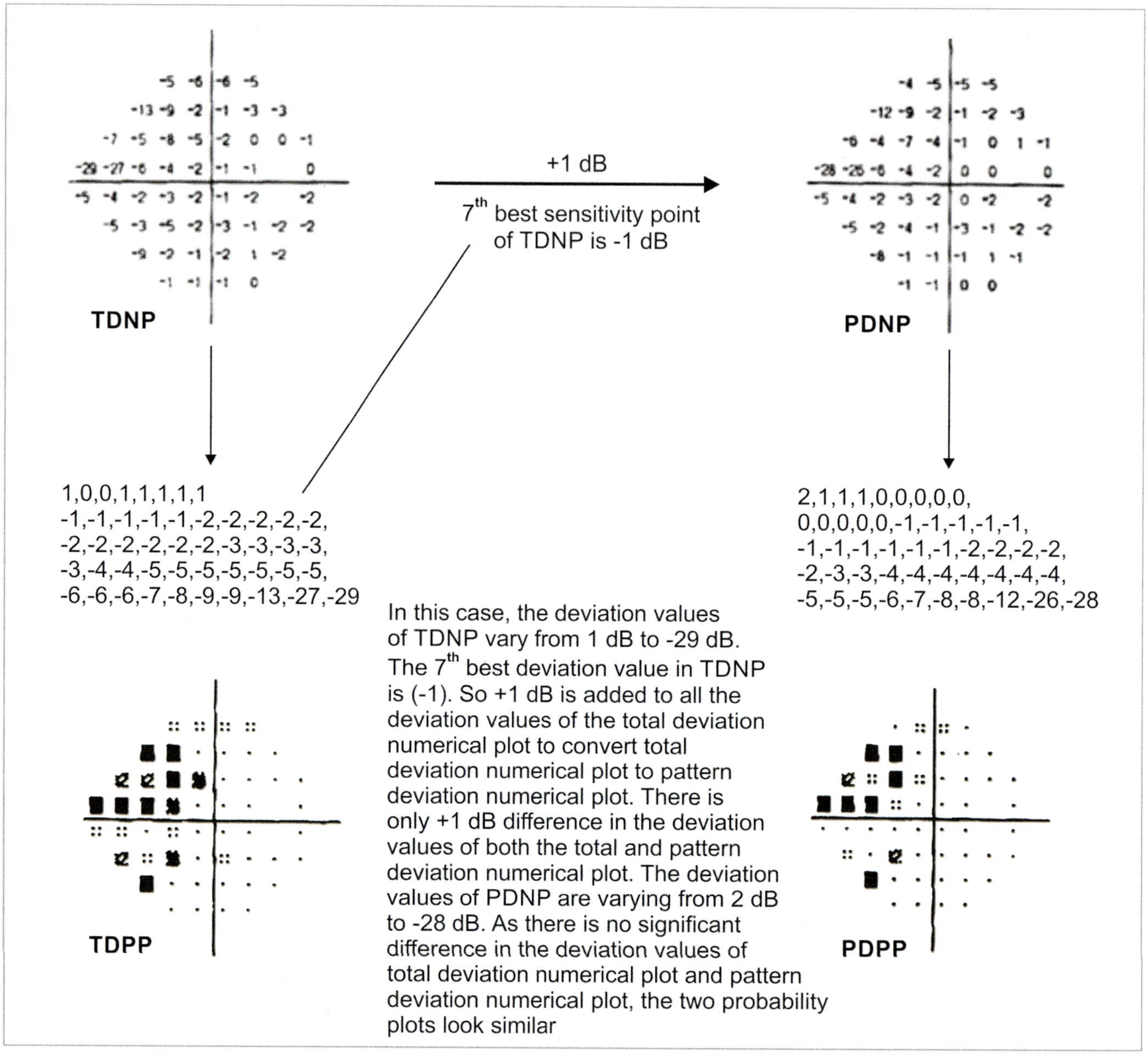

In localized scotomas the 7th best deviation point of TDNP will be close to zero (0) deviation and hence, minimal value is required to bring the 7th best deviation point to zero (0) deviation. In other words, the 7th best deviation point of TDNP is either on the normal slope of hill of vision or, just nearer to normal slope of vision. A minimal value is required to bring the 7th best deviation point to bring it to normal slope of vision. In all localized scotomas, the dB value added to all the points in the total deviation numerical plot to convert it to pattern deviation numerical plot is very minimal. So, there will not be significant difference in the numerical values of total and pattern deviation numerical plots and hence their probability plots look similar.

Summary of analysis total deviation probability plot

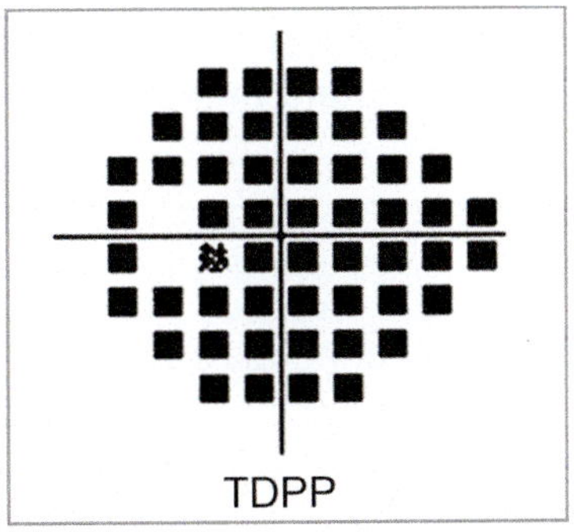

In this TDPP, there is a generalized field defect, but we do not know if it is uniform generalized field defect or irregular generalized field defect

The dB value that converts the 7th best deviation point of TDNP to (0) deviation is added to all the points of TDNP to convert it to PDNP. By elevating the sensitivity of each point of TDNP by the dB value that converts the 7th best sensitivity point to (0) deviation, we are not only eliminating the generalized depression from the TDNP but also making minimum of 7 points of the PDNP nonsignificant. So PDPP always contains minimum 7 points without symbol and hence pattern deviation plot is never a generalized depression plot. During the conversion of PDNP to PDPP, the pattern of black squares in PDPP may show localized scotoma masked by generalized depression in the TDPP (irregular generalized field defect) or no field defect, i.e. normal pattern deviation probability plot (uniform generalized field defect).

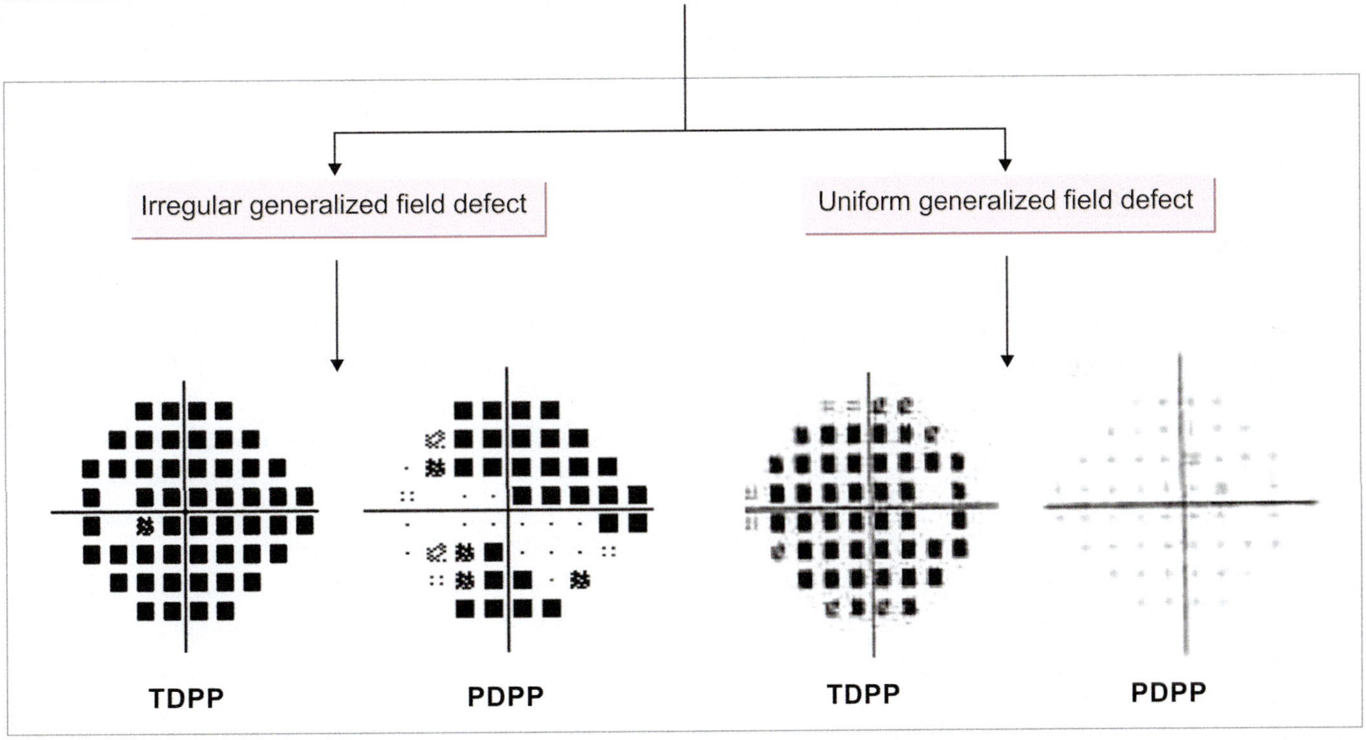

In irregular generalized field defect the total deviation probability plot shows generalized field defect and pattern deviation plot shows localized scotoma (Cataract + glaucoma)

In uniform generalized field defect total deviation probability plot shows generalized field defect and normal pattern deviation probability plot (No evidence of glaucoma in a case of cataract)

Probability plots in each type of field defect

Localized	Irregular generalized	Uniform generalized
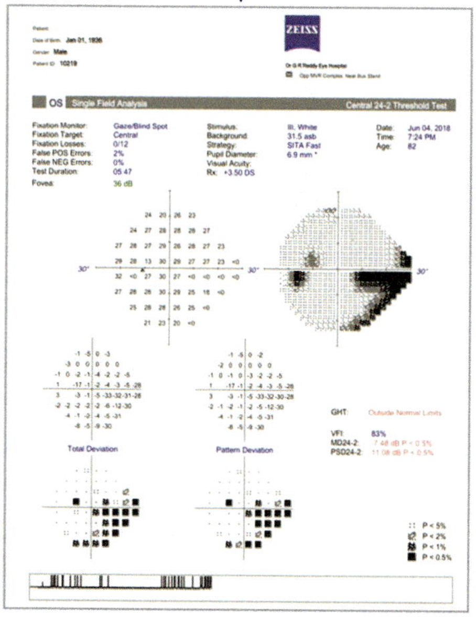	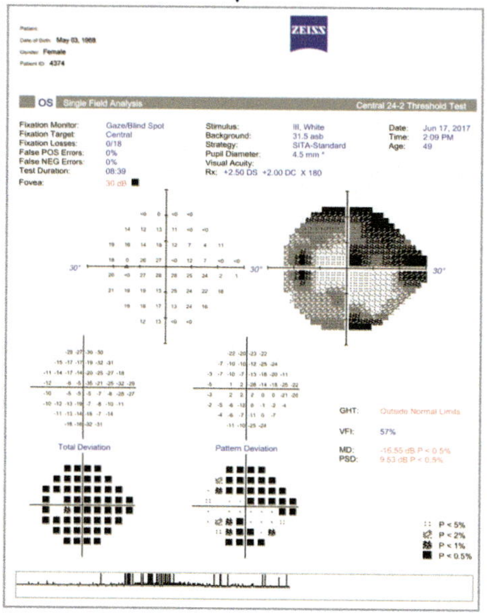	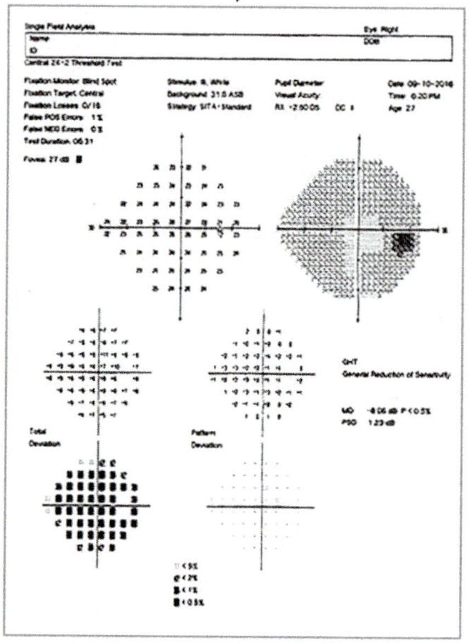
Localized field defects TDPP and PDPP almost look similar because the 7th best deviation point is either (0) or minimal deviation value. In this TDNP, the 7th best deviation point is already (0) deviation, so there is no need to add any dB value is to convert TDNP to PDNP. So TDNP and PDNP are identical. Hence TDPP and PDPP look similar.	Irregular generalized field defect shows generalized field defect in TDPP and localized field defect in PDPP. In this TDNP, the best deviation point is -5 dB, 7th best deviation point is -7 dB and the worst deviation point is -34 dB. By elevating the sensitivity of all the points by 7 dB, superficial scotomas will be eliminated and deep scotomas are highlighted in the PDPP.	Uniform generalized field defects shows generalized field defect in TDPP and normal PDPP. In this TDNP the best deviation point is -4 dB, 7th best deviation point is -7 dB and the worst deviation point is -11 dB. By elevating the sensitivity of all the points by 7 dB, all deviation values in PDNP became either 0 deviation points or close to 0 deviation points and, are not represented any symbol in the PDPP.

ZONE 9—GLOBAL INDICES

The global indices includes

1. Mean deviation (MD)
2. Pattern standard deviation (PSD)
3. Visual field index

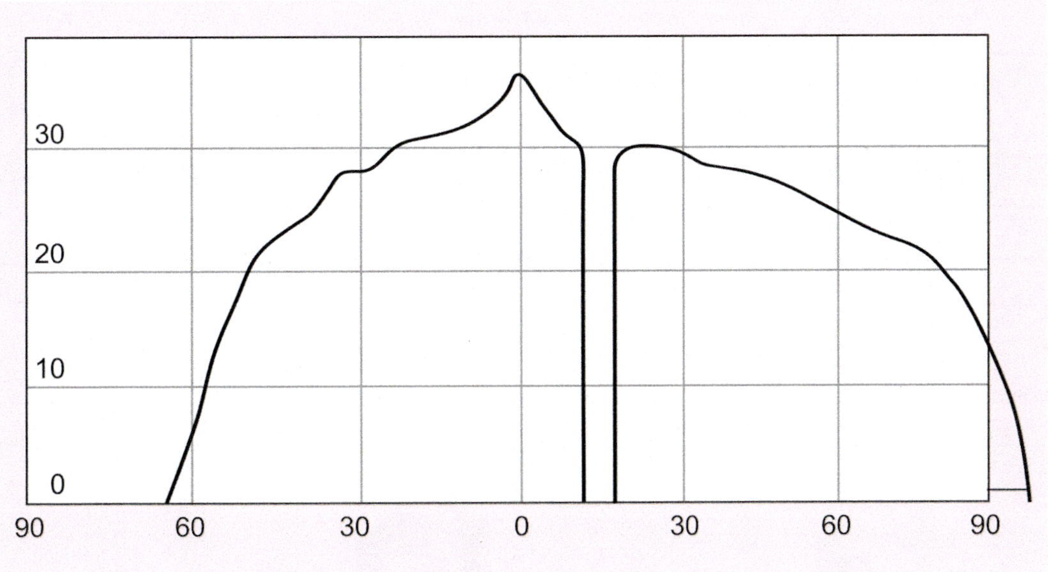

To understand global indices one should have a clear concept of the hill of vision. In the normal visual field the fovea is the highest retinal sensitivity point. The peak of the hill of vision is represented by the fovea and retinal sensitivity decreases as it moves away from the center (fovea) to the periphery. This drop of sensitivity from center to periphery gives characteristic shape and contour to the hill of vision. The slope of normal hill of vision is smooth. The loss of sensitivity can be expressed through hill of vision by two components. The two components contour and height of hill of vision are shown in the figure. Change in the sensitivity will affect the height hill of vision with or without affecting the contour to the hill of vision. Two indices (MD index and PSD) are developed to express the changes in sensitivity in terms of hill of vision. The MD index expresses the difference in the height of hill of vision between the height of hill of vision of the normative data and the height of hill of vision of the raw data and the PSD expresses the change in smoothness of the contour of the hill of vision. Basically the field defect can start either as localized field defect or as generalized field defect (uniform generalized). Some times the localized field defect may be masked in the generalized field defect (irregular generalized field defect). Now we shall discuss the role of MD index and PSD during the interpretation of the visual field printouts. As already discussed, the field defects can be divided as follows.

PSD is developed to express the contour of hill of vision. Even a small localized field defect will be seen as a dip in the contour of hill of vision. So if the contour of hill of vision is not smooth, PSD will be represented by P value.

MD index is developed to express the depth of the field defect and its value is directly proportional to the depth of the field defect.

Type of field defect

- Localized
- Irregular generalized
- Uniform generalized

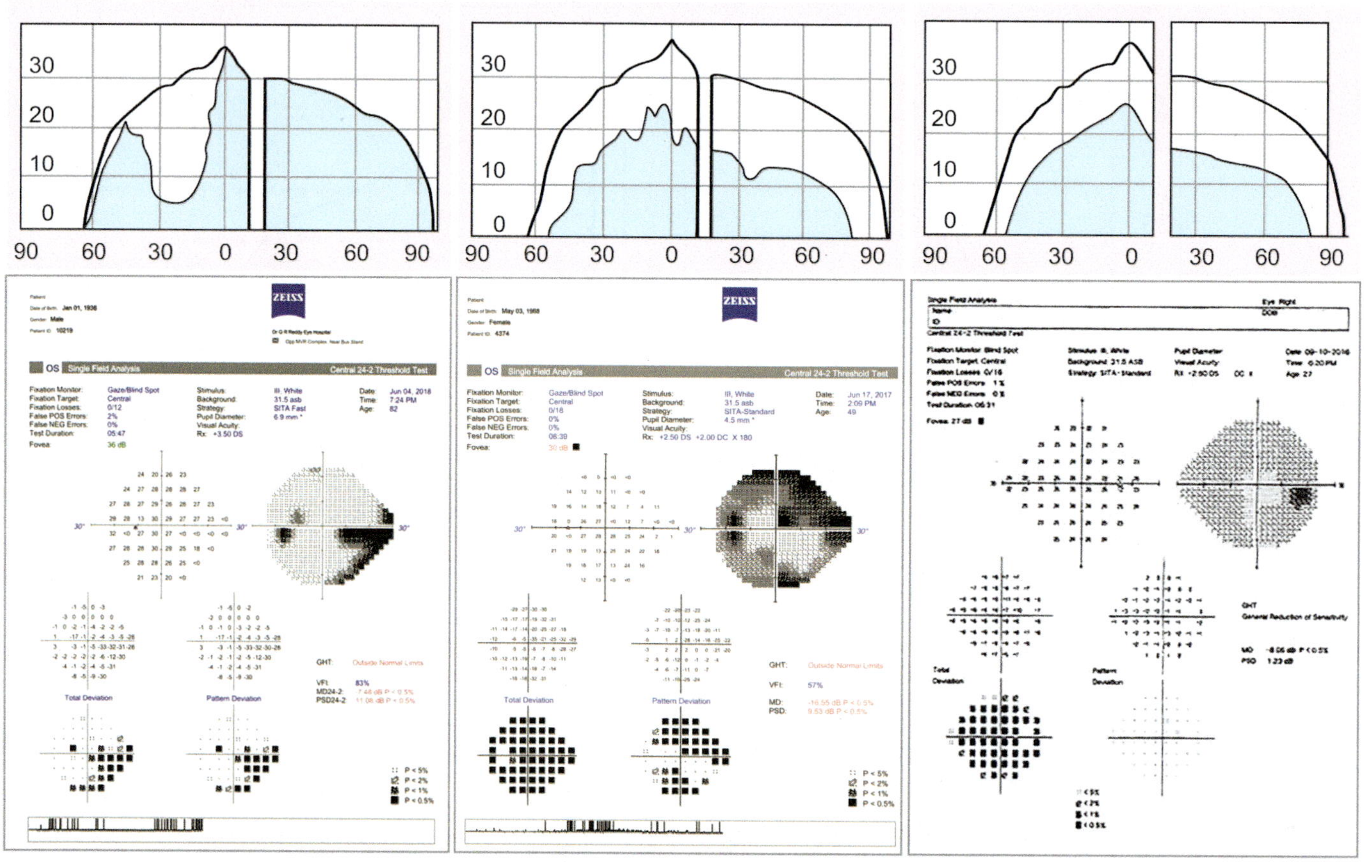

Localized: Change in contour (PSD will be significant) and change in height of hill of vision (MD index) depends on extent and depth of the localized scotoma)

PSD 11.04 dB P < 0.5%
MD 7.45 dB P < 0.5%

Irregular generalized: Significant change will be seen in both contour (PSD will be significant) and change in height of hill of vision (MD index will be significant with P value).

PSD 9.53 dB P < 0.5%
MD 16.55 dB P < 0.5%

Uniform generalized: No change in contour (PSD will be non-significant) but there is change in height of hill of vision (MD index will be significant with P value).

PSD 1.23 dB
MD 8.05 dB P < 0.5%

The most important concept regarding the value of PSD is that it is not related to height of hill of vision (the depth of the field defect) but is related to the contour of the hill of vision. In early localized scotoma PSD will be significant with minimal MD index value. In uniform generalized field defect the contour of the hill of vision is smooth and hence PSD is nonsignificant even though MD index is high. In irregular generalized field defect there will be significant change in both contour (PSD) and change in height of hill of vision (MD index). With this background we will study the MD and PSD in detail.

Mean Deviation Index

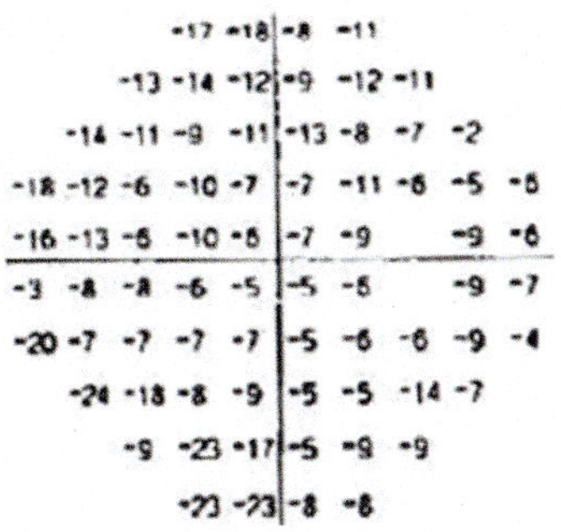

Total deviation numerical plot (TDNP)

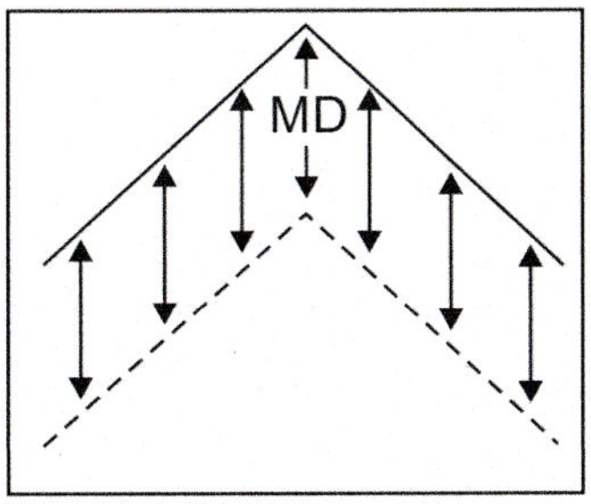

The loss of sensitivity is distributed equally to all the points

$$MD=\left(\frac{1}{n}\sum_{i+1}^{n}\frac{(x^1-N_1)}{s_{1_i}^2}\right)/\left(\frac{1}{n}\sum_{i+1}^{n}\frac{1}{s_{1_i}^2}\right)$$

Where X_i is the measured threshold at point i, N_i, is the normal reference threshold at point i, $s_{1_i}^2$ is the variance of normal field measurements at point i, and n denotes the number of test points excluding the blind spot

Formula to calculate MD index

The mean deviation index is the average of all the deviation values of the total deviation numerical plot except the deviation values of the two points in the area of the blind spot. The deviation from normal at each point is weighed according to the variance of the normal values at that location. Thus points with low variance that is, closer to fixation affects the MD value more than the eccentric points, which have a higher variance. The mean deviation is expressed in dB units with P value. The positive value indicates that the patient's overall sensitivity is better than normal observer whereas negative value indicates that the patient's overall sensitivity is worse than the average normal individual. The sensitivity profile (hill of vision) of the normal visual field is depicted by the solid diagonal lines and a general depression of visual field sensitivity is depicted by the broken line. The mean deviation (MD) is the amount of visual field depression relative to normal, as indicated by the length of the arrows. Usually, the loss of sensitivity is not exactly the same at all locations, in which case the MD is the average amount of loss. If MD is lower than that found in 10% of the normal subjects in the perimeter's database, a significant level is printed (P <10%), making it unnecessary to memorize the corresponding limits of normality. No probability statement is given for super normal findings.

Role of MD index in the diagnosis of early glaucoma: Rarely mean deviation falls outside the normal range by virtue of glaucoma without first producing one of the diagnostic signs of a localized defect. If we suspect glaucoma on the basis of IOP or asymmetry of intraocular pressure or disc cupping, the difference of mean deviation index between both the eyes should be taken as a serious clue in confirming the diagnosis of glaucoma. **(1)** 2 dB difference of mean deviation index between the two eyes. **(2)** An average 1.5 dB difference must be maintained between the two eyes on two consecutive tests. **(3)** An average difference of 1 dB must be maintained between the two eyes on four consecutive tests. Note that -1 dB difference of MD index between the two eyes in 24–2 point pattern is equal to total difference of 52 dB between the two eyes. In other words the 52 dB loss of retinal sensitivity becomes -1 dB when it is expressed in terms of MD index in 24-2 point pattern.

Role of MD index in the follow-up tests: The most important index to assess field progression is MD index. The expected change in MD index per year is -0.08 dB. More than 0.08 dB increase in MD per year should be considered as abnormal. Remember that even a small change in MD index in a case of localized field defect is significant. Confirm that the increase in MD index is not due to the following causes:

Improper refractive error correction, pupil size, high false negative errors, different point patterns and different testing strategies for the comparing tests. If the increase in MD index is not due to any of the above factors,only then we have to analyze MD index, raw data and probability plots for glaucoma progression.

Understanding of MD Index in a Localized Field Defect

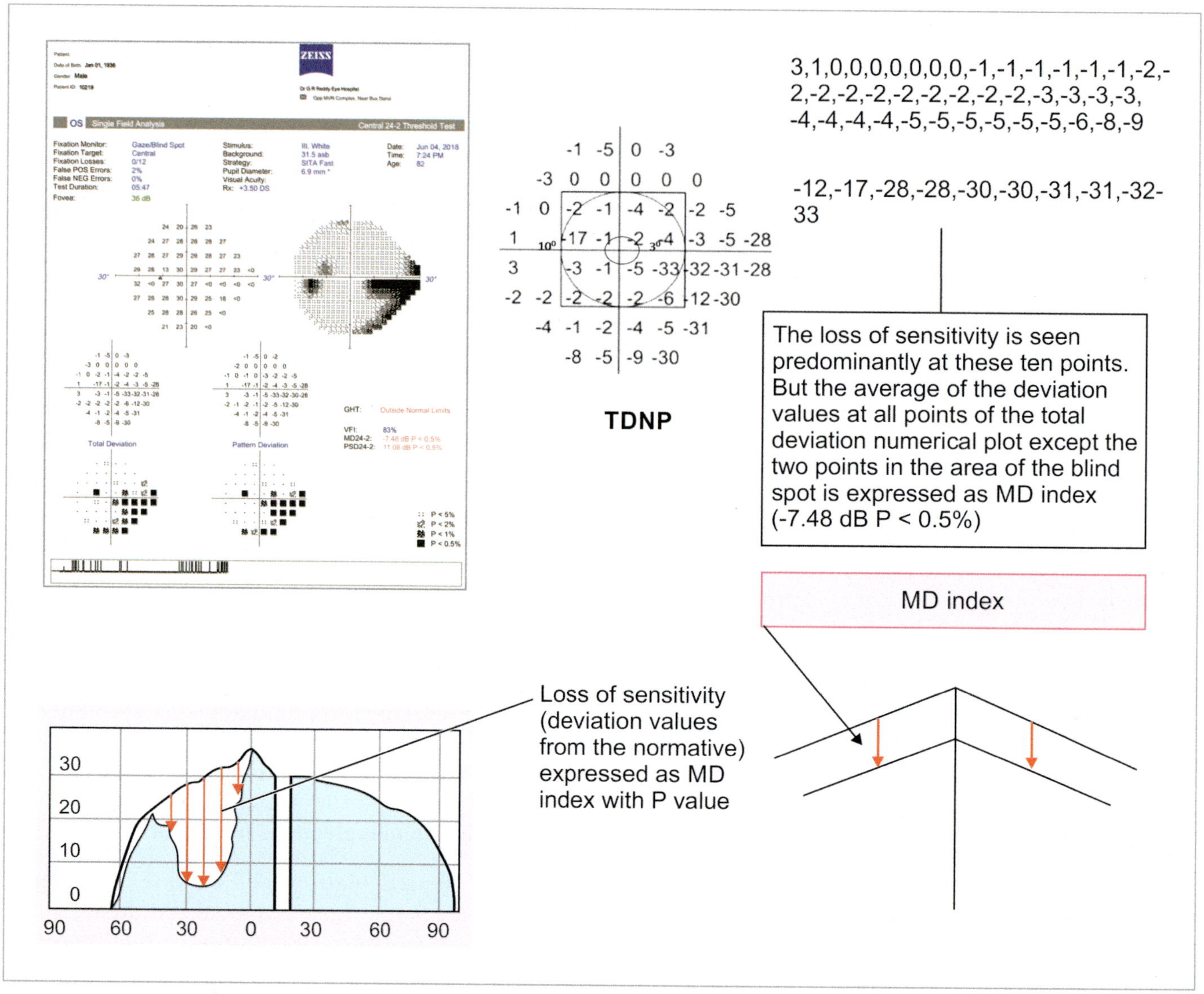

Understanding of MD index in a localized field defect is very important.

In this case, the loss of sensitivity is seen predominantly at ten points and the average loss of these points is around –30 dB but the MD index is -7.48 dB. So, one should understand that in a case of localized field defect, MD index is not true index to represent the depth of the field defect. The localized loss of sensitivity is expressed as mean deviation of all the points of TDNP in the form of MD index.

So, from this it is very clear that if the field defect is confined to one quadrant and if the MD index is – 7.00 dB, one should understand that MD index of the points in the localized field defect will be around -30 dB. If the field defect is confined to one hemisphere and if the MD index is – 7.00 dB, one should understand that MD index of the points in the localized field defect will be around -15 dB. It is very important to know that MD index does not tell the exact depth of the field defect in localized field defects. In uniform generalized field defect, MD index is true index to express the depth of the field defect and to some extent it gives true value in irregular generalized field defect.

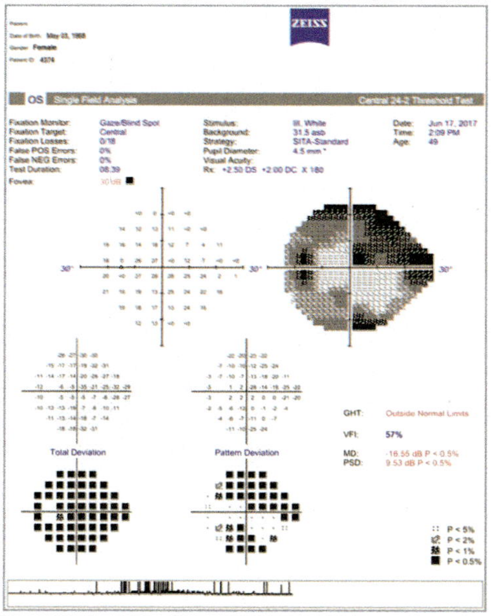

Understanding of MD index in irregular generalized field defect

		-29	-27	-30	-30			
	-15	-17	-17	-19	-32	-31		
-11	-14	-17	-14	-20	-25	-27	-18	
-12		-6	-5	-35	-21	-25	-32	-29
-10		-5	-5	-5	-7	-8	-28	-27
-10	-12	-13	-19	-7	-8	-10	-11	
	-11	-13	-14	-18	-7	-14		
		-18	-18	-32	-31			

TDNP

-5,-5,-5,-5,-6,-7,(-7) -7,-8,-8,-10,-10 -10,-11,-11,-11,-12,-12,-13,-13,-14, -14,-14-,14,-15, -17,-17,-17,18, -18,-18,-19,-19,-20,-21,-2525.-27, -27,-27,-28,-29,-29,-30,-30,-31,-31, -32,-32,-32,-35

The best deviation point is -5 dB
The worst deviation point is -35 dB
7th best deviation point is -7 dB

In irregular generalized field defect deviation values are not similar. The average (mean) of these deviation values is expressed as MD index with P value. In this printout MD index -16.55 dB P < 0.5%. In irregular generalized field defect some percentage of deviation values will be less than MD index value and some percentage of deviation values will be more than MD index value.

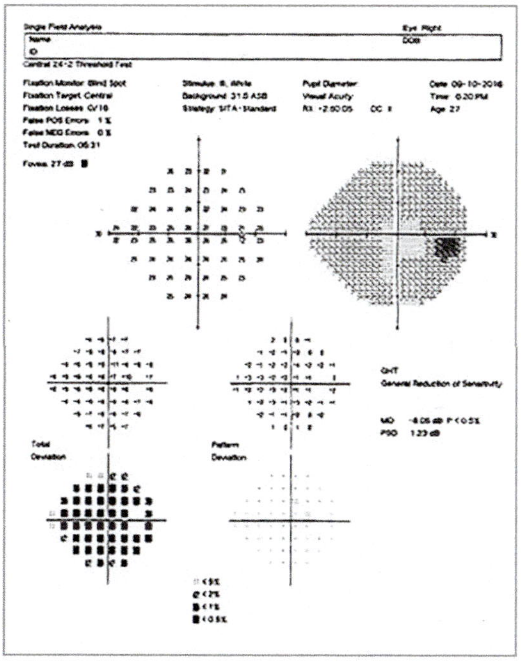

Understanding of MD index in uniform generalized field defect

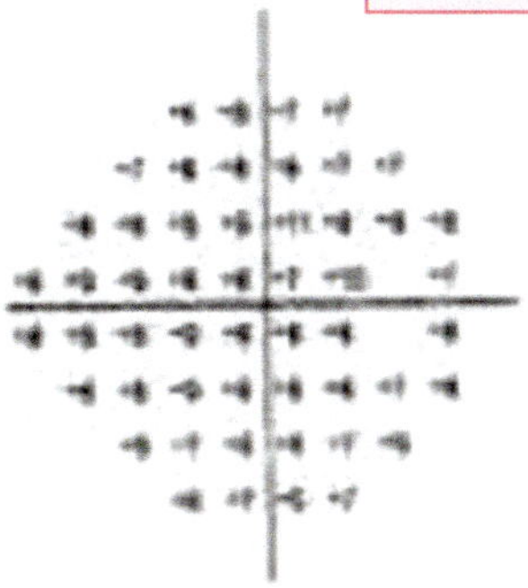

TDNP

-4,-5,-6,-6,-6,-6,(-7)-7,-7,-7,-7,-7,-7,-7,-7,-7,-7,-7,-8,-8,-8,-8,-8,-8,-8,-8,-8,-8,-8,-8,-8, -8,-8,-8,-8,-8,-8,-8,-9,-9,-9,-9 -9,-9,-9,-9,-9,-9,-9,-10,-11

The best deviation point is -4 dB
The worst deviation point is -11 dB
7th best deviation point is -7 dB

In uniform generalized field defect, deviation values are almost similar and almost equal MD index.

MD index is -8.05 dB P<0.5%

In uniform generalized field defect, the deviation values from the normative data are almost similar. So, the MD index is the true representation of loss of sensitivity at each point of TDNP. The MD index and 7th best deviation point of TDNP will be almost similar.

Role of MD Index in the Follow-up Tests: The Most Important Index to Assess Field Progression is MD Index

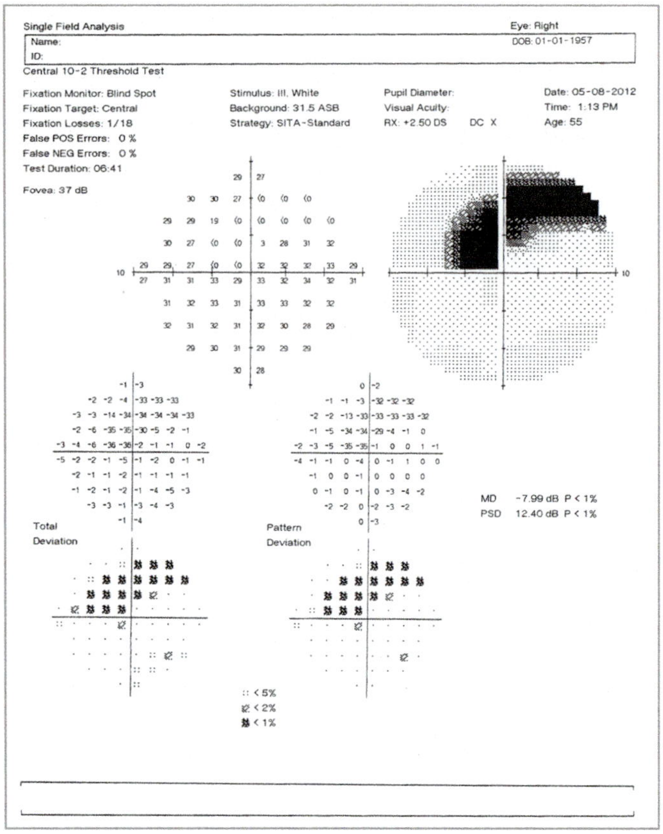

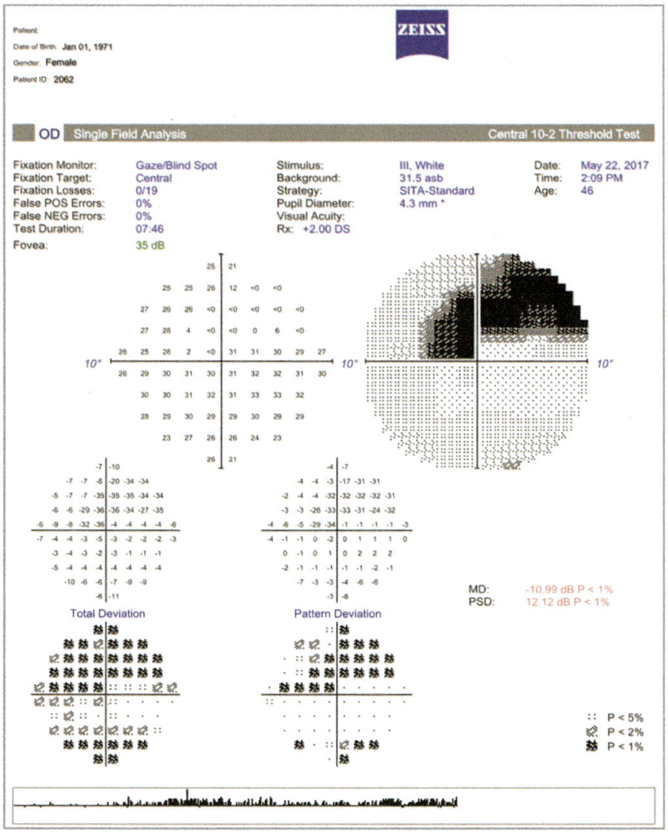

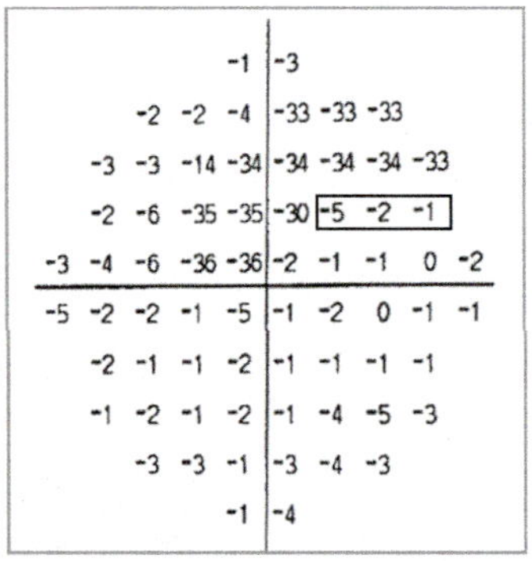

MD -7.99 dB

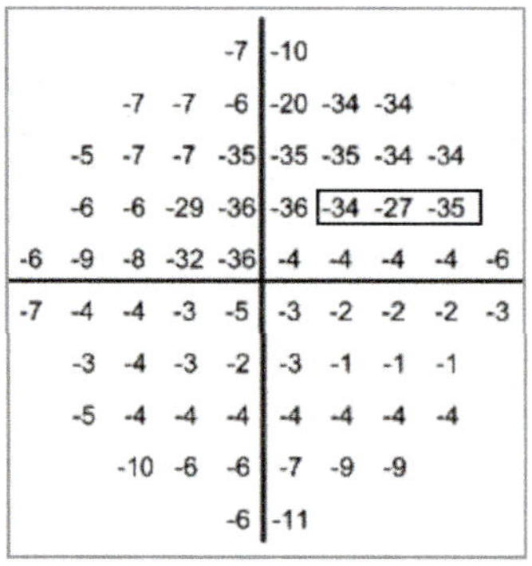

MD -10.99 dB

Here we are studying progression of glaucoma in a case of localized field defect. The MD index of the first test is -7.99 dB and MD index of the follow-up test is -10.99 dB. Change in MD is – 3.00 dB but if you see the loss of sensitivity of points adjacent to localized scotoma (points within the boxes) is not 3 dB loss at each point. They became absolute scotomas.

In a case of localized field defect, MD Index is not the true index to represent the depth of the field defect. The value of MD index is always less than the mean of the localized field defect. While assessing the progression of the field defect, we see the change in MD index between the first test and follow up test. In this example, change in MD index between these two tests is 3 dB. But, if we see the raw data, in the first test the deviation values within the box are almost normal. But in the follow-up test, they almost became absolute scotomas. So remember that the deviation values of localized scotoma will be expressed as mean of all the points of TDNP. The value of MD index is always less than the exact depth of the field defect and change in MD index is always less than the exact change.

Pattern Standard Deviation (PSD)

Pattern standard deviation (PSD) in a localized field defect.

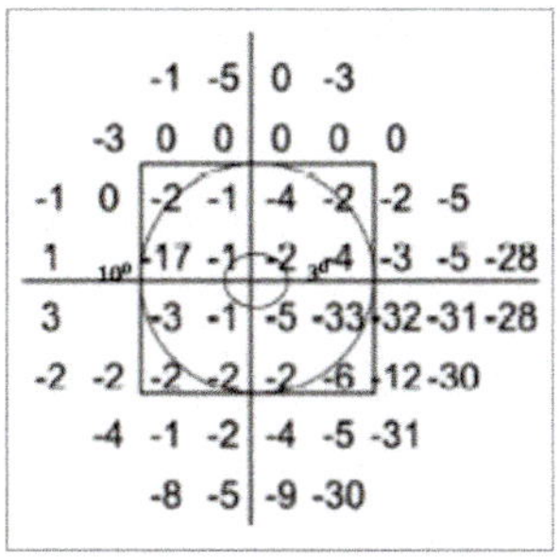

TDNP

Localized field defect

TDNP contains dissimilar deviation values. So the contour of hill of vision will be irregular and PSD will be high with significant P value.

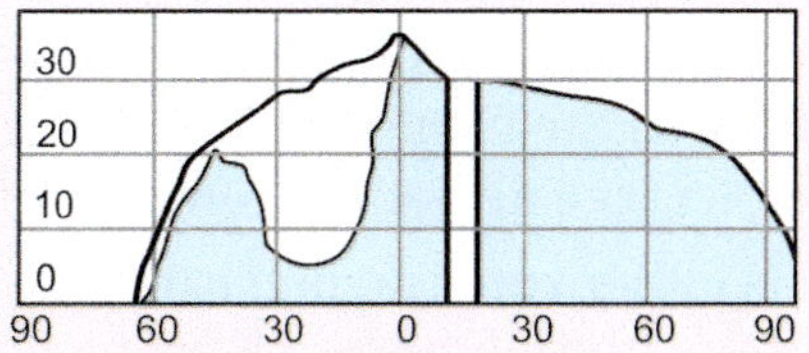

Rough contour of hill of vision PSD–high

Pattern standard deviation in irregular generalized field defect.

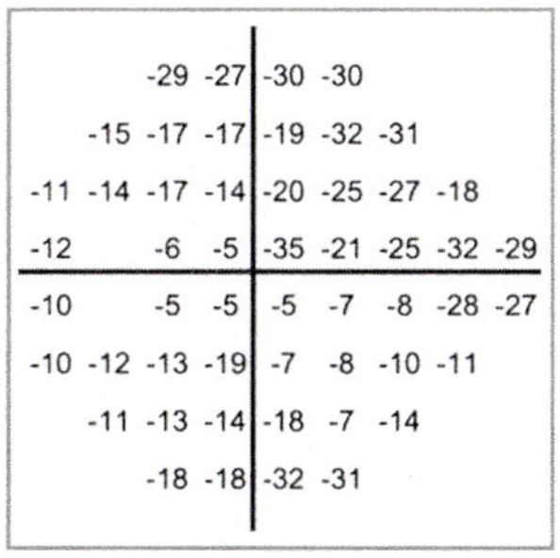

TDNP

Established case of glaucoma with irregular generalized field defect, TDNP contains dissimilar sensitivity values. So contour of hill of vision will be irregular and PSD will be high

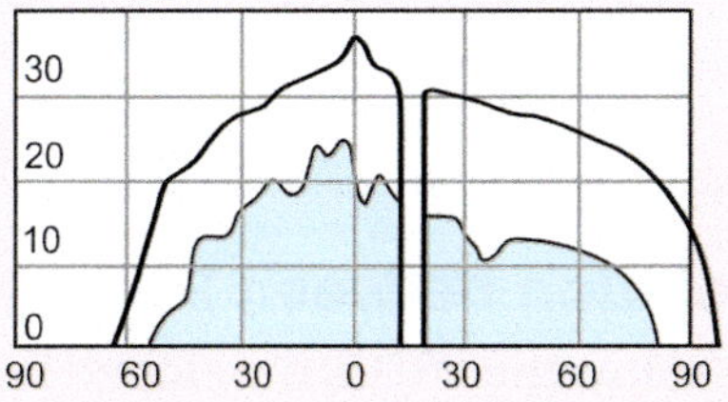

Rough contour of hill of vision PSD–high

Pattern standard deviation in uniform generalized field defect.

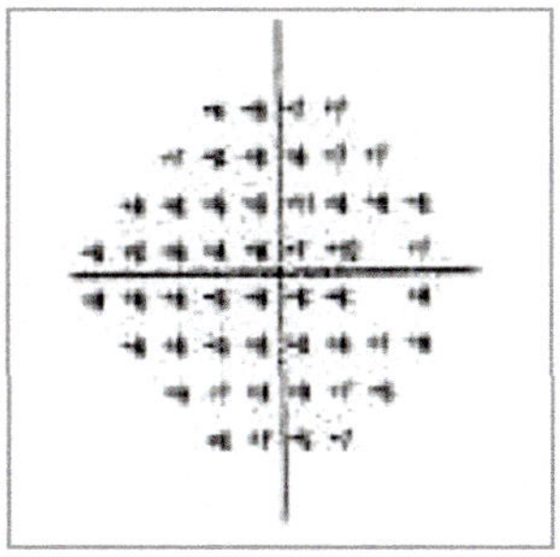

TDNP

TDNP contains similar deviation values in uniform generalized field defect. So the contour of hill of vision is smooth and PSD will be low or non-significant.

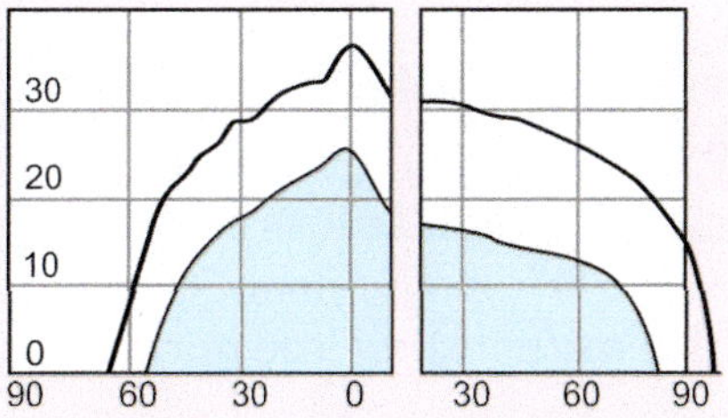

Smooth contour of hill of vision PSD low

PSD is an index which depends on the contour of hill of vision. Normal contour of hill of vision is smooth.If the contour is smooth, PSD is nonsignificant without P value. If the contour is not smooth, PSD is significant and represented by P value. In early glaucoma and established glaucoma PSD is significant and is represented by P value. In end stage of glaucoma when almost all points become absolute scotomas again PSD becomes nonsignificant. Another important point is PSD is significant even the retinal sensitivity is better than normal. The most important point is regarding PSD are—**(1)** It does not carry any symbol in front of it; **(2)** It does not tell the severity of glaucoma; **(3)** It is an index developed to pick up glaucoma at the earliest stage.

PSD is the standard deviation around the mean that constitutes the MD index and indicates the degree to which the numbers in the total deviation numerical plot are not similar to each other.

The slope of the normal visual field is quite smooth, as depicted by the upper solid diagonal lines in Figure shown here. If the visual field profile of a patient is also smooth like this, the PSD will be close to zero. The lower solid line that is irregular, depicts the visual field of a patient with localized visual field loss. The dashed line represents the adjustment of the visual field profile to account for the average or generalized deviation of the visual field from normal. Here even after adjusting the height of the visual field to account for the average deviation from normal, there are irregular departures from the normal slope.

It is either zero (no departure from the average normal slope of hill of vision) or a positive number. The higher the number the greater the deviation from the normal slope of hill of vision.

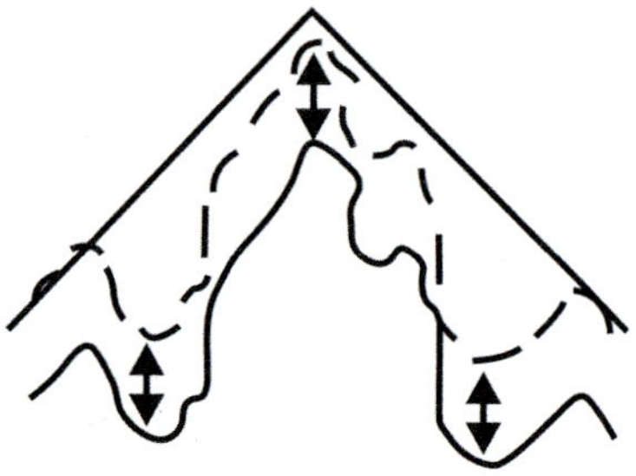

$$PSD = \sqrt{\left(\frac{1}{n}\sum_{i+1}^{n} s_{1_i}^{2}\right) + \left(\frac{1}{n-1}\sum_{i+1}^{n}\frac{(x_1 - N_i - MD)^2}{s_{1_i}^{2}}\right)}$$

Formula to calculate PSD
Where X_i is the measured threshold at point I, N_i, is the normal reference threshold at point$_i$ i, $s_{1_i}^2$, the variance of normal field measurements at point i, n denotes the number of test points, excluding the blind spot, and MD is the mean deviation

Correlation between PSD Value and Contour of Hill of Vision

As you know the PSD is developed to express the irregular loss of retinal sensitivity—higher the irregularity in the loss of sensitivity, higher the PSD value. When there is a localized field defect, the contour of hill of vision is irregular with minimal affect on the height of hill of vision (high PSD value). When there is irregular generalized field defect, the height of hill of vision is decreased and the contour of hill of vision is irregular (high mean deviation index and high PSD value). When there is uniform generalized depression (the loss of sensitivity at each point is identical), there is no dissimilarity in the loss of sensitivity and hence, the contour of hill of vision is smooth and the height of hill of vision is decreased (Low PSD and high mean deviation index).

Correlation between PSD Value and Pattern Deviation Probability Plot

The PSD values can be correlated with pattern deviation probability plot. Whenever, the PSD value is high (the sign of irregular loss of sensitivity) the pattern deviation probability plot will be abnormal. When the PSD value is nonsignificant or without P value (that is either field is normal or there is uniform generalized loss of sensitivity), we see normal pattern deviation probability plot.

Role of PSD in the Follow-up Tests

Increase in MD index and change in PSD indicate that there is progression of the field defect and it may be confined to a localized area or to a localized area in generalized depression (irregular generalized loss). Increase in MD index and no change in PSD indicate that there is progression of the field defect and it is uniform generalized type.

PSD is the index of irregular loss of retinal sensitivity which is better appreciated by the different deviation values in the total deviation numerical plot. Remember that PSD will be low and without any P value in uniform generalized field defect and PSD will be high in localized and irregular generalized field defects. PSD is not an index developed to tell the severity of field defect. It is developed to pickup dissimilar deviation values in total deviation numerical plot. For all practical purposes it is an index developed to pickup early localized field defect to diagnose glaucoma at an early stage even before we appreciate the change in the MD index due to glaucoma.

PSD in Early Glaucoma

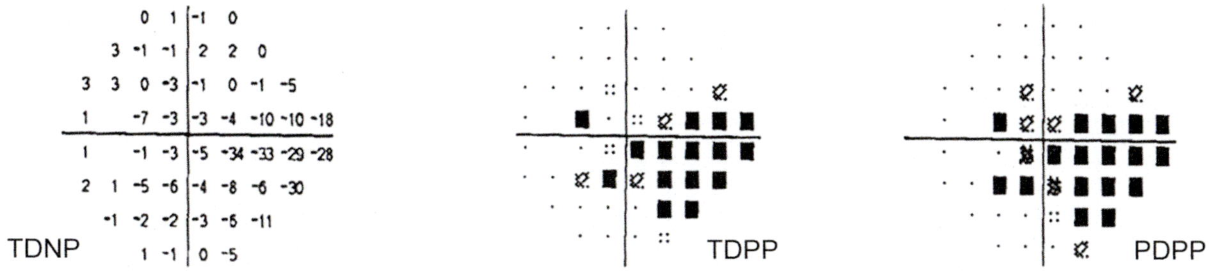

3,3,3,2,2,2,1,1,1,1,1,0,0,0,0,0,0,-1,-1,-1,-1,-1,-1,-1,-1,-2,-2,-3,-3,-3,-3,-3,-4,-4,-5,-5,-5,-5,-5,-6,-6,-6,-7,-8,-10,-10,-11,-18,-28,-29,-30,-33,-34.

MD -5.70 dB P<0.5%
PSD 10-6 dB P< 0.5%

The deviation values of TDNP are arranged according to their deviation values in a chronological order, the best deviation point (3 dB) is the first point and the worst deviation point is (-34 dB) as last point. In this example, the deviation values of TDNP are not similar to each other. The difference between the best deviation point and the worst deviation point is high and PSD is significant. PSD is 10.06 dB P < 0.5%. The PSD quantifies localized loss as a single value and is useful in identifying early defects. It is a case of early glaucoma with a localized field defect. The MD index is -5.70 dB

PSD in Advanced Glaucoma

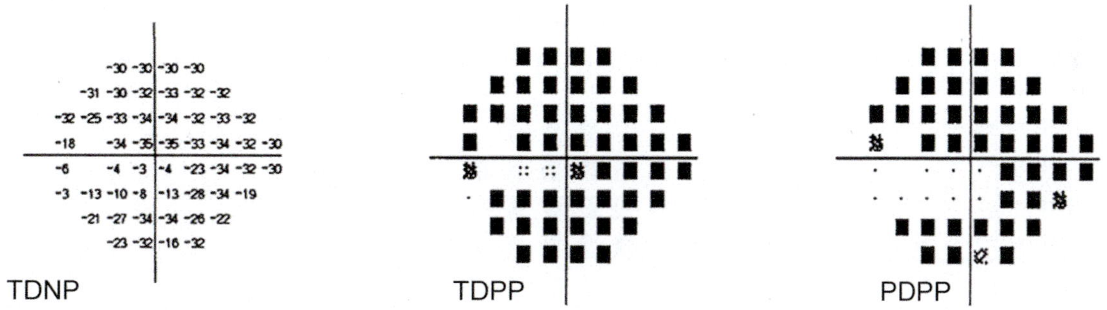

-3,-3,-4,-4,-6,-8,-10,-13,-13,-16,-18,-19,-21,-22,-23,-23,-25,-26,-27,-28,-30,-30,-30,-30,-30,-30,-31,-32,-32,-32,-32,-32,-32,-32,-32,-32,-32,--33,-33,-33,-33,--34,-34,-34,-34,-34,-34,-34,-34,--35,-35.

M.D. -25.67 dB P<0.5%
PSD11.13 dB P<0.5%

The best deviation point is (-3 dB) and the worst is (-35 dB). In this example, the deviation values are dissimilar to each other. Because the difference between the best deviation point and the worst deviation point is high, the PSD will be high. The PSD is 11.13 dB P < 0.5% and the MD index is -25.67 dB P < 0.5%.

In this example though the difference between the best deviation point and the worst deviation point is high and most of the deviational values are around -30 dB. This is the reason why the PSD is 11.13 dB P < 0.5% though the MD index is -25.67 dB. It is very important to note that there is no proportional relationship between MD index and PSD. There is no role of PSD in established and advanced cases of glaucoma as PSD is not directly proportional to the depth of the field defect. As glaucoma progresses, PSD decreases after a certain stage of glaucoma, because the dissimilarity among the deviation values will be minimum.

PSD in End Stage of Glaucoma

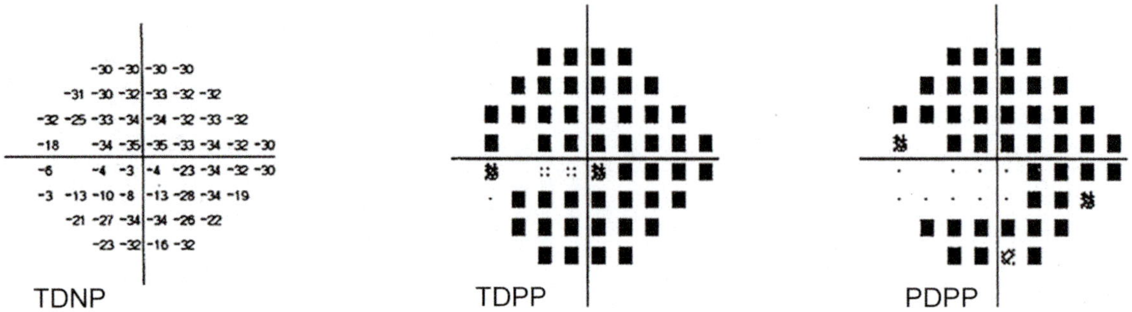

-12,-18,-21,-23,-25,-25,-26,-27,-28,-28,-30,-30,-31,-31,-31,-31,-32,-32,-32,-32,-32,-32,-32,-32,-32,-33,-33,-33,-33,-33,-33,-33,-34,-34,-34,-34,-34,-34,-34,-34,-34,-34,-34,-35,-35,-35,-35,-35,-35,-35.

M D -31.54 dB P<0.5%
PSD 4.31 dB P<0.5%

The best deviation point is -12 dB and the worst is -35 dB. Most of the points have the deviation values around -30 dB. As the dissimilarity among the points is minimal, the PSD will be low. In this case PSD is 4.31 dB P < 0.5% and the MD index is -31.54 dB P < 0.5%. PSD does not represent the severity of glaucoma. But it is an index developed to pickup early localized field defects.

This is a very advanced case of glaucoma with MD index -31.54 dB P < 0.5%. Even though the MD index 31.54 dB P < 0.5%, PSD is only 4.31 dB P < 0.5%. From this, one should understand that PSD does not represent the severity of glaucoma but depends on the degree of dissimilar values in TDNP. In the end stage of glaucoma, the loss of sensitivity of all the points will be around 30 dB and so the dissimilarity among the deviational values of TDNP will be minimum. Hence the PSD is low (4.31 dB P < 0.5%). So it is very clear that PSD has nothing to do with the depth of the field defect.

PSD in Uniform Generalized Field Defect (Cataract)

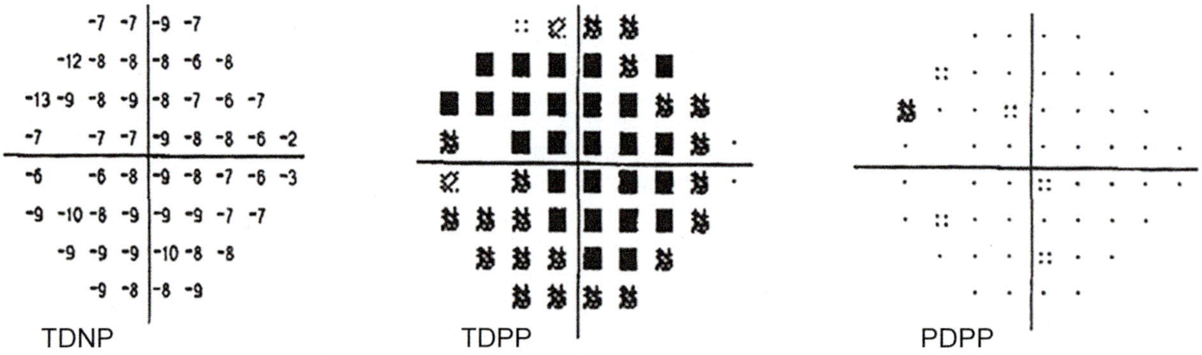

-2,-5,-6,-6,-6,-6,-6,-6,-7,-7,-7,-7,-7,-7,-7,-7,-7,-7,-7,-8,-8,-8,-8,-8,-8,-8,-8,-8,-8,-8,-8,-8,-9,-9,-9,-9,-9,-9,-9,-9,-9,-9,-9,-9,-9,-9,-10,-10,-12,-13,

The best deviation point is -2 dB and the worst is -13 dB. Most of the points have the deviation values around -8 dB. As the deviational values are similar and around -8 dB to 9 dB, PSD is 1.57 dB without P value and MD index is -7.85 dB P < 0.5%.

PSD does not represent the severity of glaucoma. But it is an index developed to pickup early localized field defect. It does not carry any sign in front of it. Please note that PSD will be without P value when there is no loss of sensitivity or uniform generalized loss of sensitivity (contour of hill of vision is smooth).

Visual Field Index (VFI)

The visual field index (glaucoma progression index) is a new perimetric index designed for two purposes

1. For calculating the rate of glaucomatous progression (glaucoma progression analysis (GPA), this is the reason why the index is also named as glaucoma progression index)
2. To reflect quality of life. So doctors may use this for educational purposes since patients can quickly perceive with minimal explanation.

VFI is expressed in percentage where 100% represents a normal visual field and 0% represents a perimetrically blind field. VFI-100% means the quality of life is not affected. The VFI cannot go beyond 100%.

Basics—to conclude

- Strongly centrally weighted (foveal test locations have more influence)
- Pattern deviation outside 5%, probability and MD > -20 dB
- Total deviation if MD < -20 dB
- Better reflects quality of life (Q-o-L), and reduces effects of cataract

Central points weighted more heavily than those on periphery

Calculate the Deviation from the Local Component and the 5% Probability of the Pattern Deviation

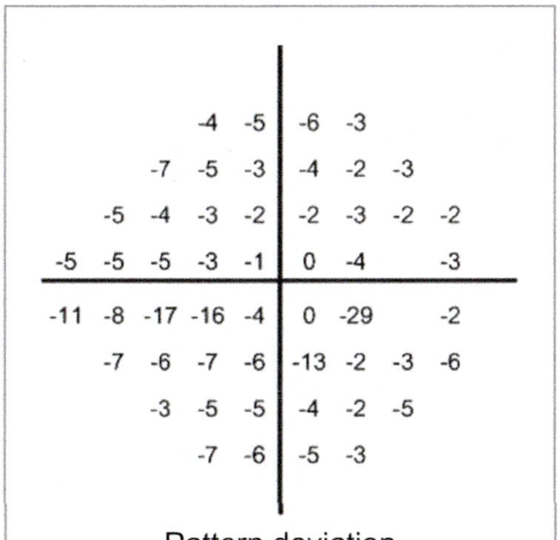

Pattern deviation numerical plot

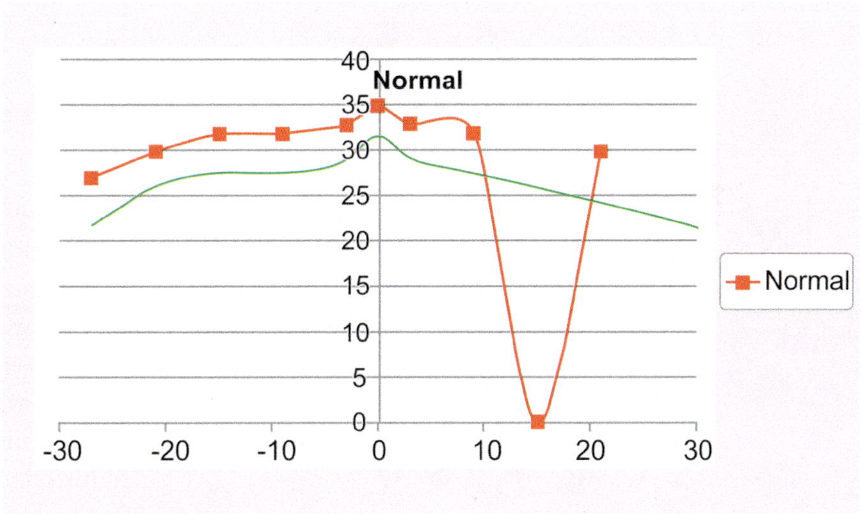

$$VFI_{principle} \ \frac{-15\ dB}{-28\ dB} = 0.54 \ = 54\%$$

This index tells the remaining percentage of strongly centrally weighted and un affected by cataract quality vision.

ZONE 10—GLAUCOMA HEMIFIELD TEST (GHT)

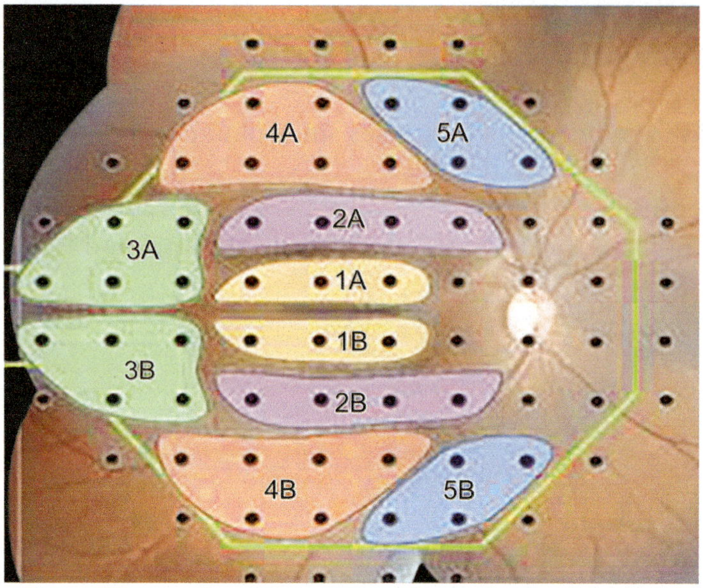

24-2 point pattern

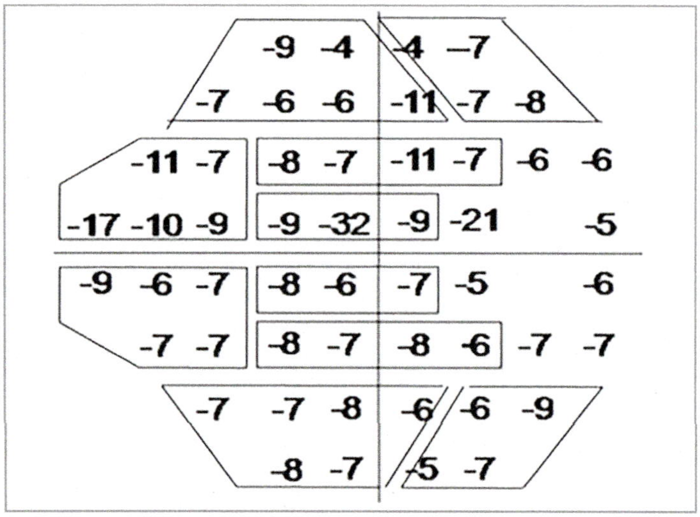

Pattern deviation numerical plot

Actually GHT can be called as a refined PSD. GHT is developed to pickup the dissimilarity among the deviation values of the corresponding points on either side of horizontal axis to diagnose glaucoma at an early stage. Glaucoma hemifield test evaluates five zones in the upper field and compares the deviation values of these zones to their mirror image zones in the lower half of the field. These zones are constructed in the approximate patterns of retinal nerve fibers, and thus GHT is directed primarily at the diagnosis of glaucomatous visual field loss and not other diseases.

A score assigned to each zone based on the location of the zones and their deviation values in the pattern deviation numerical plot. A comparison of each upper zone is made with the corresponding lower zone and the difference in scores between the upper and lower zones is calculated. The difference is compared with significant limits taken from a data base of normal subjects.

Provides the result in clear text.

The five results are:

1. Border line.
2. Outside normal limits.
3. Abnormally low sensitivity.
4. Abnormally high sensitivity.
5. And within normal limits.

Note that the outer set of points of 30-2 except the two outer most points on the nasal side are not included in the zones. Pattern deviation numerical plot is the basis for GHT.

Text Messages of GHT

Outside Normal Limits

Sensitivities in one or more of the five zones in the upper half of the field are significantly different ($P < 0.01\%$) from the sensitivities measured in the corresponding zones in the lower half of the field.

Borderline

Zones pairs differ by an amount greater than is seen in most normal subjects ($P < 0.03$), but the difference does not reach the level required for the outside normal limits message.

General Depression of Sensitivity

Test point locations are so low as to be at levels seen in only 0.5% of normal subjects will not be displayed when sensitivity differences between superior and inferior hemifields are large enough to result in an "outside normal limits" message.

Abnormally High Sensitivity

The point locations are so high as to be at levels seen in only 0.5% of normal subjects.

Within Normal Limits

Presented when none of the previous significance limits have been reached. In the absence of significant detectable deviations from the norm, a message "within normal limits" is provided. Since this message is based on statistics, the presence of pathology is not excluded and the final judgment still is the responsibility of the eye care professional.

Understanding of 0 in raw data, 0 in total deviation numerical plot and 0 in pattern deviation numerical plot.

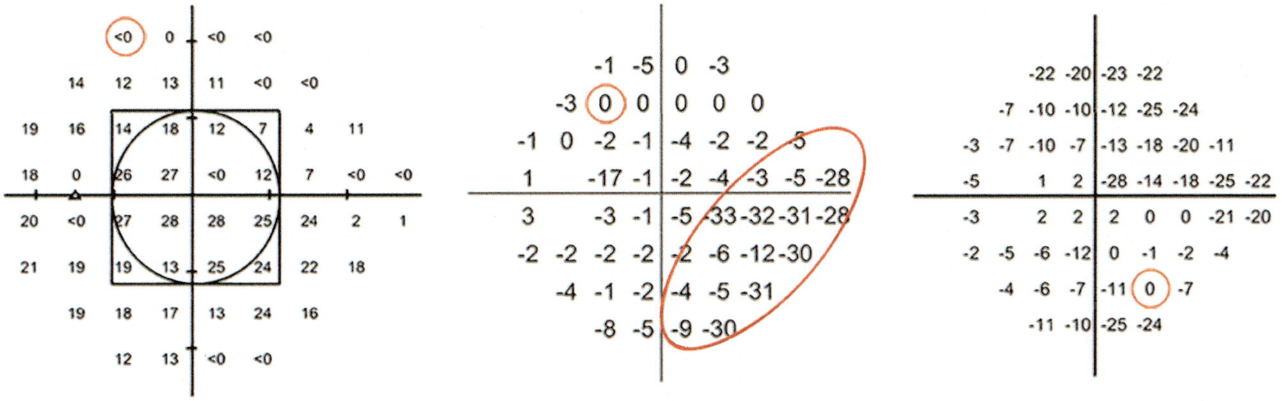

Raw data | Total deviation numerical plot | Pattern deviation numerical plot

0 in raw data is absolute scotoma

0 in TDNP is normal sensitivity point (0 deviation from normative data)

0 in PDNP corresponds to 7th best deviation point of TDNP

SUMMARY OF THE STATPAC DEPENDENT ZONES OF THE SFA PRINTOUT

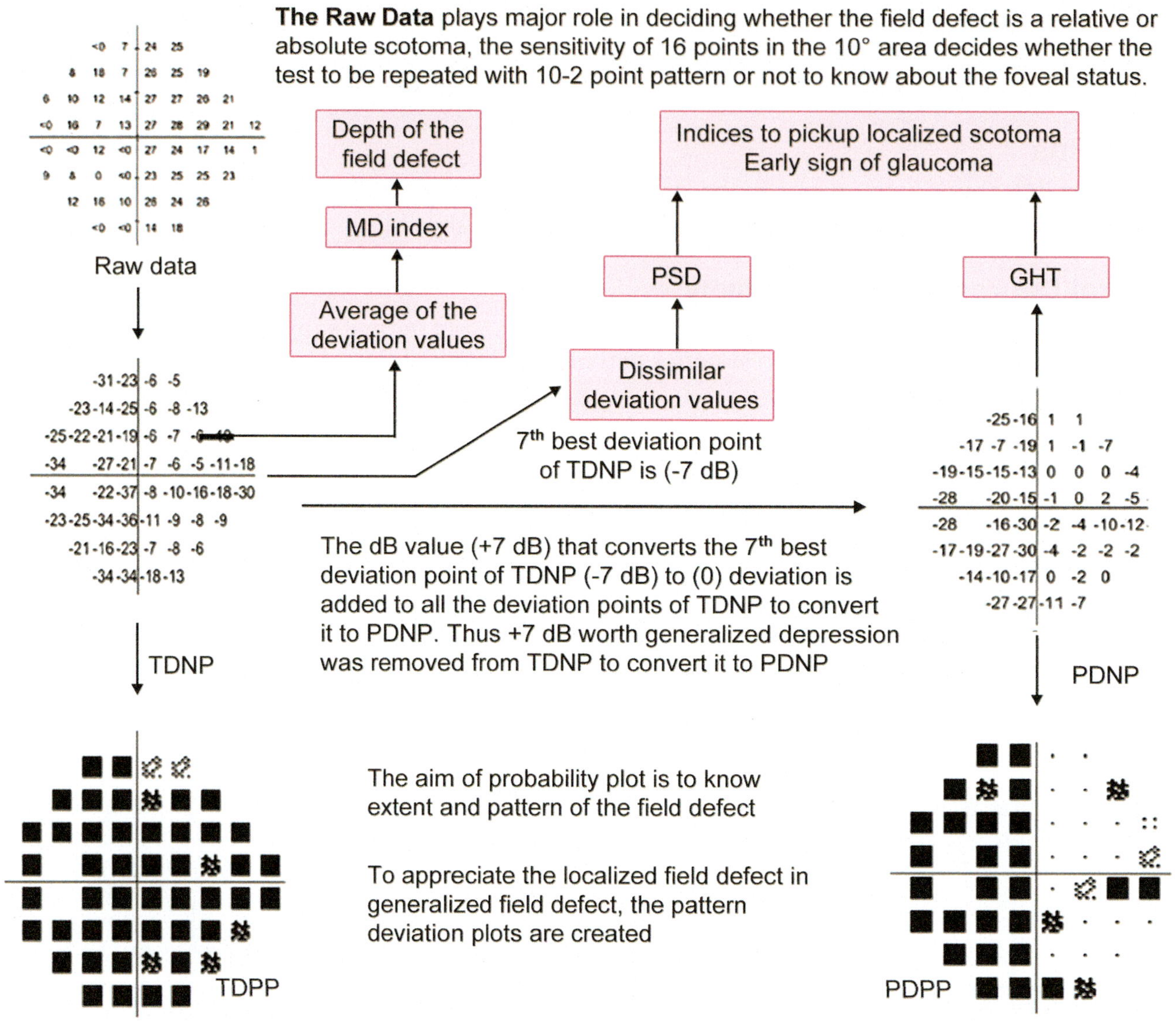

In a case of localized field defect, the pattern and extent of the field defect is known from the total deviation probability plot. When all the points in TDPP are represented by black squares, we cannot identify the type of generalized depression in TDPP.

After eliminating the generalized depression worth of the dB value that converts the 7th best deviation point of TDNP to 0 deviation from TDNP, the localized scotomas masked by generalized depression in the total deviation plots will be highlighted in the pattern deviation plots. So that the pattern of the localized field defect will be known in the PDPP. If PDPP is normal, it is a uniform generalized depression.

FEATURES OF LOCALIZED FIELD DEFECT

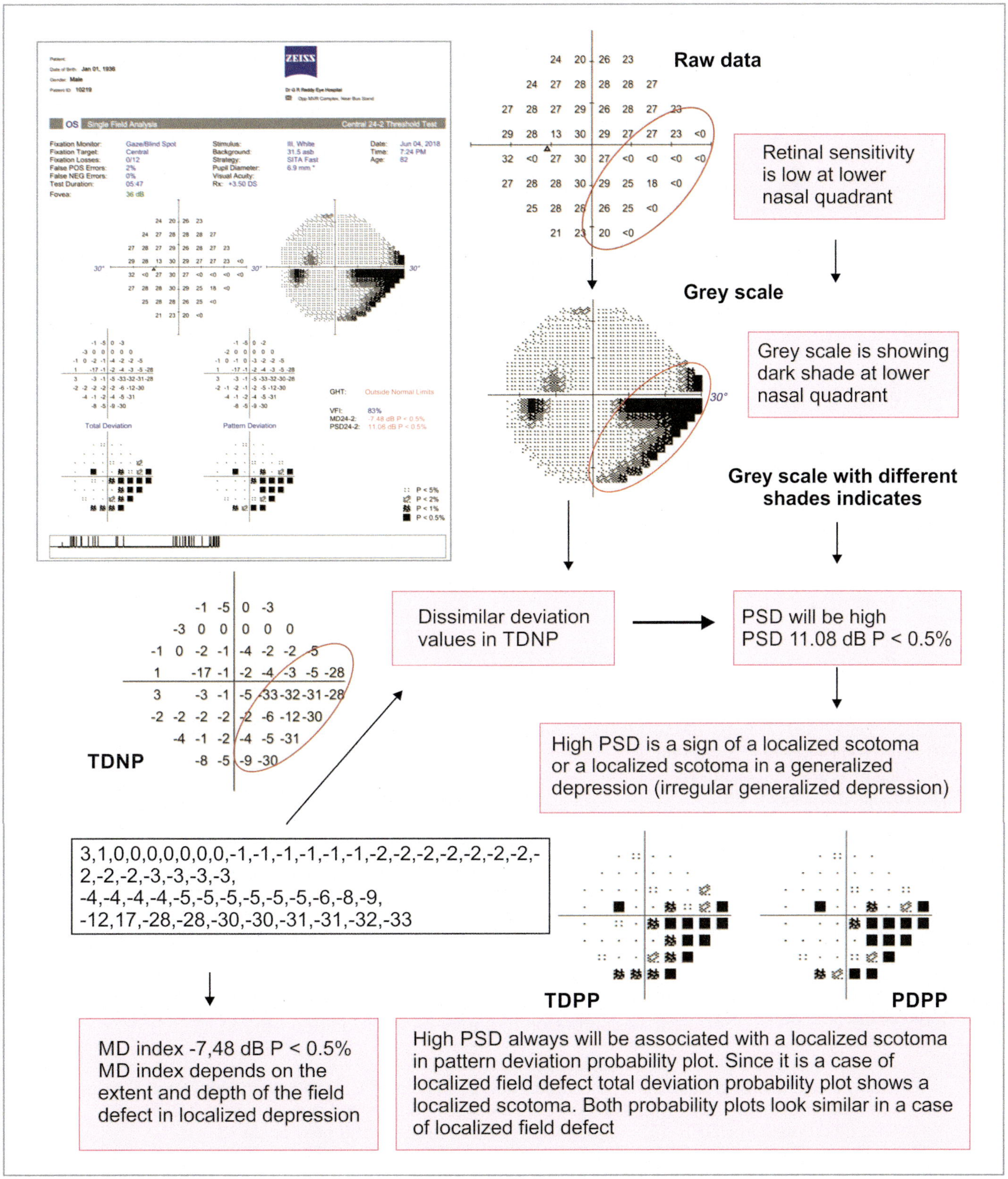

FEATURES OF IRREGULAR GENERALIZED FIELD DEFECT

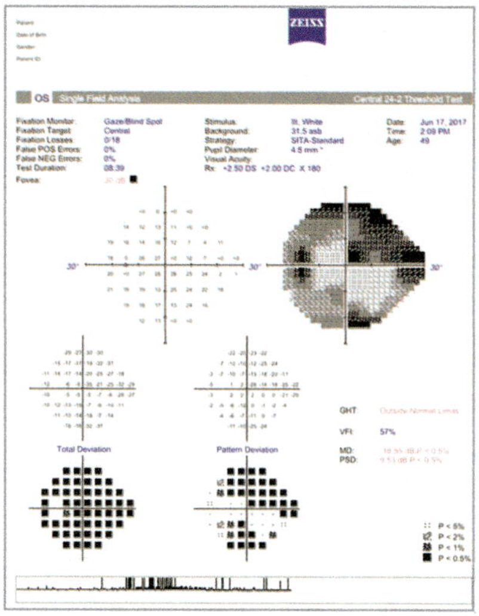

Raw data

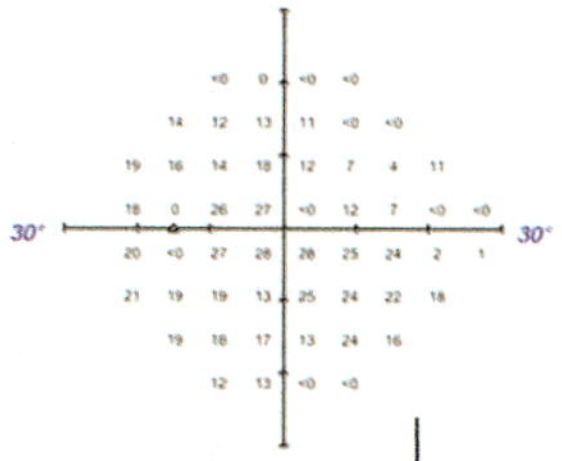

Retinal sensitivity is low at all points and some points are absolute scotomas, raw data is representing irregular generalized depression

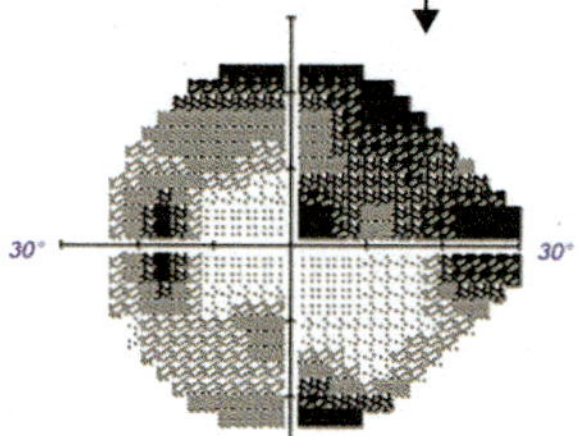

Grey scale

Grey scale is showing generalized depression with irregular shade (irregular generalized depression). Grey scale is representing raw data in shades format

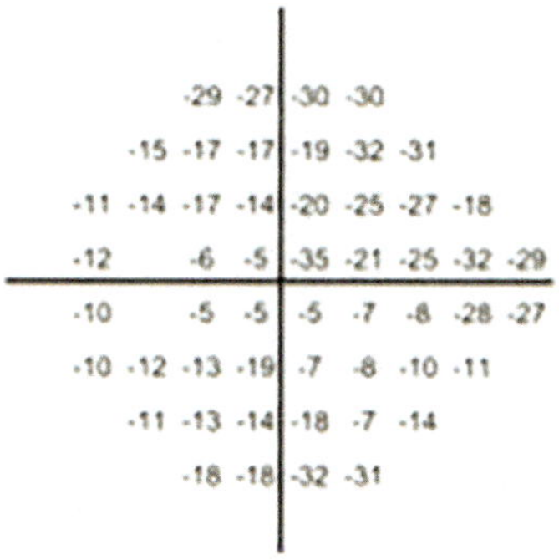

TDNP

Dissimilar deviation values in TDNP

PSD will be high
PSD 9.53 dB P < 0.5%

-5,-5,-5,-5,-6,-7,(-7) -7,-8,-8,-10,-10 -10,-11,-11,-11,-12,-12,-13,-13,-14, -14,-14-,-14,-15, -17,-17,-17,-18, -18,-18,-19,-19,-20,-21,-25 25,-27, -27,-27,-28,-29,-29,-30,-30,-31,-31, -32,-32,-32,-35

High PSD is a sign of a localized scotoma or a localized scotoma in a generalized depression (irregular generalized depression)

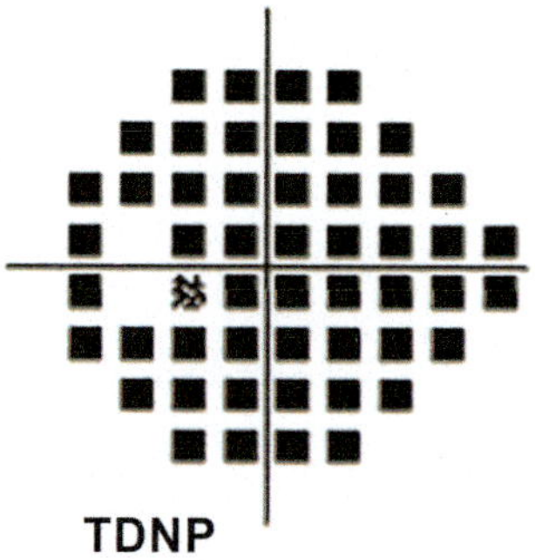

TDNP

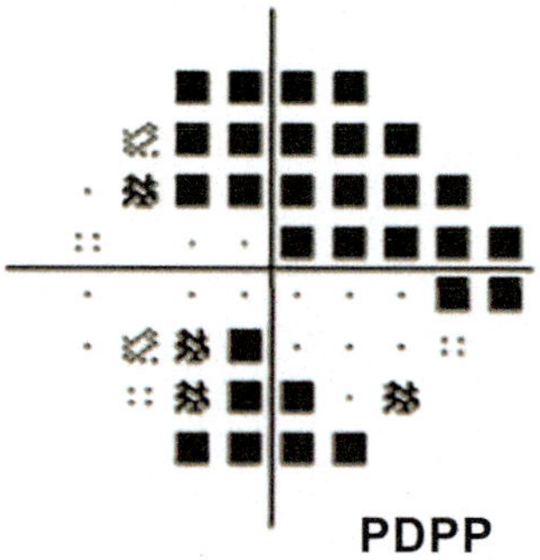

PDPP

MD index -16.55 dB P < 0.5%
Always the MD index is high with significant P value and to some extent it represents the depth of the field defect truly

High PSD always will be associated with a localized scotoma in pattern deviation probability plot. Since it is a case of generalized field defect, total deviation probability plot shows generalized depression (irregular generalized depression)

Irregular generalized field defect will be represented by (1) high PSD value with significant P value; (2) high mean deviation index with significant P value; (3) generalized depression in TDPP and localized field defect in PDPP; (4) irregular dark shaded areas in the grey scale

FEATURES OF UNIFORM GENERALIZED FIELD DEFECT

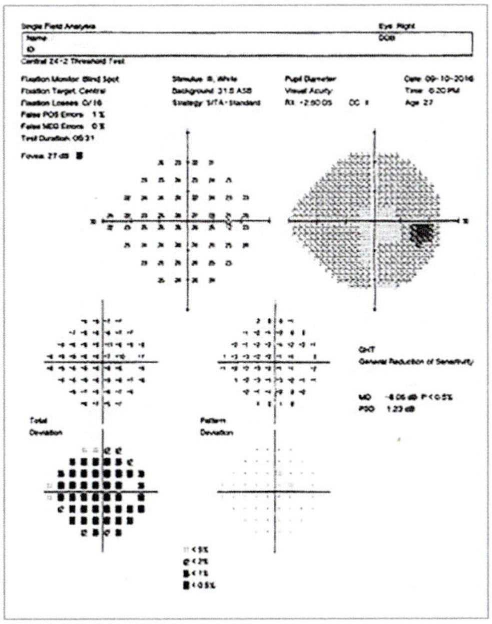

Raw data

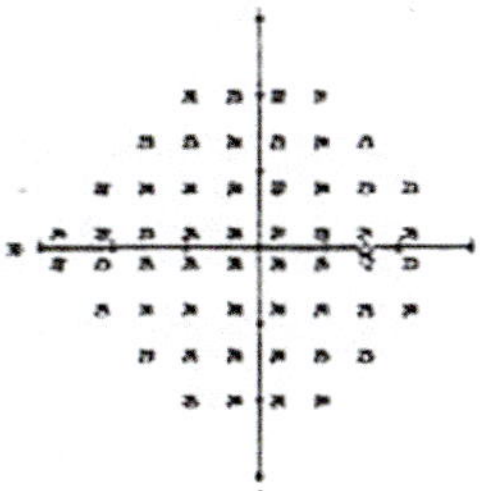

Retinal sensitivity is low at all points

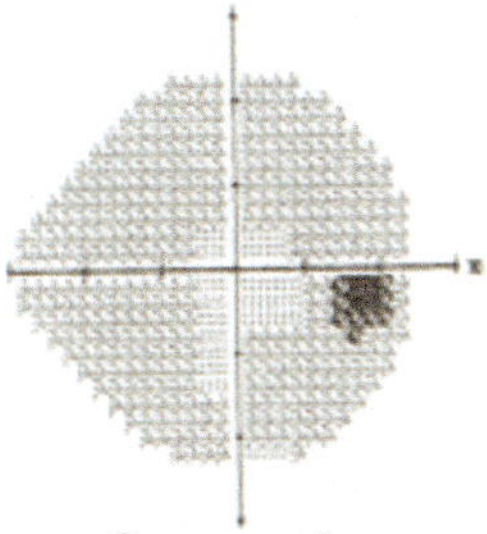

Grey scale

Grey scale shows generalized depression with uniform shades

Grey scale with uniform shade indicates

Similar deviation values in TDNP, indicates

PSD will be low or non-significant PSD 1.23 dB

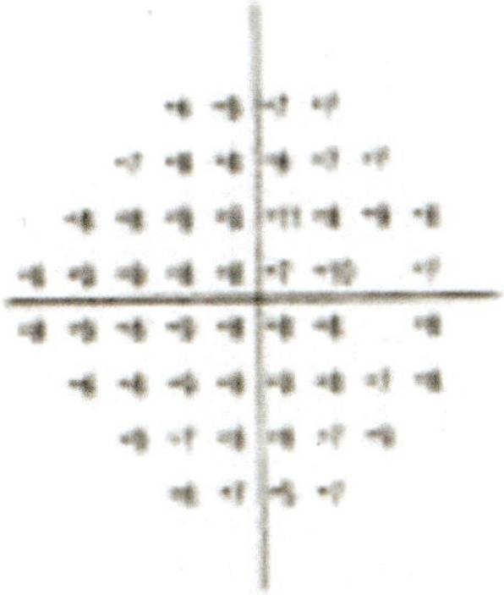

TDNP

2,1,1,1,1,0, 0, 0,0,0,0,0,0-1, -1,-1,-1,-1,-1,-1,-1,-1,-1,-1, -1,-1,-1,-1,-1,-2,-2,-2,-2,-2, -2,-2,-2,-2,-2,-2,-2,-2,-2,-2, -2,-2,-2,-3,-3,-3,-3,-3,-4,-4

Nonsignificant or low PSD is a sign of either no loss of sensitivity or uniform generalized depression

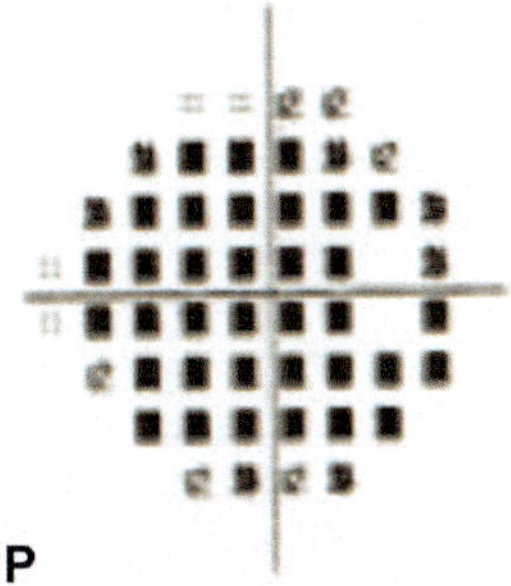

TDPP

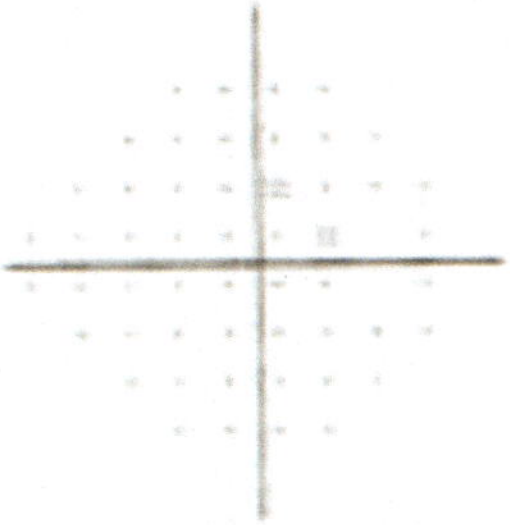

PDPP

MD -8.05 dB P < 0.5%
In uniform generalized field defect, the MD index is the true to represent the depth of the field defect and MD index and 7th best deviation point of TDNP will be almost same

Nonsignificant or low PSD always will have normal pattern deviation probability plot. It is always associated with either generalized depression in total deviation probability plot (uniform generalized field defect) or normal total deviation probability plot (no loss of sensitivity)

Analysis of total deviation probability plot and pattern deviation probability plot.

Glaucoma can present as localized field defect

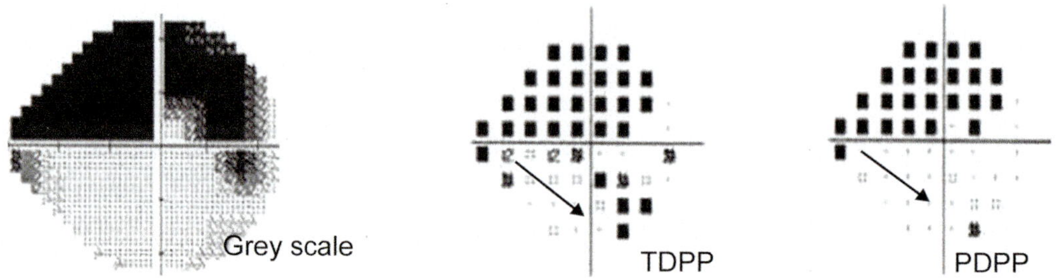

Note the recent onset scotomas in inferior field of TDPP disappear in the pattern deviation probability plot. Hence, the direction of progression will be appreciated in the TDPP with the help of PDPP. In this case the disease is progressing inferotemporally as indicated by arrow.

Glaucoma can present as irregular generalized field defect

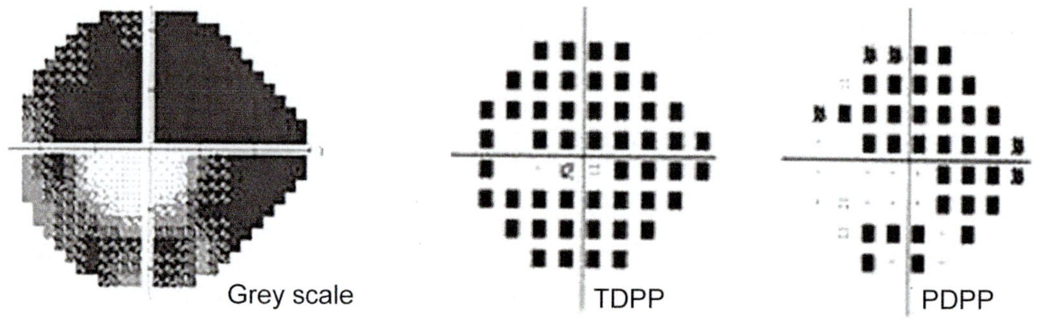

This is a case of advanced glaucoma presenting as generalized field loss in the TDPP and the deep scotomas from where glaucoma started seen in PDPP. In these situations the PDPP shows the direction of progression.

Glaucoma associated with cataract

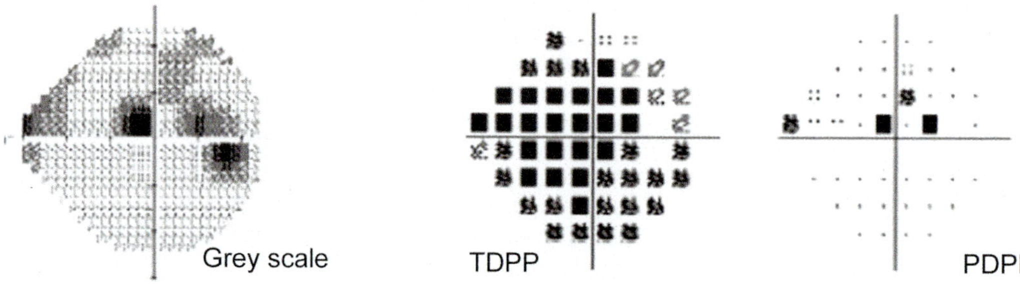

If a cataract patient develops glaucoma, the localized field defect due to glaucoma is highlighted in the PDPP.

No Evidence of Glaucoma in a Case of Cataract

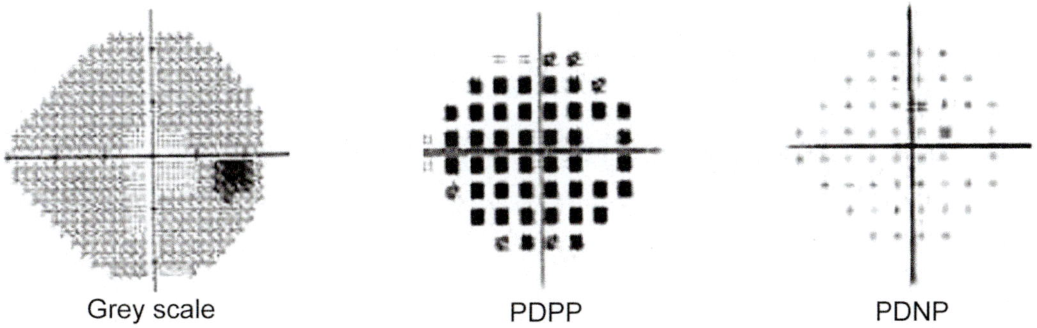

No localized field defect in PDPP. This is a case of uniform generalized depression. So there is no evidence of glaucoma.

Analysis of MD Index: Depth of the Scotoma

Interpret the value of MD index with caution especially in cases of localized field defects where MD index does not represent the exact depth of the field defect. To assess the exact loss of sensitivity at each point ,concentrate on TDNP. In a localized field defect, loss of sensitivity is confined to one area and other points are normal. In this scenario MD index is an average of normal and abnormal points. Strictly speaking, the mean deviation index should be calculated for abnormal points alone. Hence, the actual MD index in a localized scotoma would be more than the mean deviation index value printed in SFA printout.

Analysis of the Signs of Irregular Loss of Sensitivities: PSD and GHT

GHT and PSD are the two indices developed to pickup glaucoma at an early stage. These two indices will not play any significant role in established case of glaucoma. But there is a definite role of PSD in the follow-up fields. In the follow-up fields, increase in MD index with change in PSD indicates that there is progression of the field defect either as a localized field defect or as a localized field defect in generalized depression (irregular generalized loss). Increase in MD index with no change in PSD indicates that there is progression of the field defect and it is uniform generalized type.

Analysis of Raw Data

The raw data plays major role in deciding whether the test has to be repeated with 10-2 point pattern or not. Concentrate on the sensitivities of the 16 points in the 10° circle area. If there is severe loss of sensitivity even at one point among the 16 points, repeat the test with 10-2 point pattern. If the probability plot shows a black square at any point, do not come to any conclusion whether the black square is an absolute scotoma or a relative scotoma until you see the raw data. A 0 dB in the raw data indicates absolute scotoma. Macular split–Never come to a conclusion regarding the foveal status from the probability plots (even from 10-2 point pattern). Never say that there is foveal split, unless you see the 0 dB sensitivity at any of the four points on 1° circle around fixation.

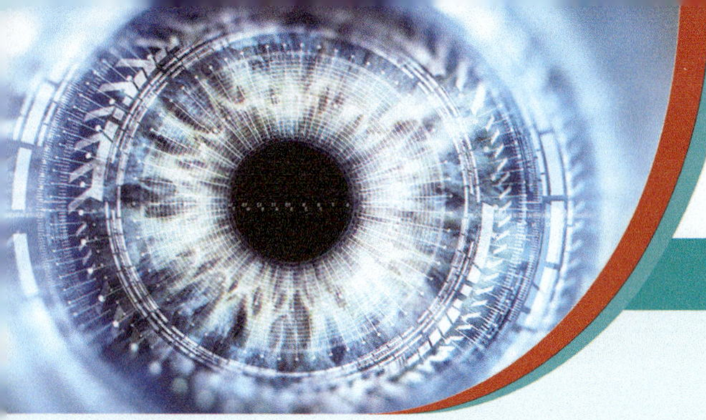

CHAPTER 4

Identification of Nonglaucomatous Field Defects and Artifacts

Verify whether the patient data and the test data are properly fed to the field analyzer by the technician. The information fed to the field analyzer should be exactly similar to that given in the order form for visual field testing.

The measured foveal sensitivity should correlate with visual acuity. It indicates that the refractive error correction for near vision is correct.

Location of blind spot. Confirm the normal position of the blind spot.

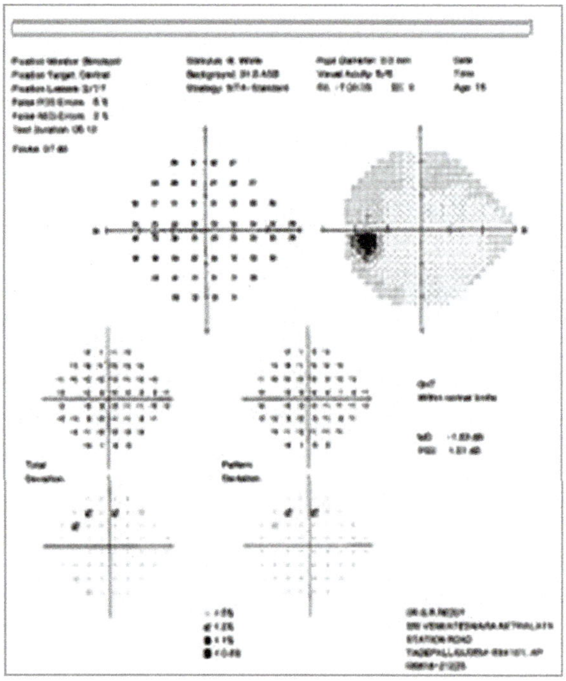

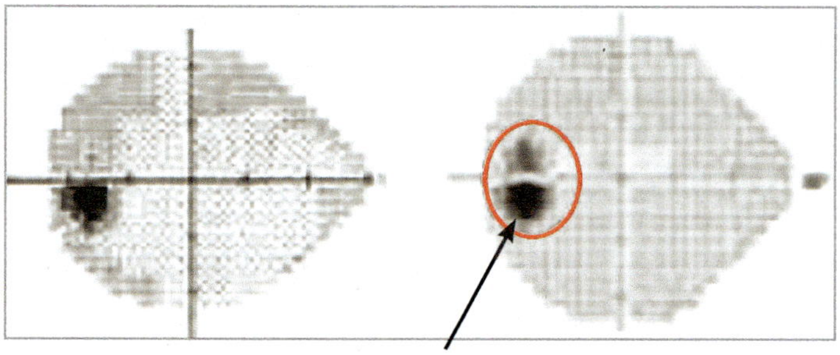

Enlarged blind spot papilledema

The blind spot will be below the horizontal meridian, the center of the blind spot being 15° temporal to fixation point. It is very important to know, how the blind spot looks in the grey scale normally to appreciate enlargement of blind spot in papilledema.

Interpreting the single field analysis printout starts with probability plots. So strictly speaking it is not the interpretation of single field analysis printout, it is actually the interpretation of probability plots.

If a field defect is seen in the probability plot, analyse the field defect as below:

Interpretation of visual fields

- *Step 1*: Identification of non-glaucomatous field defects
- *Step 2*: Identification of artifacts
- *Step 3*: Identification of glaucomatous field defects

Never interpret visual fields in isolation. It should always be correlated with fundus

STEP 1: IDENTIFICATION OF NONGLAUCOMATOUS FIELD DEFECTS

Example 1: Medullated nerve fibers (right eye)

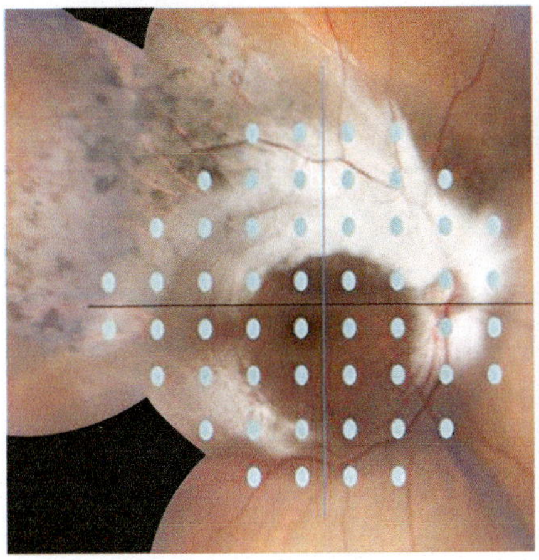

24-2 point pattern

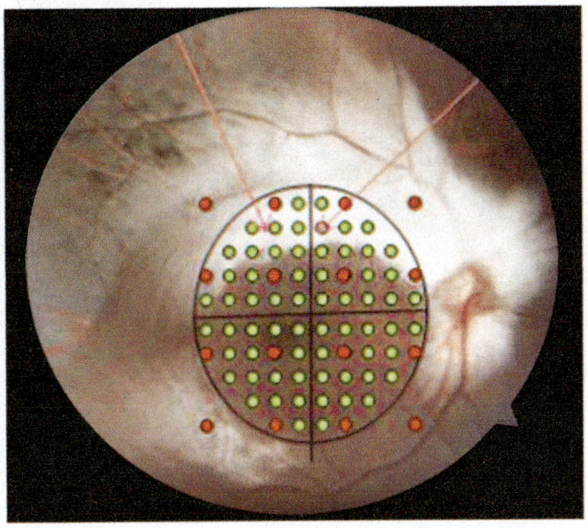

10-2 point pattern

Showing 1st example to emphasize that never interpret visual fields in isolation. It should always be correlated with fundus.

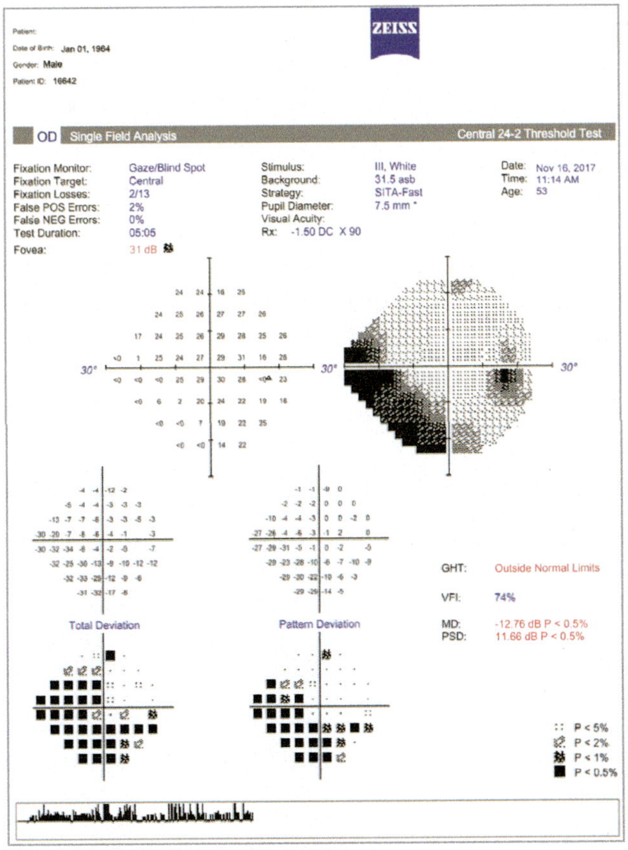

24-2 SITA Fast

FL 2/13; FP 2%; FN 0%

MD -12.76 dB P < 0.5%

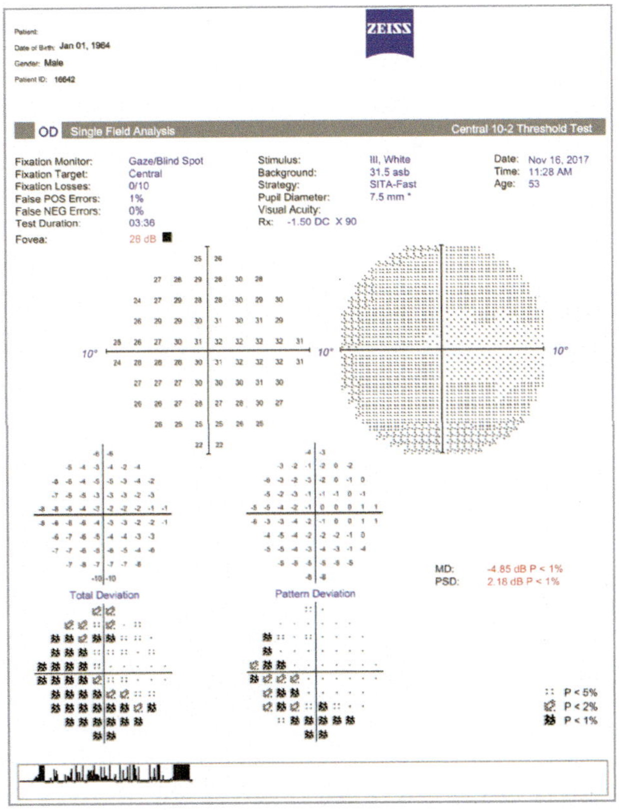

10-2 SITA Fast

FL 0/10; FP 1%; FN 0%

MD -4.85 dB P < 1%

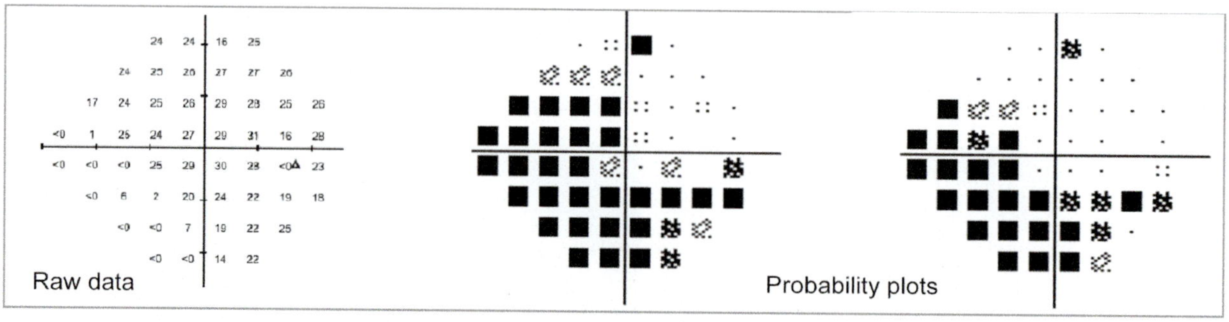

Field defect: Localized field defect involving entire lower quadrant and upper nasal quadrant with deep localized scotoma in the lower nasal quadrant. Depth of the field defect—MD 12.76 dB.

Raw data: The points of 21° and 15° circles are showing absolute scotomas, out of 16 points in the 10° circle area. The sensitivity of the 9° point in the lower nasal quadrant is 2 dB, so we have to repeat the test with 10-2 point pattern.

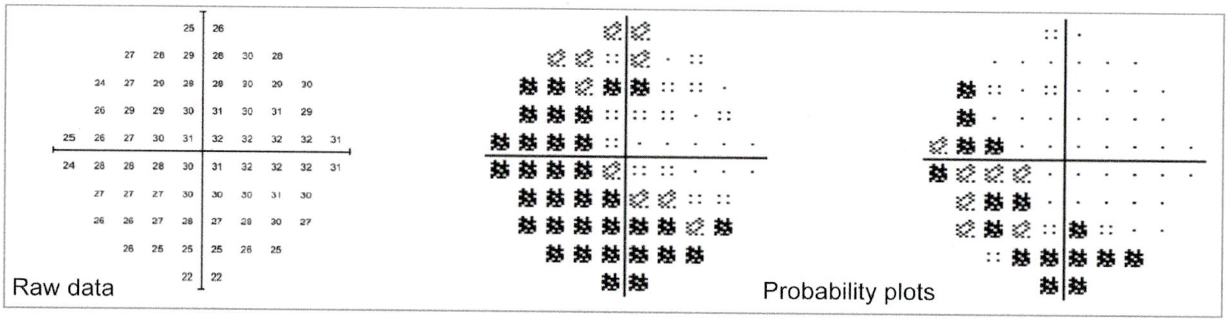

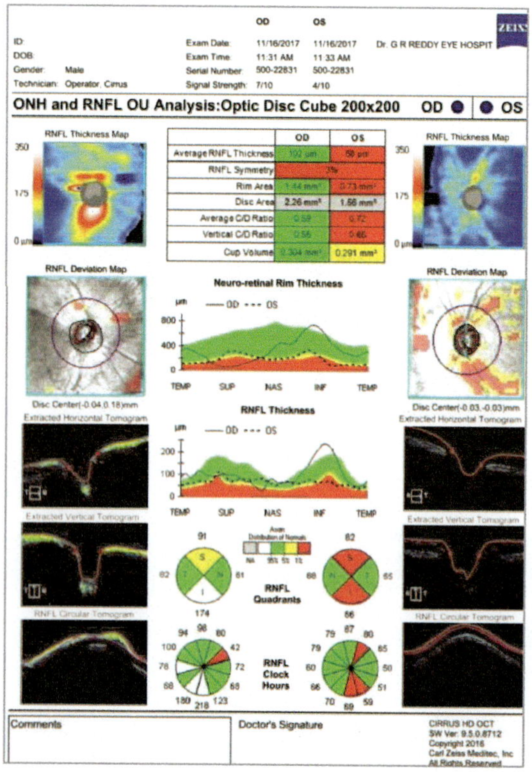

Without showing fundus picture a student should not be blamed for interpreting the field defect as a glaucomatous field defect. But one should remember not to make a diagnosis without correlating fields with fundus picture. The best student will only quantify and qualify the field defect, but never tells the diagnosis till he sees the fundus picture.

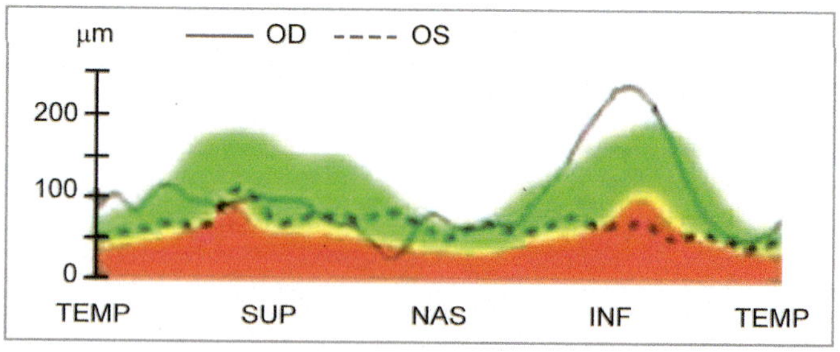

Right eye optical coherence tomography (OCT) showing thicker retinal nerve fiber layer (RNFL) in inferior quadrant than in the superior quadrant.

Example 2: Never interpret visual fields in isolation. It should always be correlated with fundus.

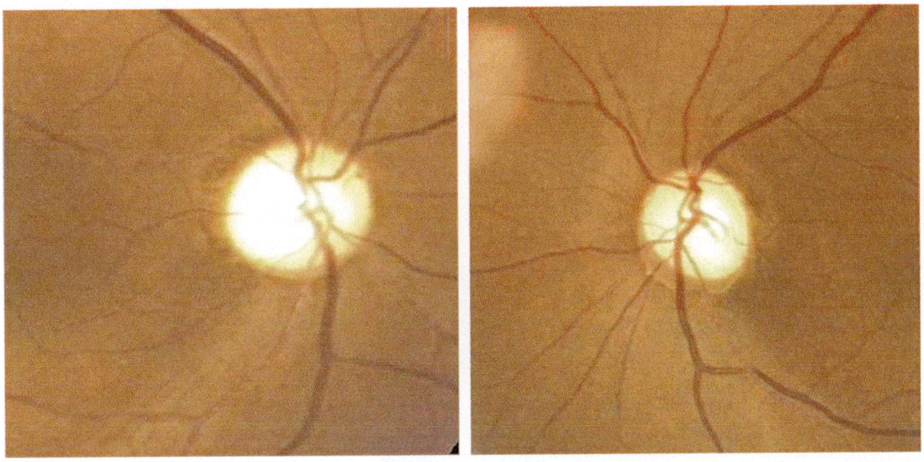

On the basis of shallow anterior chamber and visual fields, diagnosis of glaucoma is made and the patient was put on antiglaucoma medication without proper evaluation of disc and retina.

Visual fields and fundus must correlate with one another. In this example, if one evaluates the disc carefully the disc pallor is exceeding the cup pallor. If disc pallor is exceeding the cup pallor one should ask for CT or MRI to rule out intracranial pathology.

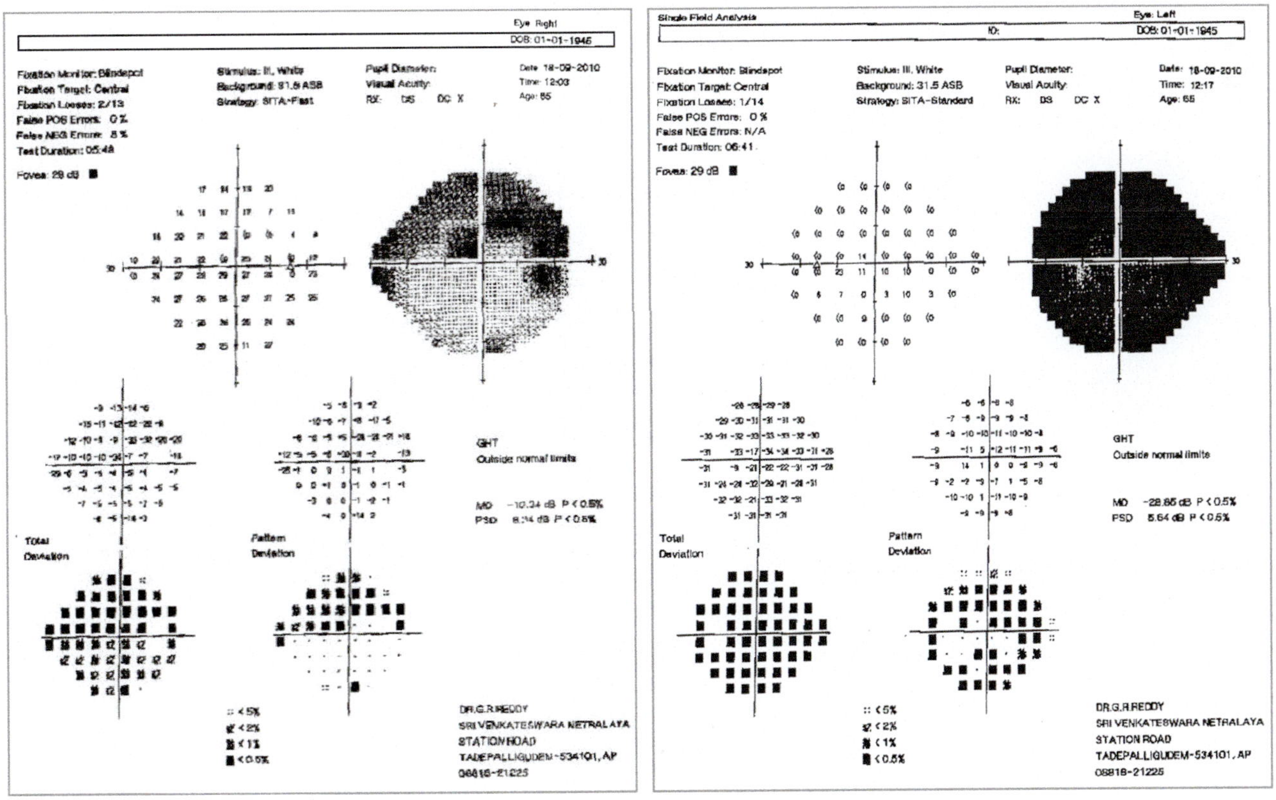

Pattern of the field defect—Both the visual field printouts are showing generalized field defects with deep scotomas in upper half of the field.

MD index—RE -28.85 dB and LE -10.34 dB.

You will not be wrong if you diagnose the case as advanced glaucoma. RE > LE from the visual field as base.

In this case disc pallor is exceeding the cup pallor. CT was advised.

Example 2: Never interpret visual fields in isolation. It should always be correlated with fundus.

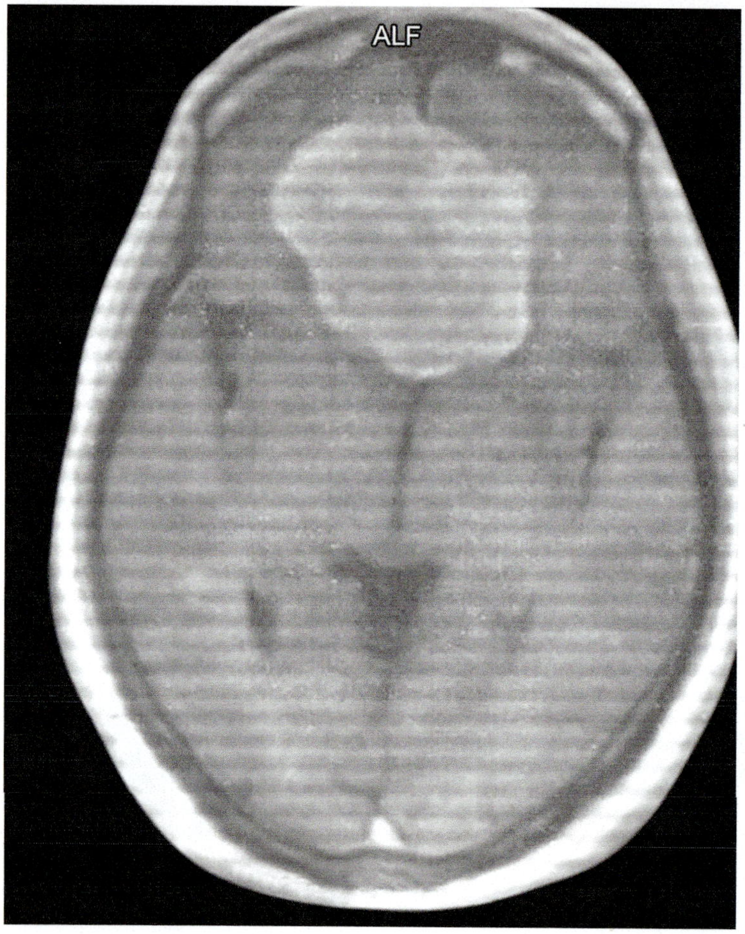

Evidence of well-defined round lobulated intensely homogeneously enhancing T1 isotense, T2/FLAIR predominantly hyperintense lesion with minimal perilesional edema noted in the midline arising from frontal convexity of the dura. Size approximately about 5.6 × 5.6 × 5.6 cm.

NEVER INTERPRET VISUAL FIELDS IN ISOLATION. VISUAL FIELDS SHOULD ALWAYS BE CORRELATED TO DISC CHANGES. YOU SHOULD NEVER MAKE A DIAGNOSIS ON THE BASIS OF VISUAL FIELDS. THE VISUAL FIELDS REPRESENT FUNCTIONAL CHANGES AND DISC REPRESENTS STRUCTURAL CHANGES.THEY MUST CORRELATE TO ONE ANOTHER.

Example 3: Never interpret visual fields in isolation. It should always be correlated with fundus: Left eye tilted disc.

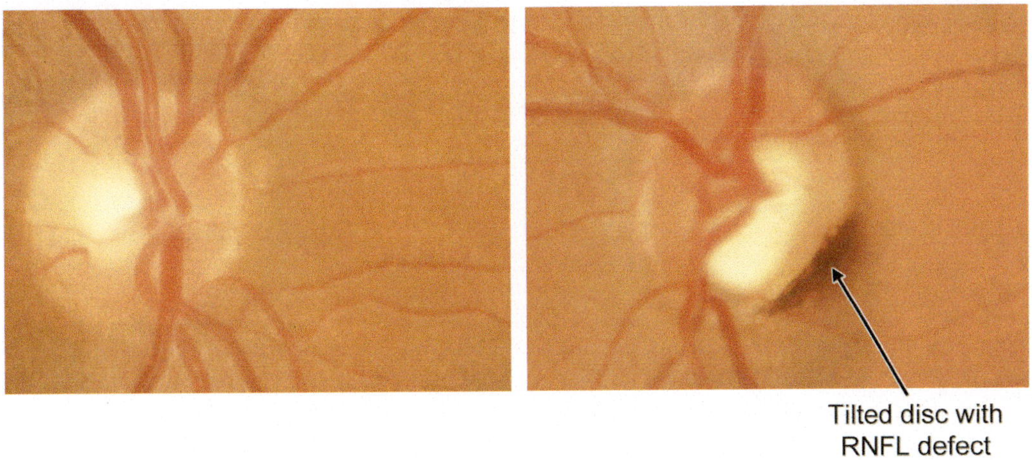

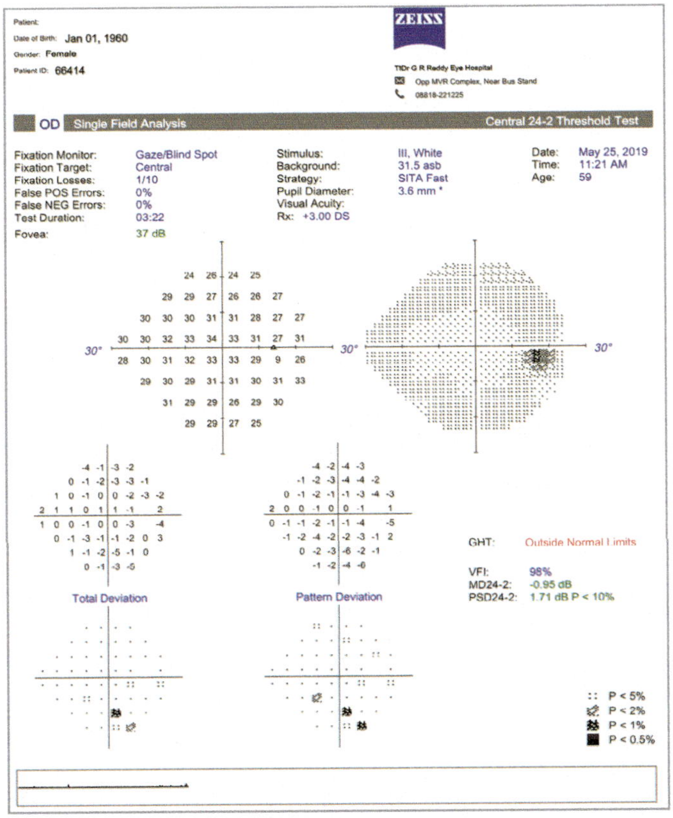

24-2 SITA Fast
FL 1/10; FP 0%; FN 0%
MD -0.95 dB; VFI 98%

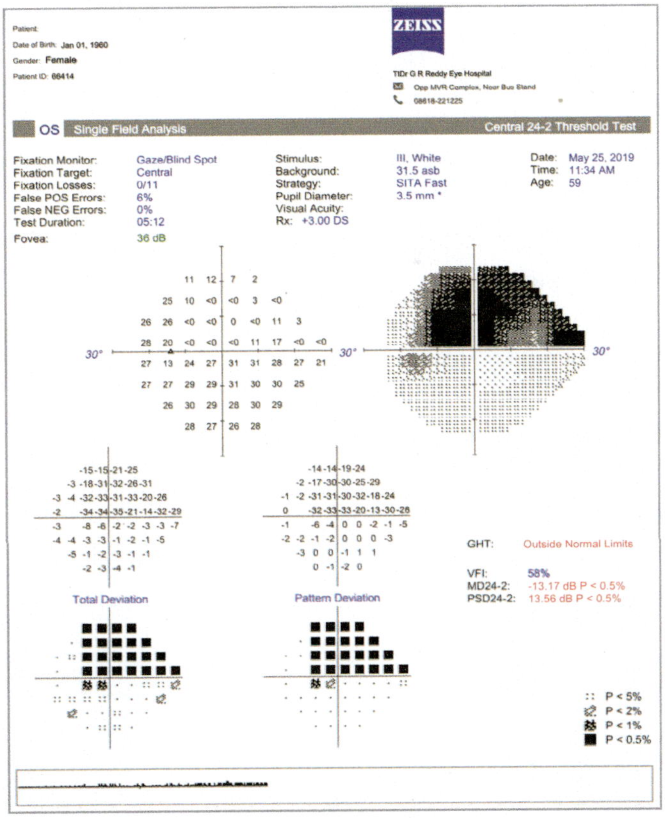

24-2 SITA Fast
FL 0/11; FP 6%; FN 0%
MD -13.17 dB P < 0.5%; VFI 58%

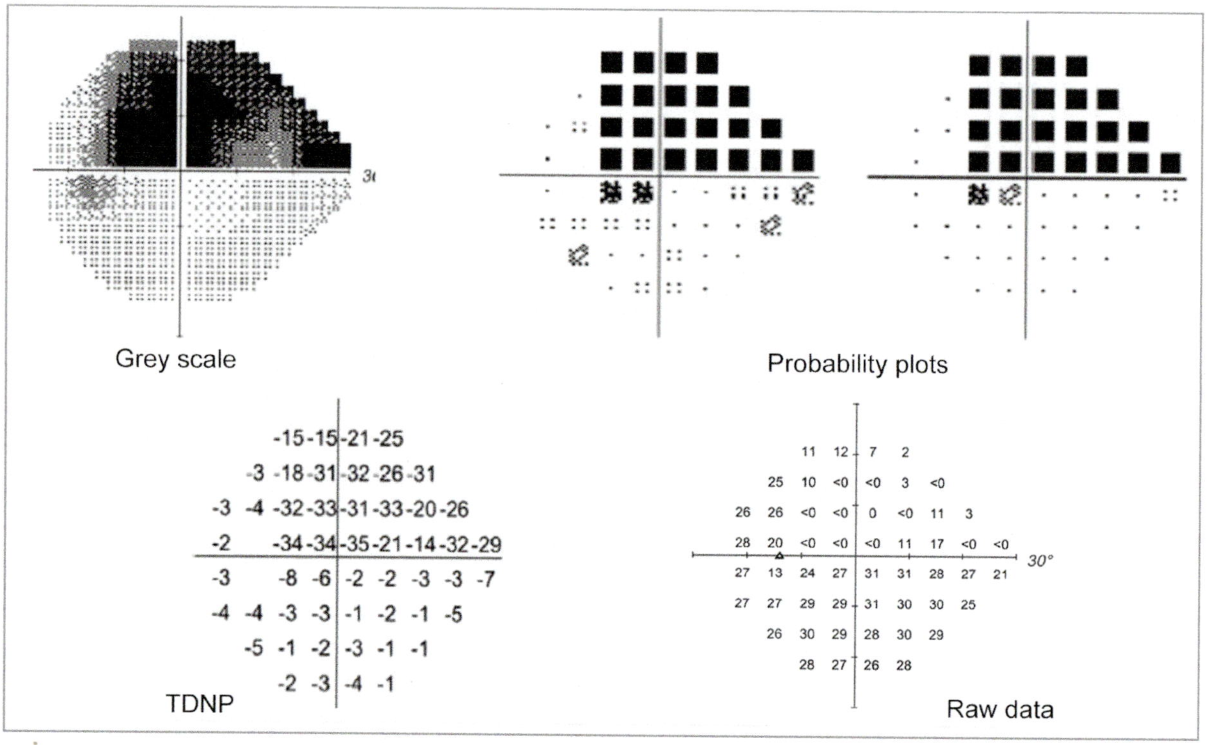

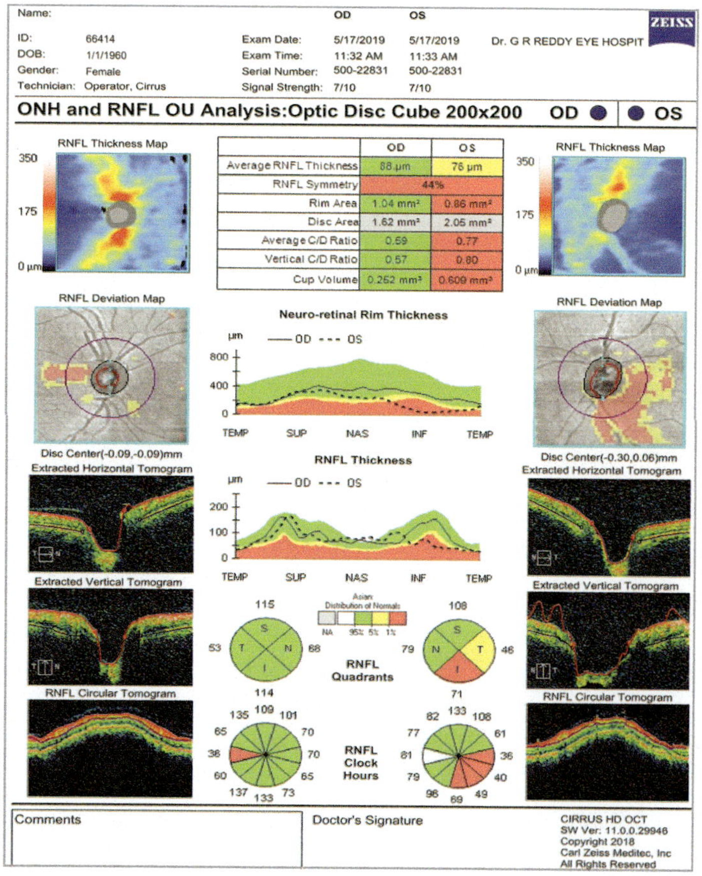

SFA in a Case of Tilted Disc

In this case, initially glaucoma is suspected by seeing LE fundus.

RE—Fundus is normal.

IOP—Normal in both the eyes.

LE—field is showing upper arcuate scotoma—Not typical of glaucoma. On careful examination of fundus, it is a case of tilted disc.

OCT is corresponding to the fundus of LE.

STEP 2: IDENTIFICATION OF THE ARTIFACTS

The art of interpretation of visual fields is the identification of the artifacts. If the scotoma in the probability plot is not due to disease, we label it as an artifact. The main factors causing artifacts are as follows:

1. The size of the pupil (The size of the pupil should be 3–4 mm)
2. Improper refractive error correction for near vision
3. Reliability indices:
   a. Fixation losses
   b. False positive errors
   c. False negative errors
4. Dim bulb
5. Rim artifacts.

The Effect of Size of the Pupil on the Visual Field

Normally the size of the pupil should be between 3–4 mm (The normative data is obtained with the pupil size of 3–4 mm). Constricted pupil is thought to give rise to diffuse visual field depression or edge scotomas. Pupil less than 2 mm is more likely to exert a significant effect on the overall level of the visual field particularly if media opacity is present in the visual axis. So it is recommended that the pupil less than 2 mm size should be dilated before conducting the test. To note the size of the pupil is very important particularly in the follow-up tests. Before interpreting the follow-up field test always see that the size of the pupil of the present test and previous test. The size of the pupil must be within the normal limits (3–4 mm), otherwise there is a chance for misinterpretation.

It is very important to know how exactly the size of the pupil influences its effect on the visual field examination. As you know the visibility of the stimulus depends on the contrast between the stimulus intensity and the background illumination. The light intensity of the stimulus and the background illumination change in proportion by the size of the pupil. So the contrast is unaffected. The visibility also depends on the total amount of light reaching retina. This is affected by the size of the pupil, the optical properties of the central part of the lens and the optical correction for near vision.

In general, testing of the visual field will be done with the normal size of the pupil and pupil should not be dilated unless there is a definite indication. All the Humphrey normal data are collected from the subjects with undialated pupil. So, finally the clinician must decide whether to dilate the pupil before subjecting the patient to perimetry. A subcapsular cataract that seriously impedes vision in the undilated state is an example of an exception. So, the clinician should take necessary precaution when to dilate the pupil.

Figure 1: Single field analysis printout with 2 mm pupil (Pilocarpinized pupil).The probability plots are showing edge scotomas and most of them are absolute scotomas.

Figure 2: The field test was repeated with 30-2 point pattern and size of the pupil 3 mm (after cessation of Pilocarpine). Even in 30-2 field with 3 mm pupil, there were no edge scotomas which were seen when the pupil size was 2 mm. Always remember that even the edge scotomas of 24-2 point pattern should not be taken into consideration when pupil size is less than 3 mm.

The Effect of the Size of the Pupil on the Visual Field Printout

Figure 1 SFA with 2 mm pupil

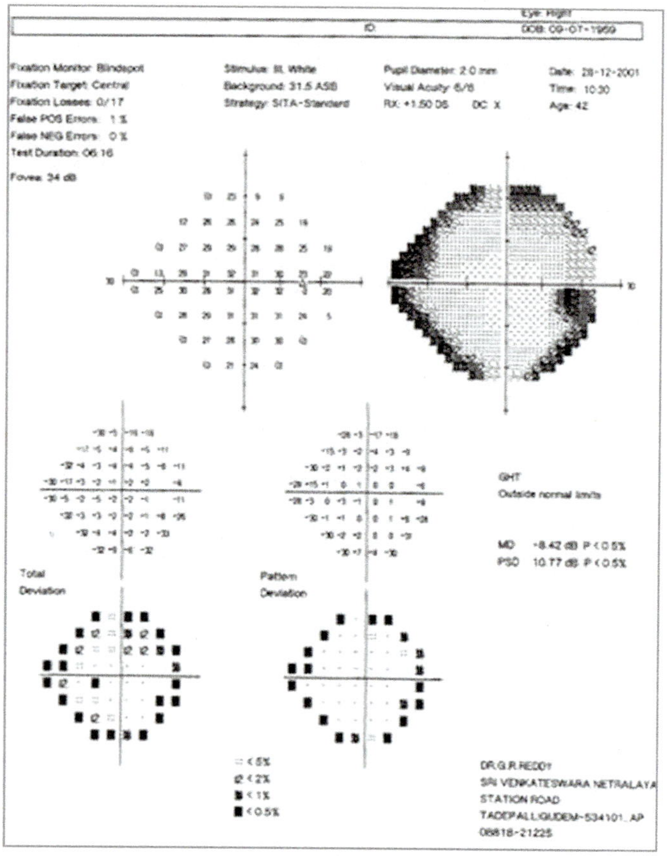

Fig. 1: 24-2 point pattern.
Edge scotoms with 2 mm pupil

Figure 2 SFA with 3 mm pupil

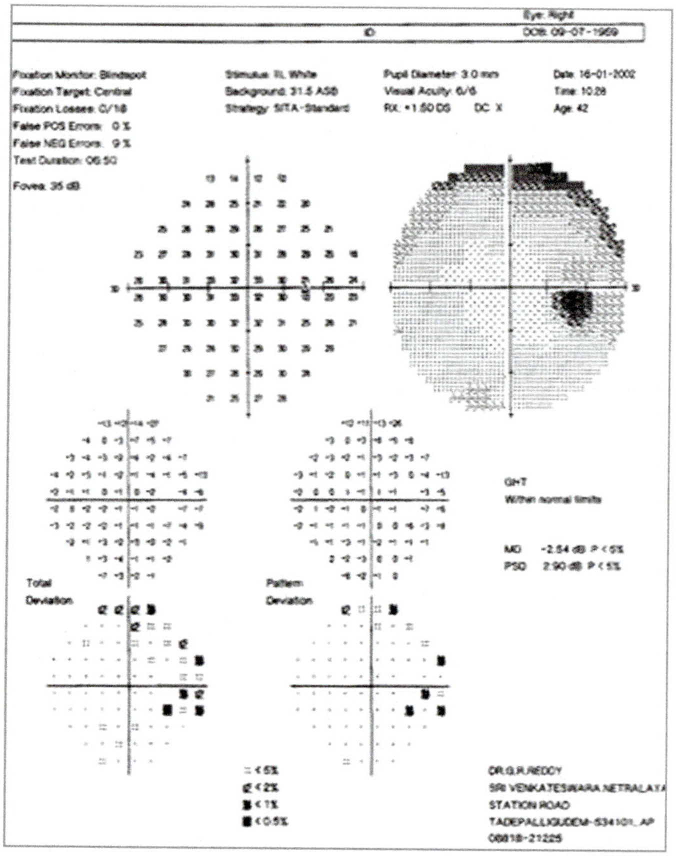

Fig. 2: 30-2 point pattern.
No edge scotoms with 3 mm pupil even in 30-2 point pattern

Figure 1 SFA with 2 mm pupil: The probability plots are showing the edge scotomas (the scotomas of the outer most set of points are called as edge scotomas) and are represented by significant P < 0.5%. Whenever there are edge scotomas, remember that these scotomas may be due to small pupil, high FN (-ve) errors, or lens rim artifacts.

The most important point one should notice is with 3 mm pupil size the edge points of 30-2 (the edge points of 30-2 are the points on 27° circle) became normal along with the edge points of 24-2 (the edge points of 24-2 are the points on 21° circle). When the pupil is of 2 mm size, the edge points 24-2 (the points on 21° circle) are with significant P value.

Importance of Proper Refractive Error Correction on Visual Field Printouts

While performing the test one should check for the proper placement of the lens in the trail lens which might cause edge defects if improperly placed. Also check for accurate refractive correction for near. Improper near vision correction might cause a generalized depression in total deviation probability plot (TDPP). If foveal threshold and visual acuity correlate with each other, it indicates accurate refractive correction for near was given during the test. Improper refractive error correction will not have any effect on the pattern deviation plots. But will produce generalized depression in total deviation probability plot. Then scotomas in the pattern deviation probability plots should be taken into consideration and can ignore the generalized depression in TDPP. If the pattern deviation probability plot is normal, we can ignore the generalized depression of TDPP also caused by improper refractive correction.

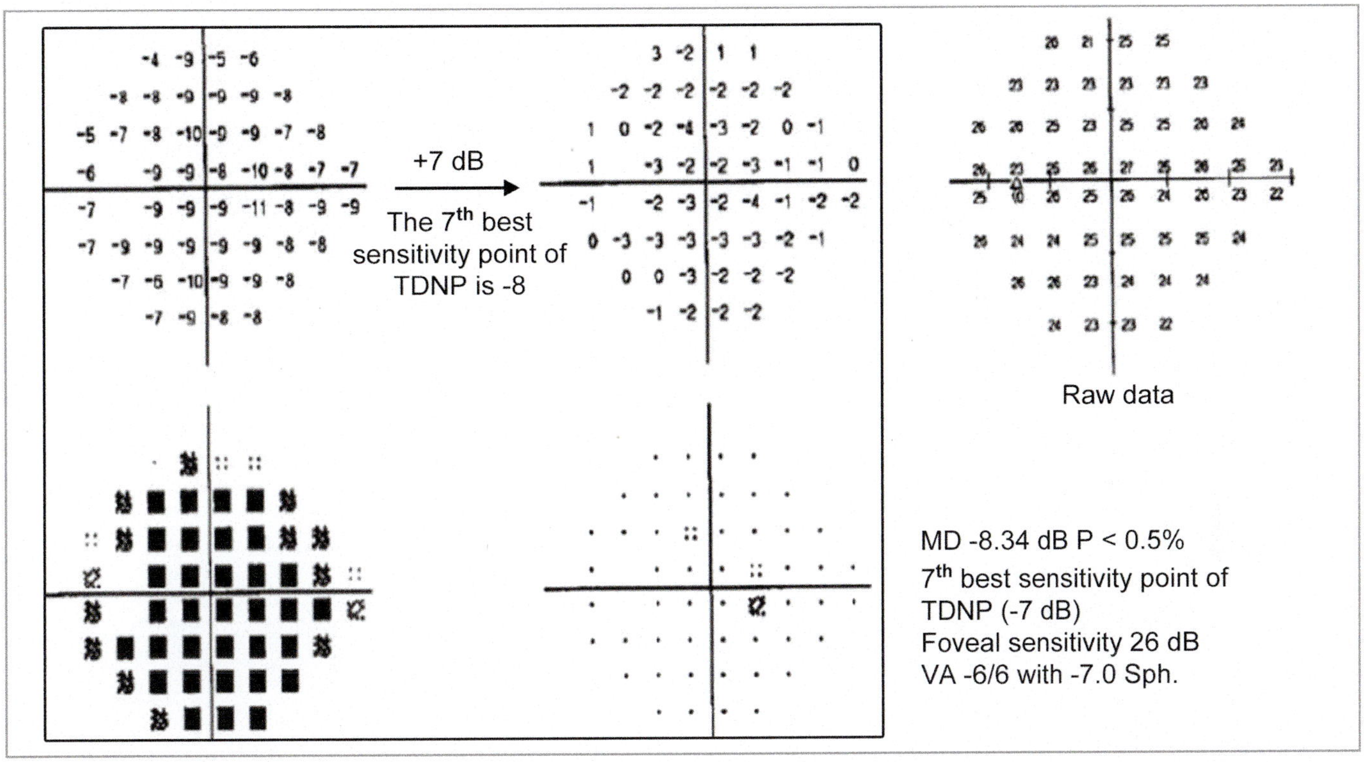

In this case, visual acuity (VA) is 6/6 with correction and if the field testing was done with proper refractive correction the measured foveal threshold should be around 36 dB. In this case the measured foveal threshold is 26 dB. Hence, VA and foveal sensitivity were not correlating with each other, indicating two possibilities, either the patient did not understand how to do the test or proper refractive error correction was not given. In this case proper refractive error correction was not given. This is the reason why foveal sensitivity is 26 dB. During the test always the foveal sensitivity will be measured first. If VA and foveal sensitivity correlate with each other, one can proceed with the test or else repeat the test. In this case, we can come to conclusion that the generalized depression in the total deviation probability plot is due to improper optical correction. When the test was repeated with proper optical correction the total deviation probability plot became normal.

Effect of Refractive Error Correction on Visual Field Printouts

The visual field analysis printout performed (Fig. 1) without refractive error correction for a known patient of -7.00 DSph. In the patient data VA and refractive error correction were not fed to the field analyzer and the test was done without refractive error correction.

Foveal sensitivity 26 dB MD -8.34 dB. The total deviation probability plot is showing generalized depression with P < 0.5% for most of the tested points.

SFA without refractive error correction
Fig. 1

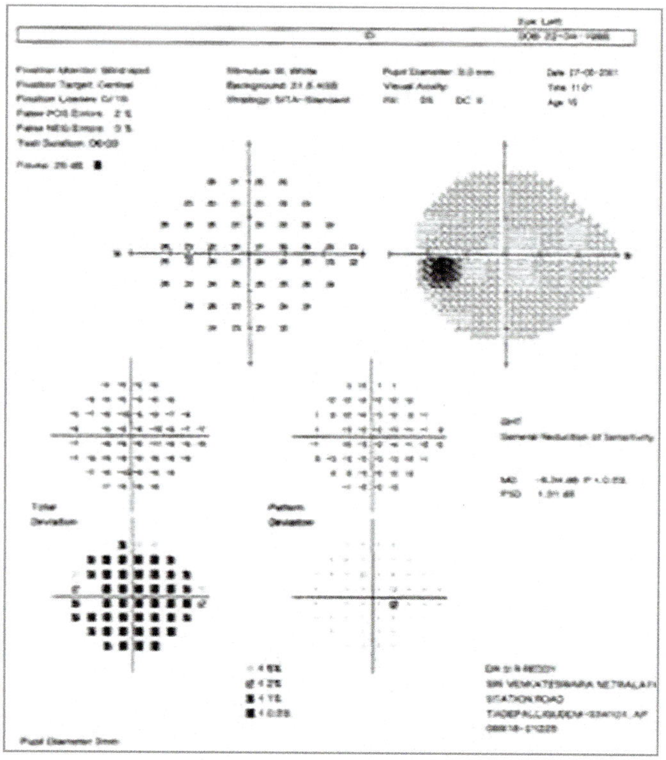

SFA with refractive error correction
Fig. 2

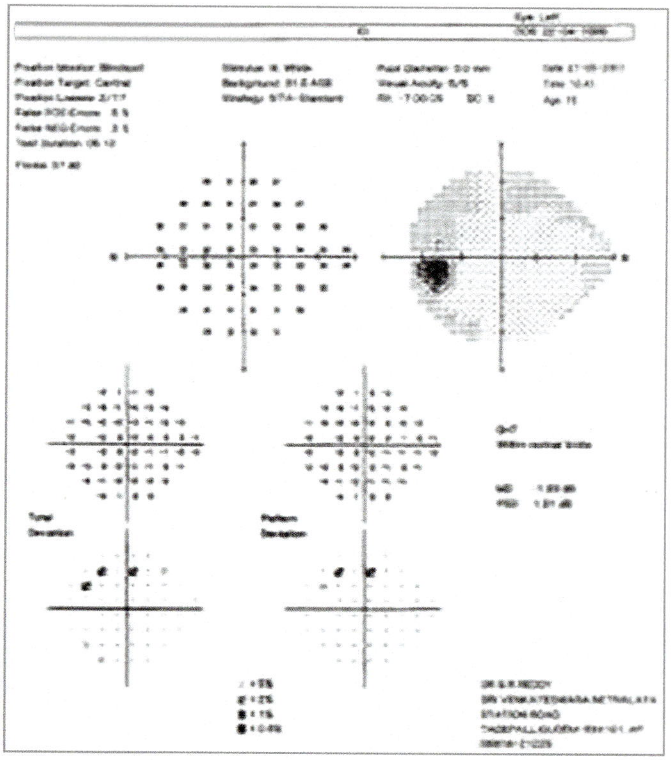

Always correlate VA and foveal sensitivity before interpretation of the SFA print. As this information is not mentioned in the printout, get the information either from the records or from the patient. From the patient's record:

Refractive error BE -7.00 DSph.
VA is - B.E. 6/6 with correction.

A person with 6/6 vision must have foveal sensitivity better than 35 dB. The test was repeated with refractive error correction (Fig. 2).

The foveal sensitivity 37 dB.
MD -1.53 dB

Total deviation probability plot—Normal.

> From this example, it is very clear that it is very important to correlate VA and foveal sensitivity before interpreting the printout and proper refractive error correction for near should always be given while performing the field test

Effect of Reliability Indices on the Measured Retinal Sensitivity

Reliability indices include fixation losses, false (+)ve errors and false (-)ve errors. Often one gets a doubt regarding what (%) of false (-), false (+) and fixation losses should be considered normal.

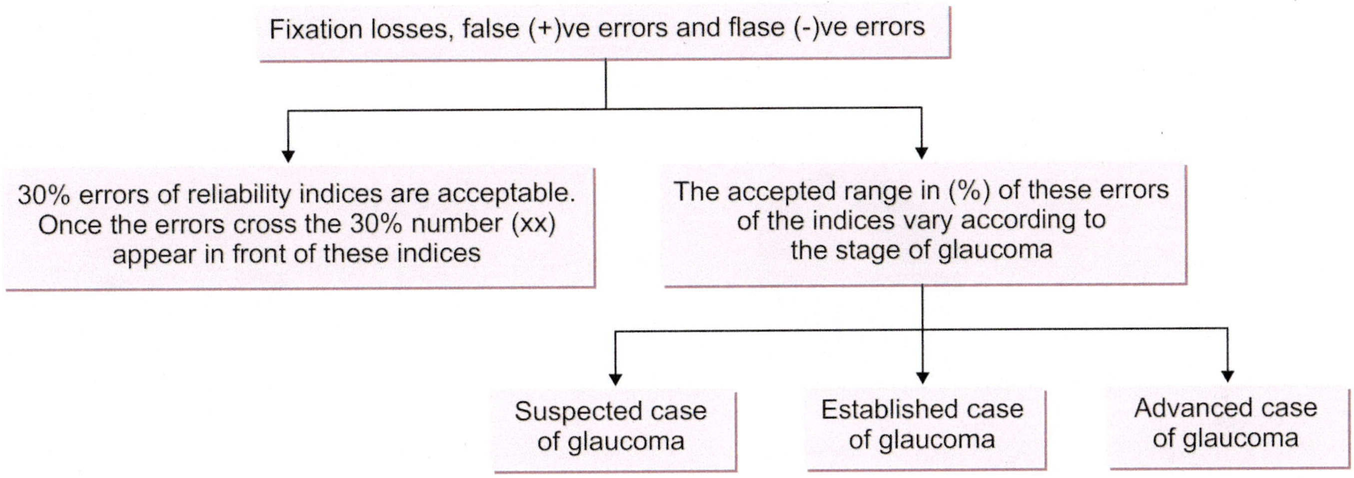

Even 1% fixation loss or 1% false positive errors or 1% false negative errors may affect the field in such a way that the localized scotoma can be labeled as glaucoma field defect on the basis of Anderson's criteria. In suspected cases of glaucoma the fixation losses, false positive and false negative errors should be nearer to 0%. In other words, the performance of the test should be 100% perfect. In established and advanced cases of glaucoma, the false (+)ve errors can be up to 15% and fixation losses up to 20%. FN rate estimates are elevated in glaucomatous visual field tests even in highly attentive patients. If the reliability indices cross 33%, then the test becomes unreliable.

In circumstances when we get high fixation losses, false (+)ve errors and false (-)ve errors even though a patient is well-instructed, it is better to change the test parameters to:

1. Change the testing strategy from SITA Standard to SITA Fast.
2. Change the central fixation target to small diamond or big diamond.
3. Change the stimulus size III to stimulus size V.

Effect of High Fixation Losses on Visual Field Printouts

SFA with high fixation losses—7/15xx (Fig. 1)

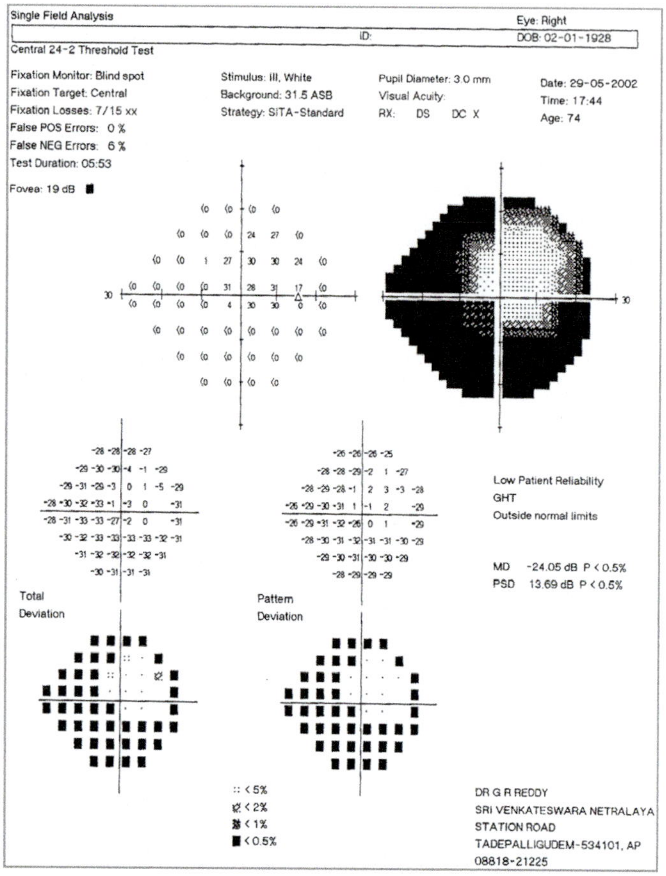

24-2 SITA Standard
Reliability indices—FL 7/15 xx
FP 0%

SFA with fixation losses—2/16 (Fig. 2)

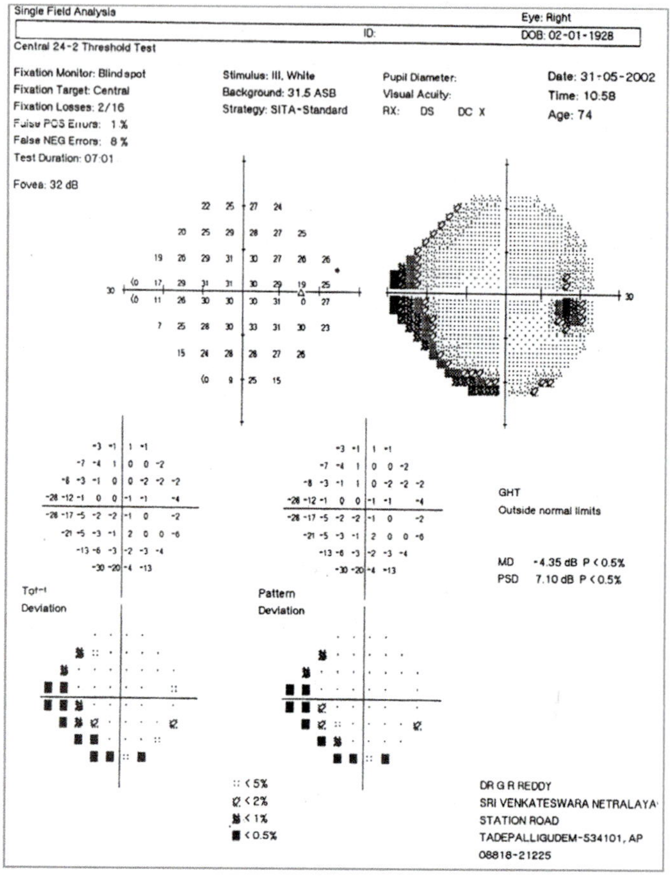

24-2 SITA Standard
Reliability indices—FL 2/16
FN 8%

Interpretation: Advised to repeat the test because of high fixation losses (7/15xx).

The test was repeated after the patient was well explained how to do the test without changing the test parameters, point pattern and testing strategy.

Note the difference between the two visual field analysis printouts. Having failed to notice high fixation losses, the defect would have been labeled as advanced glaucomatous field defect.

Effect of High Fixation Losses on Visual Field Printouts

SFA with high fixation losses—13/18xx (Fig. 1)

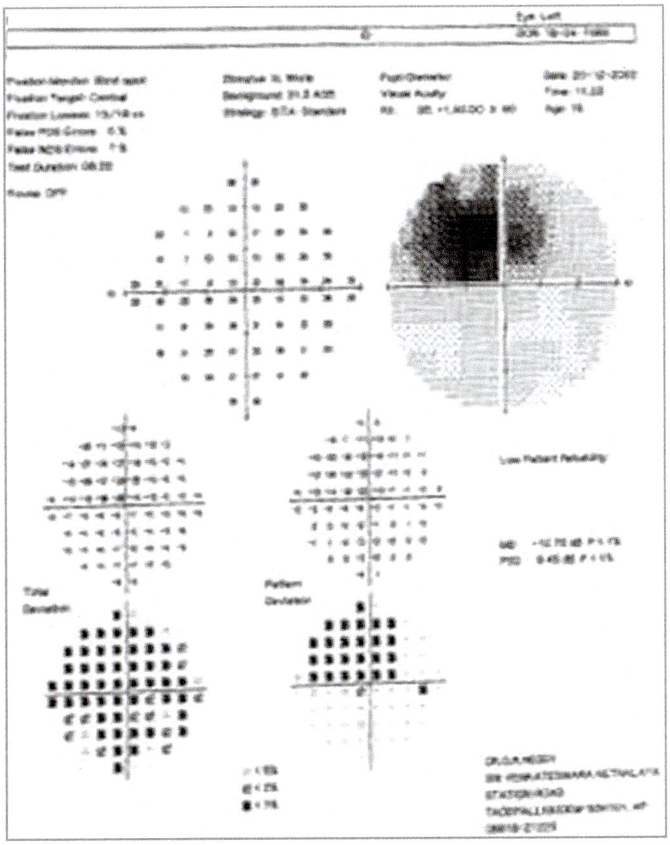

10-2 SITA Standard
Reliability indices—FL -13/18 xx; FP 0%; FN -7%

SFA with fixation losses—0/0 (Fig. 2)

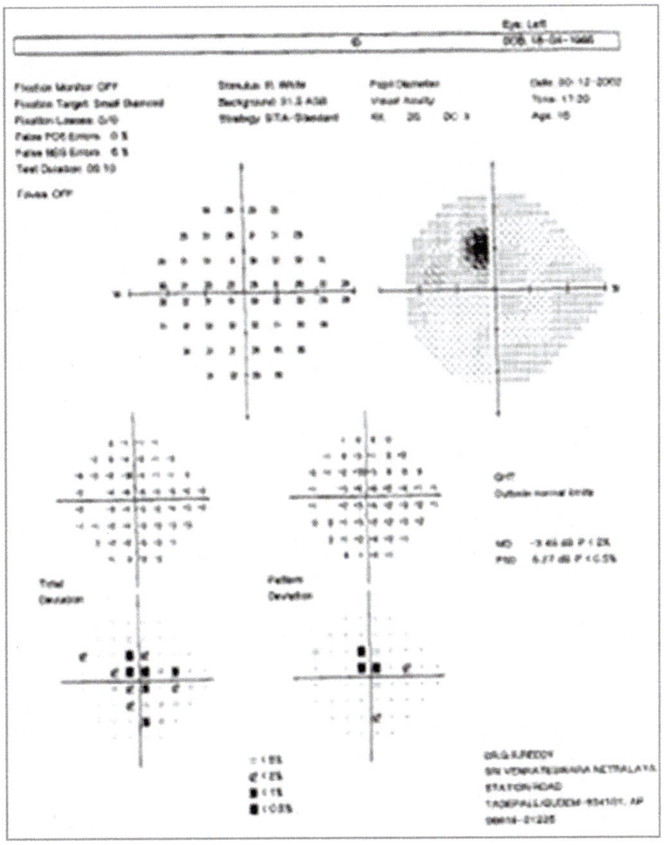

24-2 SITA Standard
Reliability indices—FL 0/0; FP 0%; FN-6

In cases of macular pathology, there will be poor central vision. To reduce high fixation losses in such cases, change the fixation target from central to either small diamond or big diamond.

Note the difference when the test is repeated with fixation target small diamond.

In Figure 1, TDPP shows central scotoma with fixation losses 13/18 xx. These scotomas disappeared when the fixation losses came down to zero on repeating the test with small diamond. This shows the importance of performing a test with small diamond in cases of macular pathology.

False Positive Response Errors

The false positive (FP) response error score measures the tendency of patients to press the response button even when no stimulus was projected ("trigger-happy" patients). The FP index is the most important and useful of the three available indices. Though FP errors up to 20% is accepted, it is better to repeat the test if FP error's exceed 15%.

Normally we see more black squares in the total deviation probability plot than in the pattern deviation probability plot. But in the SFA printout with high FP errors, more number of black squares are seen in the pattern deviation probability plot than in the total deviation probability plot. In the SFA printout with high FP errors, the sensitivity of some of the points will be measured as high values and the 7th best deviation point will be more than the mean normal value of the same age group of the patient with the measured retinal sensitivity being better than normal, black squares not seen in TDPP shown below.

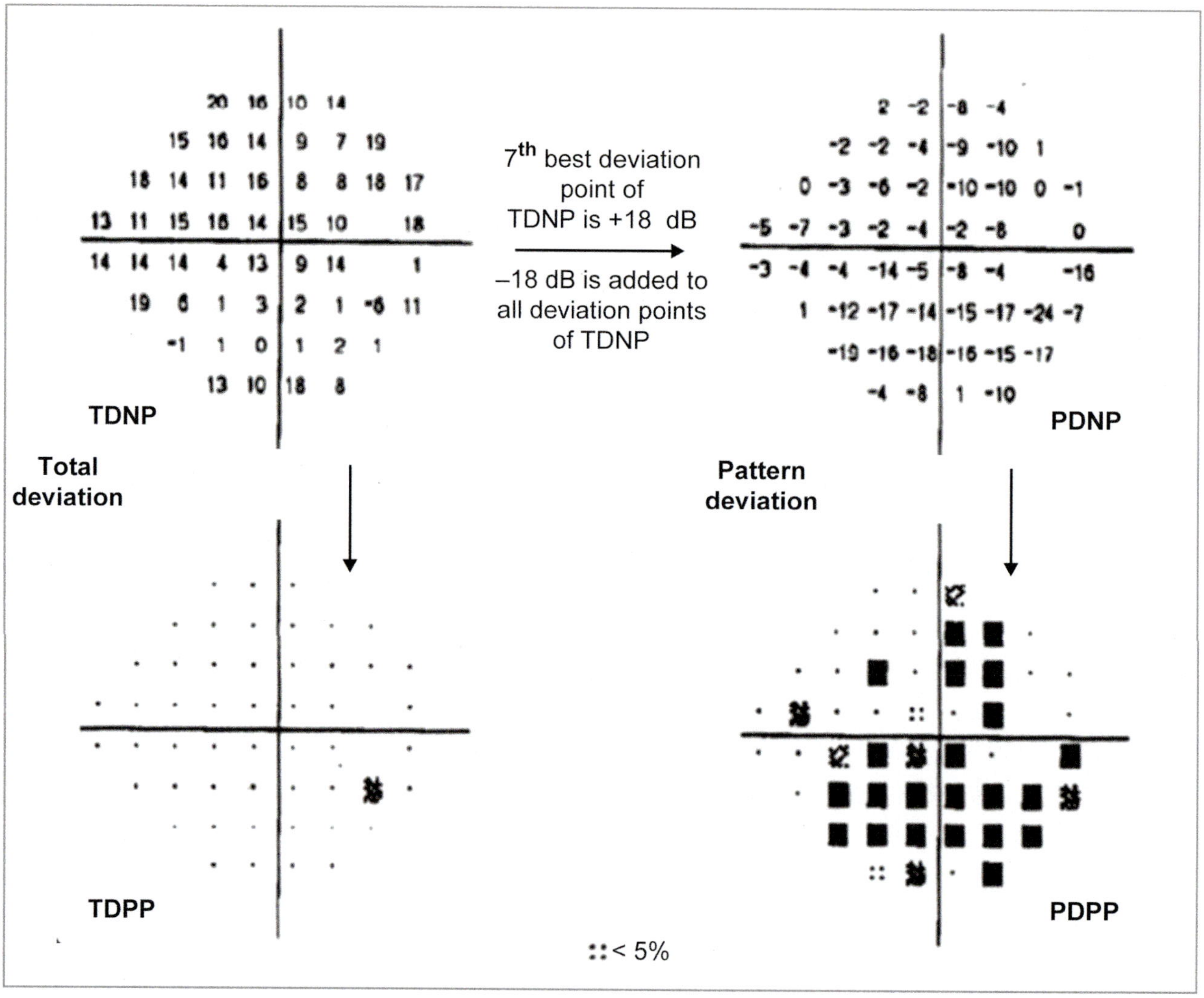

Single Field Analysis Printout with High FP Errors

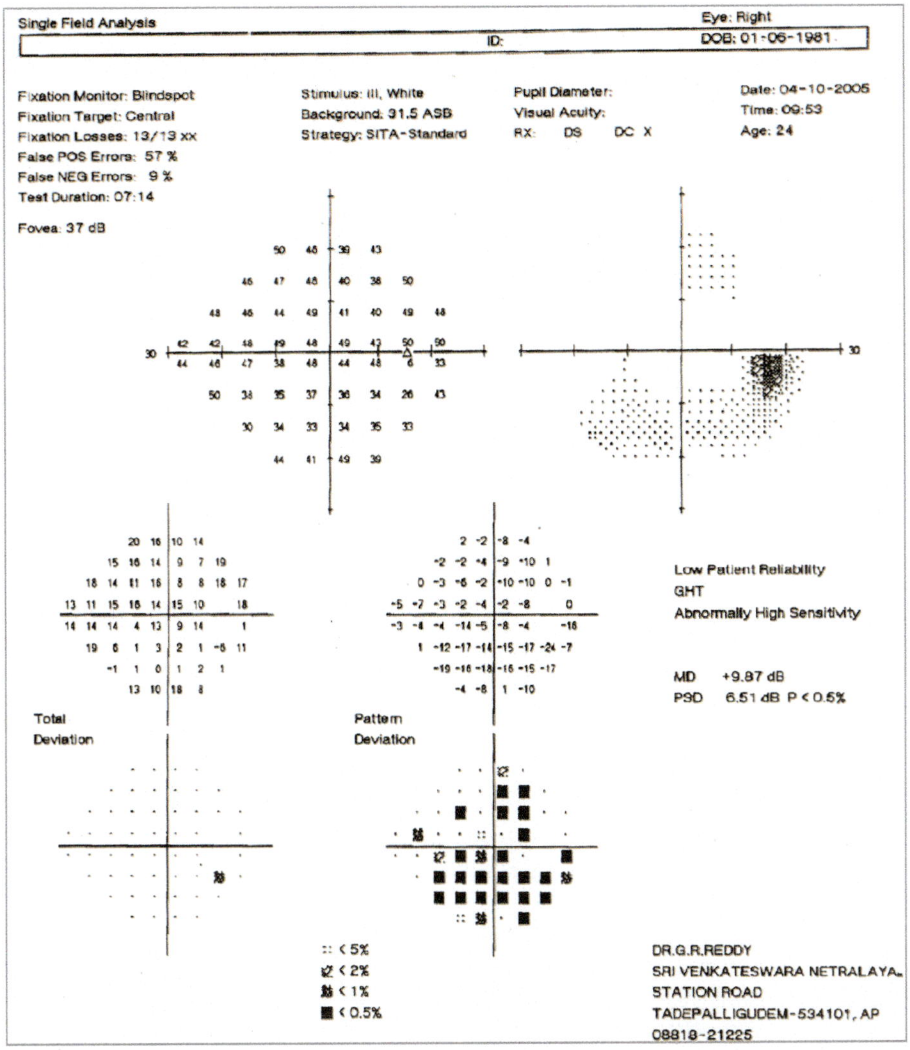

Point pattern and testing strategy 24-2 SITA Standard

Reliability indices.
Fixation losses 13/13 xx
FP errors ------57%
FN errors-------9%
7th best deviation point of TDNP +18 dB

Interpretation: Advised to repeat the test, because of high false (+)ve errors > 57% and fixation losses 13/13. Usually we do not use the grey scale printout for diagnosis, but fields with false (+)ve errors may produce characteristic changes in the grey scale printout. As shown in the grey scale of above figure, multiple white areas the so called white scotomas are seen. Some of the measured decibel values are in the high 30's and 40's. The white scotomas should draw your attention to identify high false (+)ve responses.

Features of high **FP errors.**
White scotomas in grey scale.
More black squares in PDPP than TDPP.
GHT shows abnormally high sensitivity.

There are more number of scotomas in the pattern deviation probability plot than in the total deviation probability plot. Why? Example 1.

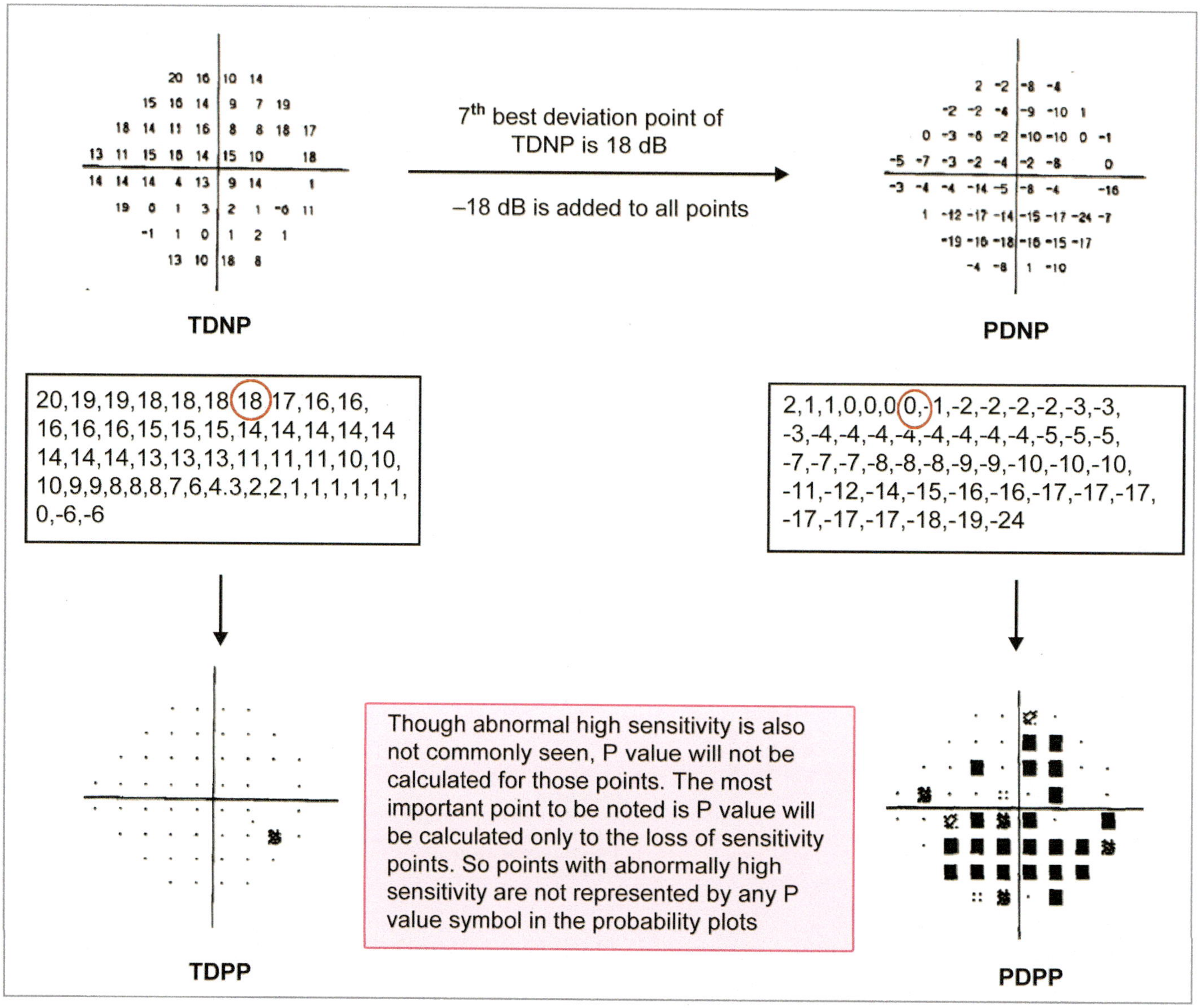

The 7th best deviation point of total deviation numerical plot (TDNP) is +18 dB. Now -18 dB is added to all the points in TDNP to convert it to pattern deviation numerical plot (PDNP). Normally during the conversion of TDNP to PDNP, the sensitivity of each point in the TDNP will be elevated to eliminate the generalized depression from TDNP. But in this example, since the 7th best deviation point of TDNP is +18 dB (better than normative data), the sensitivity of each point in TDNP is decreased by 18 dB or in other words a generalized depression worth of (-18 dB) is added to TDNP during its conversion to PDNP. As there is decrease in sensitivity at all the points in PDNP, we see more number of black squares in the PDPP than the TDPP.

Single Field Analysis Printout with High FP Errors

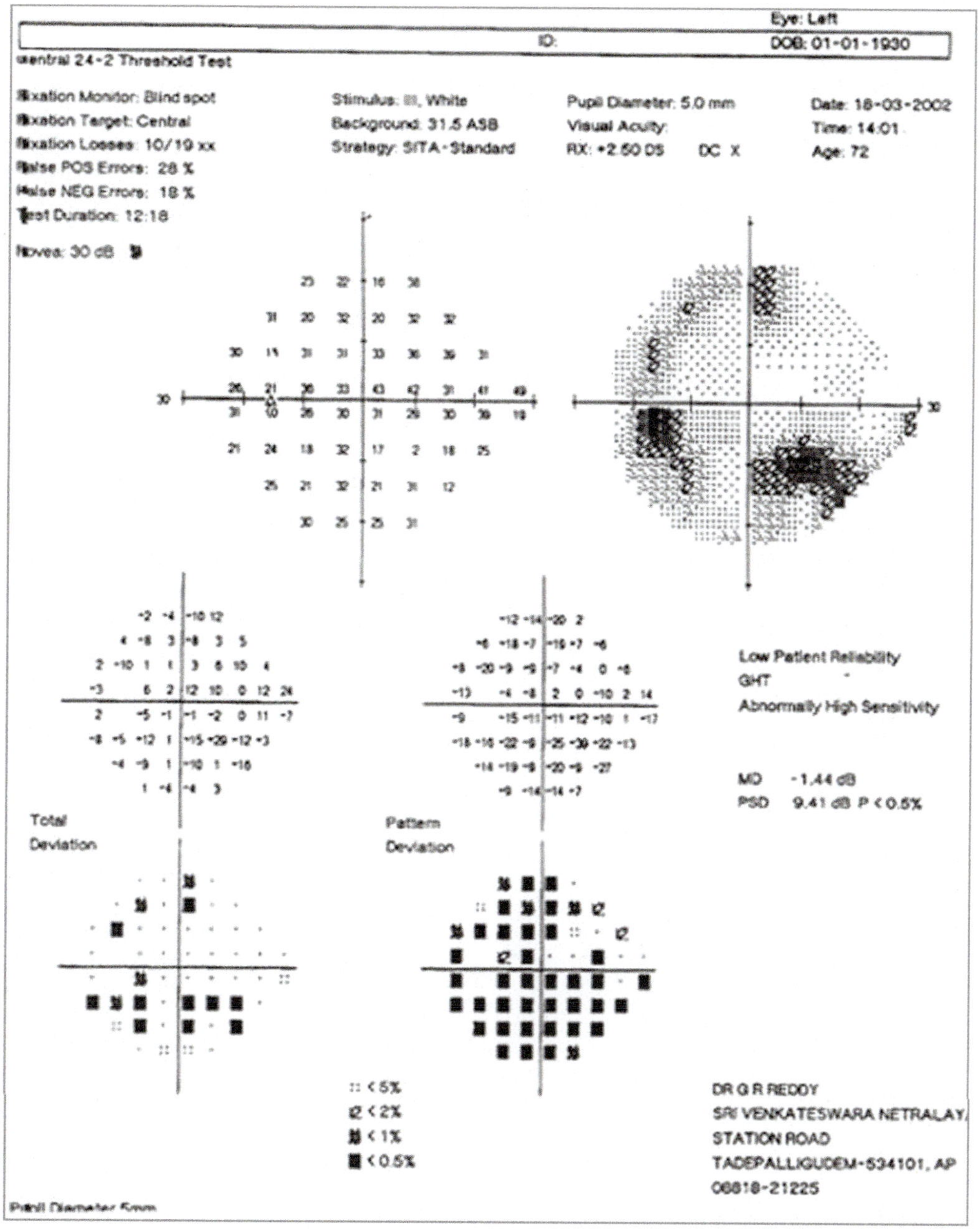

Reliability indices	FL 10/19 xx; FP 28%; FN 18%
Foveal sensitivity	30 dB
7th best sensitivity point of	TDNP +10 dB

Point pattern and testing strategy—24-2-Point pattern

SITA Standard -Testing strategy

There are more number of scotomas in the pattern deviation probability plot than in the total deviation probability plot. Why? Example 2

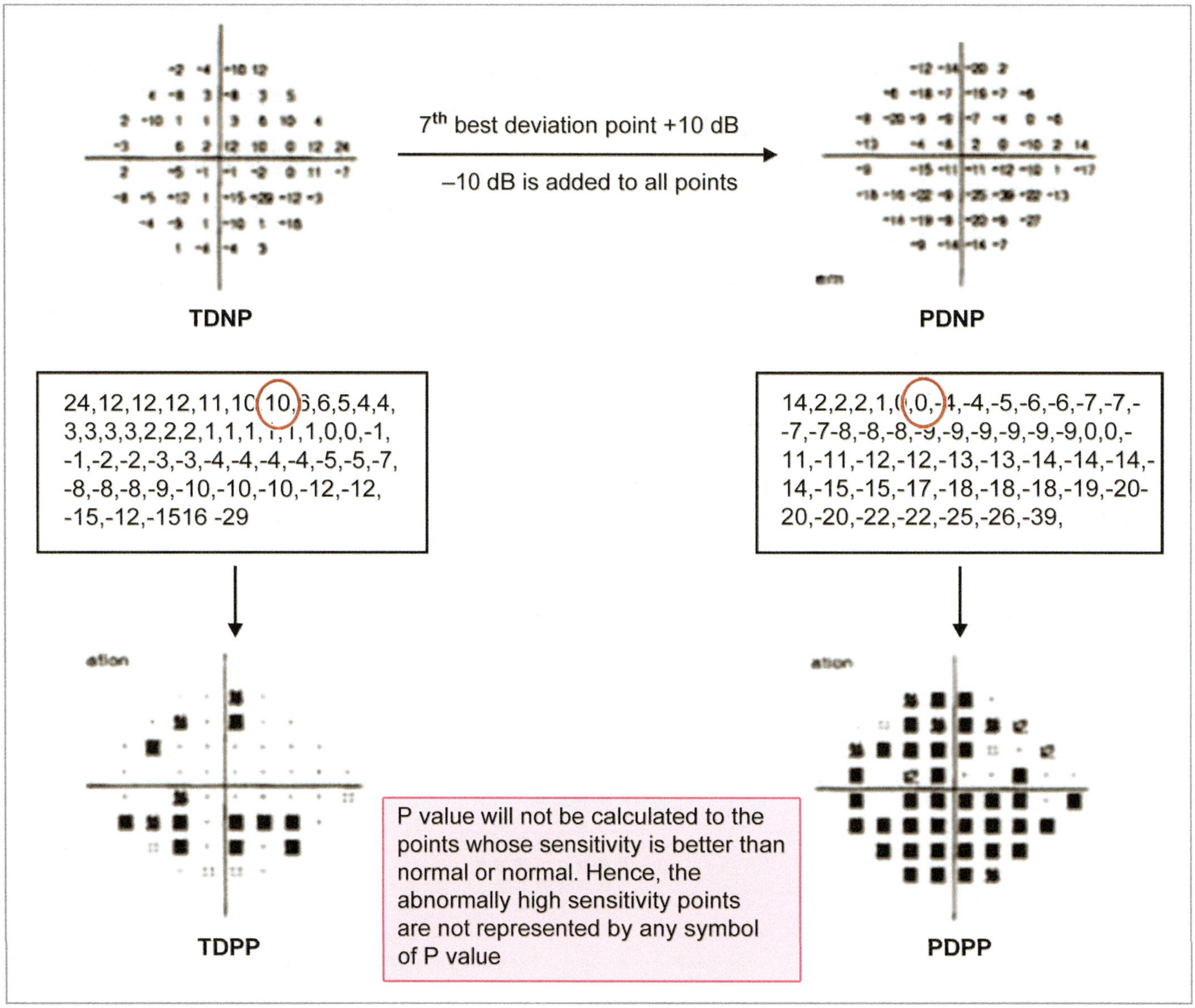

The 7th best deviation point of TDNP is +10 dB. -10 dB is added to all the points in TDNP to convert it to PDNP. In this example, since the 7th best deviation point of TDNP is +10 dB (better than normative data), the sensitivity of each point in TDNP is decreased by 10 dB or in other words a generalized depression worth of (-10 dB) is added to TDNP during its conversion to PDNP. As there is decrease in sensitivity at all the points in PDNP, we see more number of black squares in the PDPP than the TDPP.

False Negative Response

The tested area will be retested with a brighter stimulus to which the candidate should actually respond; failure to respond to this brighter stimulus is a false negative response. The false negative responses are expressed in (%) SITA strategies. High false negatives may indicate lack of attentiveness, fatigue or hypnosis. In general, greater than 20% of false negative response is considered to be abnormal though the machine defaults to 33%. Fields should not be considered unreliable based solely upon a false negative response rate, particularly if there is a great deal of pathology. In patients with advanced glaucomatous optic nerve damage we may get more than 50% false response which can be attributed to small shifts in fixation.

The grey scale shows the typical CLOVER LEAF PATTERN fairly characteristic of a fatigue field with high false negatives. Here, initially the patient performs well and then becomes progressively less responsive. When we get edge scotomas, we should always check the false negative error index, size of the pupil and position of the correcting lens. Usually edge scotomas are due to high false negative responses or small pupil or due to edge of the refractive error correction glasses. The peripheral points will be tested after testing the central points. This is the reason why we see edge scotomas in fatigued patients because of high false negative errors.

Single field analysis printout with high false negative (FN) Errors

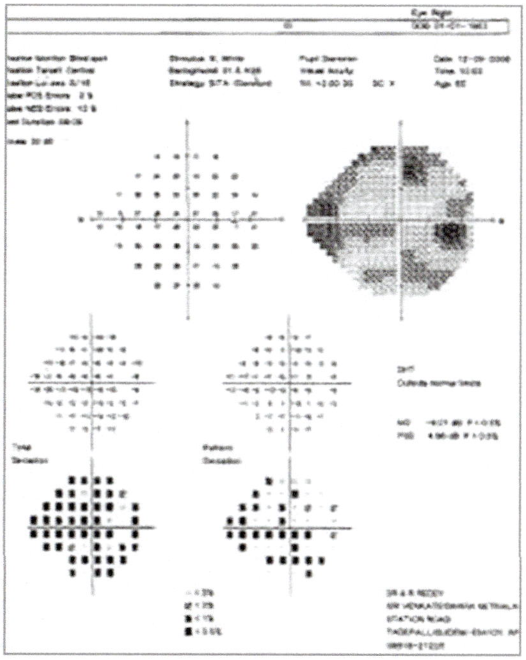

24-2 SITA Standard

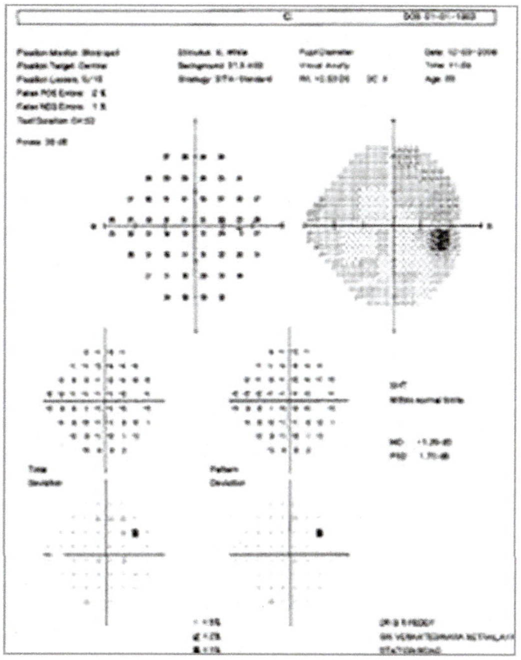

24-2 SITA Standard

1st test: Reliability indices—FL 0/16, FP 2%, FN 13%.

Take enough time to explain the patient how to do the test and here the test was repeated without changing the parameters.

2nd test: Reliability indices—FL 0/15; FP 2%, FN 1%.

You can see clearly the effect of FN 13% on MD, PSD and probability plots and grey scale.

SINGLE FIELD ANALYSIS PRINTOUT WITH HIGH FN ERRORS

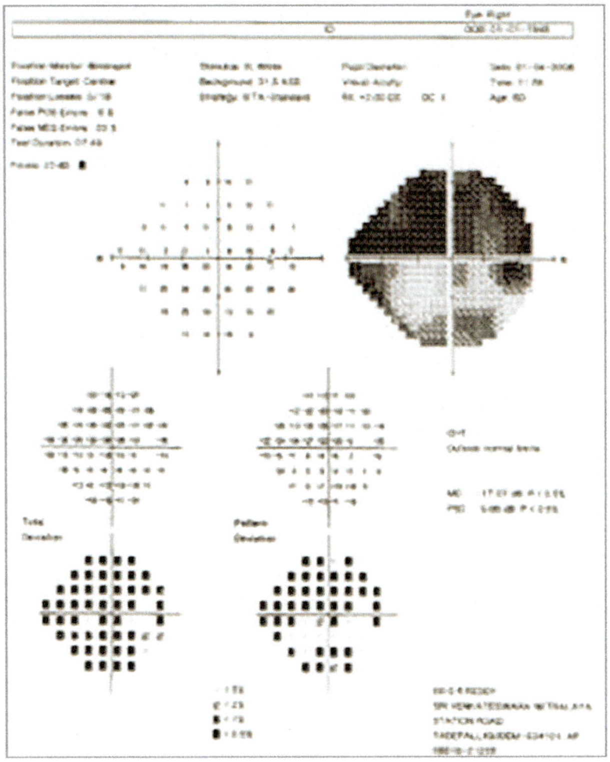

Point pattern and testing strategy—24-2 SITA Standard

Reliability indices	
FL	0/18
FP	5%
FN	33%

Advised to repeat the test with SITA Fast strategy to reduce high false (-)ve errors.

↓

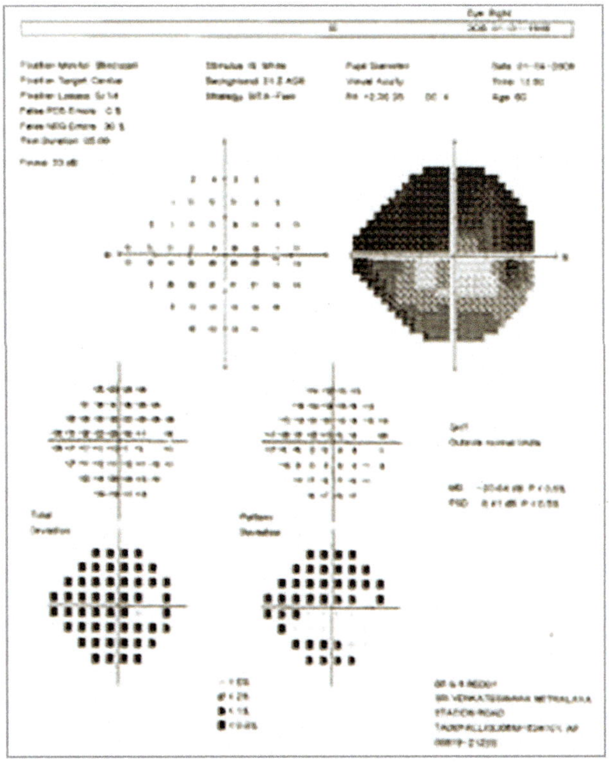

Point pattern and testing strategy 24-2 SITA Fast.

Reliability indices	
FL	0/14
FP	0%
FN	30%

↓

Even with SITA Fast strategy the high false (-)ve errors did not come down.

Advised to repeat the test with stimulus size V with FASTPAC strategy to reduce high false (-)ve errors.

24-2 FASTPAC

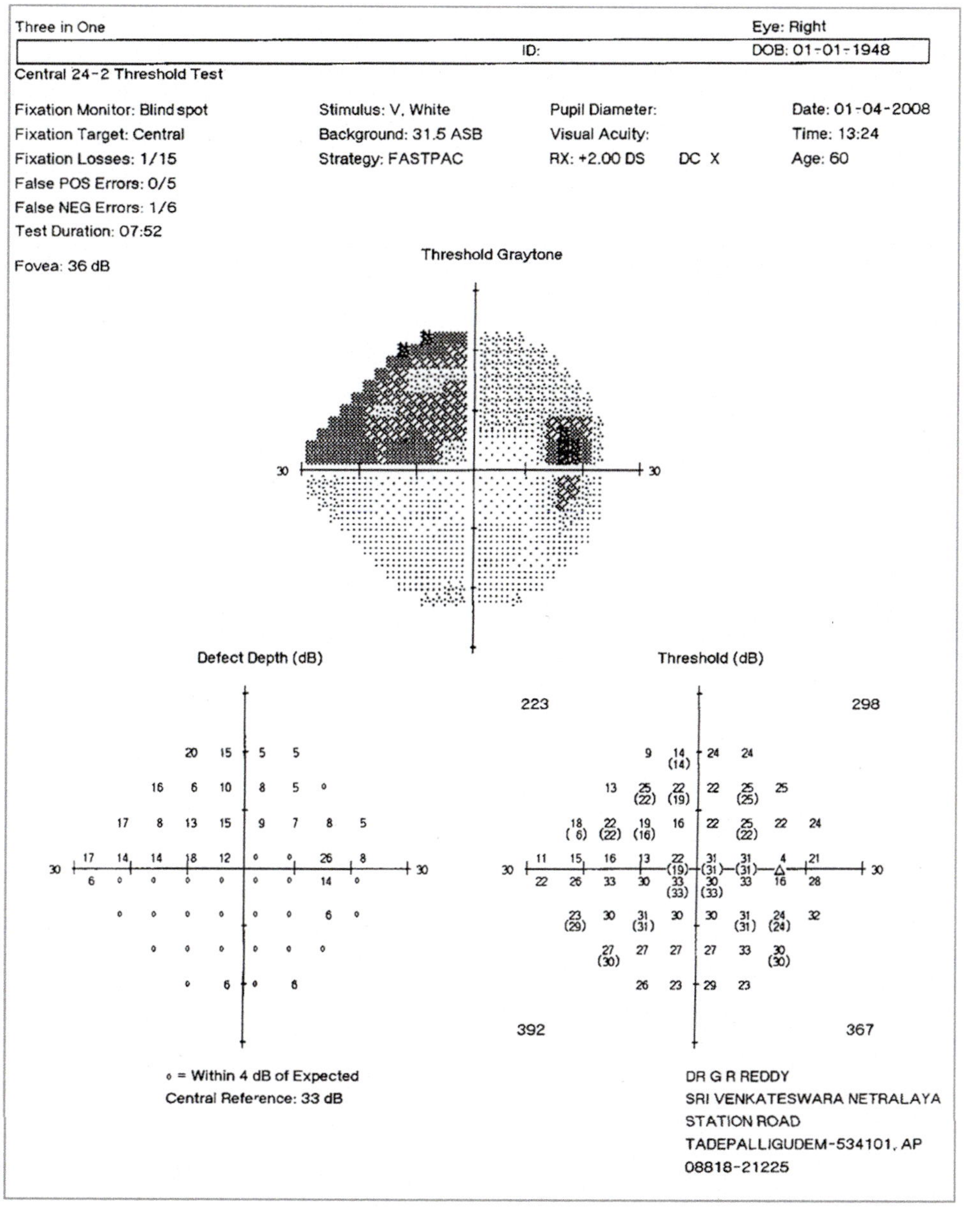

Reliability indices—FL1/15, FP 0/5, FN 1/6

Foveal sensitivity 36 dB.

By changing the stimulus size III to V, the false (-) ve errors are brought down to 1/6.

As there is no normative data to stimulus size V, we do not get a single field analysis printout. We get a 3 in 1 printout. As SITA strategies are not available for the test parameters which do not have normative data, the test is repeated with FASTPAC strategy. This is the reason why the reliability indices are expressed in ratios.

Different methods to reduce high fixation losses, high false (-)ve errors, high false (+)ve errors:

1. *Strategy*: Repeat the test with fast strategy—SITA Fast.
2. *Fixation target*: Change the fixation target central to small diamond or big diamond.
3. *Stimulus size*: Change the size of the stimulus from III to size V.

Lens Rim Artifacts

The most important point one should know is lens rim artifacts are common. It is very important to recognize these artifacts.

i. Typical lens rim artifacts are easily recognized because they tend to be absolute and sharply demarcated. Sometimes, arcuate scotomas starting from blind spot may appear due to lens rim and usually they do not widen on the nasal side of its course and will disappear on subsequent tests with appropriate positioning of the lens.
ii. When the lens is too far from the eye or not properly centered, its rim can produce a sharply demarcated absolute defect.
iii. If the lens is not placed sufficiently close to eye, it may produce sometimes double arcuate scotoma.

From these points we understand the importance of positioning the lens in the most appropriate position to avoid these rim artifacts.

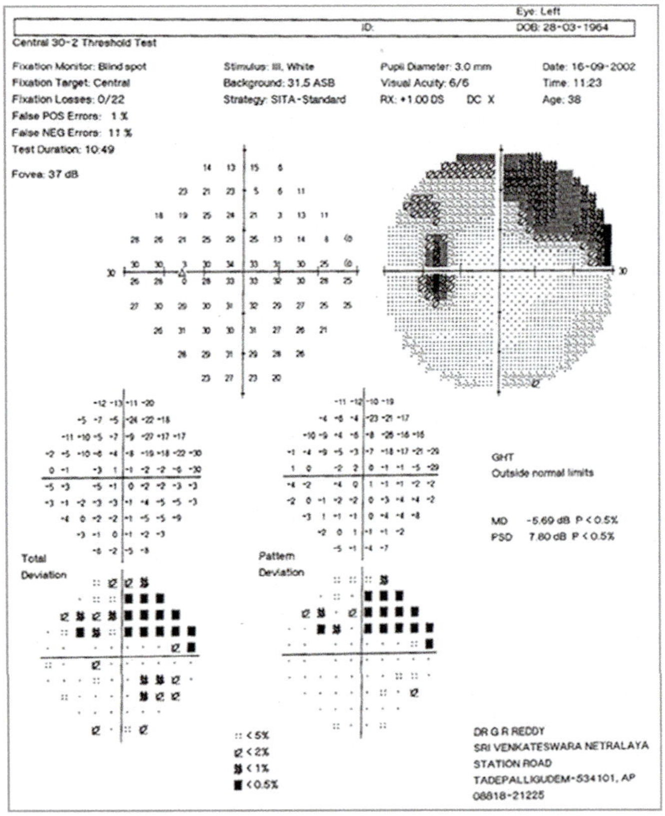

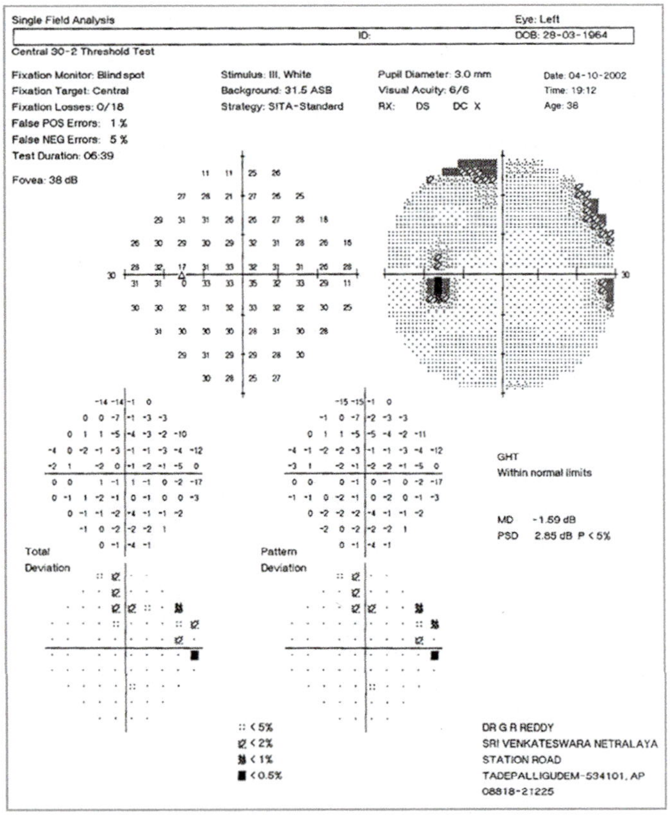

(Fig. 1) 30-2 SITA Standard (FL 0/22, FP 1%, FN 11%) (Fig. 2) 30-2 SITA Standard, FL 0/18, FP 1%, FN 5%

The superior scotoma in Figure 1 disappeared in Figure 2. The localized scotomas are not in the locations where we usually see, and when the field changes are not corresponding to the disc changes, one should not diagnose glaucoma on visual field defects alone.

Thinking that the scotoma in the first field might have been be due to the rim of the correcting lens, the repeated test was conducted without near vision correction as the patient's age is 38. The superior scotoma in Figure 1 disappeared in Figure 2.

Case of glaucoma suspect. Strong family history of POAG. C/D disparity of both eyes. Corrected IOP around 20 mm Hg.

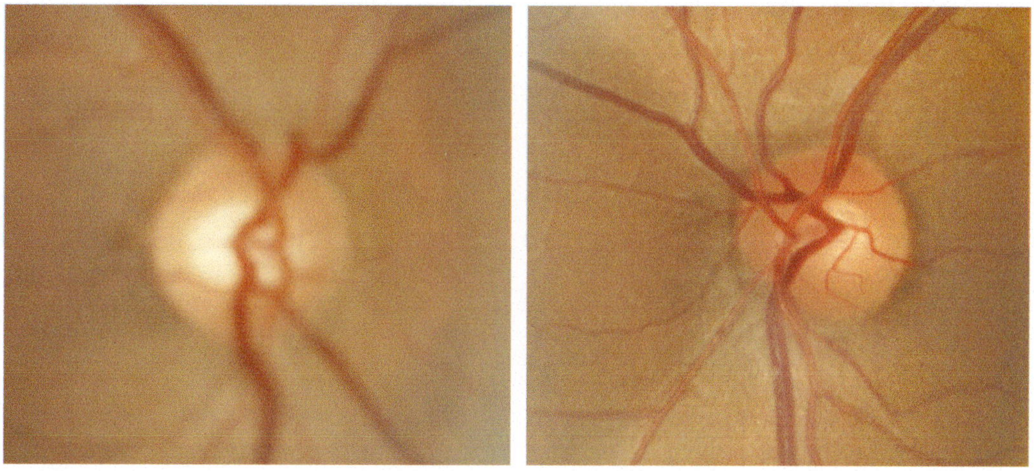

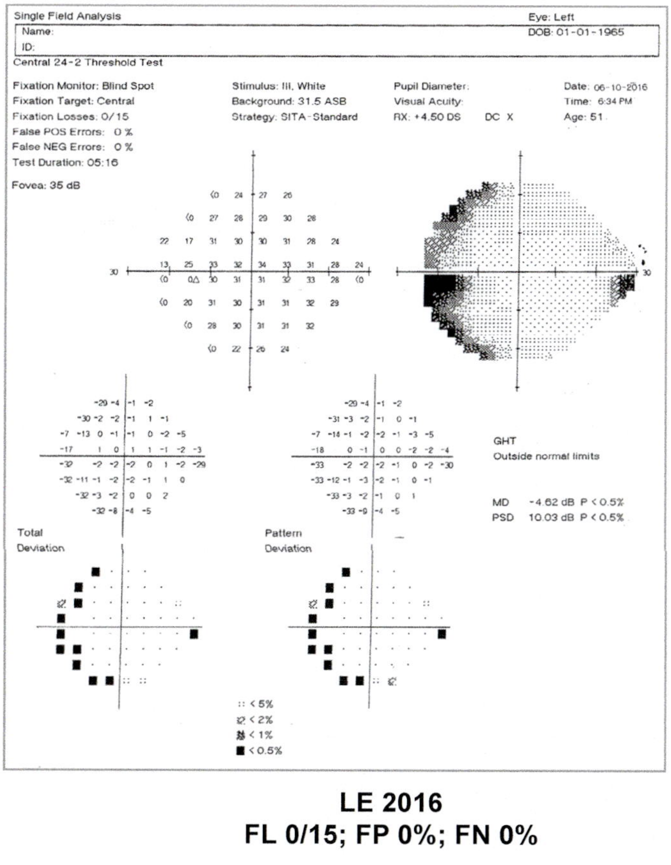

LE 2016
FL 0/15; FP 0%; FN 0%

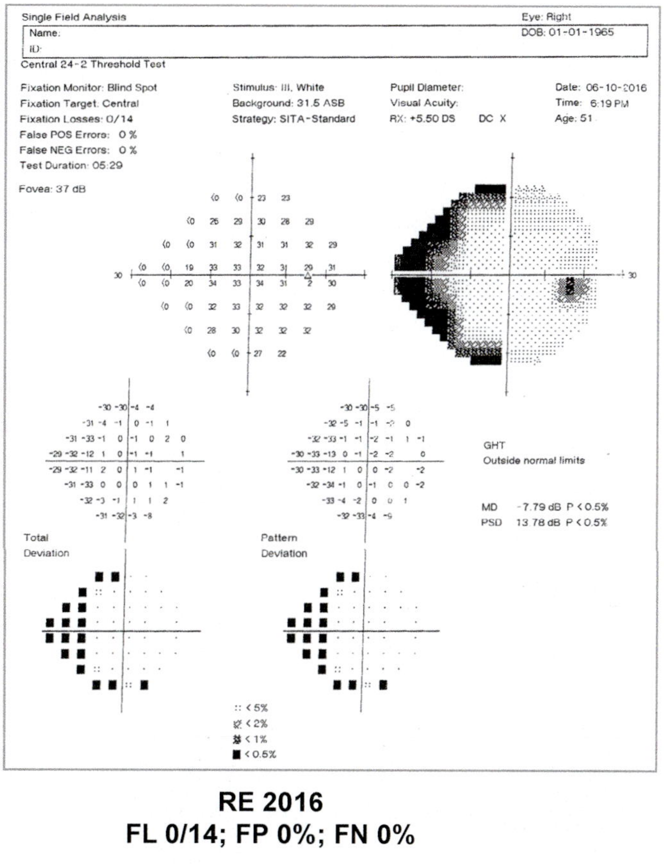

RE 2016
FL 0/14; FP 0%; FN 0%

The most important point to notice in this example is that the reliability indices are 100% perfect in both the printouts, all the scotomas are edge and absolute scotomas. Since they are absolute and edge scotomas, we can consider them as rim artifacts. Because of strong family history and C/D disparity, the patient was kept under observation and repeated the test after one year.

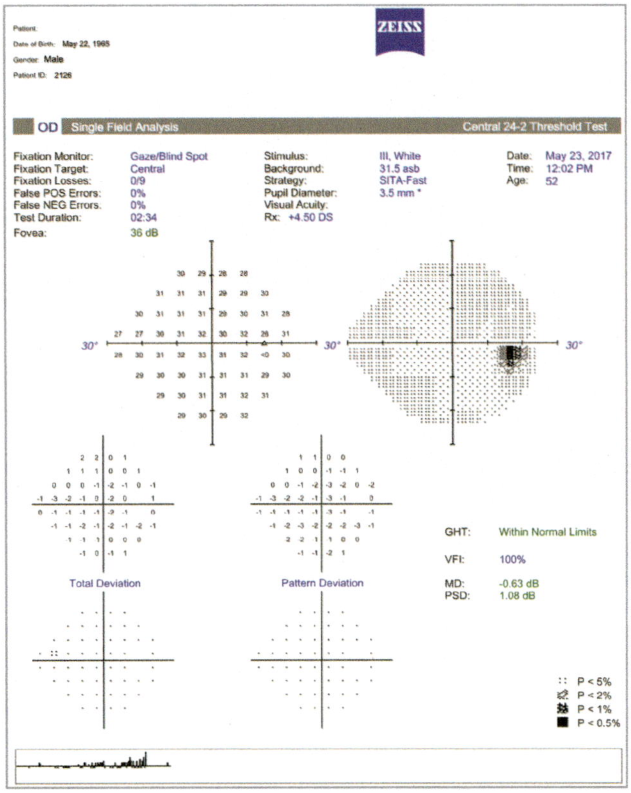

RE 2017
FL 0/9; FP 0%;
FN 0%; PSD 1.08 dB
GHT—Within Normal Limits

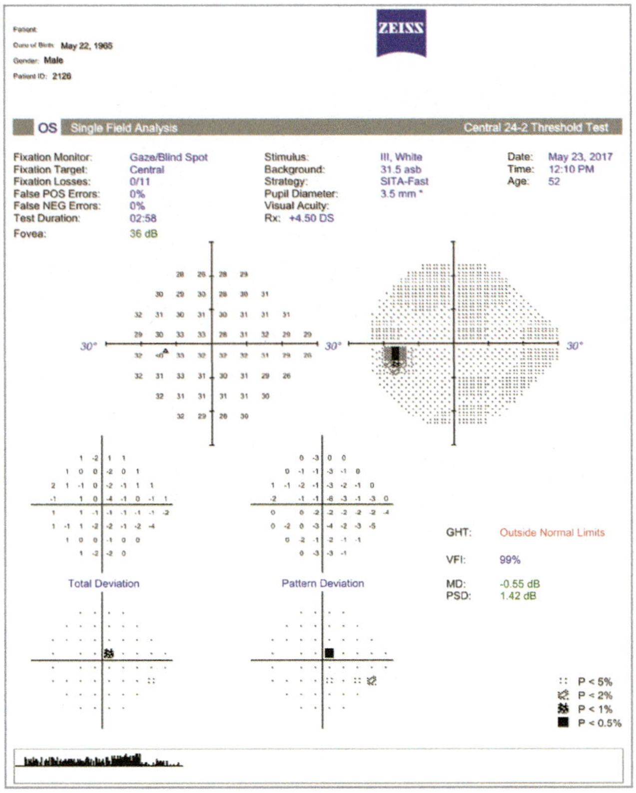

LE 2017
Fixation Losses: 0/11
False POS Errors: 0%
False NEG Errors: 0%
PSD 1.42 dB
GHT—Outside Normal Limits.

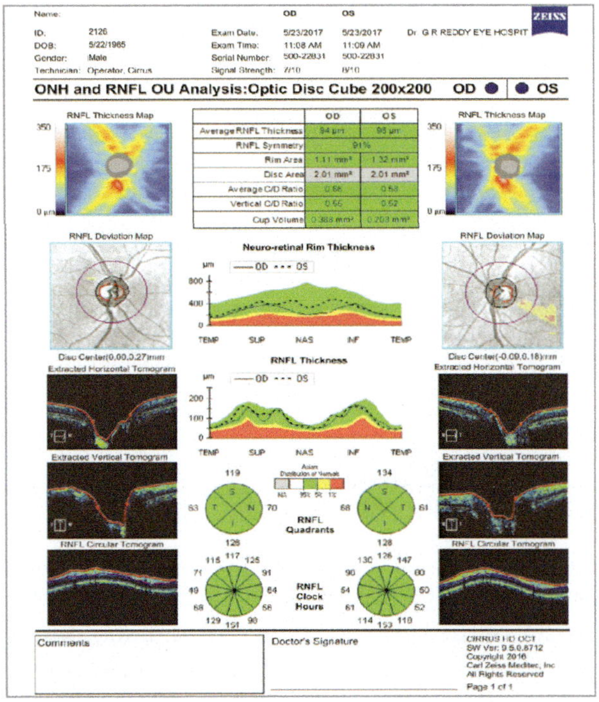

In repeated test also the reliability indices in both the printouts are 100% perfect and all the scotomas which were seen in 2016 were not seen in 2017 printout.

In this situation OCT plays a major role. If OCT is also normal, we can safely keep the patient under observation. The OCT is normal.

Single Field Analysis Printout with Dim Projecting Bulb

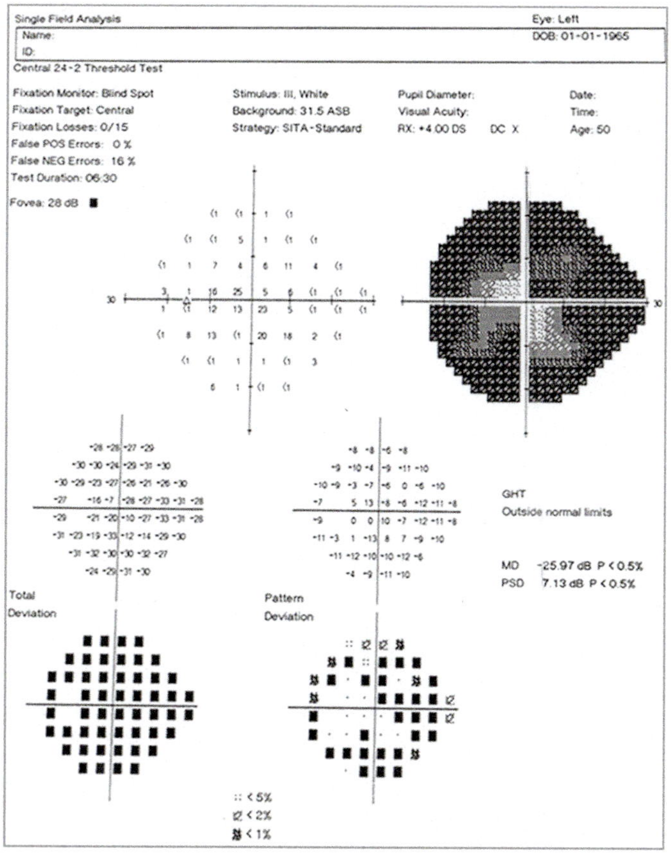

SFA printout with dim bulb

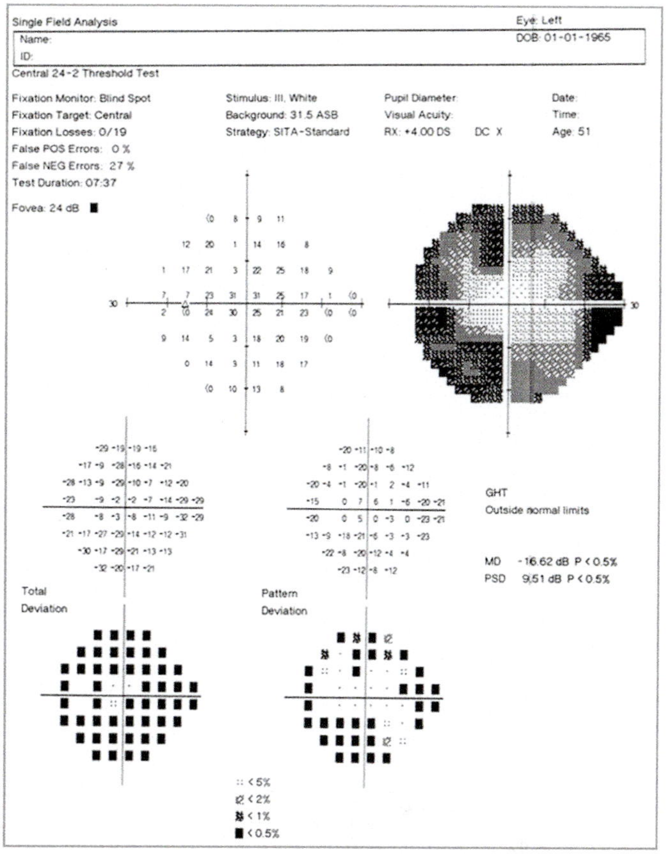

SFA printout after replacing the bulb

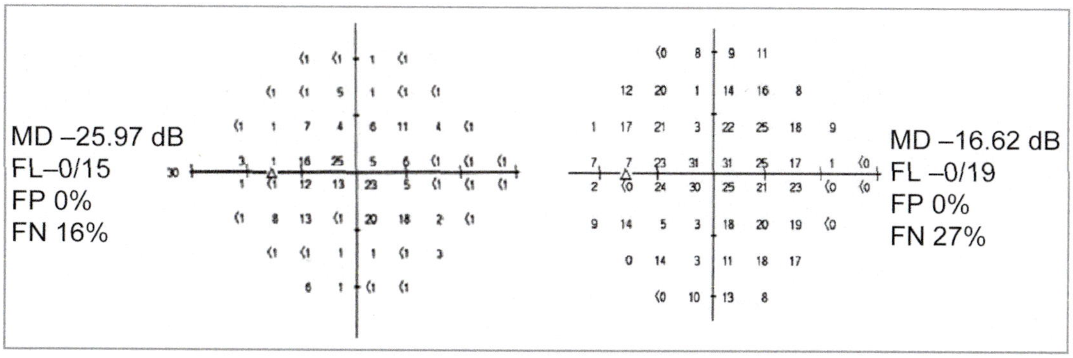

The MD index is -25.97 dB with 16% FN errors in the SFA printout of dim bulb. After replacing the bulb, the MD index is -16.62 dB with 27% FN errors. Normally the MD index should be more with 27% FN errors than with 16 % FN errors. This information gives a clue that the raw data is not reliable. We should always see the raw data before start interpreting the printout to know the functioning capacity of the bulb. If the raw data does have (<) sign in front 0, it indicates the function of the bulb is perfect and if (<) sign appears infront of any numerical value, it indicates that the bulb is not projecting the maximum intensity of light.

SFA with dim projecting bulb **SFA after replacing the bulb**

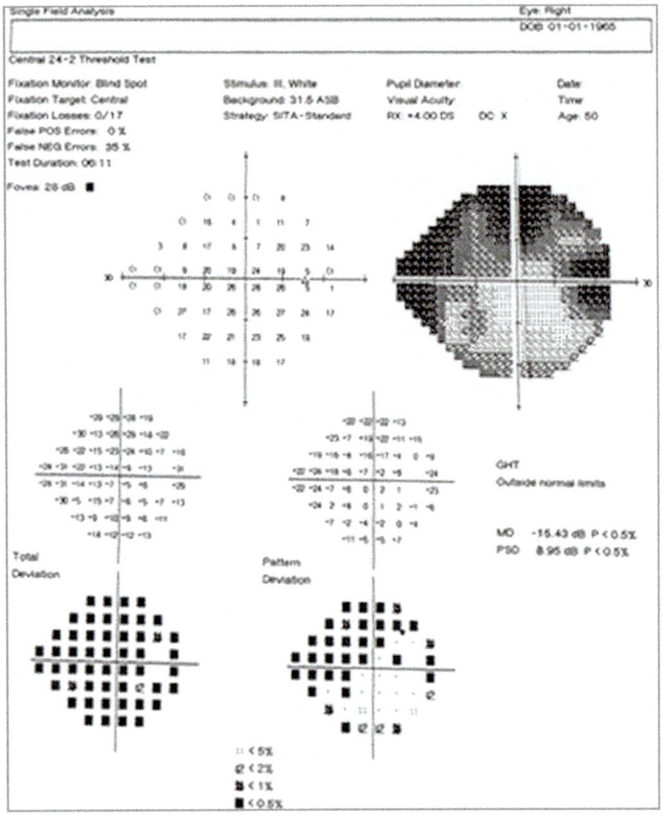

SFA printout-1

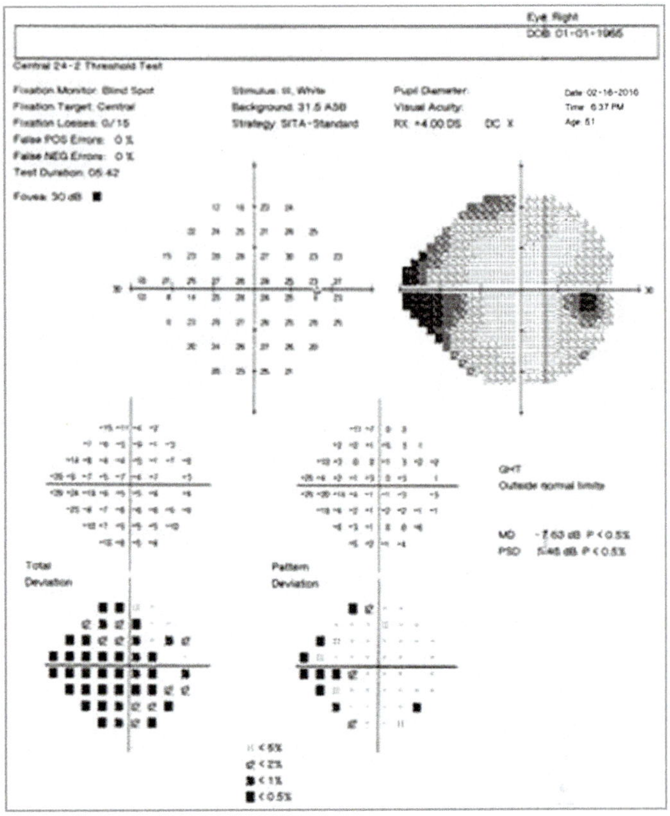

SFA printout after replacing the bulb

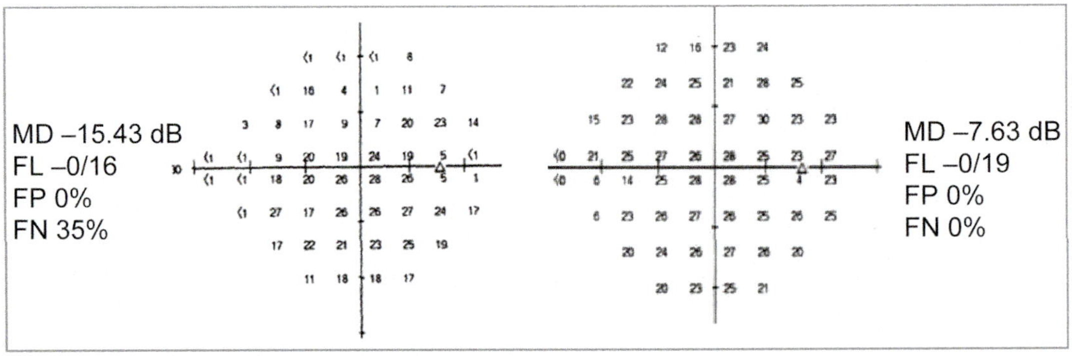

The raw data of the SFA printout has (<) sign infront of numerical value 1 dB. An (<) sign in front of any digit other than 0 indicates that the bulb is becoming dim and it is time to replace the bulb or it should be recalibrated. The raw data should have either absolute scotoma (0) or (<) sign in front of any numerical value. Then only we know the functioning capacity of the bulb. If the raw data has no absolute scotoma or no (<) sign in front of any numerical value, then it is not possible to tell about the functioning capacity of the bulb. If the raw data does not contain absolute scotoma or no (<) sign infront of any numerical value, we presume the functioning of the bulb is perfect.

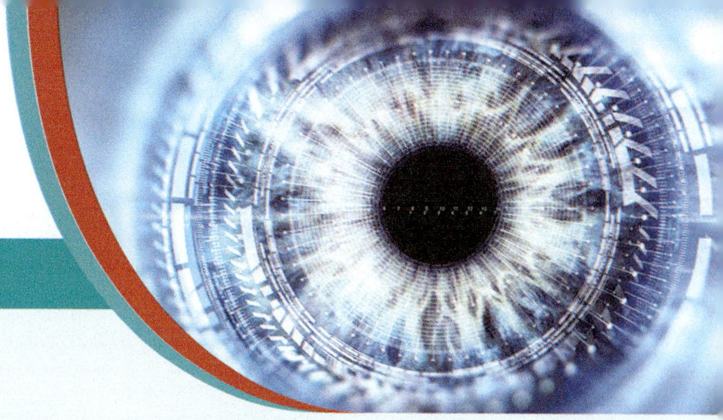

CHAPTER

5

Classification of Primary Open-angle Glaucoma

CLASSIFICATION OF PRIMARY OPEN-ANGLE GLAUCOMAS

The new concept in the classification of open-angle glaucomas is based on the location of the field defect. Perimetry helps to classify open-angle glaucomas into 3 types.

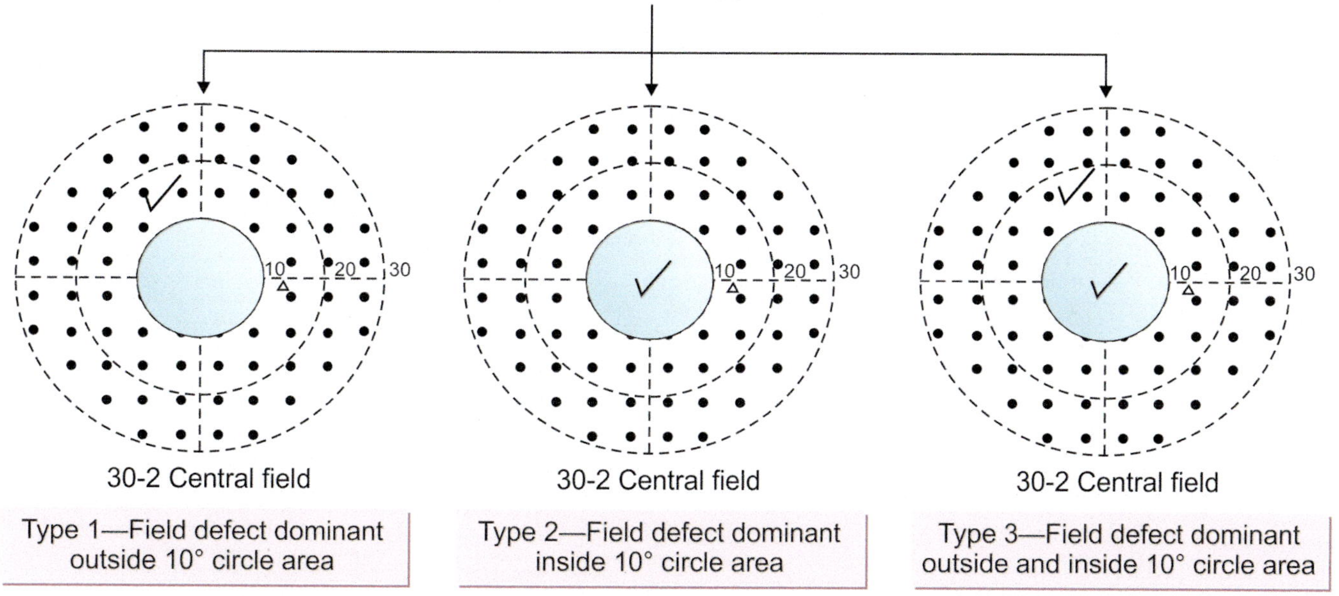

In each type of glaucoma again there are 2 stages of glaucomas—suspicious stage and established stage. Normally, we suspect open-angle glaucoma when we come across some important clinical situations in our daily clinical practice are as follows:

- Disc clinically looking normal with intraocular pressure (IOP) >20 mm Hg.
- Disc clinically looking suspicious with IOP <20 mm Hg.
- Disc clinically glaucomatous with IOP >20 mm Hg (established glaucoma).
- Disc clinically glaucomatous with IOP <20 mm Hg (normal tension glaucoma).
- C/D disparity between the two eyes with either normal or increased IOP.

When we suspect glaucoma, the first test we ask is visual fields to confirm diagnosis of glaucoma. **Selection** of the test is **the point pattern—30-2 (or) 24-2** and strategy SITA Standard. SITA Fast will be selected in situations when the patient is either old or when we think that patient cannot concentrate for a long time. The visual printout helps to diagnose glaucoma and decides the type of glaucoma.

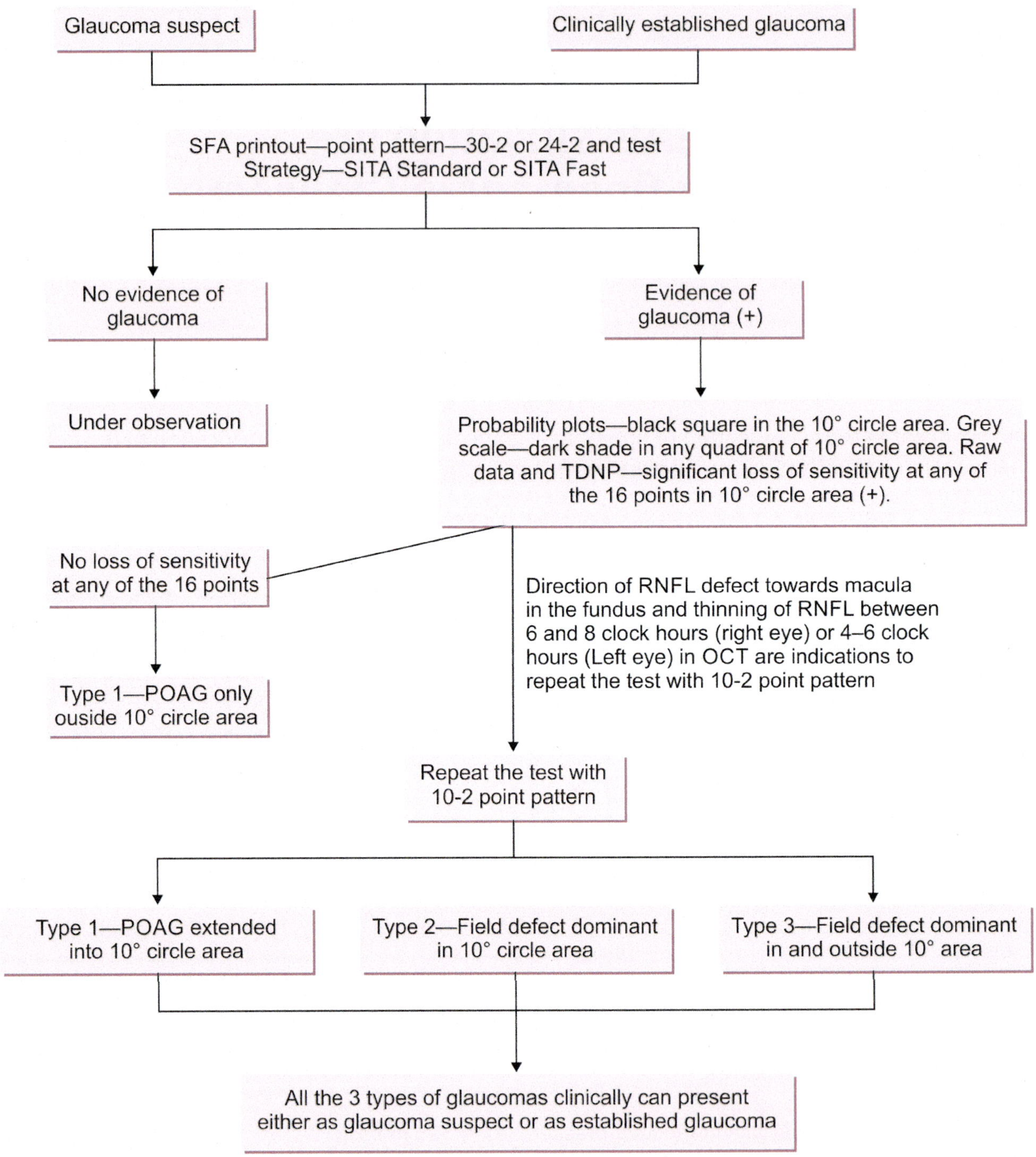

From this flowchart, it is very clear that when we see a suspected or established case of open-angle glaucoma, we ask for the visual field testing. It starts with 30-2 or 24 -2 point pattern. On the basis of single field analysis (SFA) printout the diagnosis and type of glaucoma will be decided or the person may remain as glaucoma suspect. So again in each type of glaucoma there will be glaucoma suspect and established glaucoma. Interpretation of SFA printout in a suspected case of glaucoma will be different from that of an established case of glaucoma.

Interpretation of Visual Field Defect in a Suspicious Case of Glaucoma

The main object of visual field testing in a case of glaucoma suspect is to know whether glaucoma is present or not (diagnosis of glaucoma).

Reliability indices FL, FP, FN and gaze tracking) should be nearer to 100% perfection.

Identification of the artifacts is the most important step during the interpretation of SFA printout in a suspected case of glaucoma.

Reproducibility—The field defect must be reproducible and should correlate with disc and retinal findings and it must fulfill Anderson's criteria to label the field defect as glaucomatous field defect. If the field defect correlates with fundus and fulfills Anderson's criteria then glaucoma suspect becomes an established case of glaucoma.

Any localized scotoma to be labeled as glaucomatous field defect, it must fulfill certain **criteria**. These criteria are called as **Anderson's criteria**. So one should know about **Anderson's criteria.**

Localized field defect: Concentrate on the total deviation probability plot (TDPP)
Generalized field defect: Concentrate on the pattern deviation probability plot (PDPP)

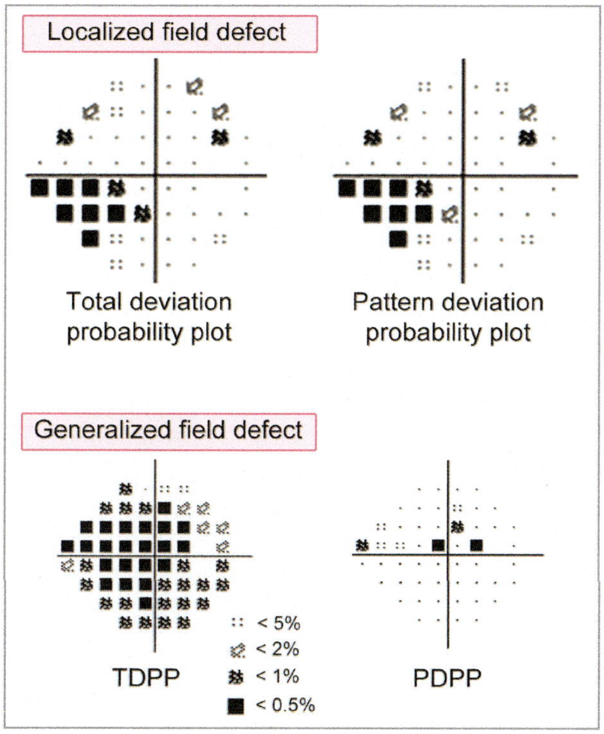

Anderson's criteria 1: Probability Plots

There should be a minimum of three nonedge adjacent or cluster points in an expected locations usually where glaucoma starts, with significant P values either in total deviation probability plot (localized field defects) or in pattern deviation probability plot (in generalized field defect). The P values of these three points should be as follows:

P value of two points should be <5% and the remaining one point should have the P value <1%.

The location of the field defect should correspond to the disc changes.

Anderson's criteria 2: PSD P < 5%

Anderson's criteria 3: GHT—outside normal limits

The edge scotomas in 30-2 fields will not be considered as defective. The edge scotomas of 24-2 should be considered with a great caution if they exist without nonedge scotomas. In the single field analysis printout, glaucoma hemifield test (GHT) and pattern standard deviation (PSD) are developed to pickup early focal defects. This is the reason why, they are included in Anderson's criteria. So they should be abnormal.

If the field defect correlates with fundus and fulfills Anderson's criteria, then glaucoma suspect will become established case of glaucoma. Always take the help of OCT while evaluating the suspected case of glaucoma.

Not fulfilled Anderson's criteria → Keep under observation

Fulfilled Anderson's criteria → It becomes established case of glaucoma

Interpretation of Visual Field Defect in an Established Case of Glaucoma

Once the diagnosis of glaucoma is confirmed then the aim is to set the target IOP to arrest progression and to prevent onset of new glaucomatous damage elsewhere. The most important features of field defect which determines the target IOP are as follows—Location, extent of the field defect, direction of progression of the field defect (Probability plots) depth of the field defect (Total deviation numerical plot), macular status and foveal split (Raw data).

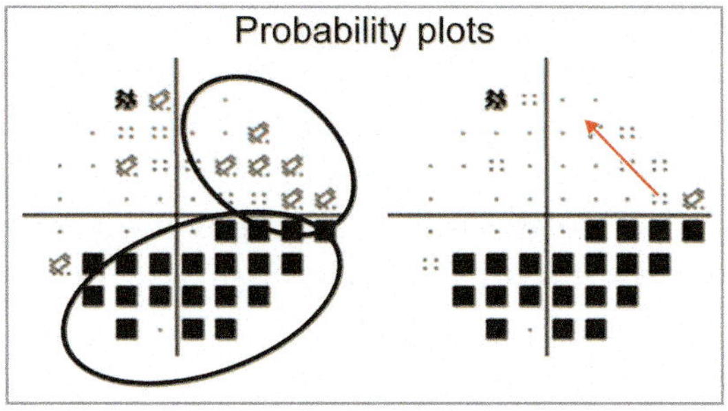

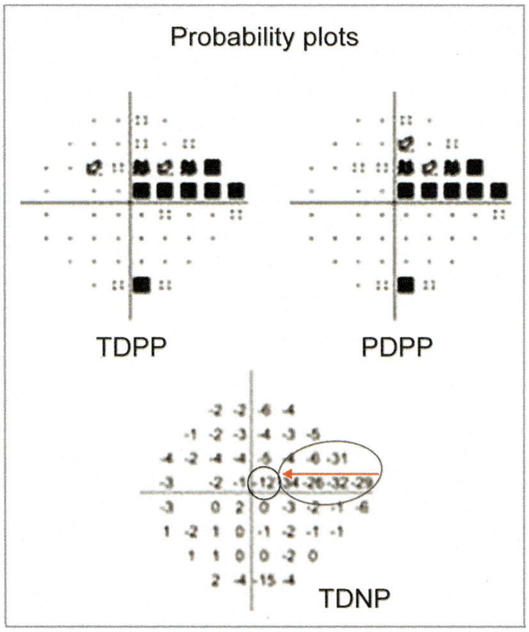

Interpretation of visual field defect in an established case of glaucoma starts with probability plots—From the probability plots we know location, extent and direction of progression of the field defect:

Direction of progression of the field defect—The pattern deviation probability plot gives the direction of progression of glaucoma. During conversion of total deviation plots to pattern deviation plots, the recent onset scotomas of TDPP will disappear in PDPP. From this we know the direction of progression of the field defect. As in this case we can identify the superficial scotomas in the TDPP through P value symbols.

Direction of progression—When both the probability plots look similar and if all the points are represented by black squares, it is difficult to tell the direction of progression of the field defect through probability plots. In this situation, the total deviation numerical plot (TDNP) and grey scale help in knowing the direction of progression of the field defect.

TDNP (Depth of the scotoma)—From the TDNP, it is very clear that the field defect started outside 10° circle area and progressing towards fixation because the loss of sensitivity at the points outside 10° circle around 30 dB and the loss of sensitivity at 3° nasal point is -12 dB. So we have to correlate both the probability plots and TDNP to know the direction of progression of the field defect.

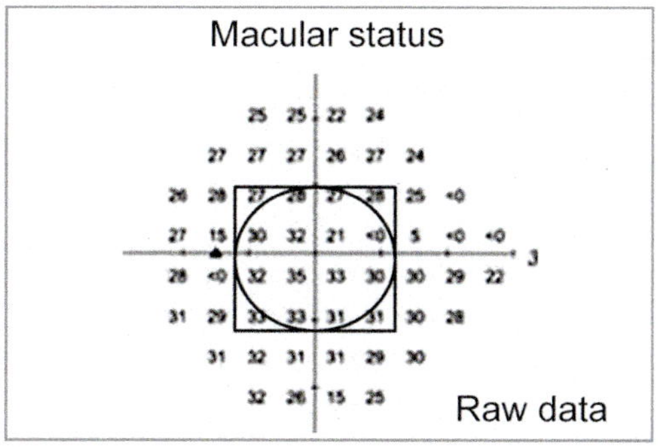

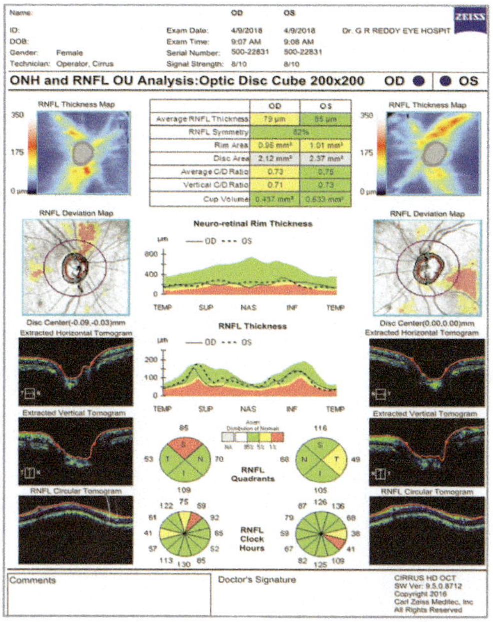

The loss of sensitivity at some of the points is around 30 dB and at most of the points it is around 5 dB, MD index -4.97 dB $P < 0.5\%$.

TDNP gives deviation value from normative data at each point and MD index gives the average of the deviation values of all the points in the TDNP.

The measured retinal sensitivity at each point of the point pattern will be known only from raw data. From the raw data only we know whether the field defect is absolute or relative or combination of both.

Depending on the sensitivities of the 16 points in the 10° circle area of raw data it will be decided whether we have to repeat the test with 10-2 point pattern or not to know the foveal status. The functioning status of the projecting bulb will be known from the raw data.

Optical coherence tomography (OCT) plays a major role in a case of glaucoma suspect. In many a times SFA printout will not be 100% perfect and not able to come to definite conclusion to say that it is a case of glaucoma. In the circumstances where there is strong clinical suspicion with border line IOP then if OCT correlates with fundus finding, we can make the diagnosis of glaucoma.

Visual field dependent factors to set target IOP

1. *Location and extent of the field defect*: If glaucomatous field defect is either started outside 24° and extended into 10° circle area or the started within 10° circle we should aim at low target IOP.
2. *Direction of the field defect*: If the direction of progression is towards fixation, we should aim at low target IOP.
3. *Depth of the field defect*: After the location and extent of the field defect, depth of the field defect is very important. MD index represents the depth of the field defect. Depending on the value of MD index we should not grade glaucoma. If the field defect is within 10° circle area and the direction of progression is towards fixation, even though the MD index is not high we should aim at low target IOP. If the field defect is outside 10° circle area and the direction of progression is not towards fixation, even though the MD index is high we need not aim at low target IOP. Presence of absolute scotoma (nonedge point), aim for low target IOP.

CHAPTER

6A

Interpretation of Single Field Analysis Printouts of Type 1 Primary Open-angle Glaucoma

TYPE 1 PRIMARY OPEN-ANGLE GLAUCOMA WITH FIELD DEFECT OUTSIDE 10° CIRCLE AREA

I will be presenting six cases of Type 1 glaucoma (Field defect outside 10° circle area). All the six cases are glaucoma suspects. Normally open-angle glaucomas will be suspected either from fundus appearance or by increased intraocular pressure (IOP). In these six cases, the disc is almost looking normal. The only clue to suspect glaucoma is C/D disparity between the two eyes or doubtful notch and majority of these cases are associated with risk factors like increased IOP, strong family history of glaucoma, high myopia, pseudoexfoliation, etc.

Case 1

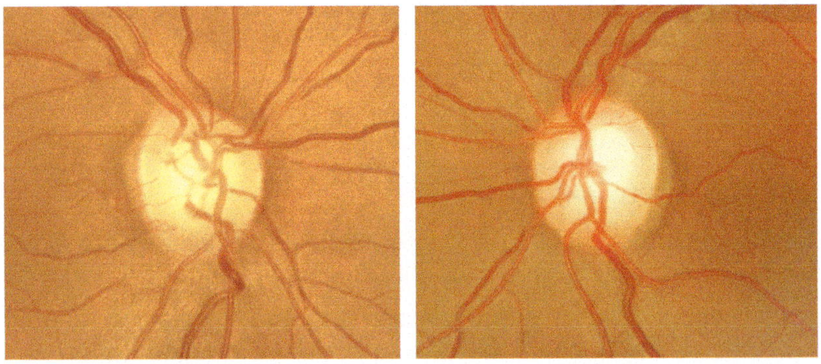

Case 2

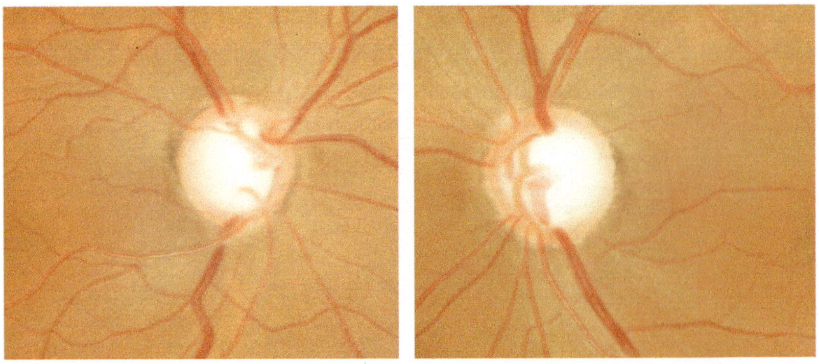

Case 3

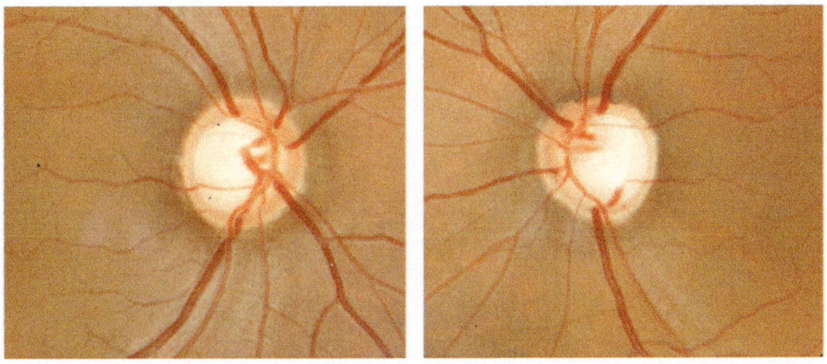

Case 4

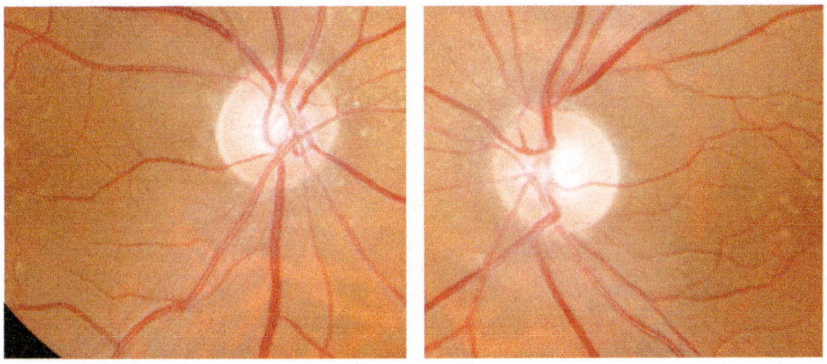

Case 5

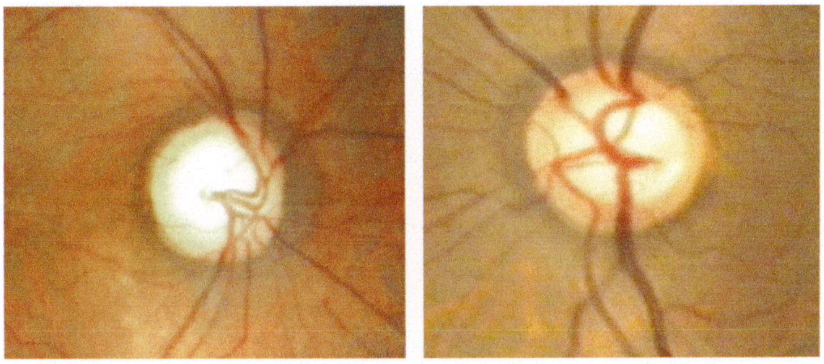

Case 6

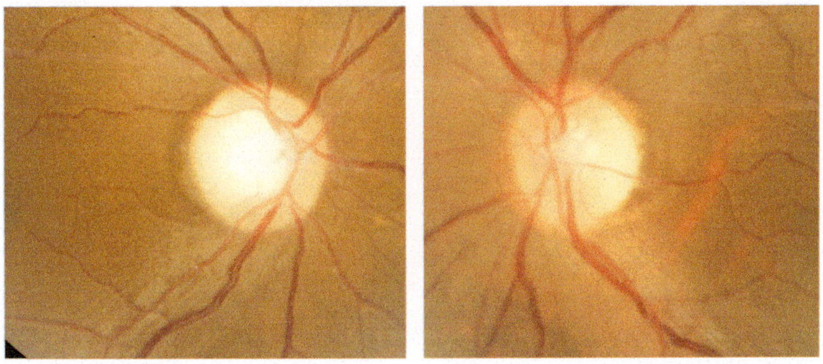

Case 1 Right Eye (RE)

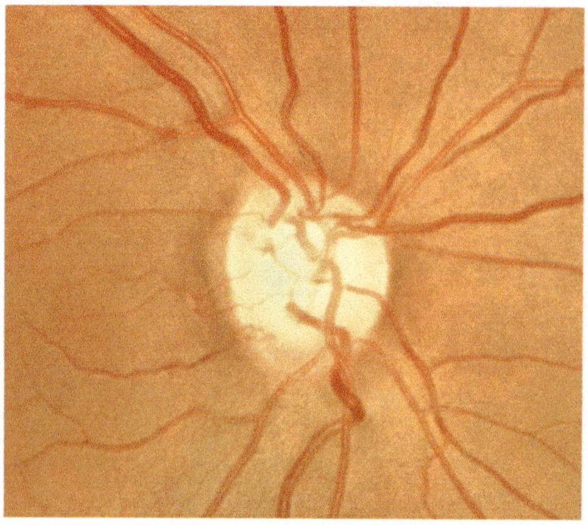

Case 1 Left Eye (LE)

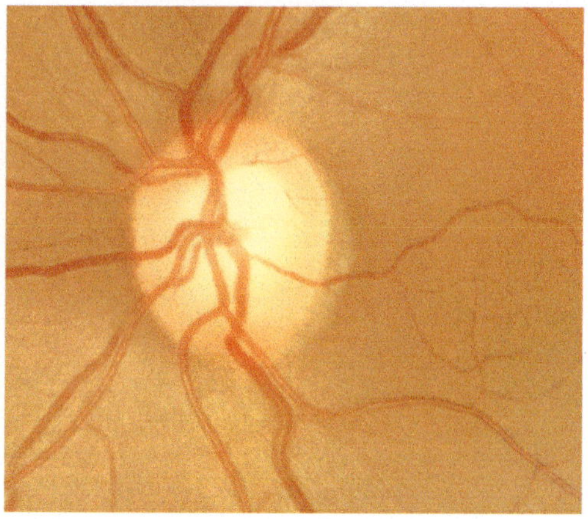

Glaucoma is suspected because of increased IOP (21 mm Hg). No clue from disc to label it as glaucomatous disc except for C/D disparity between the two eyes.

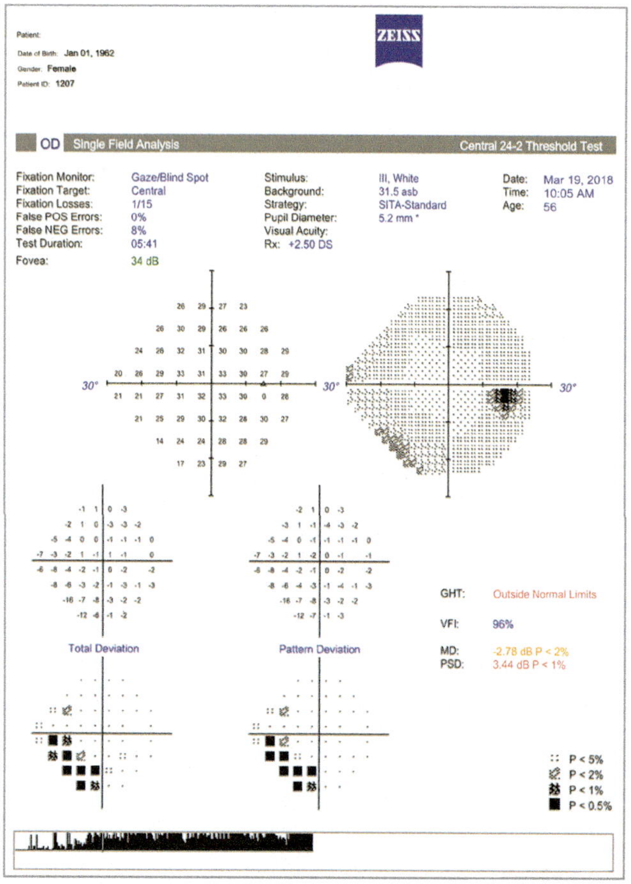

FL 1/15; FP 0%; FN 8%; Fovea 34 dB
2018-MD -2.78 dB P < 2%; PSD 3.44 dB P < 1%
GHT-ONL; VFI 96%

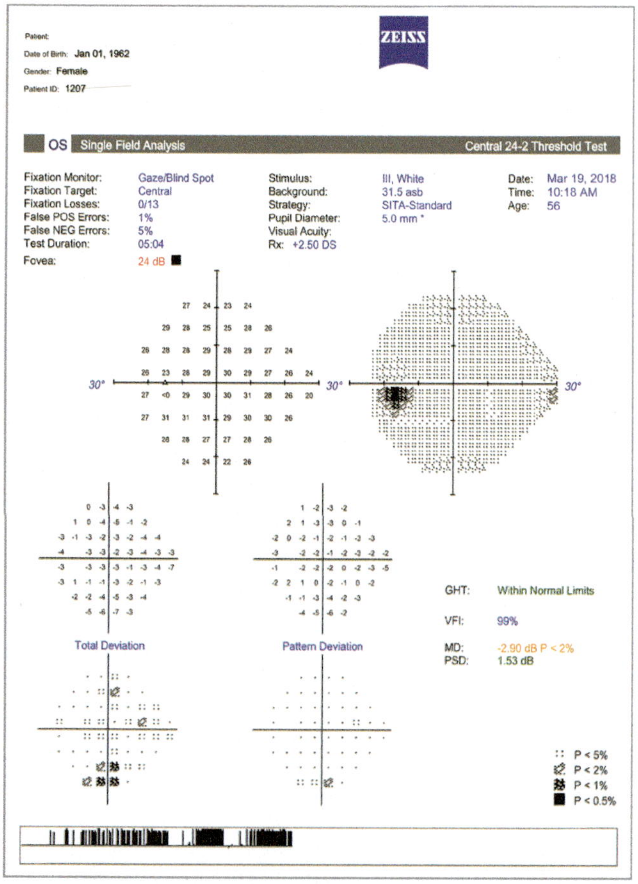

FL 0/13; FP 1%; FN 5%; Fovea 24 dB
MD -2.90 dB P < 2%; PS 1.53 dB
GHT-WNL; VFI 99%

Case 1 RE

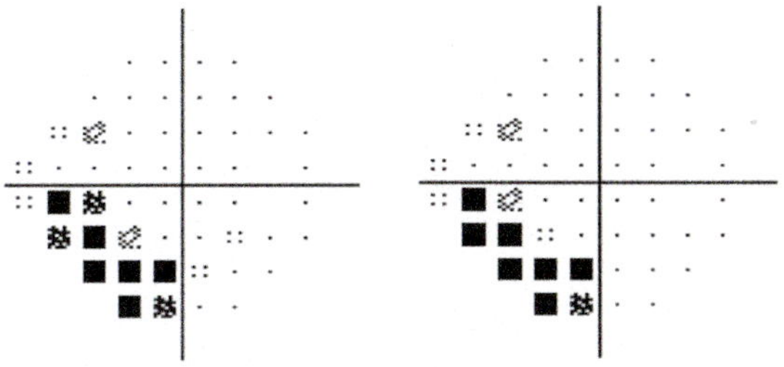

TDPP PDPP

MD -2.78 dB P < 2%
PSD 3.44 dB P < 1%

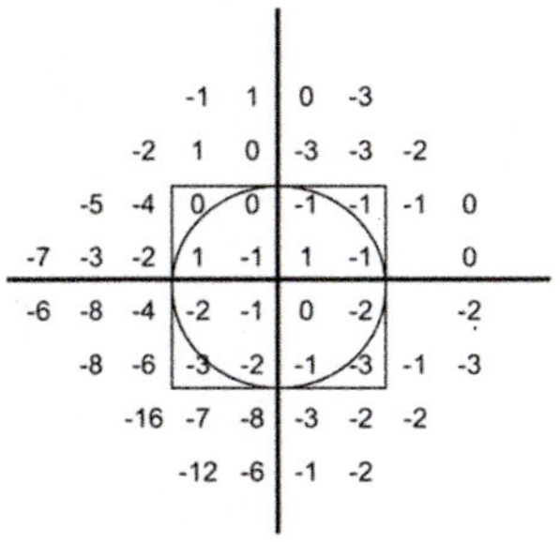

TDNP

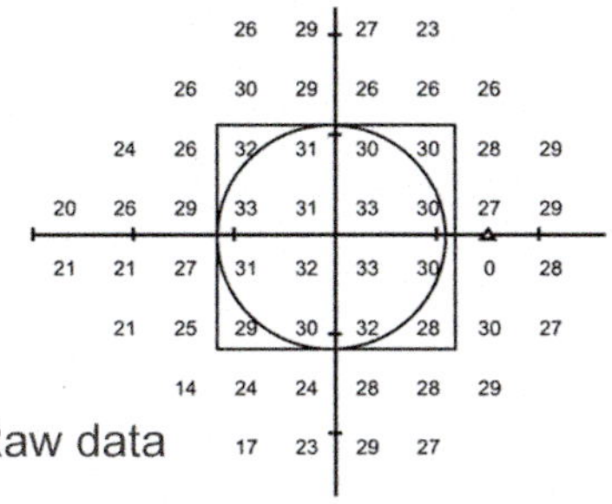

Raw data

Location and extent of the field defect: Localized scotoma in the lower nasal quadrant in the total deviation probability plot (TDPP).

Depth of the field defect: It is a relative scotoma with highest loss of sensitivity point is 16 dB. Probability plots, pattern standard deviation (PSD) and glaucoma hemifield test (GHT) are fulfilling Anderson's criteria to label the **localized scotoma as glaucomatous field defect.**

> In a case of glaucoma suspect the aim is to diagnose the case. Reproducibility of the field defect is very important. The patient was put on antiglaucoma medication and repeated the field test after 1 year. The repeated field (2019 SFA) also showed the field defect.

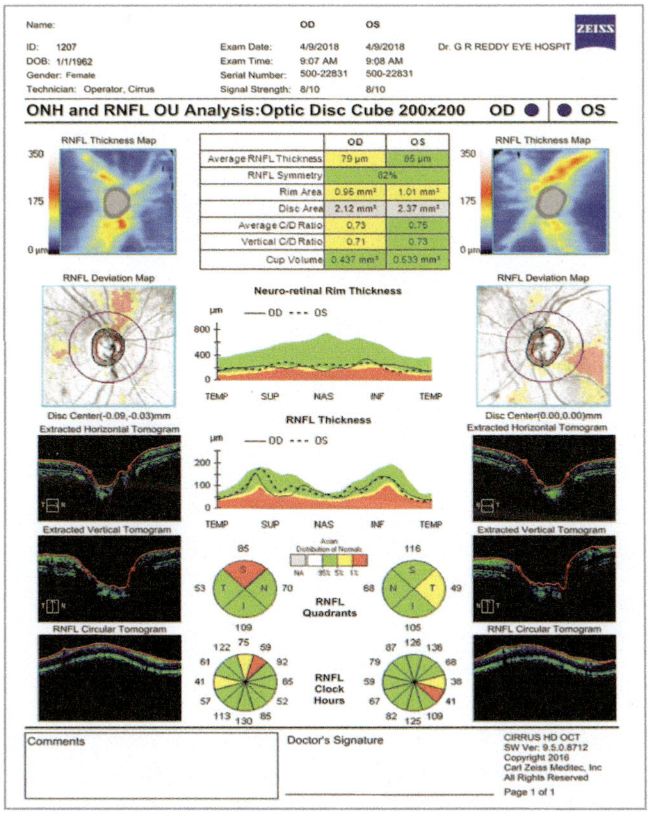

Interpretation of single field analysis (SFA) printout in a case of glaucoma suspect. Point pattern and testing strategy should be 30-2 and 24-2 and SITA Standard respectively. Reliability indices should be close to 100% perfect. The localized field defect should fulfill Anderson's criteria and the field defect should be reproducible.

When there is no clue to label the disc as glaucomatous disc or no RNFL defects and IOP is around 20 mm Hg, but the field defect is fulfilling **Anderson's criteria**, then OCT plays a major role to diagnose glaucoma.

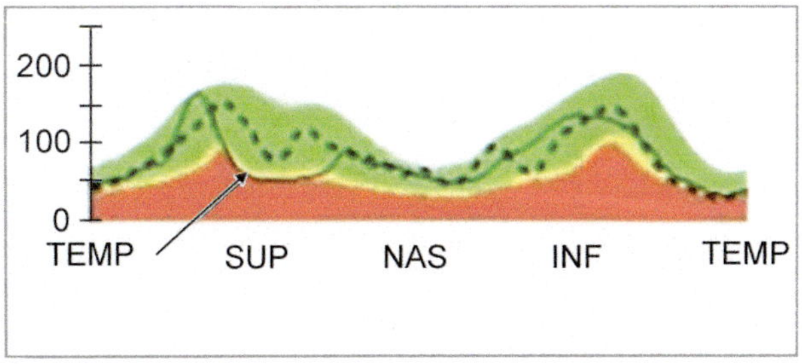

If **OCT findings correlate with field defects**, it gives strength to label glaucoma suspect as a case of glaucoma.

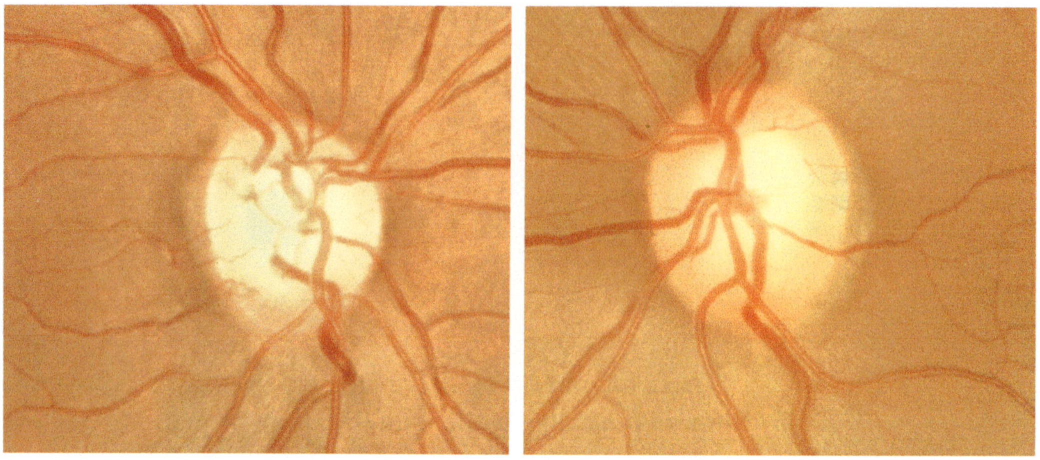

Case 1: Follow-up after one year. The target—IOP is maintained around 15 mm Hg. (Initial IOP is 21 mm Hg in both the eyes).

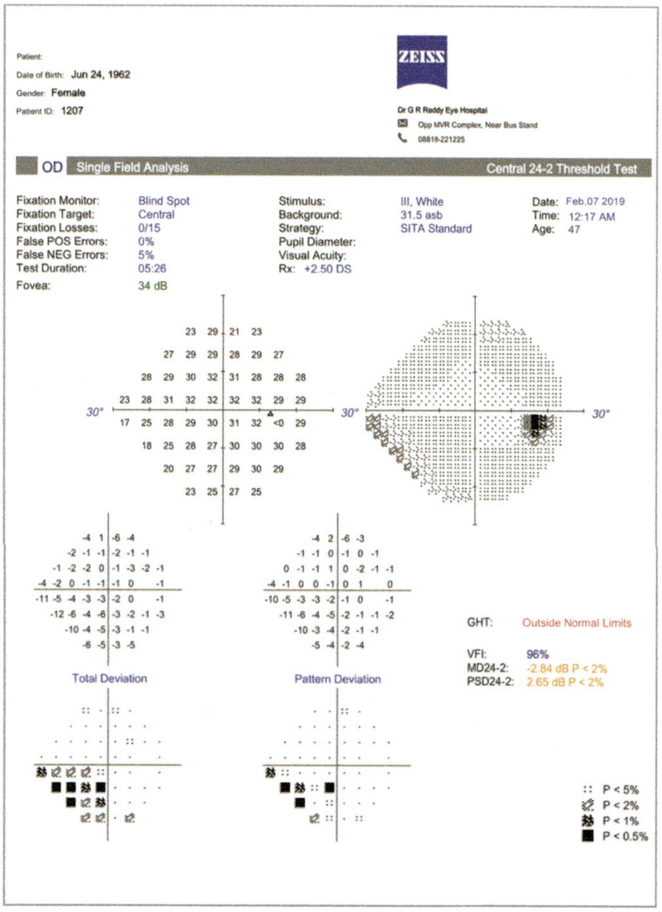

FL 0/15; FP 0%; FN 5%
Fovea 34 dB; GHT-ONL; VFI 96%
MD -2.84 dB P < 2%; PSD 2.65 dB P < 2%

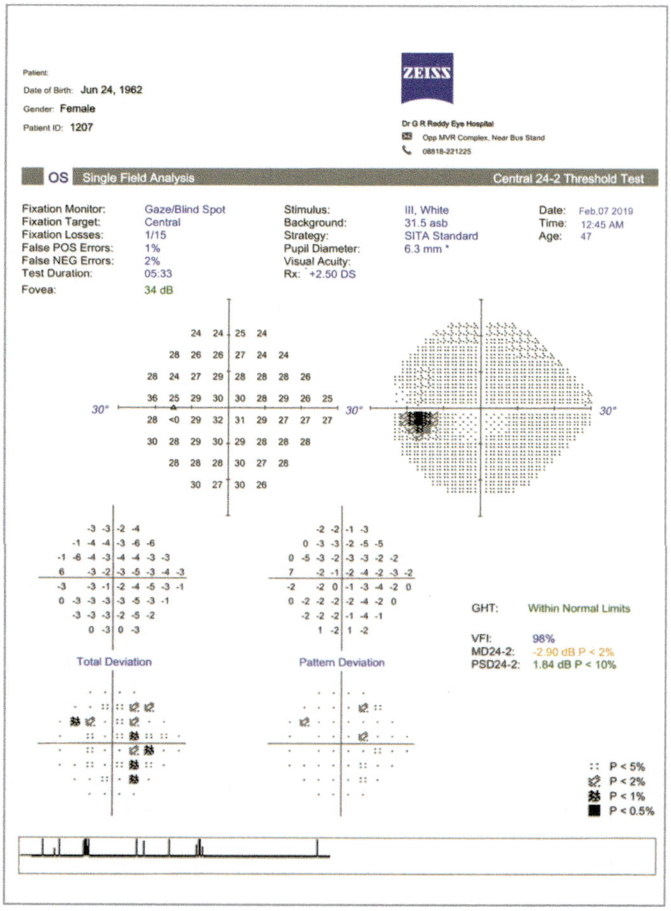

FL 1/15; FP 1%; FN 2%
Fovea 34 dB; GHT-WNL; VFI 98%
MD -2.90 dB P < 2%; PSD 1.84 dB P < 10%

Case 1: Follow-up after one year (RE)

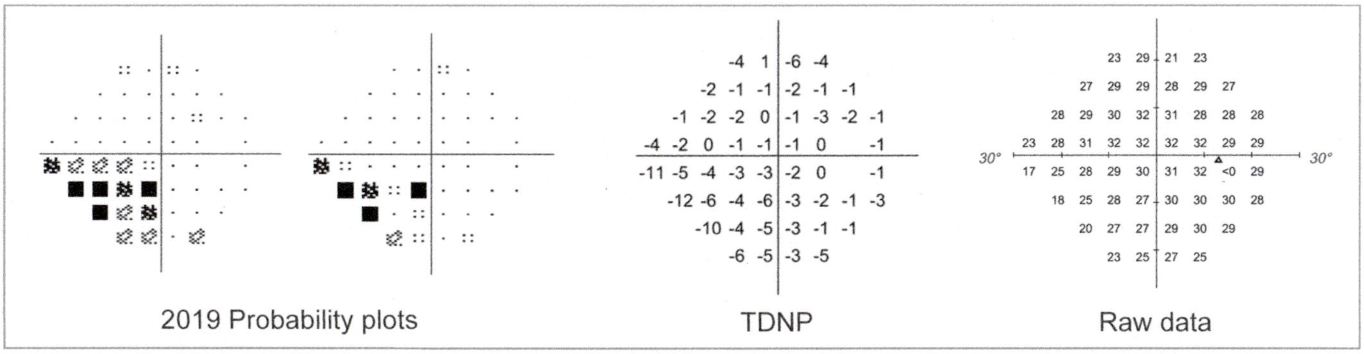

GHT-ONL; VFI 96%
MD -2.84 dB P < 2%
PSD 2.65 dB P < 2%

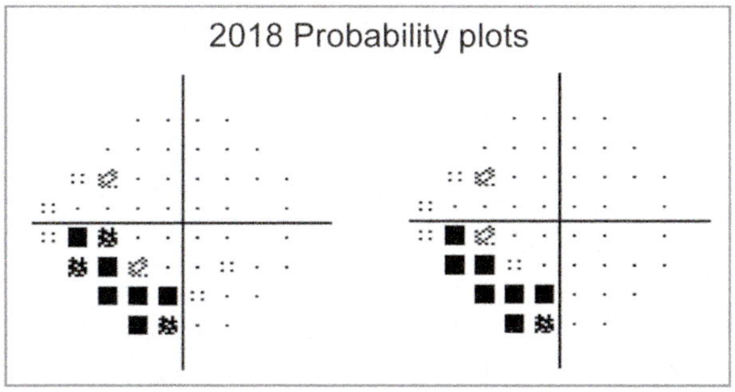

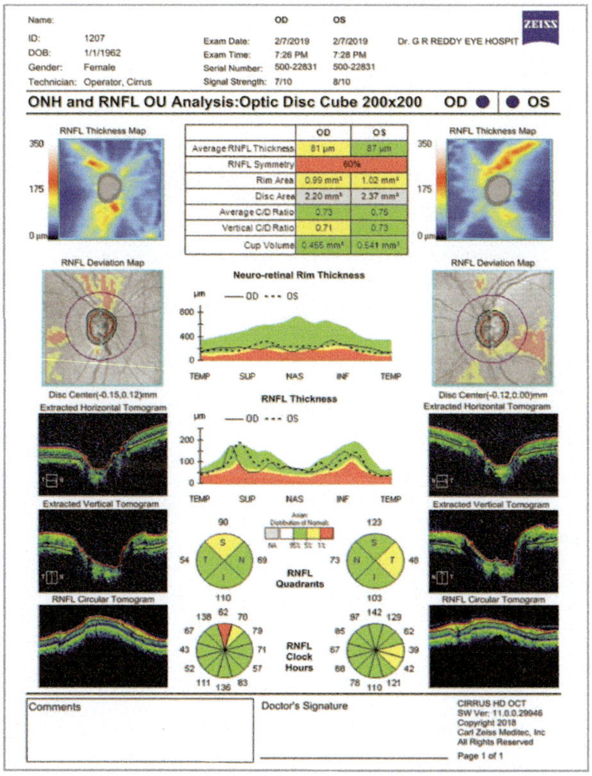

In a case of glaucoma suspect reproducibility of the field defect is very important. The field defect persisted in the followup field after one year and the field defect, OCT findings are correlating with 2019 fields.

In glaucoma suspect the important facts are as follows:

1. Point pattern should be either 30-2 or 24-2
2. Testing strategy should be SITA Standard
3. Reliability—FL, FP and FN should be near 100% perfect.
4. OCT should correlate to fundus and fields.
5. Reproducibility of the field defect in the follow-up tests.

If the peripheral fibers are involved the RNFL, clock hour map shows the thinning either at 6° clock or 12° clock, OCT is correlating with fundus and visual fields.

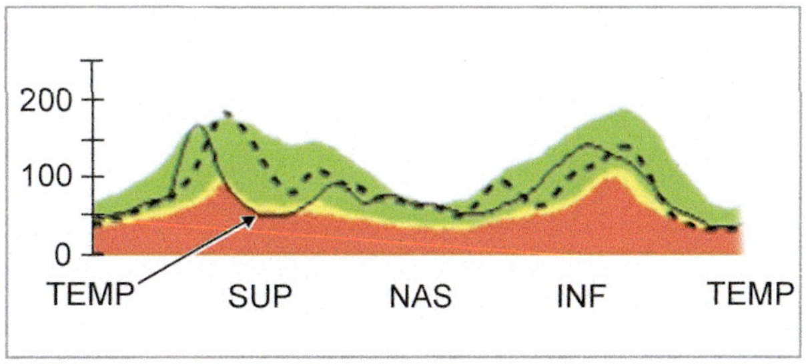

Note the dip is superior and nasal.

Case 2 RE 2017 | **CASE 2 LE 2017**

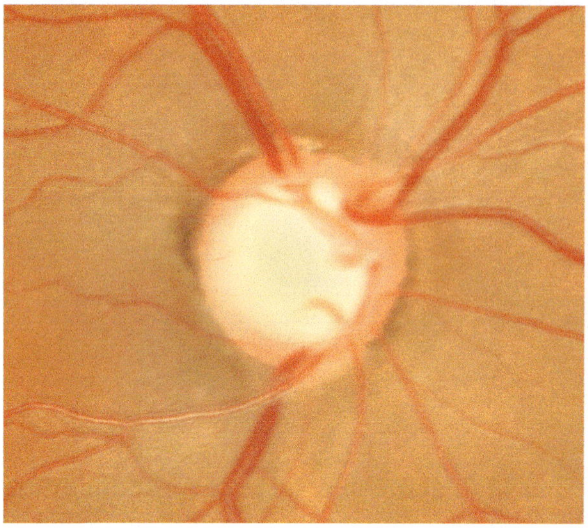

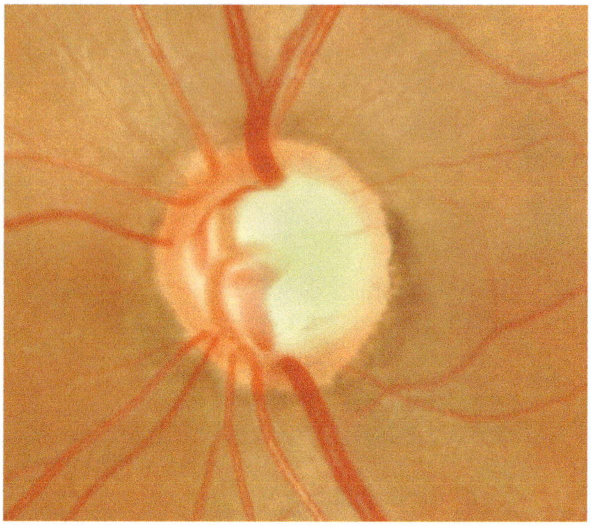

No definite clue from fundus to label it as glaucomatous disc. Glaucoma is suspected on the basis of IOP which is around 20 mm Hg.

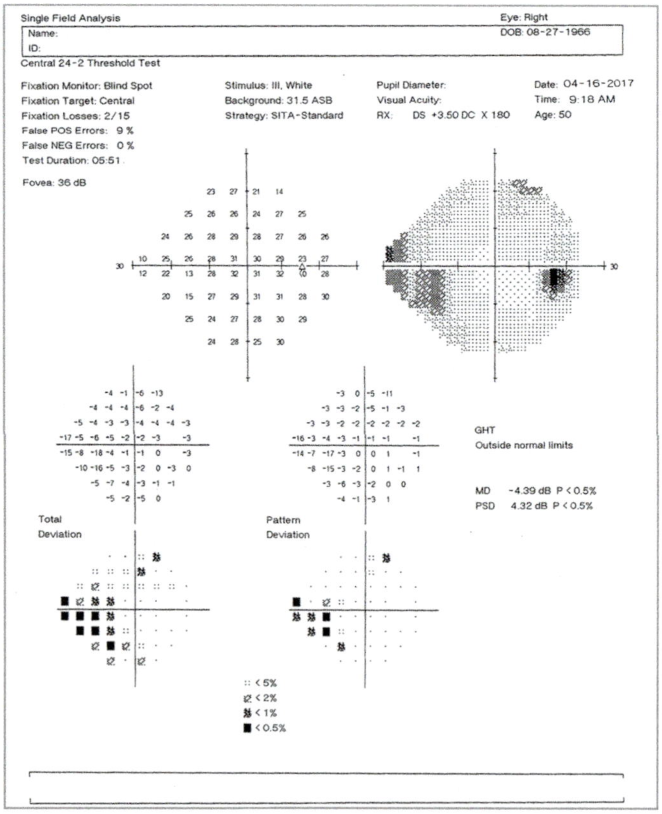

FL 2/15; FP 9%; FN 0%
Fovea 36 dB; GHT-ONL
MD -4.39 dB P < 0.5%; PSD 4.32 dB P < 0.5%

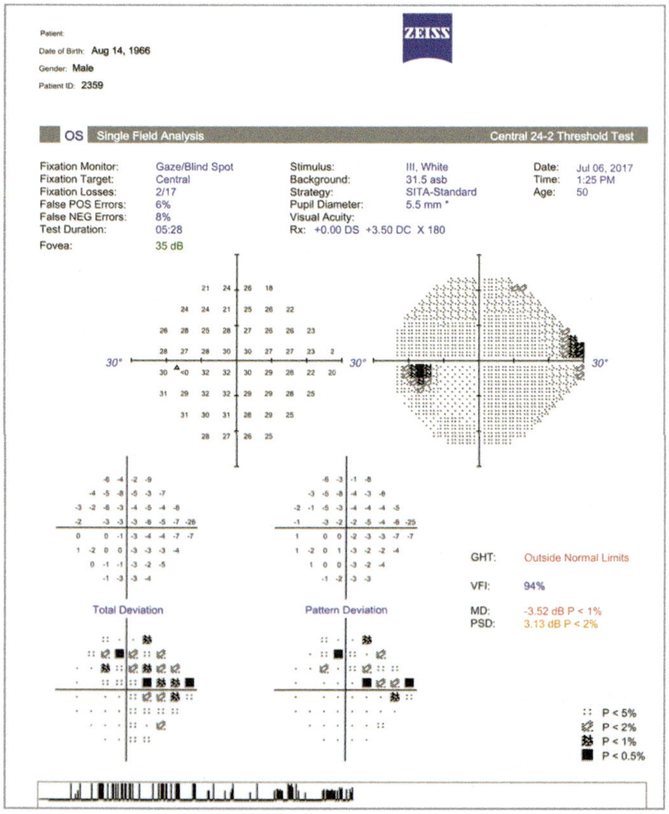

FL 2/17; FP 6%; FN 8%
Fovea 35 dB; GHT-ONL; VFI 94%
MD -3.52 dB P < 1%; PSD 3.13 dB P < 2%

Case 2 RE 2017

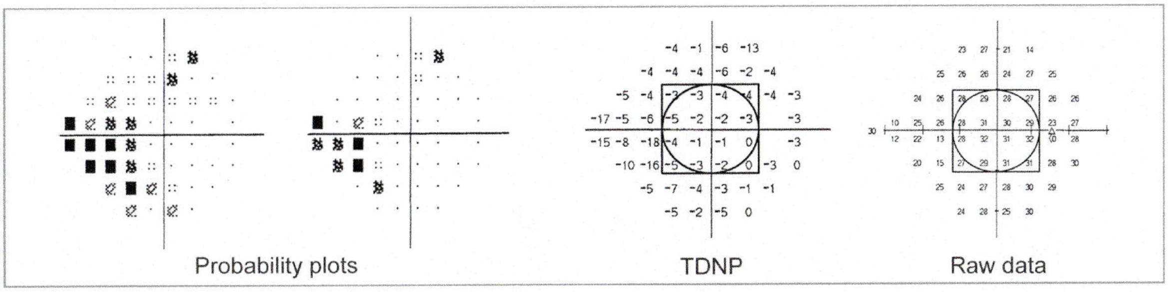

Right eye—Lower arcuate relative scotoma in the nasal quadrant with maximum loss of sensitivity point is 17 dB with good sensitivity in the 10° circle area.

GHT-ONL PSD 4.32 dB P < 0.5%.

The localized scotoma, PSD and GHT are fulfilling the Anderson's criteria to label the scotoma as glaucomatous field defect. **MD -4.39 dB P < 0.5 %.**

Case 2 LE 2017

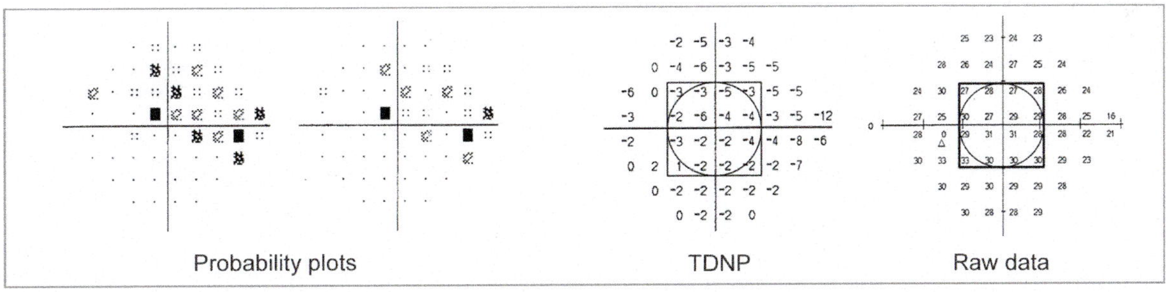

Left eye—Upper arcuate relative scotoma in the nasal quadrant with maximum loss of sensitivity point is 12 dB with good sensitivity in the 10° circle area. **GHT-ONL PSD 3.13 dB P < 2%. The localized scotoma, PSD and GHT are fulfilling the Anderson's criteria to label the scotoma as glaucomatous field defect. MD -3.52 dB P < 1%.**

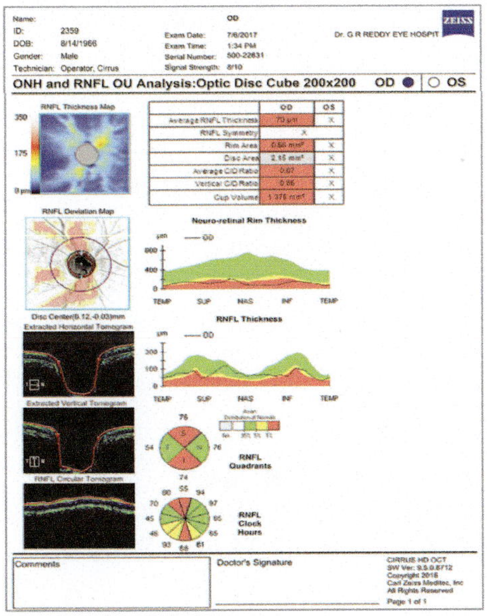

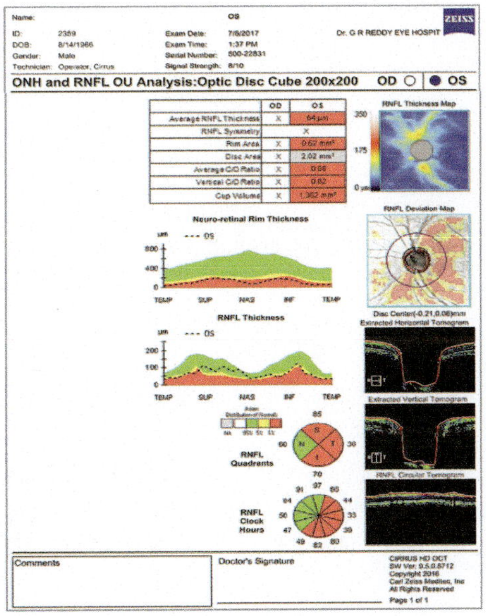

This is one of the cases where OCT is not correlating with fundus and fields.

Case 2 RE 2018

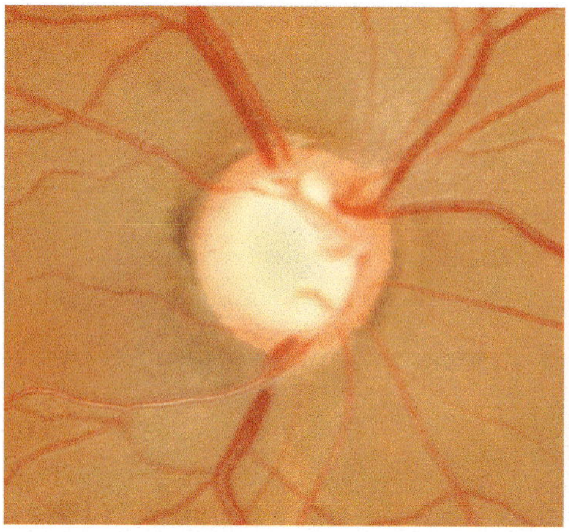

Case 2 LE 2018

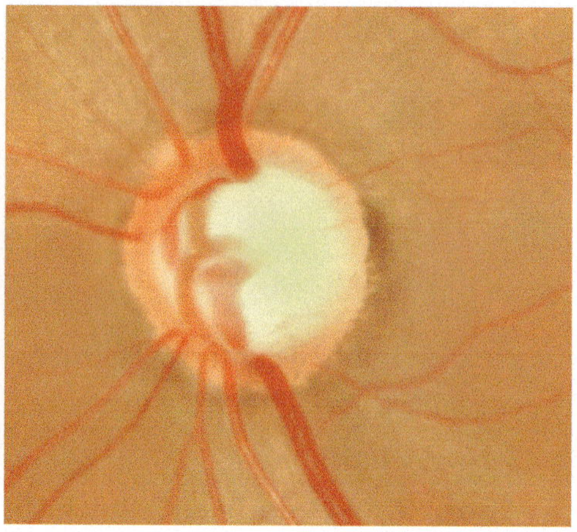

Case 2: Follow-up after 1 year. No definite clue from fundus to label it as glaucomatous disc. Glaucoma is suspected on the basis of IOP which is around 20 mm Hg.

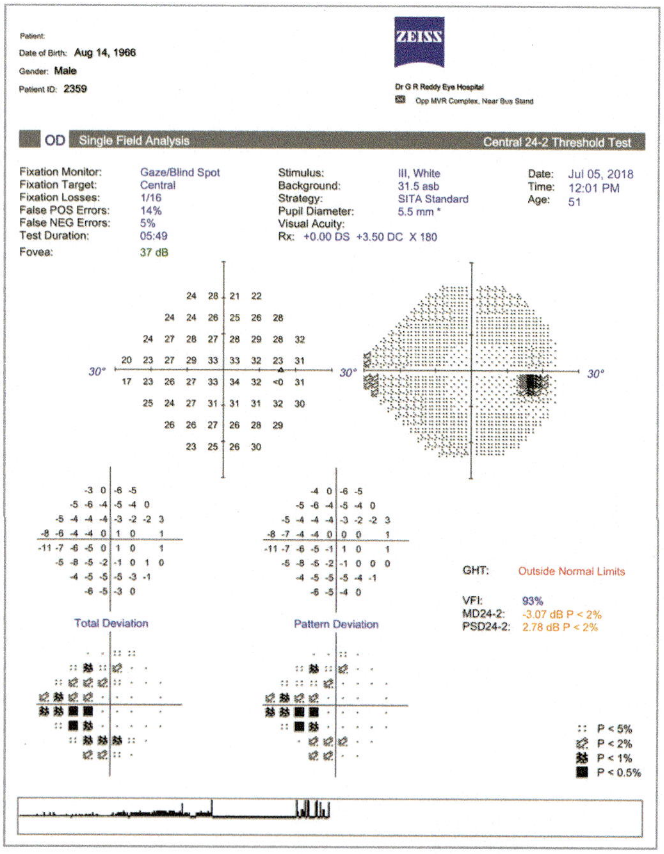

FL 1/16; FP 14%; FN 5%
Fovea 37 dB; GHT-ONL; VFI 93%
MD -3.07 dB P < 2%; PSD 2.78 dB P < 2%

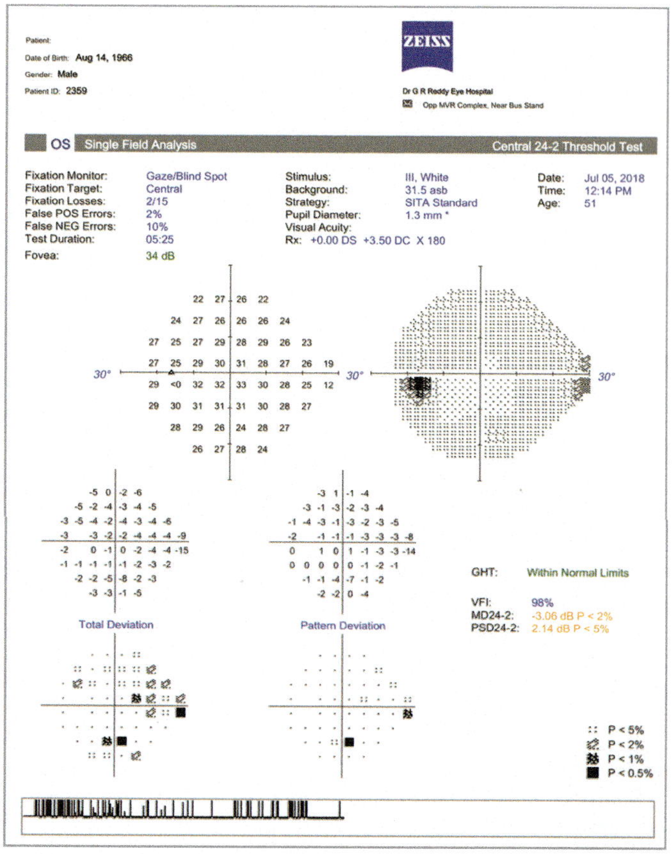

FL 2/15; FP 2%; FN 10%
Fovea 34 dB; GHT-WNL; VFI 98%
MD -3.06 dB P < 2%; PSD 2.14 dB P < 5%

Case 2 RE 2018

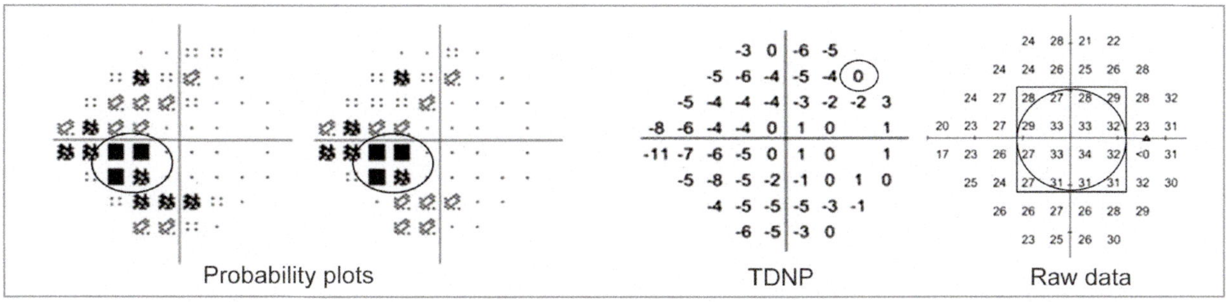

Right eye—Biarcuate relative scotoma in the nasal half of the field with maximum loss of sensitivity point is 17 dB with good sensitivity in the 10° circle area.

GHT ONL-PSD 2.78 dB P < 2%

The localized scotoma, PSD and GHT are fulfilling the Anderson's criteria to label the scotoma as glaucomatous field defect. **MD -3.07 dB P < 2%**

Case 2 LE 2018

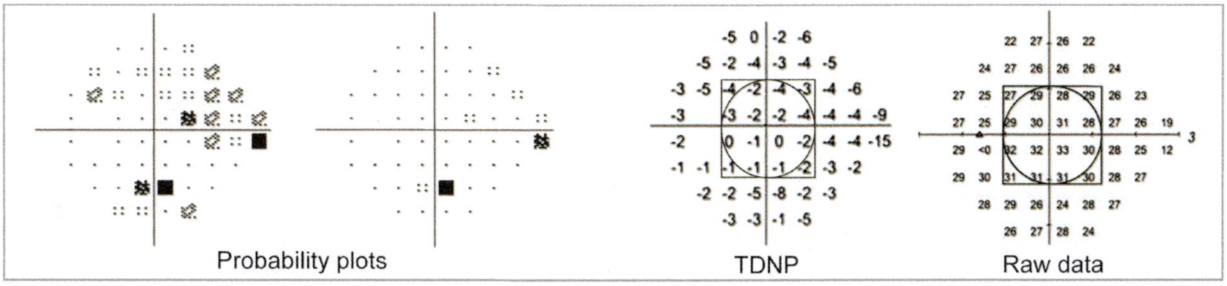

Left eye—Upper arcuate relative scotoma in the nasal half of the field with loss of sensitivity at most of the points is around 4 dB with maximum loss of sensitivity point is 15 dB with good sensitivity in the 10° circle area. **MD -3.07 dB P < 2%.**

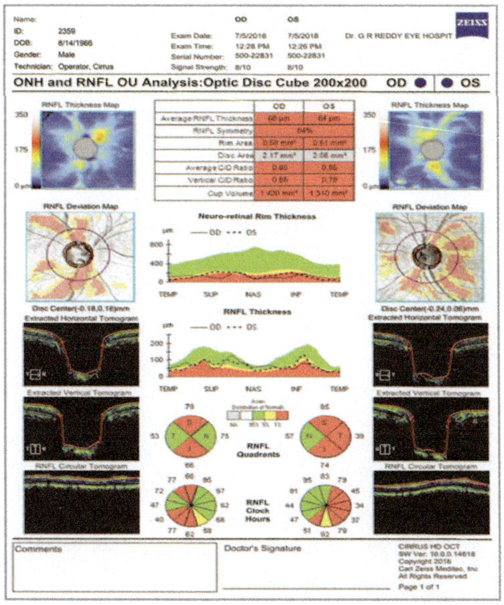

The localized scotoma, PSD and GHT are fulfilling the Anderson's criteria to label the scotoma as glaucomatous field defect.

In a suspected case of glaucoma, reproducibility of the field defect is very important.

This is one of the cases where OCT is not correlating with fundus and fields.

Case 3 RE 2017

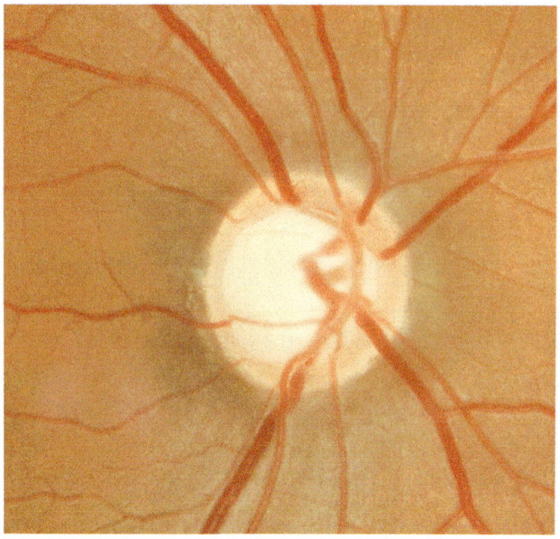

Case 3 LE 2017

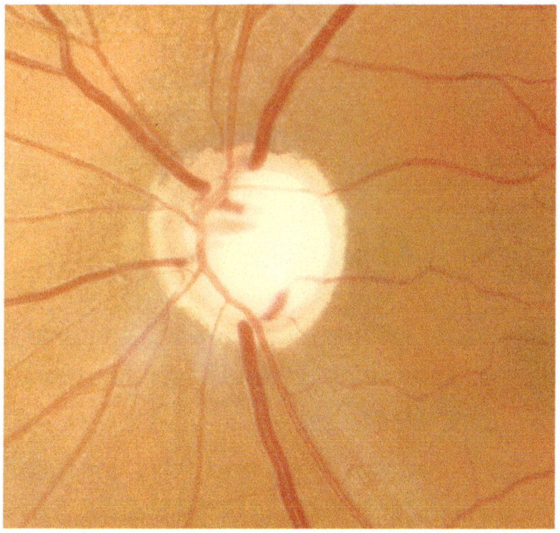

IOP 20 mm Hg. No definite clue from the discs of both the eyes except for suspicious notch at 6-0-clock position of left eye.

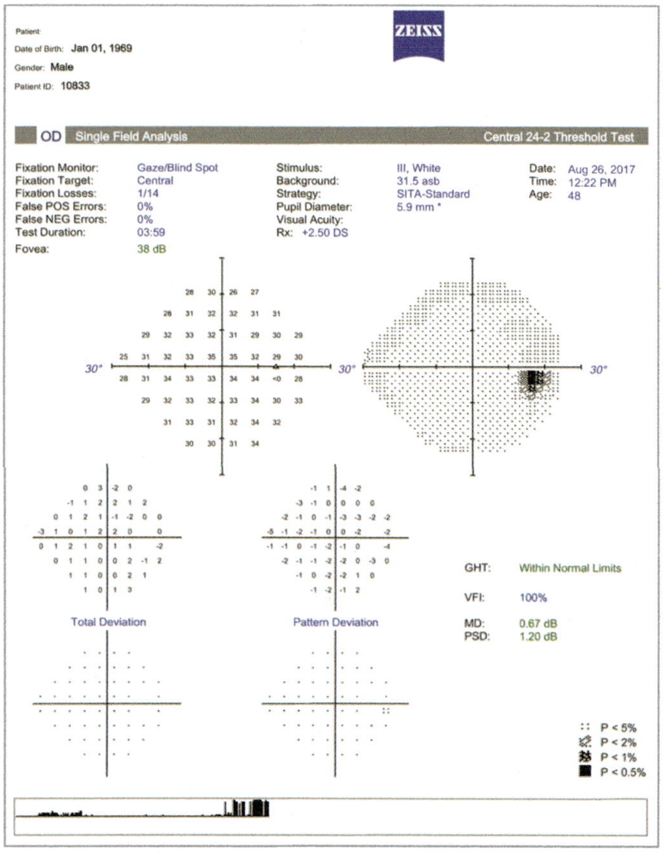

FL 1/14; FP 0%; FN 0%
Fovea 38 dB; GHT-WNL; VFI 100%
MD 0.67 dB; PSD 1.20 dB

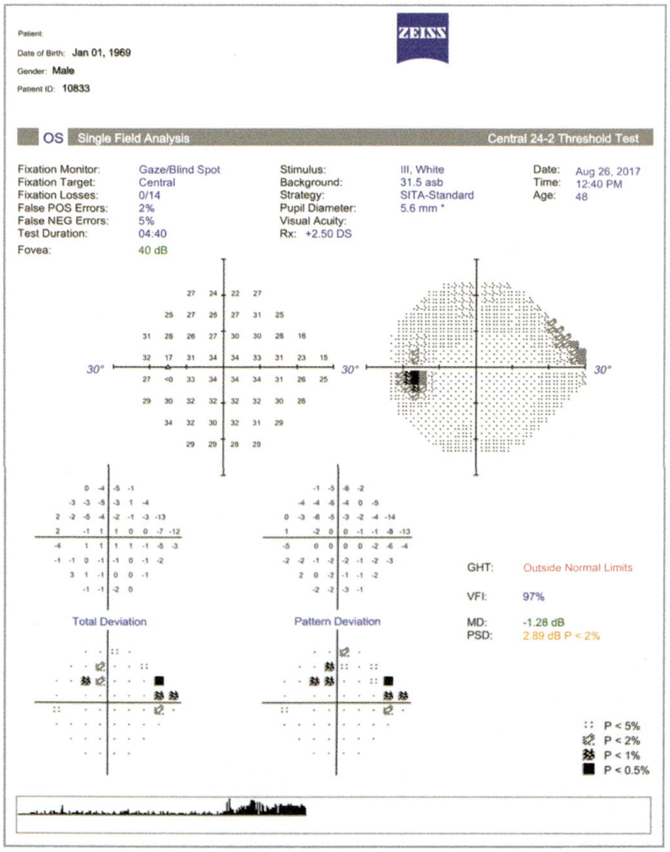

FL 0/14; FP 2%; FN 5%
Fovea 40 dB; GHT-ONL; VFI 97%
MD -1.28 dB; PSD 2.89 dB P < 2%

Case 3 RE 2017

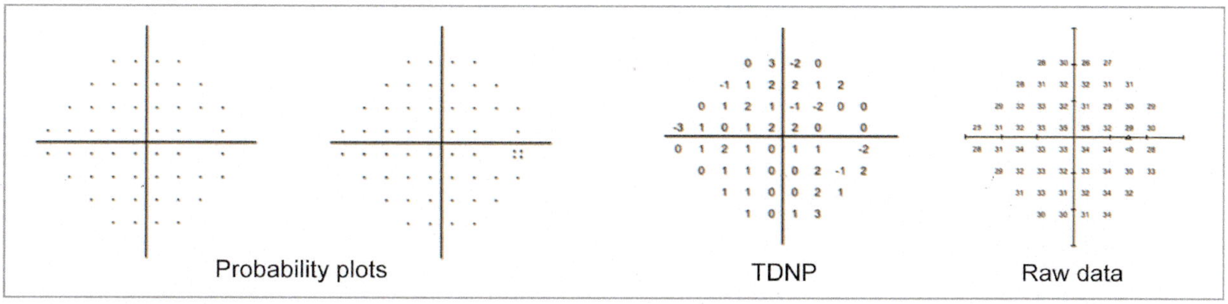

FL 1/14; FP 0%; FN 0%
Fovea 38 dB; GHT-WNL; VFI 100%
MD 0.67 dB; PSD 1.20 dB

RE field—no evidence of glaucoma.

Case 3 LE 2017

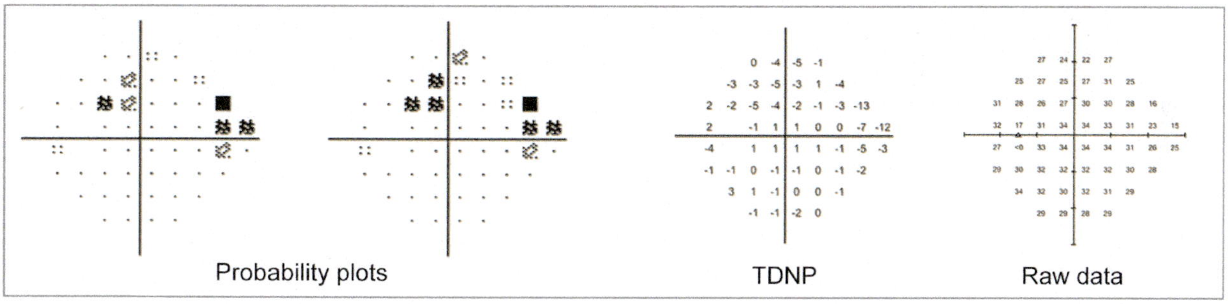

Left eye—Two localized relative scotomas are seen in upper nasal quadrant (nasal step) and in upper temporal quadrant. The loss of sensitivity, at most of the points is around 4 dB except at two points. The maximum loss of sensitivity point is 13 dB. The localized scotoma, PSD and GHT are fulfilling the Anderson's criteria to label the scotoma as glaucomatous field defect.

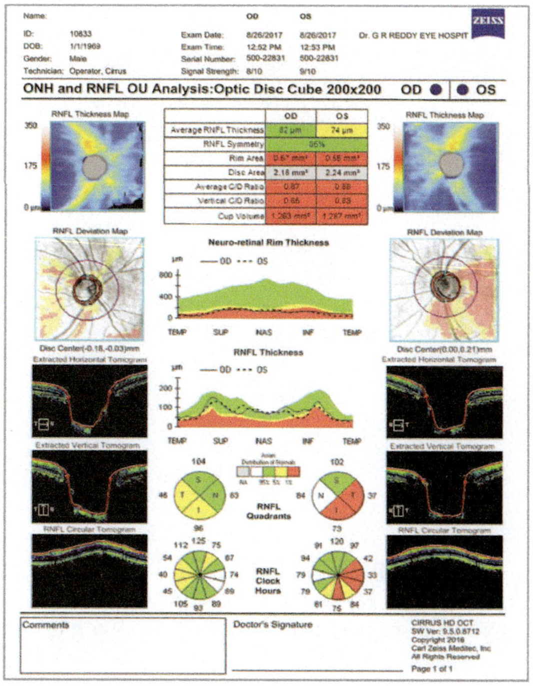

Right eye: OCT is correlating with fundus and fields and the left eye OCT is not correlating with fundus and fields. OCT is showing more damage which was not seen either in the fundus or in the fields.

In the right eye the fundus, visual fields and OCT are looking normal.

Case 3 RE 2019 **Case 3 LE 2019**

Follow-up after 18 months

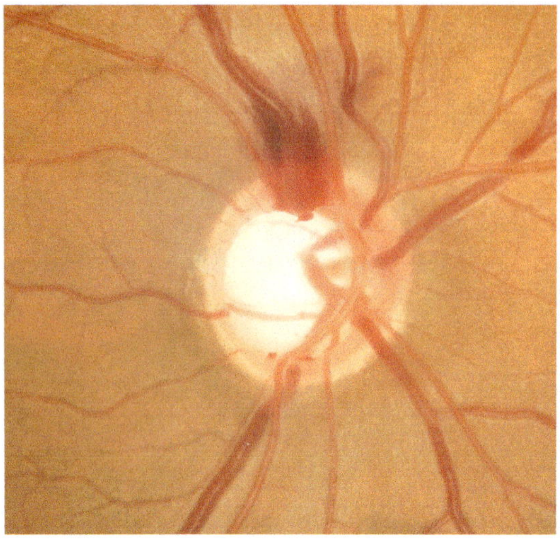

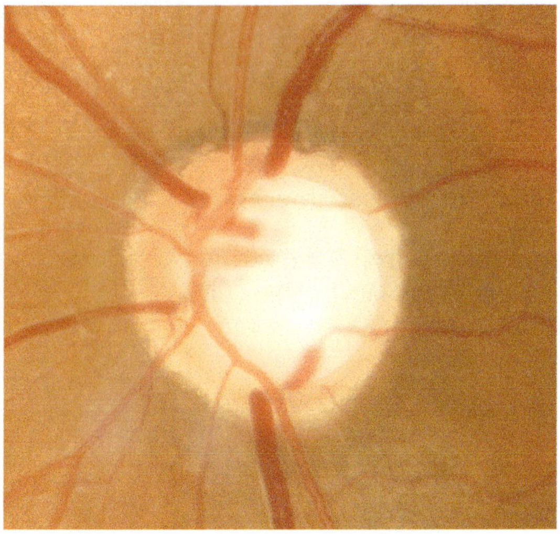

Patient who is on antiglaucoma treatment presented with RE—disc hemorrhage.

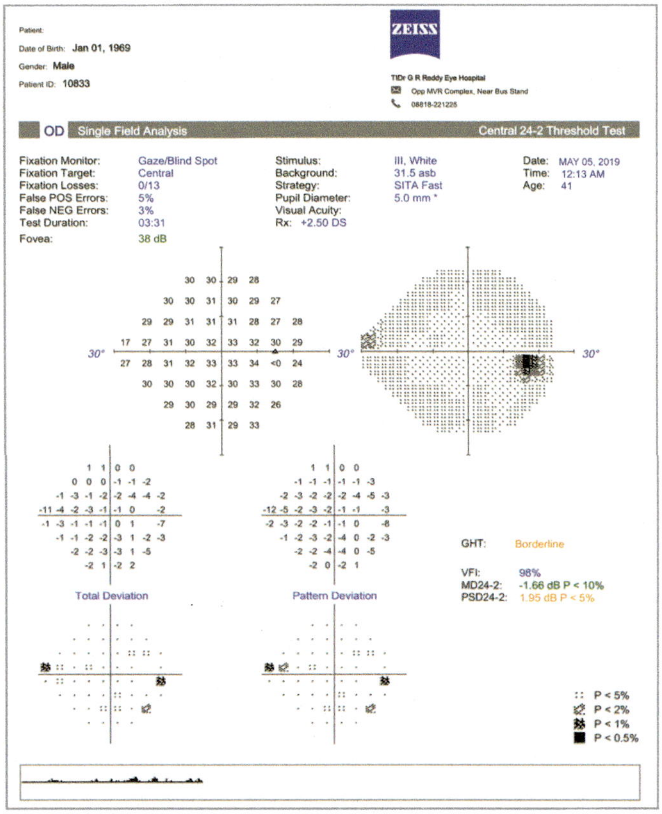

FL 0/13; FP 5%; FN 3%
Fovea 38 dB; GHT-BLL; VFI 98%
MD -1.66 dB P < 10%; PSD 1.95 dB P < 5%

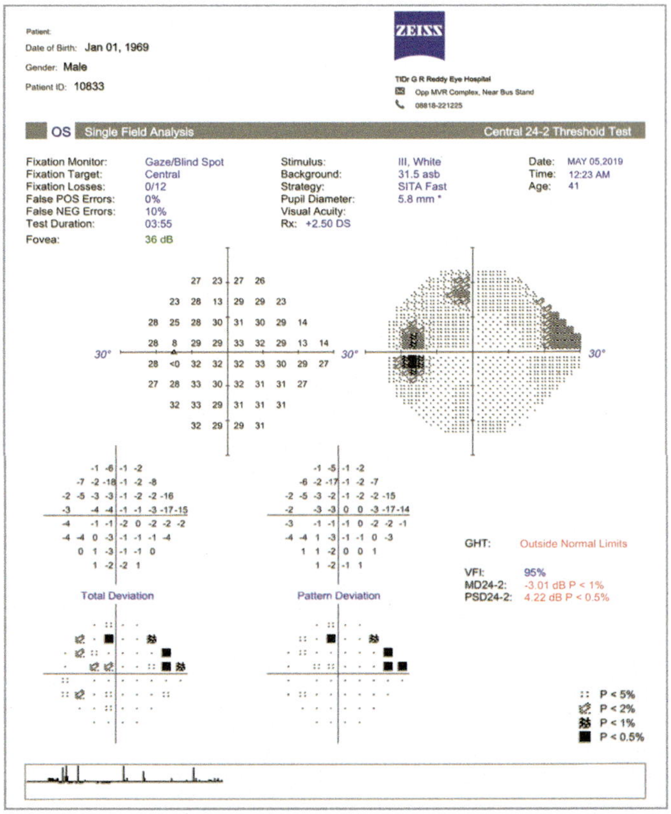

FL 0/12; FP 0%; FN 10%
Fovea 36 dB; GHT-ONL; VFI 95%
MD -3.01 dB P < 1%; PSD 4.22 dB P < 0.5%

Case 3 RE 2019

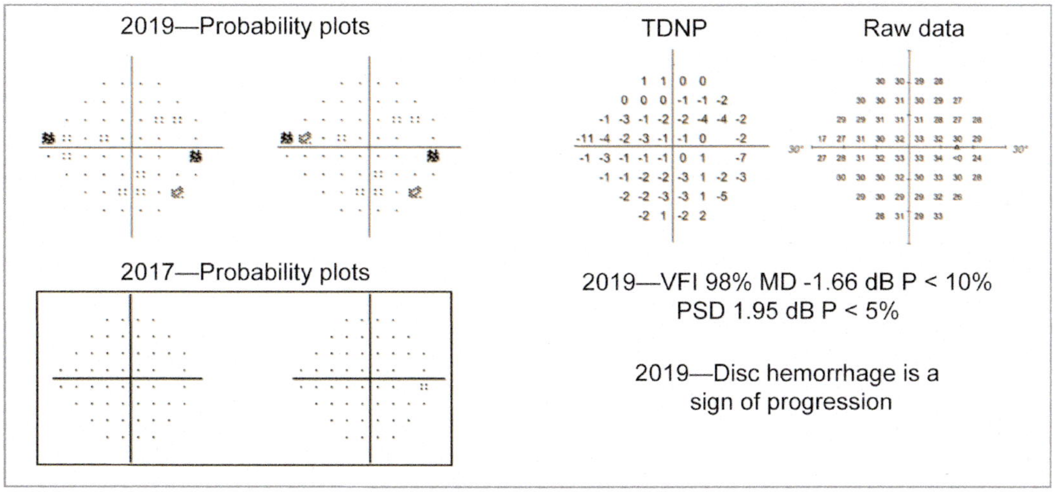

Case 3 LE 2019

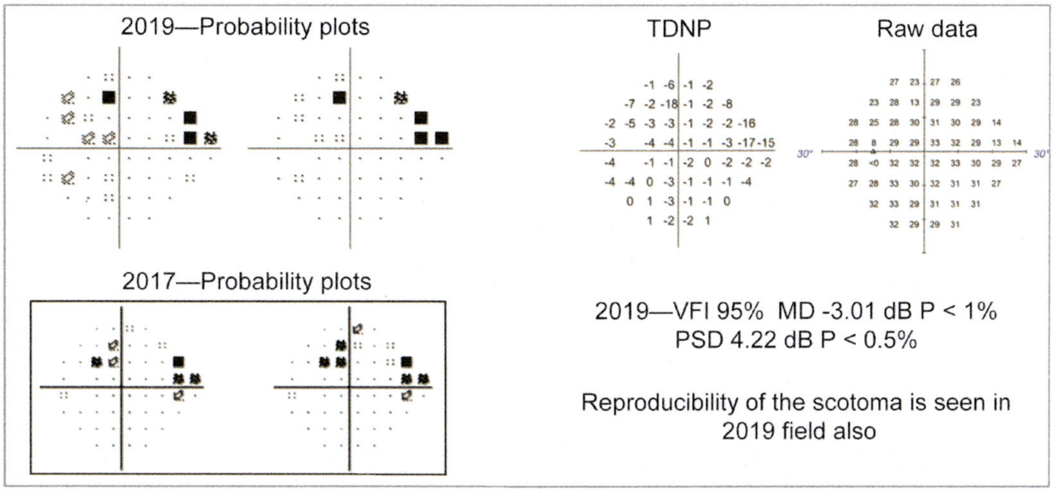

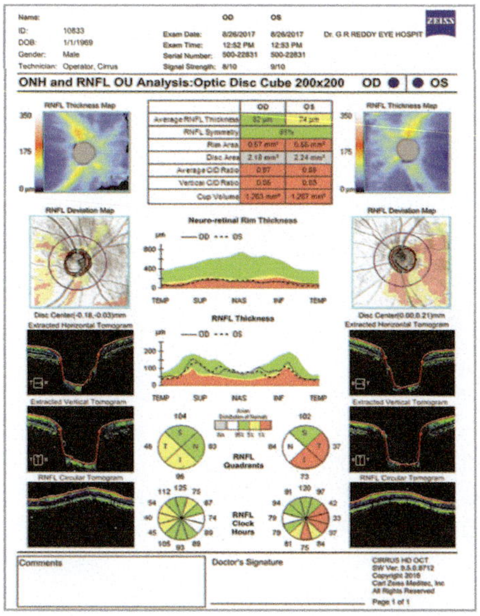

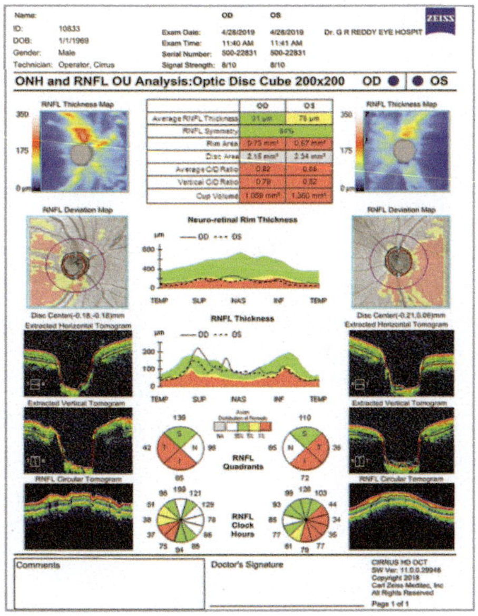

Left eye OCT is not correlating with fundus and fields. OCT is showing more damage which was not seen either in the fundus or in the fields.
Right eye 2017 SFA and OCT are normal. 2019 SFA and OCT are showing the change at the same time. One should note that it is not always true that RNFL defect will be picked by OCT earlier to fields.

Case 4 RE

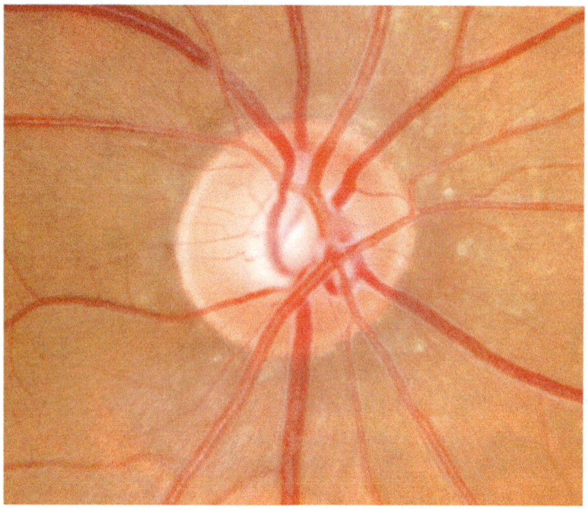

Case 4 LE

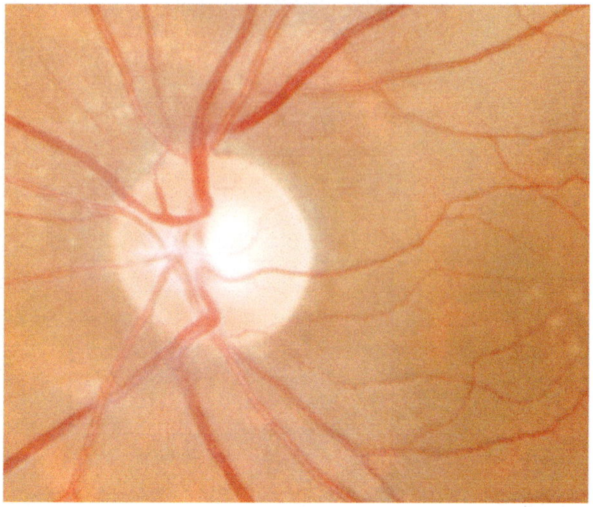

No clue from disc to label it as glaucomatous disc except for C/D disparity between the two eyes.

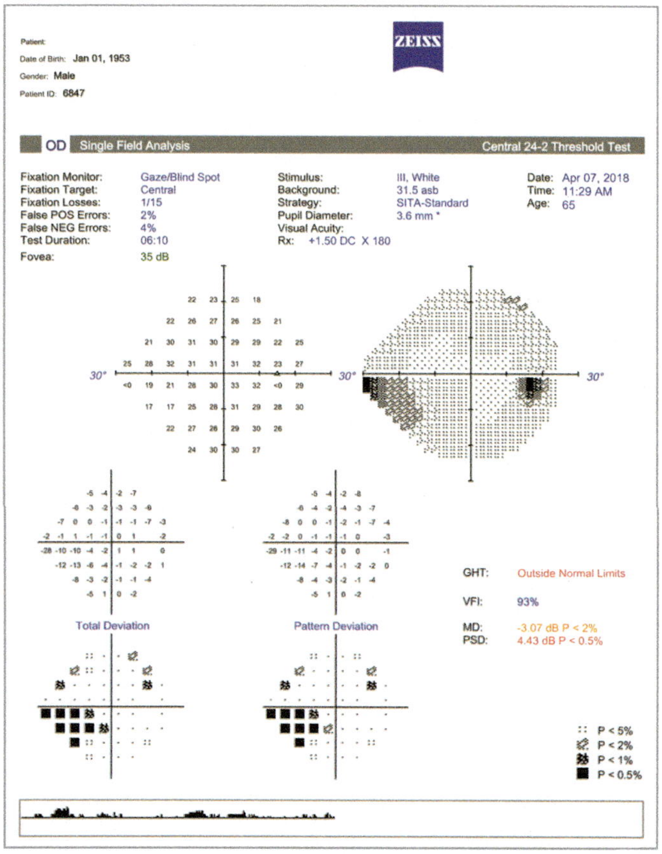

FL 1/15; FP 2%; FN 4%
Fovea 35 dB; GHT-ONL; VFI 93%
MD -3.07 dB P < 2%; PSD 4.43 dB P < 0.5%

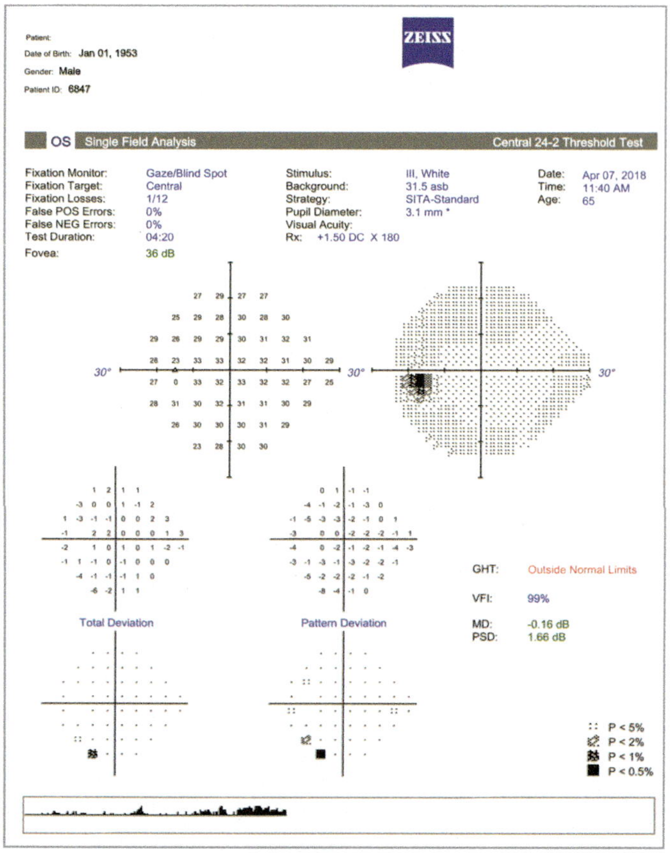

FL 1/12; FP 0%; FN 0%
Fovea 36 dB; GHT-ONL; VFI 99%
MD -0.16 dB; PSD 1.66 dB

Case 4 RE

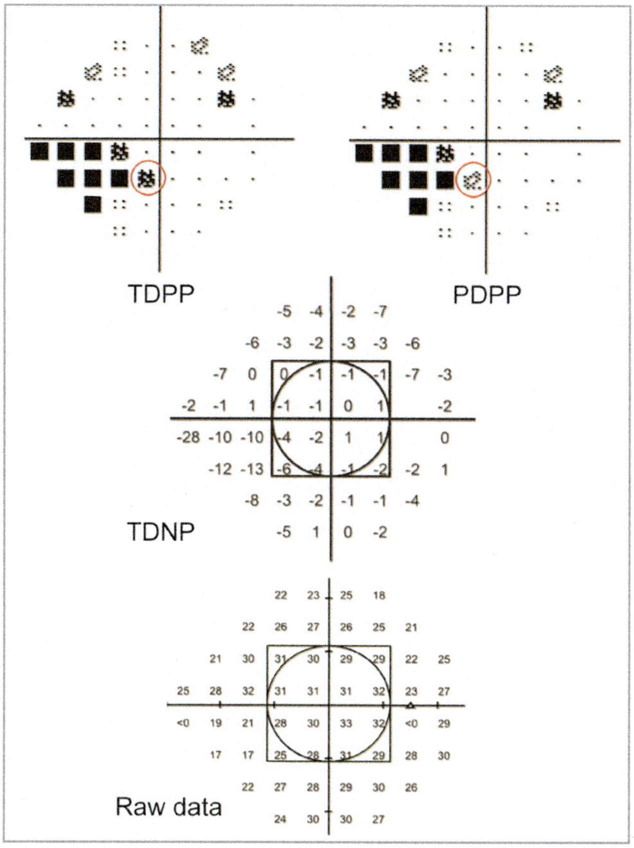

Location and extent of the field defect: Localized scotoma in the lower nasal quadrant in the TDPP. Almost all the points in the field defect are represented by black squares (P < 0.5%). The direction of progression is looking like towards fixation also. In the follow-up tests concentrate on this area.

Depth of the field defect (TDNP): The loss of sensitivity is in the range of -13 dB to -4 dB. MD -3.07 dB P < 2% PSD 4.43 dB P < 0.5%.

We see raw data to know if any of the black square is an absolute scotoma or not. The 27° point in the lower nasal quadrant is showing absolute scotoma. Since it is edge scotoma we can ignore it. The sensitivities of the 16 points in the 10° circle area are good and no need to repeat the test with 10-2 point pattern. Since we noticed the direction of progression could be towards fixation, we have to concentrate on the sensitivities of the points in the 10° circle area in the follow-up fields.

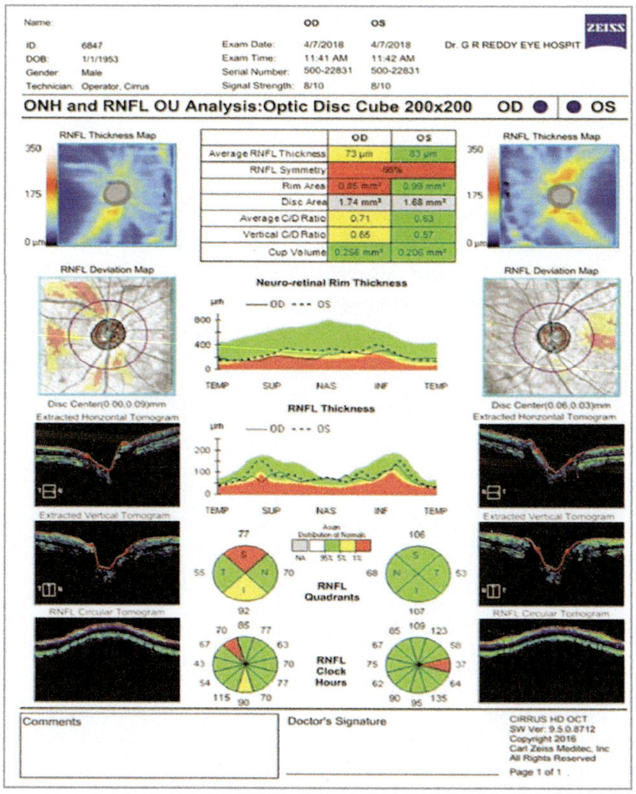

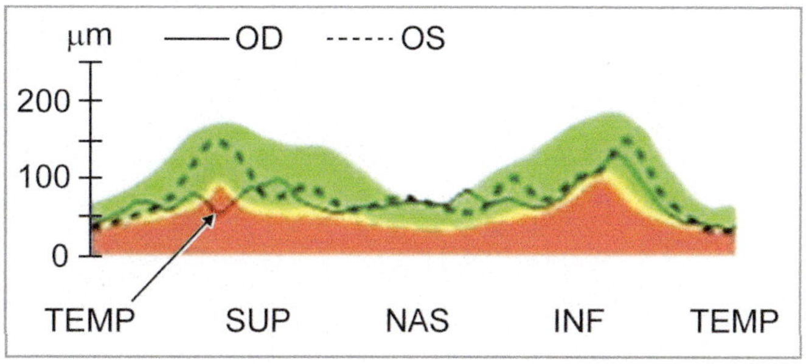

When we diagnose glaucoma on the basis of IOP and probability plots (no clue from fundus to diagnose glaucoma) OCT plays a major role to diagnose glaucoma. In this case OCT and field defect are correlating with each other.

Case 5 RE **Case 5 LE**

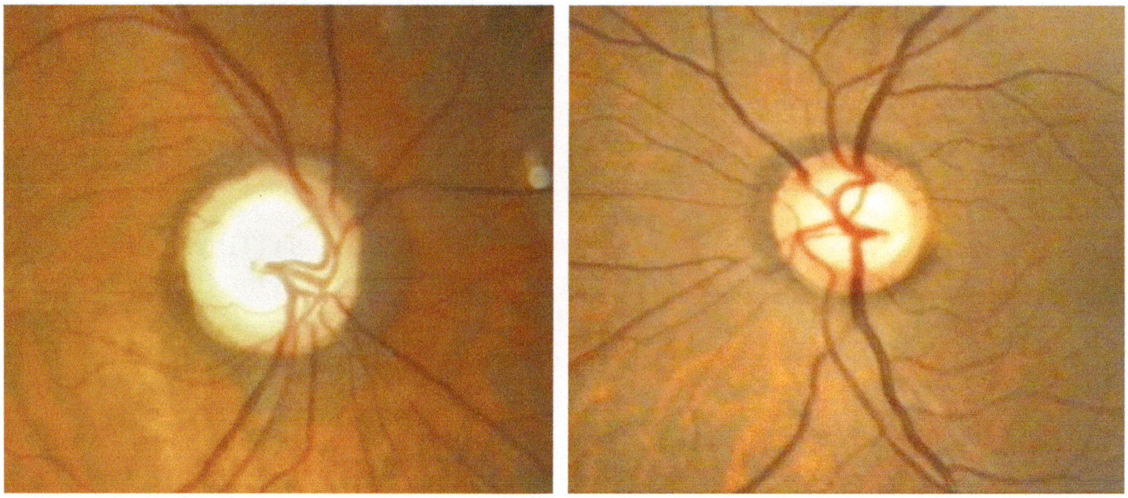

Glaucoma is suspected because of IOP 21 mm Hg. No clue from disc to label it as glaucomatous disc except for C/D disparity in C/D ratio between the two eyes. (Disparity in the size of the disc is also present.)

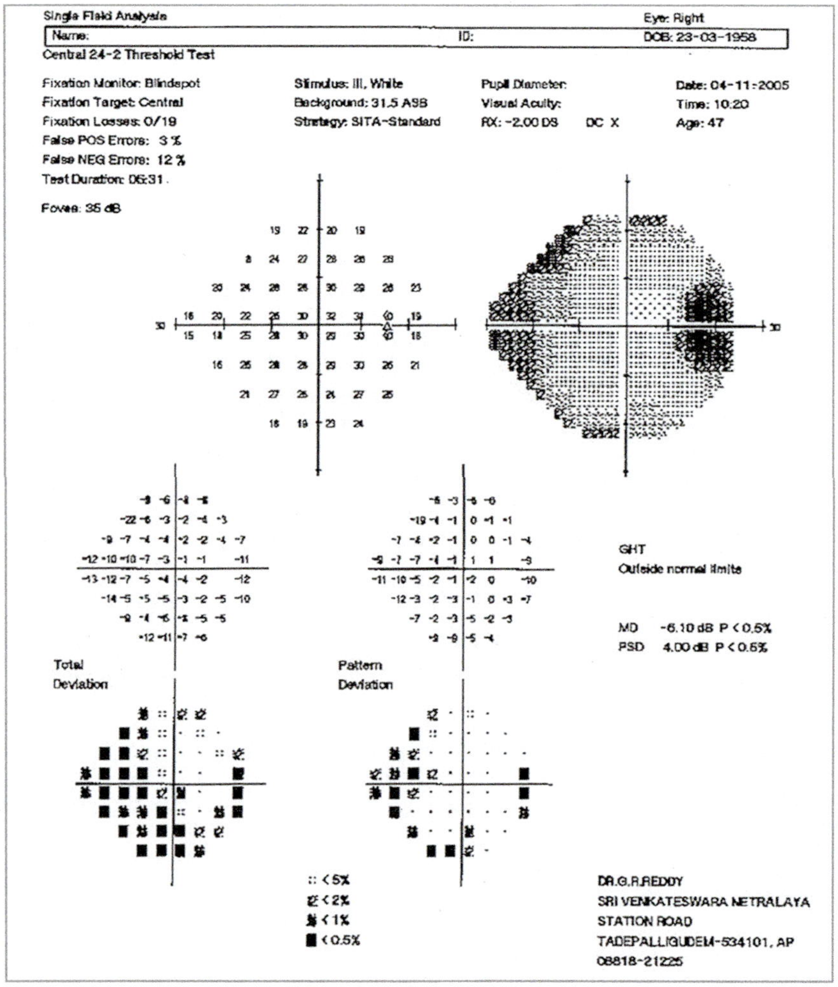

FL 0/19; FP 3%; FN 12%
Fovea 36 dB; GHT-ONL
MD -6.10 dB P < 0.5%
PSD 4.00 dB P < 0.5%

Case 5 RE 2019

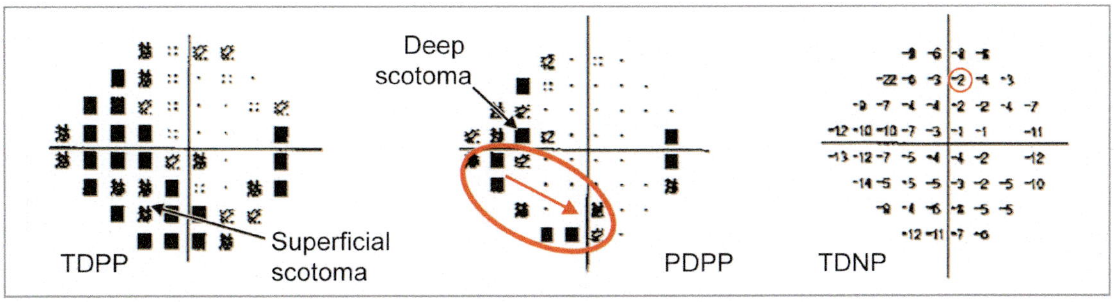

Location and extent of the field defect: Probability plots—the TDPP is showing biarcuate scotoma in the nasal field. Most of the points in the arcuate scotoma are represented by black squares.

The direction of progression: During the conversion of total deviation plots to pattern deviation plots, the superficial scotomas (lower arcuate field defect) are eliminated and the deep scotoma (upper arcuate field defect) are highlighted in the pattern deviation probability plot. From this we can tell that the glaucomatous damage started in the upper nasal quadrant and is progressing towards lower nasal quadrant and towards fixation point.

Depth of the field defect (TDNP) **MD -6.10 dB P < 0.5%.**

Probability plots, PSD and GHT are fulfilling Anderson's criteria to label the localized scotoma as glaucomatous field defect.

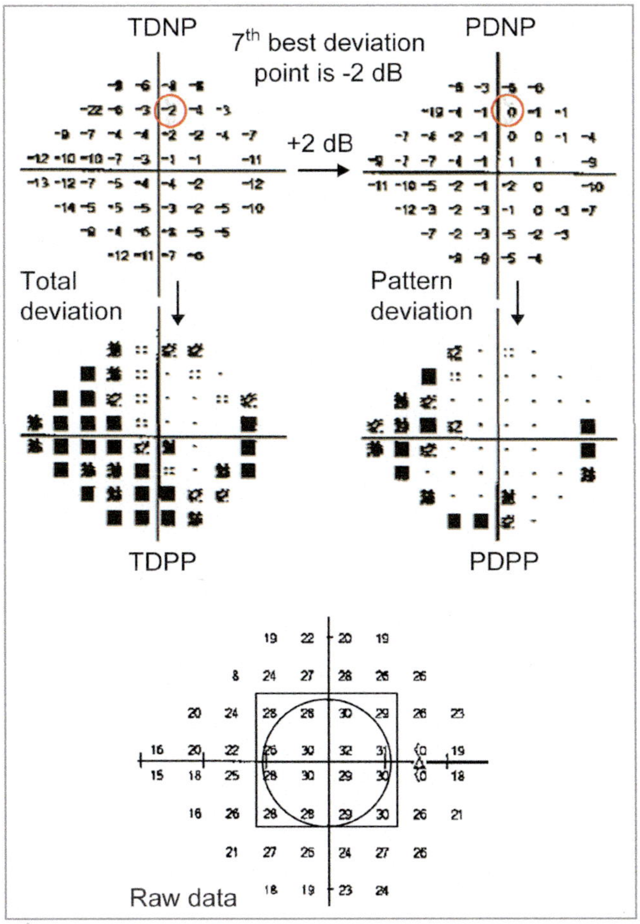

7th best deviation point is -2 dB

By adding 2 dB to all the points in the TDNP only the points in the upper nasal quadrant retained the P value and remaining points became normal (points without P value). During the conversion of total deviation plots to pattern deviation plots, the superficial scotomas (lower arcuate field defect) in localized field defect disappeared in the pattern deviation probability plot. The superficial scotomas represent recent onset field defects and hence they tell direction of progression.

Always see the raw data to know whether any point in the field defect is represented by 0 dB (0 dB in raw data is an absolute scotoma). The loss of sensitivity of the 16 points in the 10° circle area is not severe and hence there is no need to repeat the test with 10-2 point pattern.

Case 5 RE

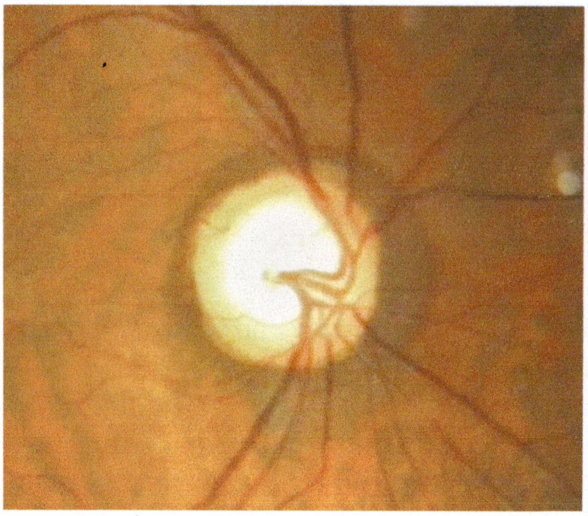

Case 5 LE

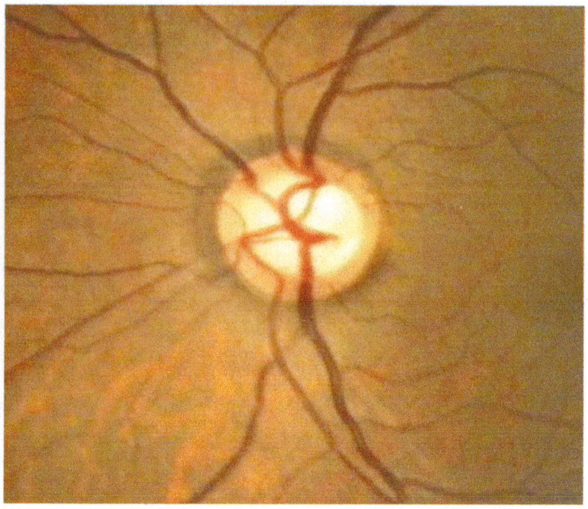

No clue from disc to label it as glaucomatous disc except for C/D disparity in C/D ratio between the two eyes. (Disparity in the size of the disc is also present.)

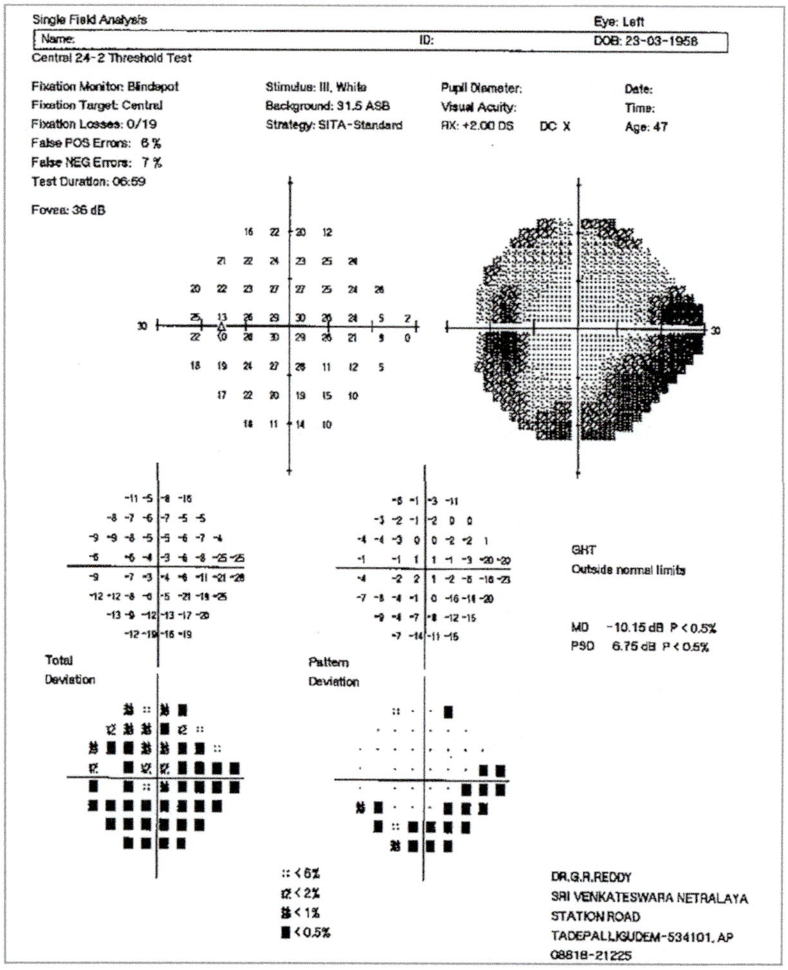

FL 0/19; FP 6%; FN 7%
Fovea 36 dB; GHT-ONL
MD -10.15 dB P < 0.5%
PSD 6.75 dB P < 0.5%

Case 5 LE

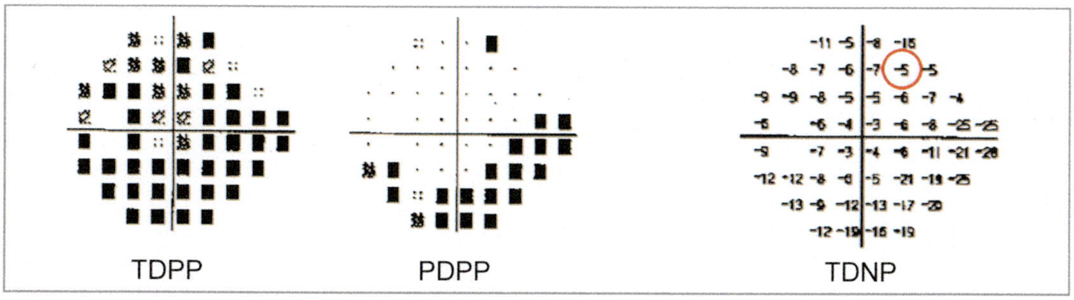

Location and extent of the field defect (Probability plots): The TDPP is showing generalized depression. Most of the points in the lower half of the field and 50% of the points in the upper half of the field are represented by black squares. PDPP is showing a localized scotoma in the lower nasal quadrant in an arcuate pattern and extending to lower temporal quadrant. Since all the points are affected due to glaucoma. From this we can tell that the glaucomatous damage started in the lower nasal quadrant (deep scotoma) quadrant and progressing in all the directions. Since the foveal sensitivity is 36 dB, the generalized depression is not due to cataract.

Depth of the field defect (TDNP)—**MD -10.15 dB P < 0.5%.**

Highest deviation point is -29 dB and the lowest deviation point is -3 dB. So, PSD is high **(PSD 6.75 dB P < 0.5%**).

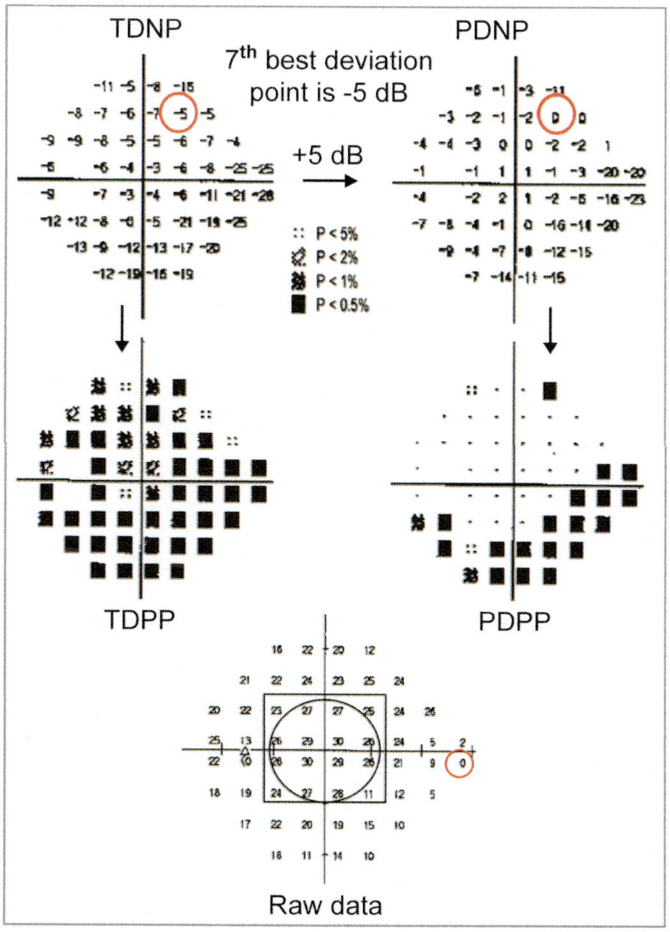

Conversion of total deviation plots to pattern deviation plots

7th best deviation point is -5 dB.

By adding 5 dB to all the points in the TDNP only the points in the lower nasal quadrant retained the P value and remaining points became normal (points without P value). During the conversion of total deviation plots to pattern deviation plots, the superficial scotomas (upper half of the field) in the generalized field defect disappeared in the pattern deviation probability plot. The superficial scotomas represent recent onset field defects and hence indicates the direction of progression.

Only the encircled point is absolute scotoma. So, basically, it is a relative scotoma. The sensitivity of the 16 points in the 10° circle area is good. So we need not repeat the test with 10-2 point pattern.

Case 6 RE

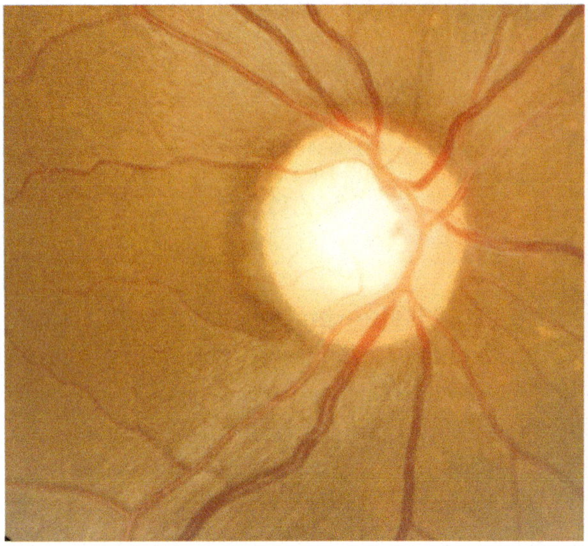

Case 6 LE

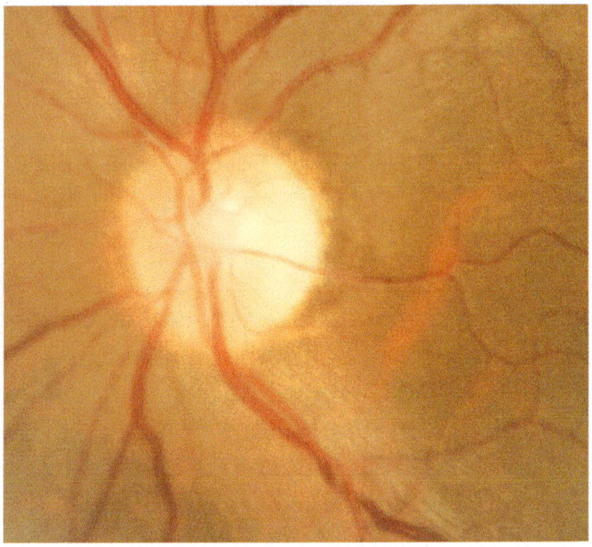

Only clue from disc to label it as glaucomatous disc is C/D disparity in C/D ratio between the two eyes.

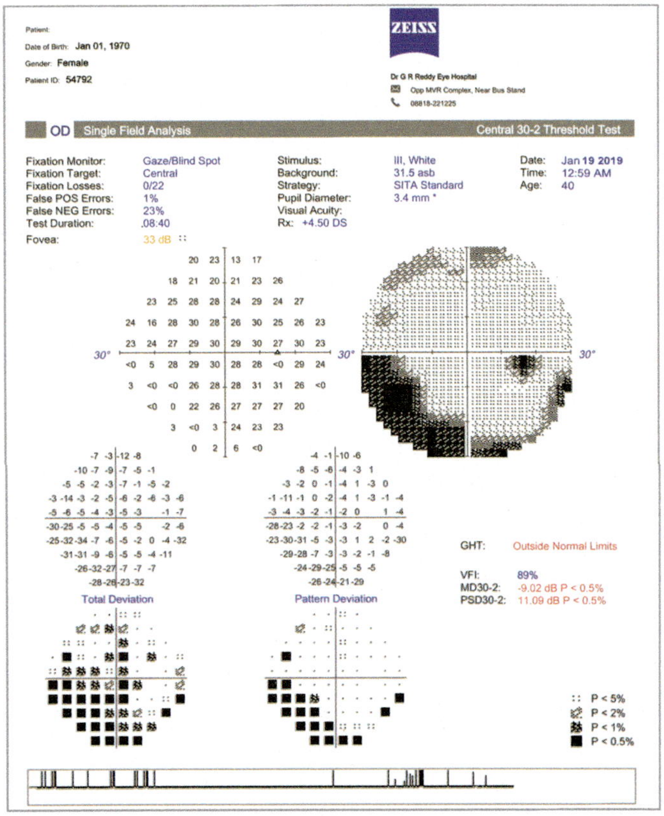

FL 0/22; FP 1%; FN 23%
Fovea 33 dB; GHT-ONL; VFI 89%
MD -9.02 dB P < 0.5%
PSD 11.09 dB P < 0.5%

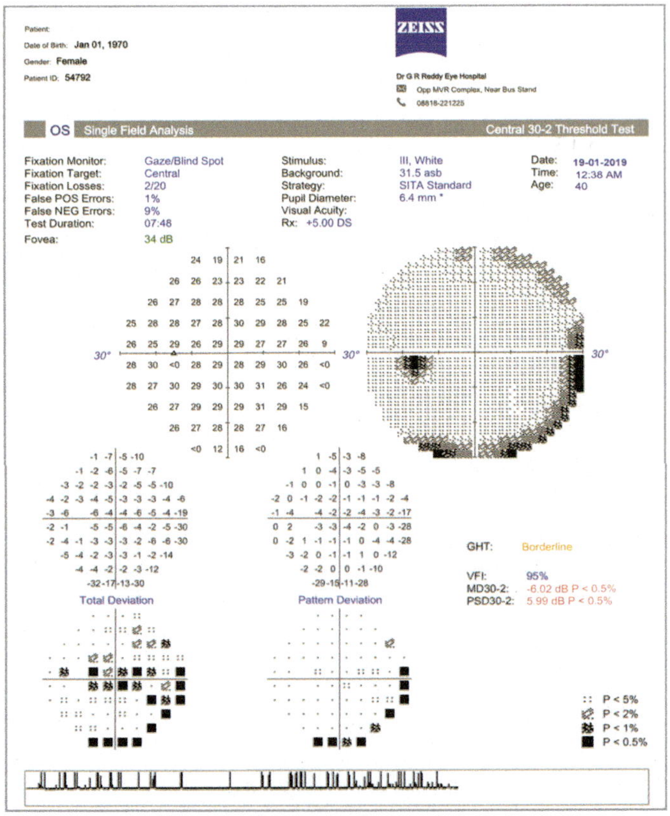

FL 2/20; FP 1%; FN 9%
Fovea 34 dB; GHT Border line; VFI 95%
MD -6.02 dB P < 0.5%
PSD 5.99 dB P < 0.5%

Case 6 RE

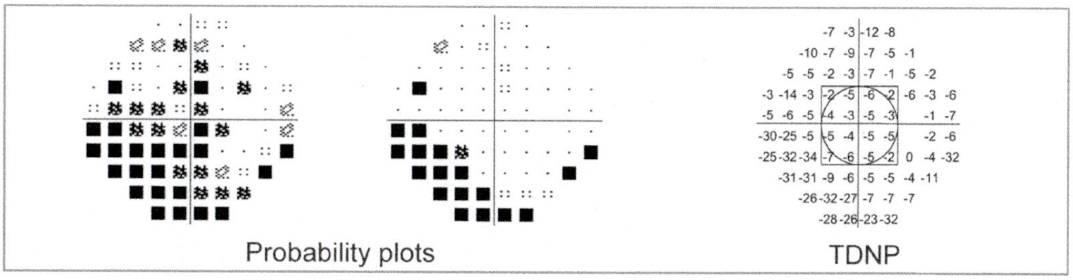

Location and extent of the field defect: Probability plots—TDPP is showing localized scotoma in the lower nasal quadrant of the field extending to both lower temporal quadrant and upper nasal quadrant. Most of the points in the scotoma are represented by back squares.

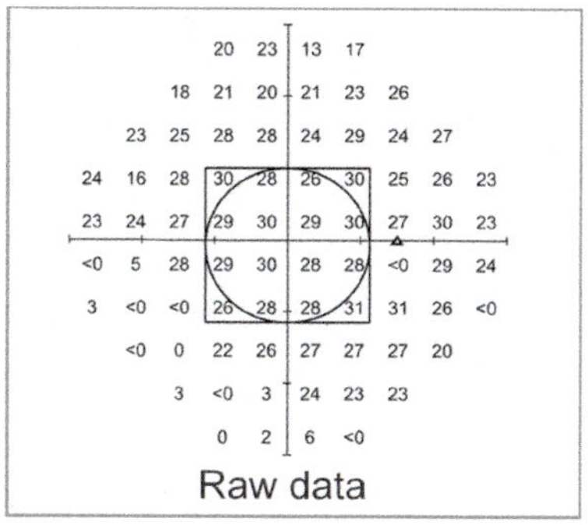

The direction of progression: During the conversion of total deviation plots to pattern deviation plots, the superficial scotomas are eliminated and the deep scotomas (lower arcuate field defect) are highlighted in the pattern deviation probability plot. Deep scotomas tell the location from where the ganglion cell damage started. The ganglion cell damage started in the lower nasal quadrant (deep scotoma) superficial scotomas which disappeared in the PDPP tells the direction of progression. The direction of progression in this case is towards fixation also.

TDNP: We know the depth of the scotoma from TDNP. The loss of sensitivity is more than 25 dB at most of the points in the lower nasal quadrant (Deep scotomas or black squares in the PPDP) and at most of the remaining points, the loss of sensitivity is between 5 dB to 15 dB; MD index is -9.02 dB P < 0.5%.

The foveal sensitivity is 33 dB. The sensitivity at 8 points is 0 dB (absolute scotoma). The sensitivities of the 16 points in the 10° circle area are good. So there is no need to repeat the test with 10-2 point pattern. As the extent, depth is significant and scotoma is also progressing towards fixation, we have to aim for low target IOP.

Case 6 LE

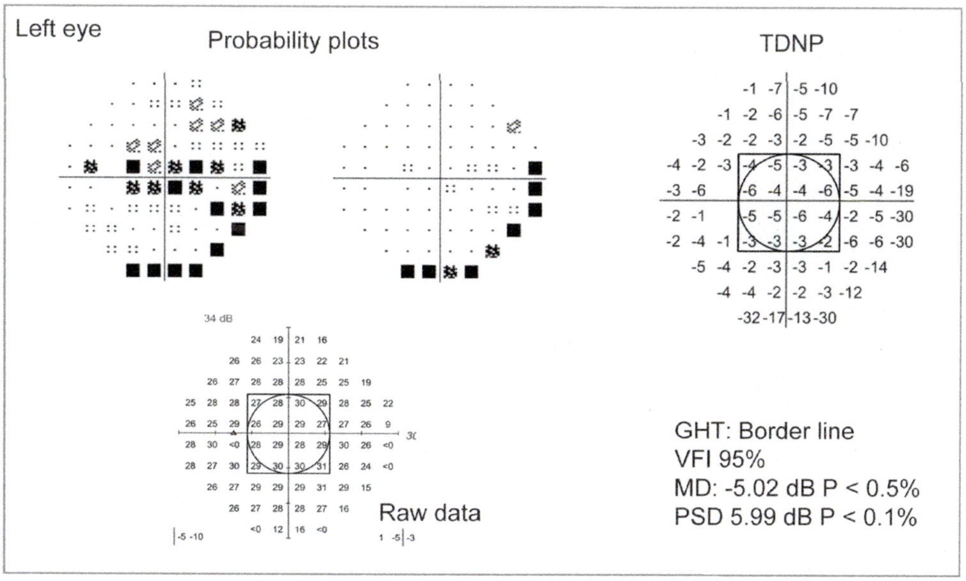

Case 6 RE **Case 6 LE**

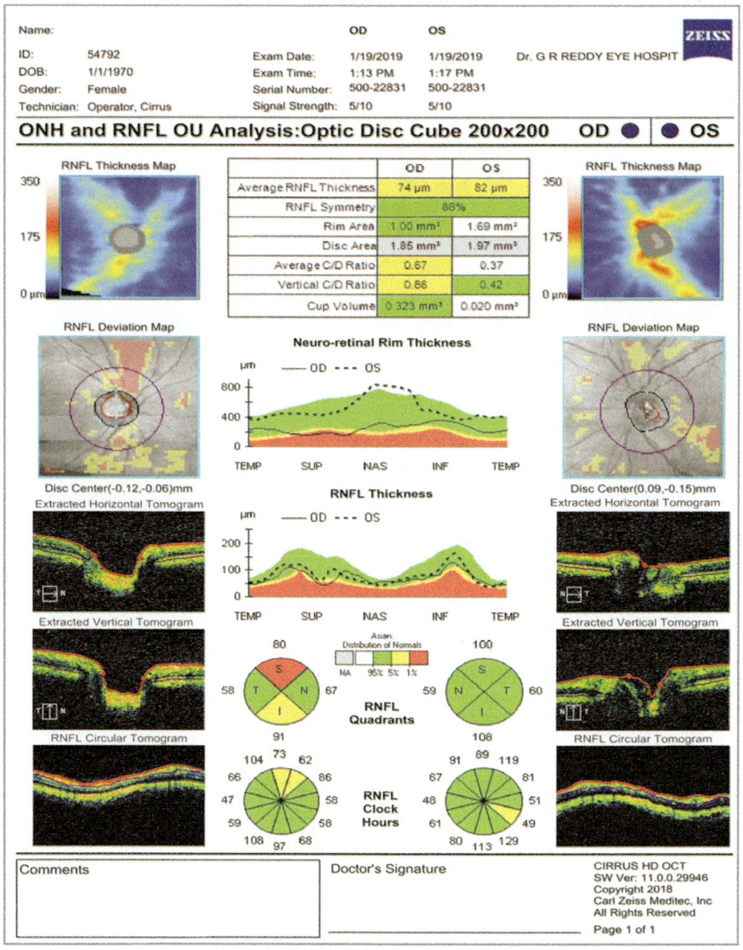

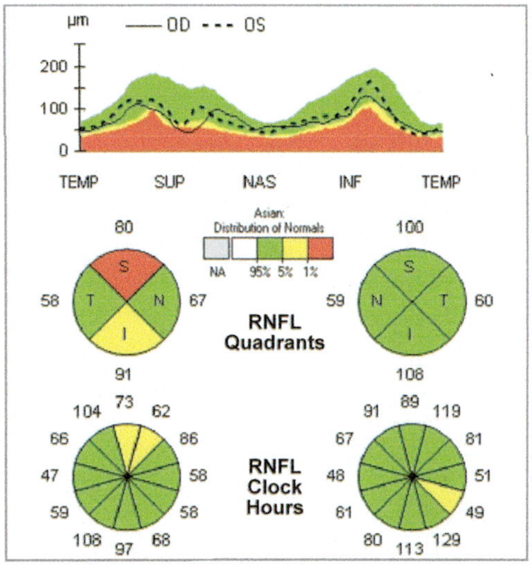

When we diagnose glaucoma on the basis of IOP and probability plots (No clue from fundus to diagnose glaucoma). OCT plays a major role to diagnose glaucoma.

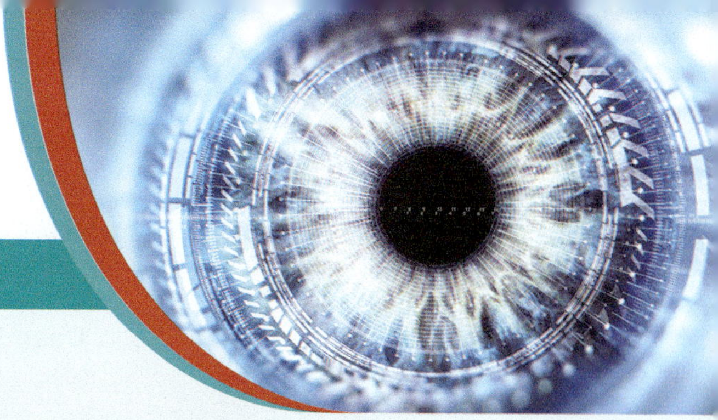

CHAPTER

6B

Interpretation of Single Field Analysis Printouts of Type 1 Primary Open-angle Glaucoma

TYPE 1 PRIMARY OPEN-ANGLE GLAUCOMA: FIELD DEFECT DOMINANT OUTSIDE 10° CIRCLE AREA WITH OR WITHOUT INVOLVING 10° CIRCLE AREA

I will be presenting 6 cases of **clinically established** open-angle glaucomas (field defect outside 10° circle with or without involving 10° circle area). In all these cases there are definite clinical signs from the fundus as definite notch or retinal nerve fiber layer (RNFL) defect or disc hemorrhage and raised intraocular pressure (IOP) in most of the cases. The aim of visual fields in this group is to set the target IOP to arrest progression and prevention of onset of new field defects starting elsewhere. The direction of the RNFL defect gives us a clue regarding the location of the field defect. In some cases the direction of RNFL defect is towards fixation (macula) and in some cases the direction is away from fixation. Another most important point to be remembered is even relative scotomas can be associated with RNFL defect. In other words, absolute scotomas are not required to produce RNFL defect.

Case 7 Disc hemorrhage

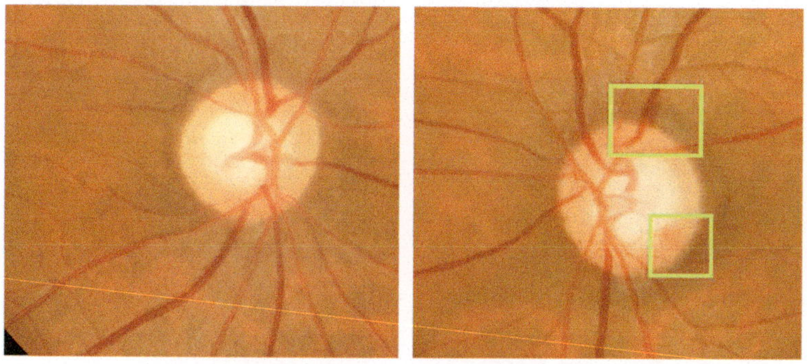

Case 8 RNFL defect in one eye

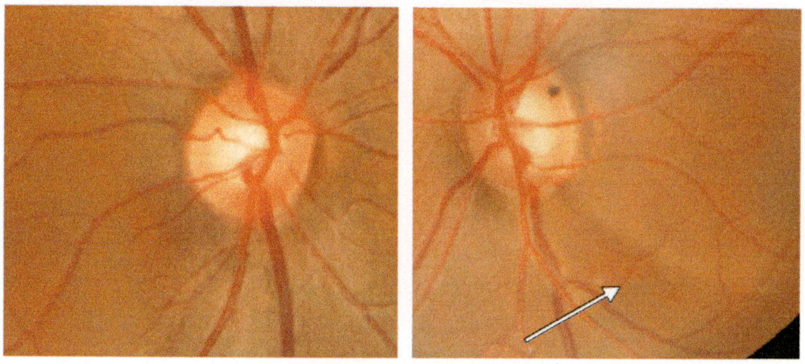

Case 9 RNFL defect in both the eyes

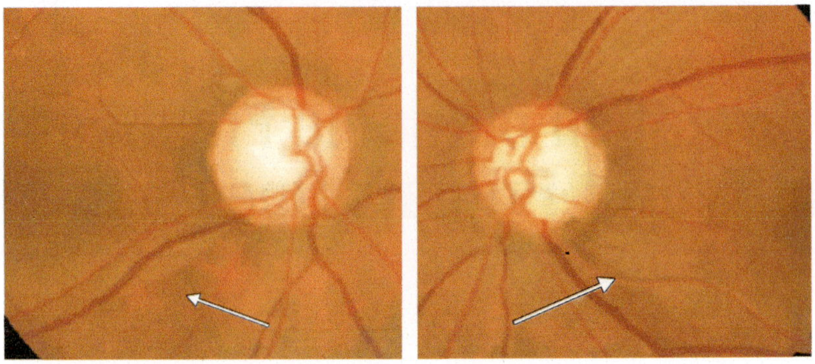

Case 10 RNFL defect in both the eyes

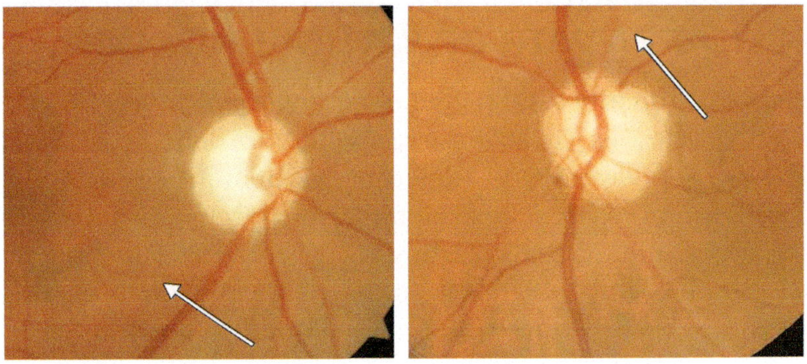

Case 11 RNFL defect in both the eyes

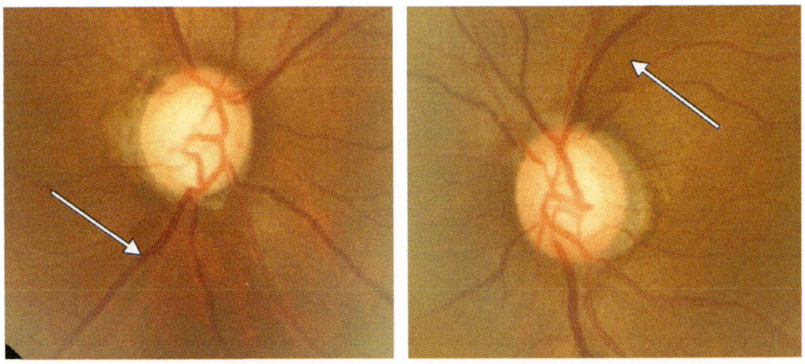

Case 12 RNFL defect in both the eyes

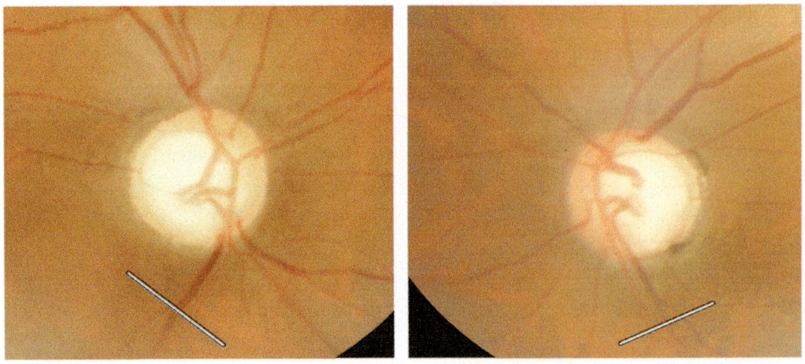

Case 7 RE **Case 7 LE**

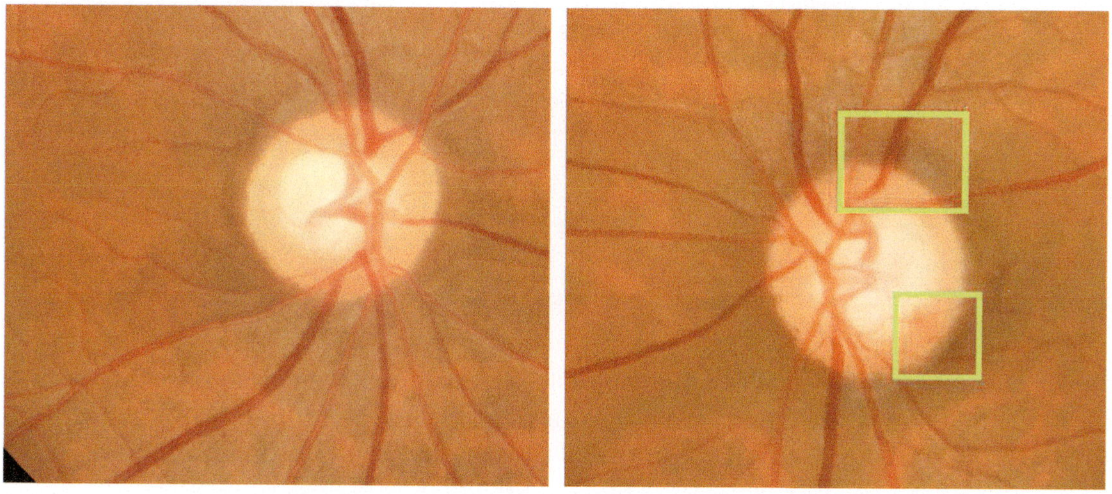

Left eye: Disc hemorrhage is the only clue to suspect glaucoma.

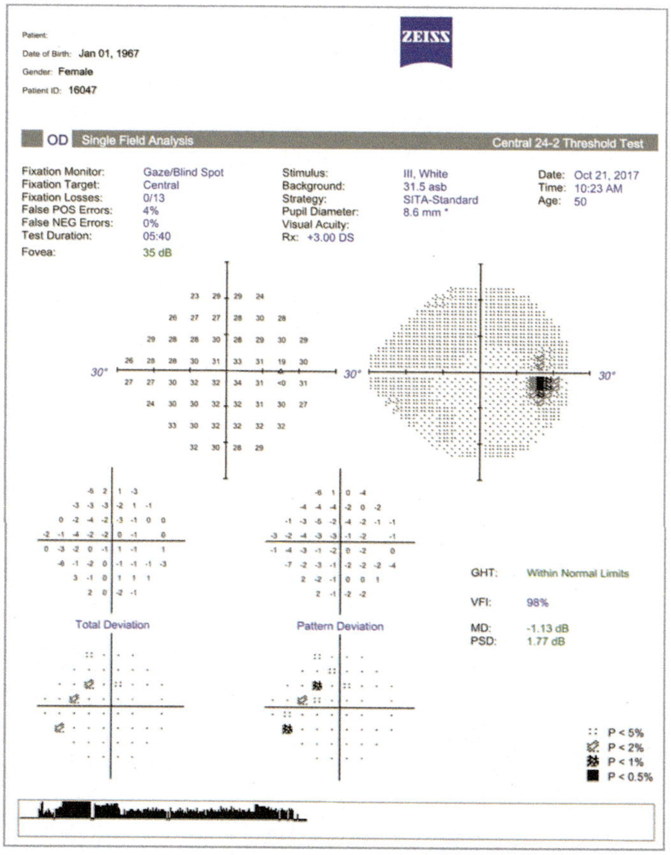

FL 0/13; FP 4%; FN 0%
Fovea 35 dB; GHT-WNL; VFI 98%
MD -1.13 dB; PSD 1.77 dB

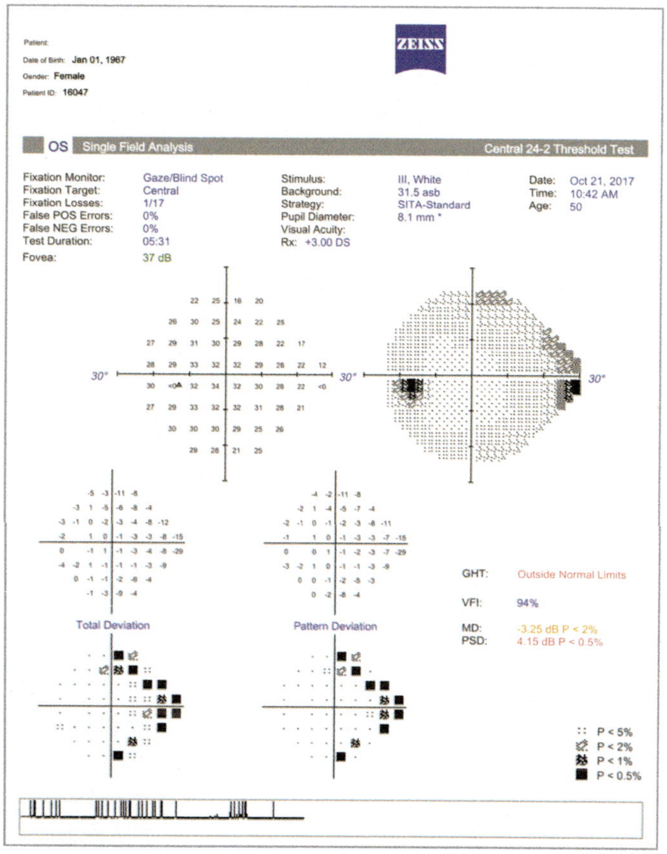

FL 1/17; FP 0%; FN 0%
Fovea 37 dB; GHT-ONL; VFI 94%
MD -3.25 dB P < 2%; PSD 4.15 dB P < 0.5%

Case 7 LE

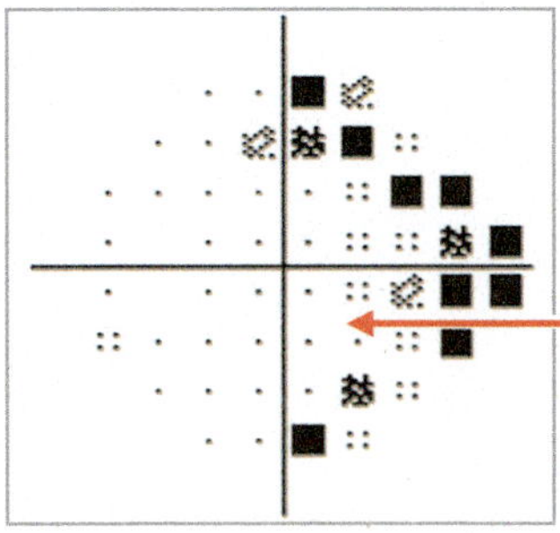

TDPP

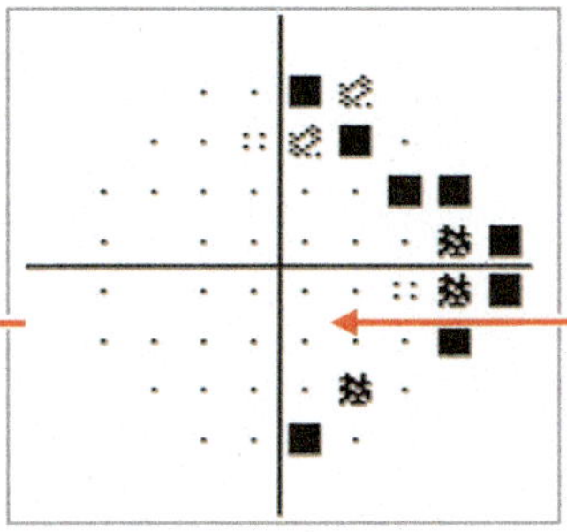

PDPP

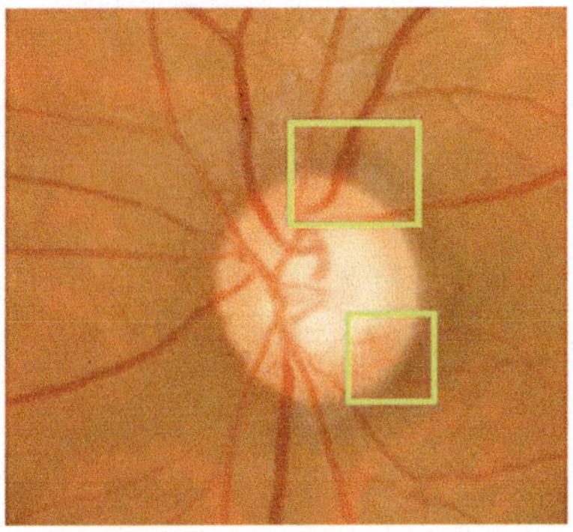

Location and extent of the field defect: Probability plots—Biarcuate scotoma in the nasal half of the field. Most of the points in the field are represented by black squares and both the probability plots are almost looking similar because the 7th best deviation point is normal (0 deviation from normative data).

Direction of progression: Normally the deep scotomas indicate the location from where the disease process started and the superficial scotomas indicate the recent origin field defects. By identifying the recent origin field defects we will be knowing the direction of progression. During the conversion of total deviation plots to pattern deviation plots, some points retain their P < 0.5% and some points change their P values to P < 1%, P < 2%, P < 5% or to without P value in the PDPP. So from the probability plot it is evident that the disease process started as a nasal step and is mainly progressing in an upper arcuate pattern and also towards fixation. This is very important information to set the target IOP. As there is an indication that the direction of progression is towards fixation also, we should concentrate on the 16 points in the 10° circle area in the raw data of follow up fields.

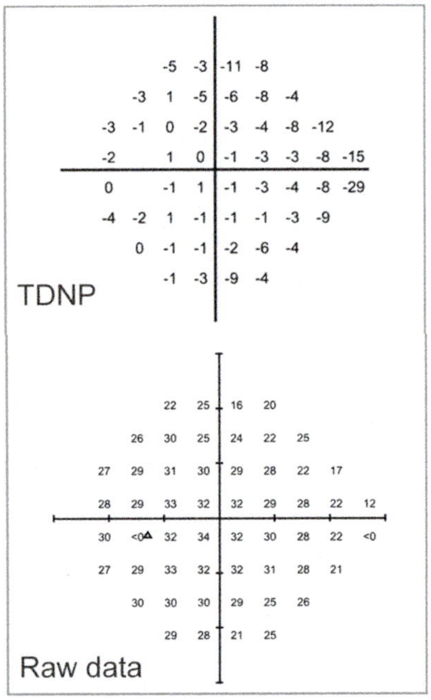

TDNP—(Depth of the scotoma): The loss of sensitivity is around 8 dB at most of the points in the scotoma. MD -3.25 dB P < 2%, PSD 4.15 dB P < 0.5 % and GHT are fulfilling Anderson's criteria to label the localized scotoma as glaucomatous field defect. Optical coherence tomography (OCT) is correlating with the field defect and fundus.

There is no absolute scotoma in the raw data. So the localized scotoma is a relative scotoma.

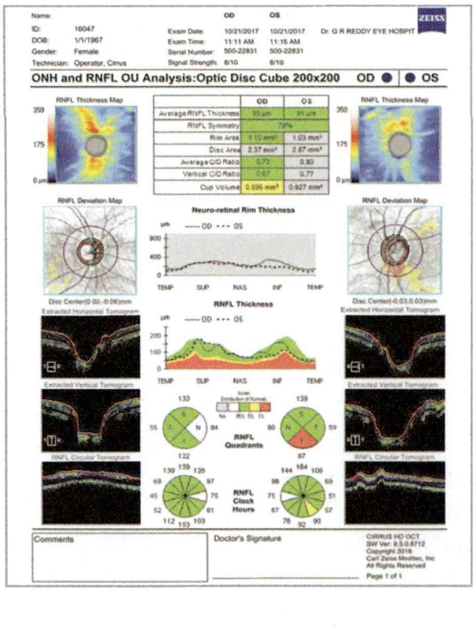

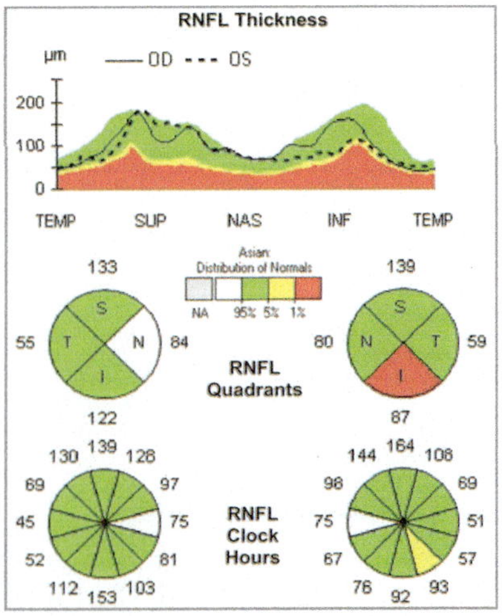

OCT is correlating with fundus and the field defect.

Case 8 RE **Case 8 LE**

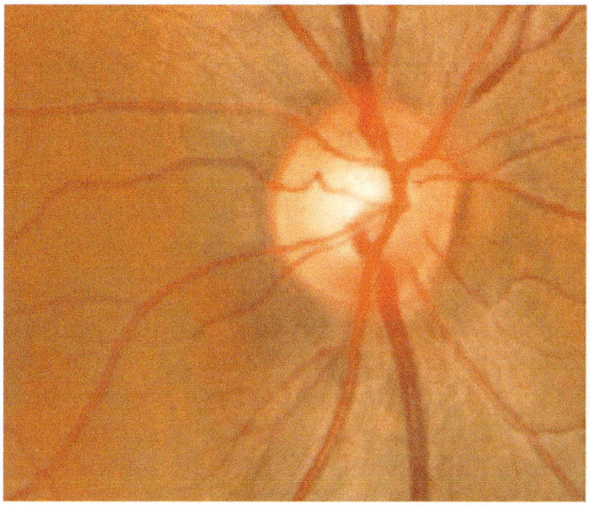

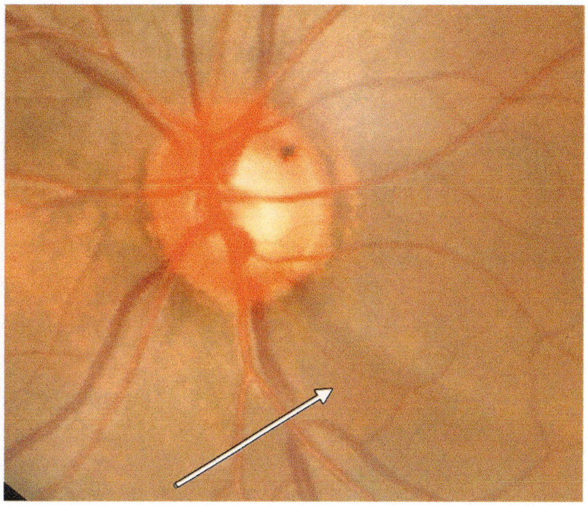

RNFL defect in left eye.

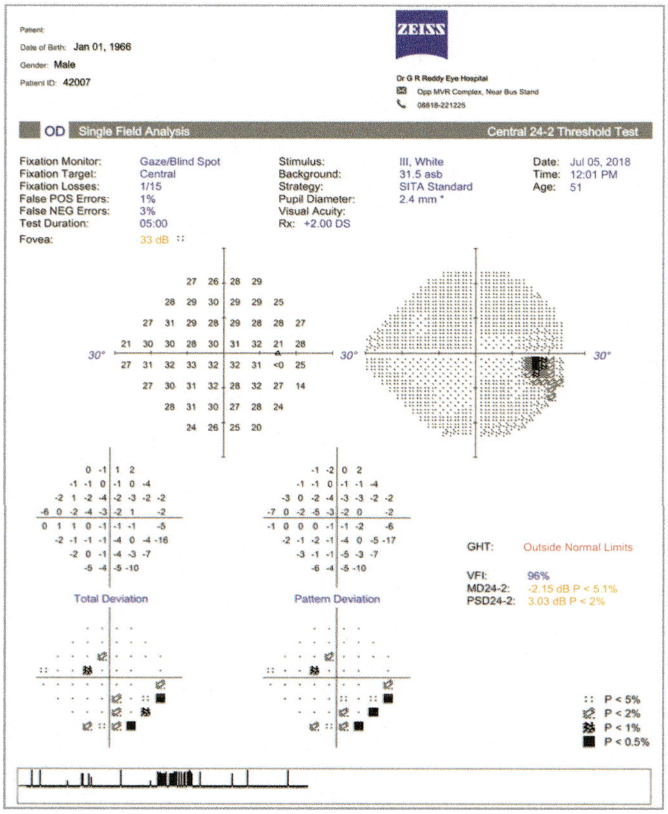

FL 1/15; FP 1%; FN 3%
Fovea 33 dB; GHT-ONL; VFI 96%
MD -2.15 dB P < 5.1%; PSD 3.03 dB P < 2%

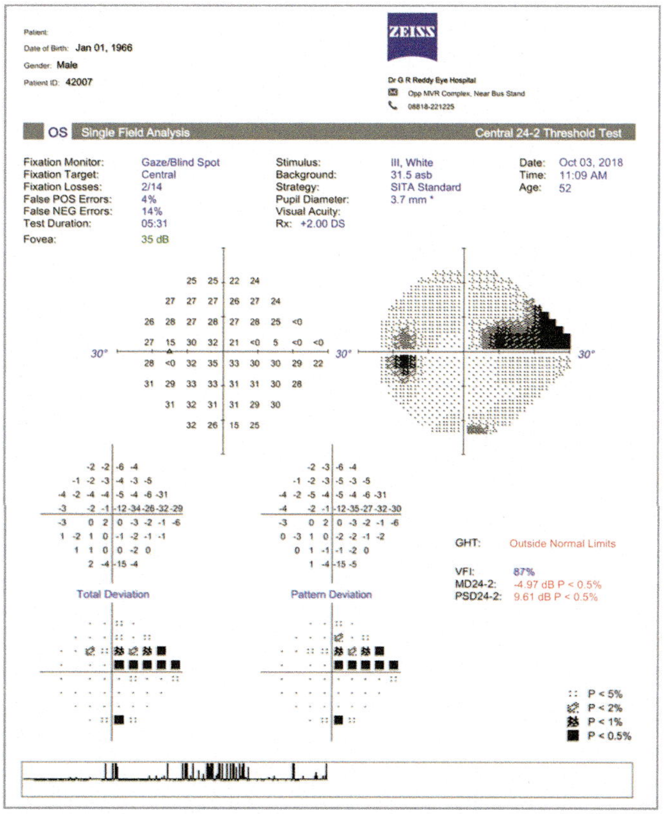

FL 2/14; FP 4%; FN 14%
Fovea 35 dB; GHT-ONL; VFI 87%
MD -4.97 dB P < 0.5%; PSD 9.61 dB P < 0.5%

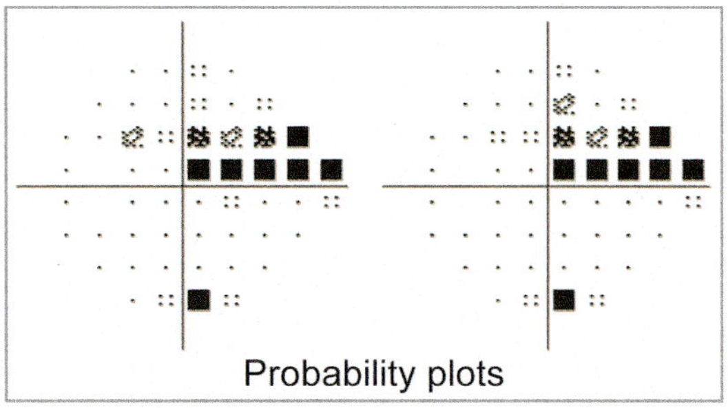

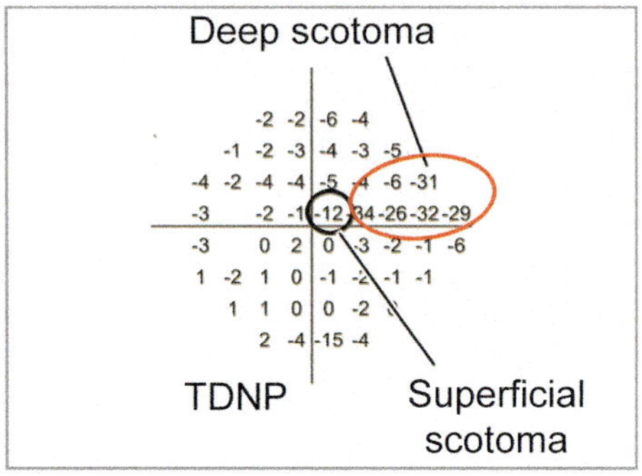

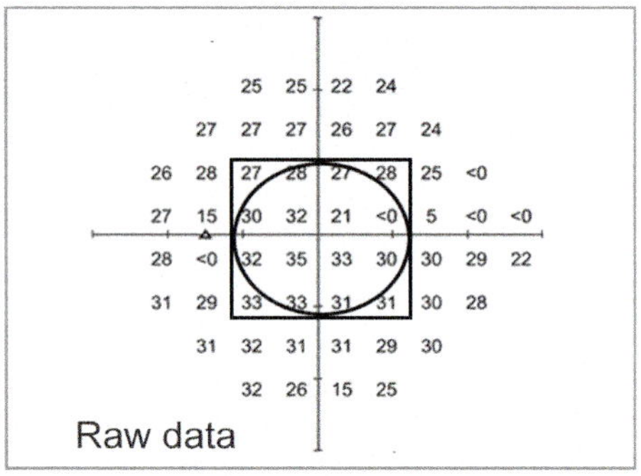

Case 8 LE

Location, extent and direction of progression of the field defect: Localized scotoma in the upper nasal quadrant with most of the points are represented by P < 0.5% (black square). Both the probability plots are looking similar because the 7th best deviation point of TDNP is (0) deviation from normative data. When both probability plots look similar and all points are represented by black squares, it is difficult to tell the direction of progression from the probability plots. Then we have to take the help of TDNP to know the direction of progression.

TDNP (direction of progression): From the TDNP it is very clear that the field defect started outside 10° circle area and is progressing towards fixation because the loss of sensitivity at the points outside 10° circle around 30 dB and the loss of sensitivity at 3° nasal point is 12 dB. So we have to correlate both the probability plots and TDNP to know the direction of progression of the field defect. The direction of progression of the field defect towards fixation is not a good sign. We have to aim for low target IOP.

Depth of the scotoma: Few points have loss of sensitivity around 30 dB and at most of the points the loss of sensitivity is < 5 dB. **PSD 9.61 dB P < 0.5% and** MD index -4.97 dB P < 0.5%.

Foveal sensitivity and raw data: Foveal sensitivity is 35 dB and absolute scotomas (<0) are seen at three points in the localized scotoma (<0) in raw data represents absolute scotoma. There is one absolute scotoma among the 16 points in the 10°circle area. So we should repeat the test with 10-2 point pattern to know the sensitivity of the points in the macular area.

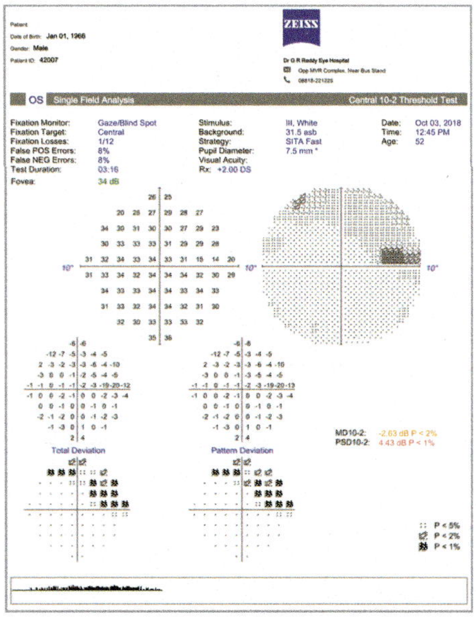

10-2 point pattern

In this case though the MD index is -4.97 dB P < 0.5%, the IOP is causing absolute scotomas and direction of progression is towards fixation and keeping the age of the patient (52 year) in mind, we have to aim for low target IOP.

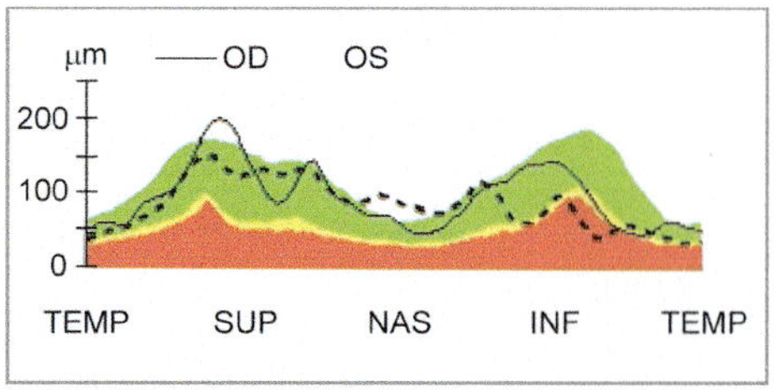

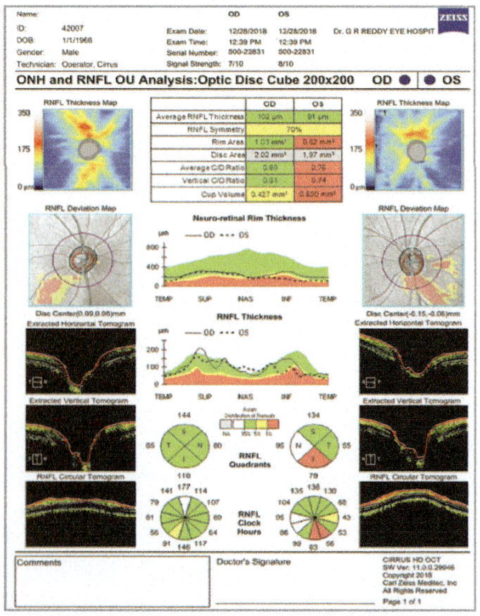

OCT is correlating to the fundus and field defect.

Case 9 RE

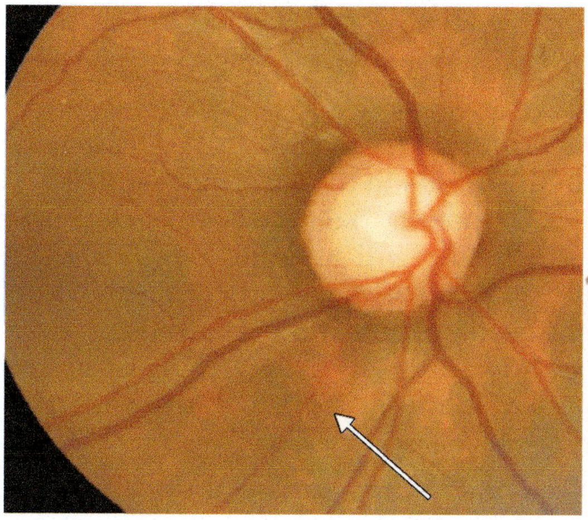

Case 9 LE

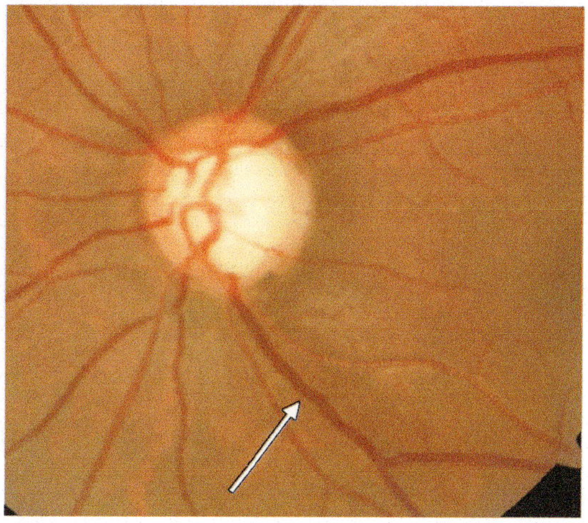

RNFL defect in both the eyes.

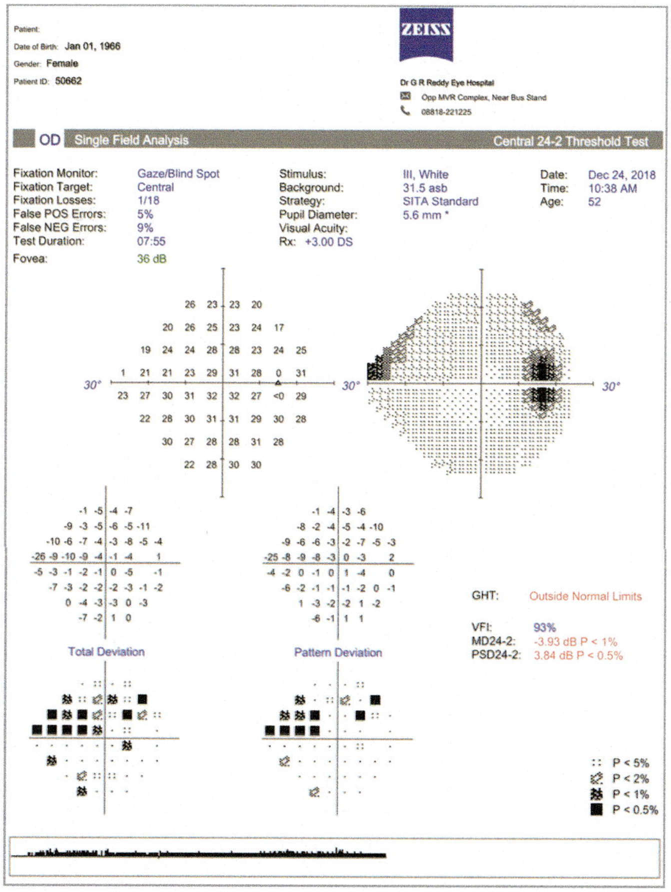

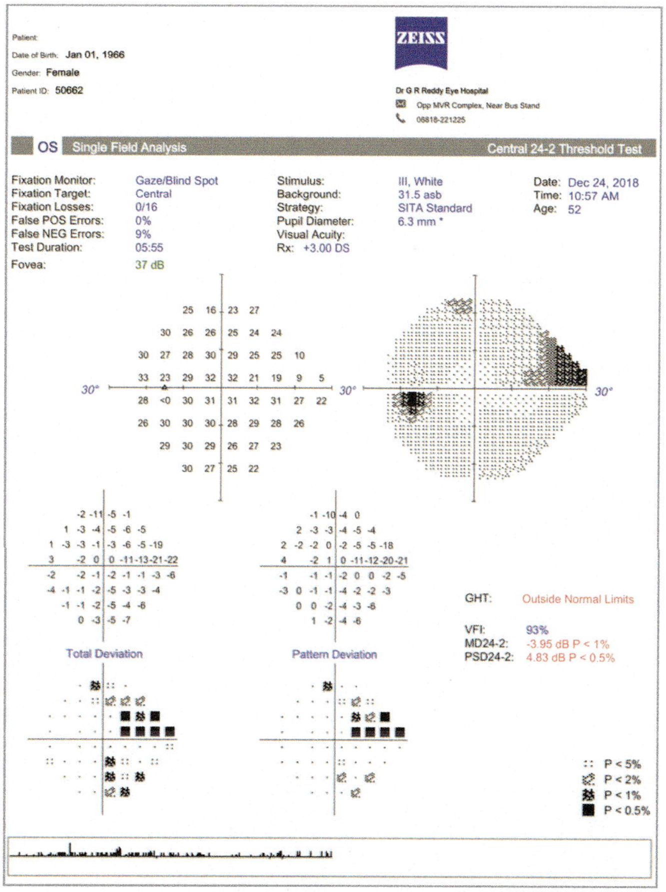

FL 1/18; FP 5%; FN 9%
Fovea 36 dB; GHT-ONL; VFI 93%
MD -3.93 dB P < 1%; PSD 3.84 dB P < 0.5%

FL 0/16; FP 0%; FN 9%
Fovea 37 dB; GHT-ONL; VFI 93%
MD -3.95 dB P < 1%; PSD 4.83 dB P < 0.5%

Case 9 RE

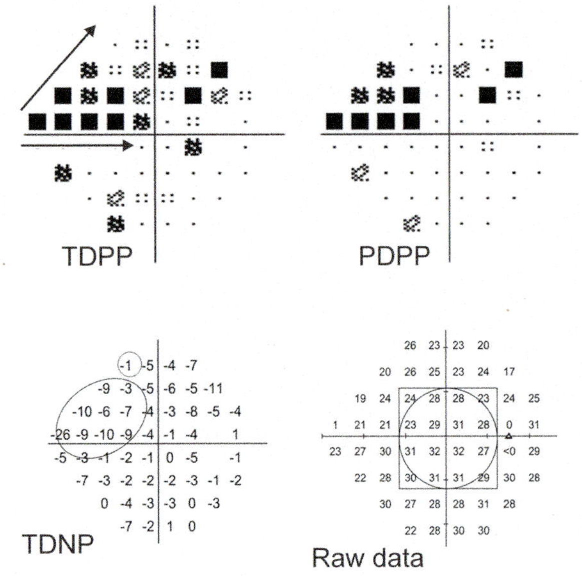

Location, extent and direction of progression of the field defect: Localized scotoma in the upper nasal quadrant and it is progressing upwards and towards fixation.

TDNP (Depth of the scotoma): The loss of sensitivity at most of the points in the localized scotoma is around 10 dB. The MD index is -3.93 dB P < 1%. In localized scotomas MD index value will not represent the average of the deviation values of the points of the field defect, but it gives the average of the deviation values of all the 54 points (24-2 point pattern) in the TDNP. This is the reason why MD index value is always less than the actual depth of the field defect.

The localized scotoma is a relative scotoma. Note that a relative field defect is associated with RNFL defect. The sensitivity values of the 16 points are good in 10° area and there is no need to repeat the test with 10-2 point pattern.

Case 9 LE

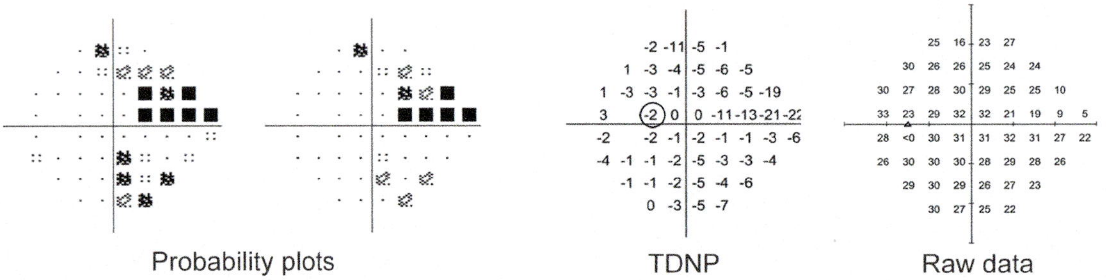

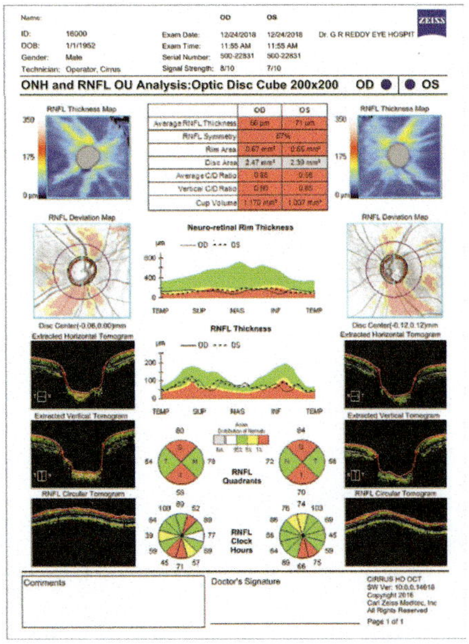

Location, extent and direction of progression of the field defect: Localized scotoma in the upper nasal quadrant with more than 50% of the points are represented by black squares (P < 0.5%).

The most alarming point in this field chart is that the field defect is progressing towards fixation. The loss of sensitivity at the point 9° from the vertical axis and 3° away from horizontal axis in the upper nasal quadrant is 11 dB. It indicates the progression of the field defect is also towards fixation point. In the follow-up fields we have to concentrate on this area. The MD index is -3.95 dB P < 1%.

Target IOP: Though the field defect is a relative scotoma, confined to one quadrant and MD index is -3.93 dB P < 1% we have to aim for low target IOP as the field defect is progressing towards fixation.

OCT is correlating to the fundus and field defect.

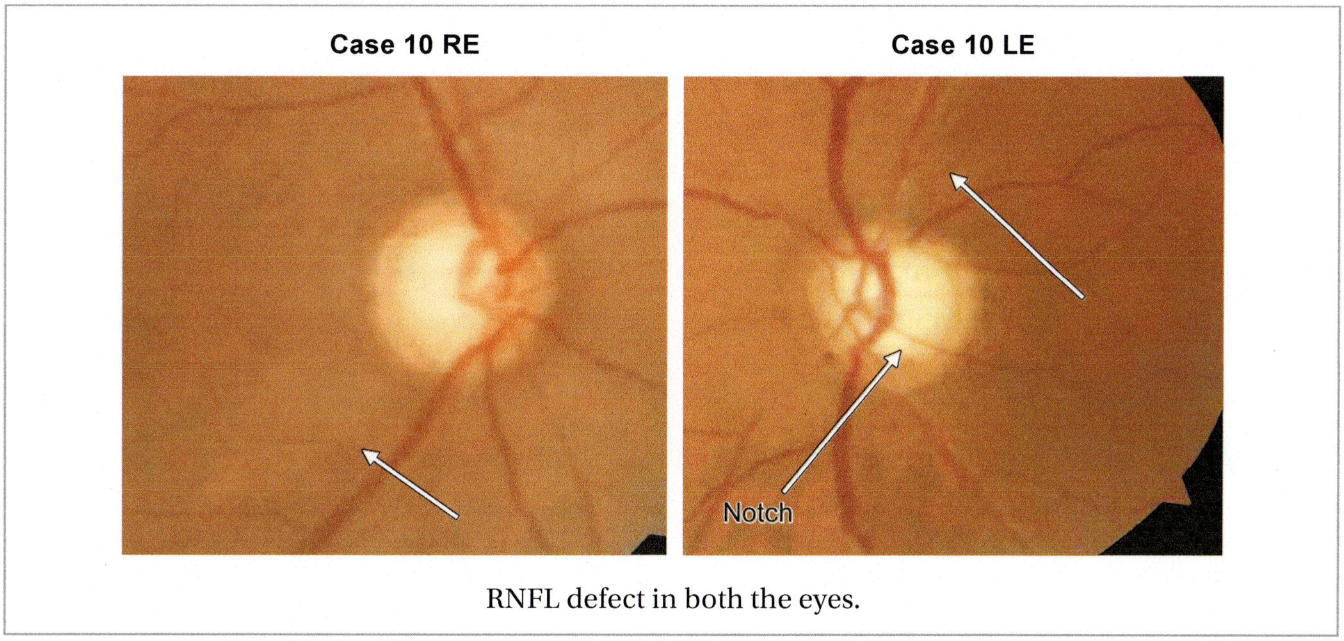

RNFL defect in both the eyes.

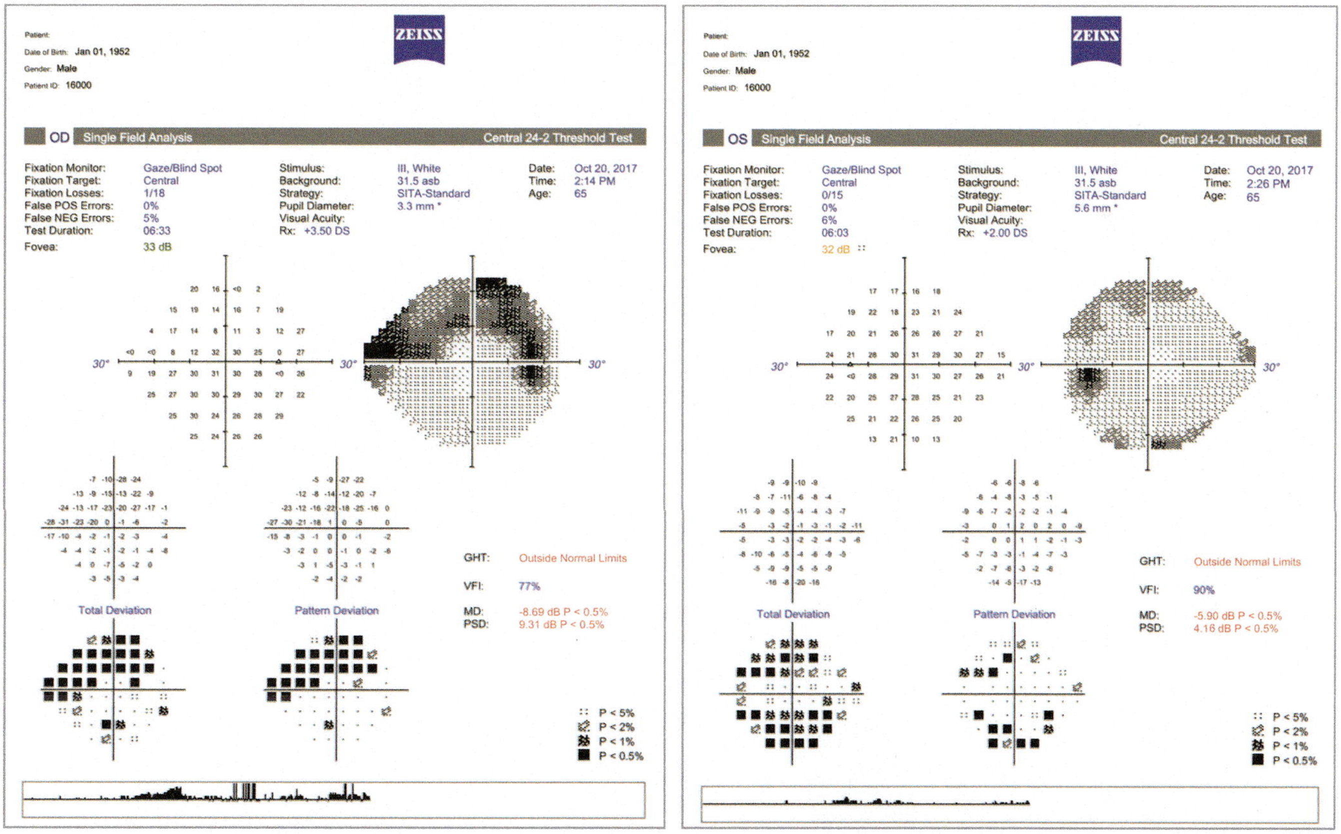

FL 1/18; FP 0%; FN 5%
Fovea 33 dB; GHT-ONL; VFI 77%
MD -8.69 dB P < 0.5%; PSD 9.31 dB P < 0.5%

FL 0/15; FP 0%; FN 6%
Fovea 32 dB; GHT-ONL; VFI 90%
MD -5.90 dB P < 0.5%; PSD 4.16 dB P < 0.5%

Case 10 RE

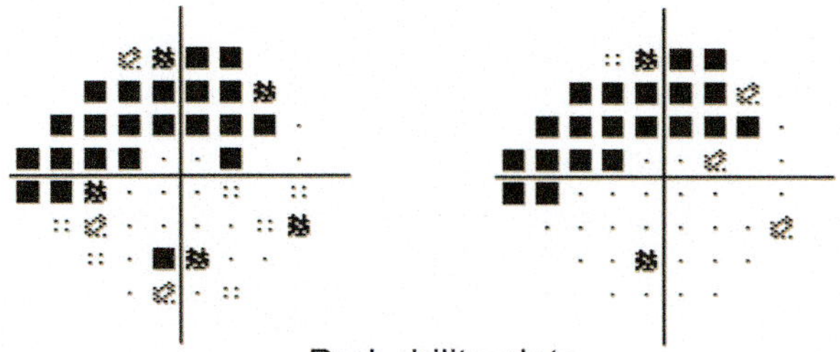

Probability plots

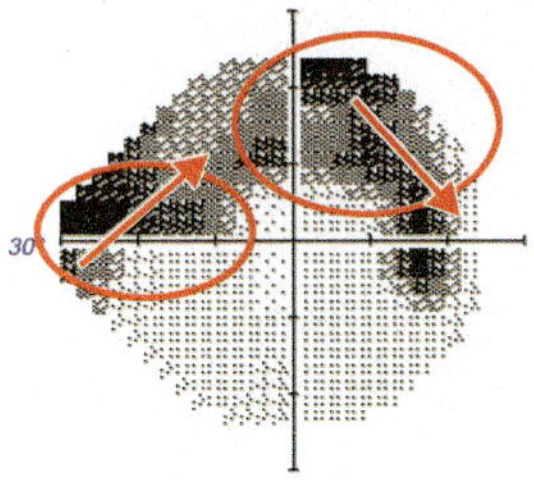

Grey scale

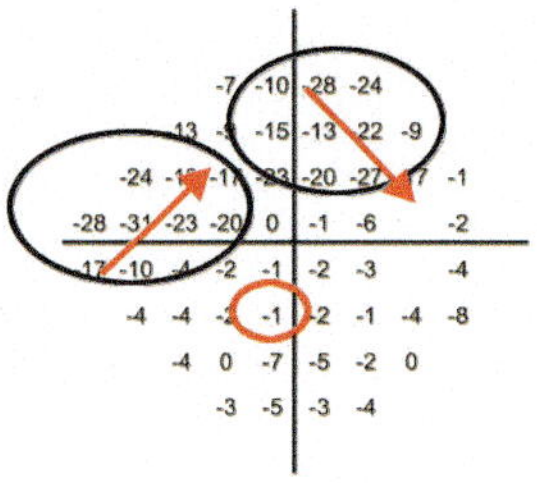

TDNP

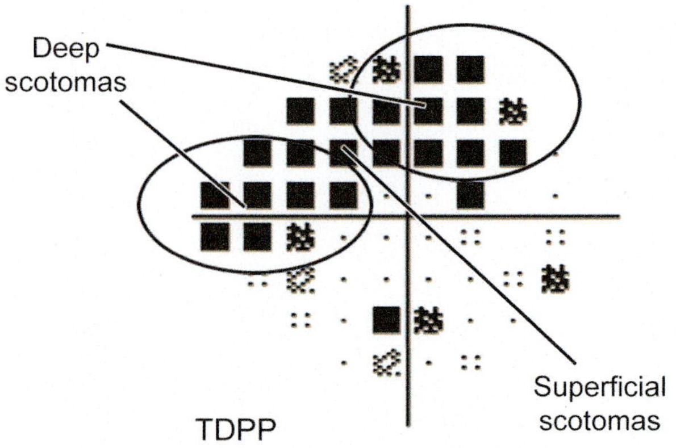

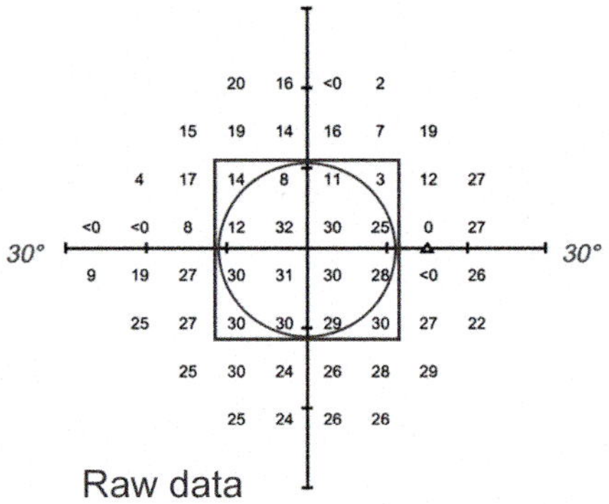

Raw data

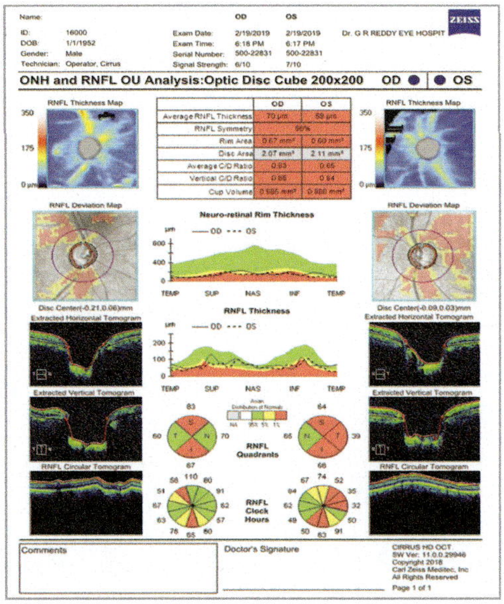

Location and extent of the field defect: Localized scotoma occupying the upper half of the field with more than 90% of the points are represented by black squares (P < 0.5%).

From the probability plots the field defect is looking as a single field defect, but from the grey scale it is clearly evident that the ganglion cell damage started at two locations. One location is in the upper nasal quadrant close to horizontal axis and the second location is in the upper temporal quadrant close to vertical axis away from fixation and their direction of progression is depicted by arrows.

Depth of the field defect (TDNP): The highest loss of sensitivity point in the scotoma is 31 dB. **MD -8.69 dB P < 0.5%. In a localized field defect MD index does not represent the exact depth of the field defect.** The field defect started outside 10° circle and slowly progressing towards fixation. Raw data—Only two points are absolute scotomas among the black squares.

Target IOP: The presenting IOP in this case is 22 mm Hg. The target IOP aimed is around 17 mm Hg.

There is no need to ask OCT in this case as it is an established case of glaucoma. In future, if the patient cannot perform the field test well, this OCT printout will be helpful for progression analysis.

Case 10 LE

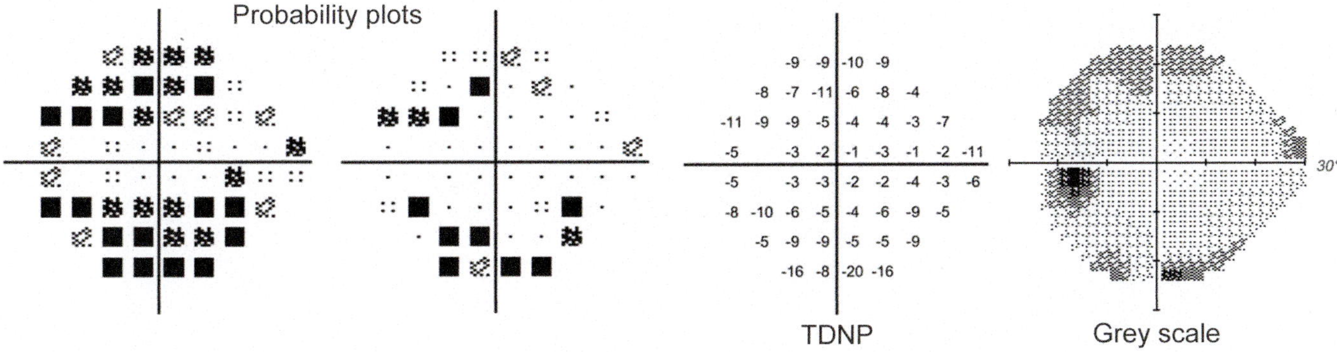

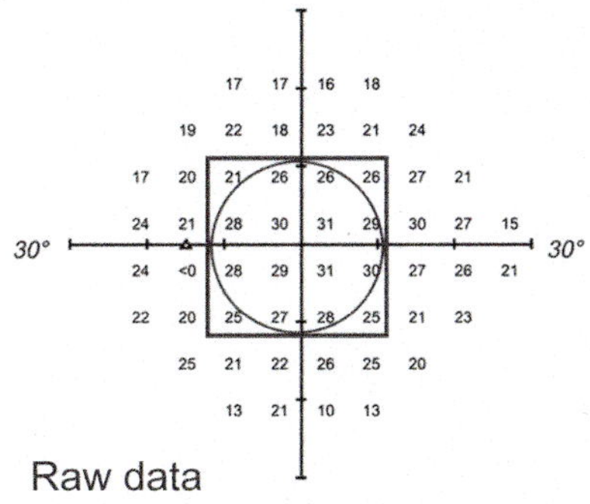

Location and extent of the field defect: (Probability plots) Total deviation probability plot (TDPP) is showing two localized scotomas. One is occupying the upper temporal quadrant and part of upper nasal quadrant, not involving points 3° away from the horizontal axis. The second localized scotoma is in the lower half of the field not involving the points 3° away from the horizontal axis. Always get the habit of seeing probability plots and grey scale simultaneously. From the grey scale, we will have an idea regarding the depth, direction of progression and origin of field defects as either single or multicentric origin. In this case by seeing the grey scale we can tell that the depth of the field defect is not severe and the field defect started from the periphery.

TDNP: Depth of the scotoma. The highest loss of sensitivity in the upper localized scotoma is 11 dB and 20 dB in the lower localized scotoma and at most of the points the loss of sensitivity is around is 4 dB. **MD -5.90 dB P < 0.5%, PSD 4.15 dB P < 0.5%.**

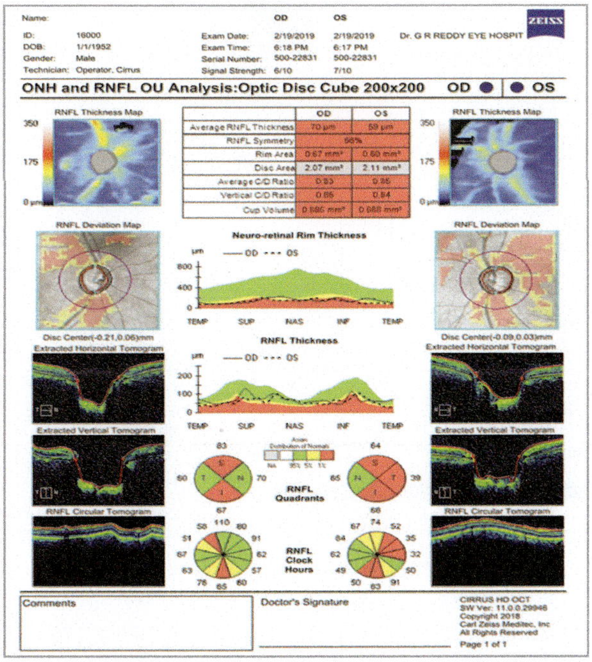

Target IOP: There is no absolute scotoma in both the localized scotomas. It is a relative scotoma. The sensitivities of the 16 points in the 10° circle area are good and no need to repeat the test with 10-2 point pattern.

RE 24-2; VFI 77%
MD -8.69 dB P < 0.5%
LE 24-2; VFI 90%
MD -5.90 dB P < 0.5%

Glaucoma is more advanced in RE than LE. OCT is also showing more damage in the RE.

Case 11 RE

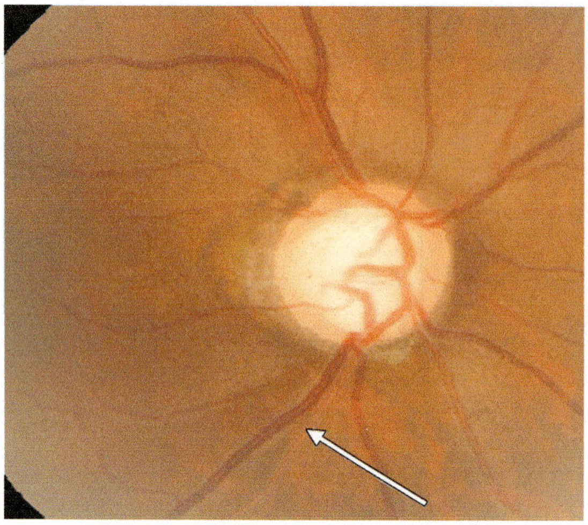

Case 11 LE

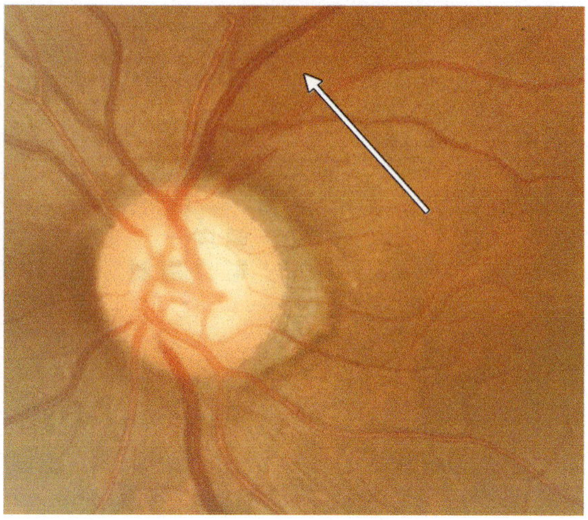

RNFL defect in both the eyes.

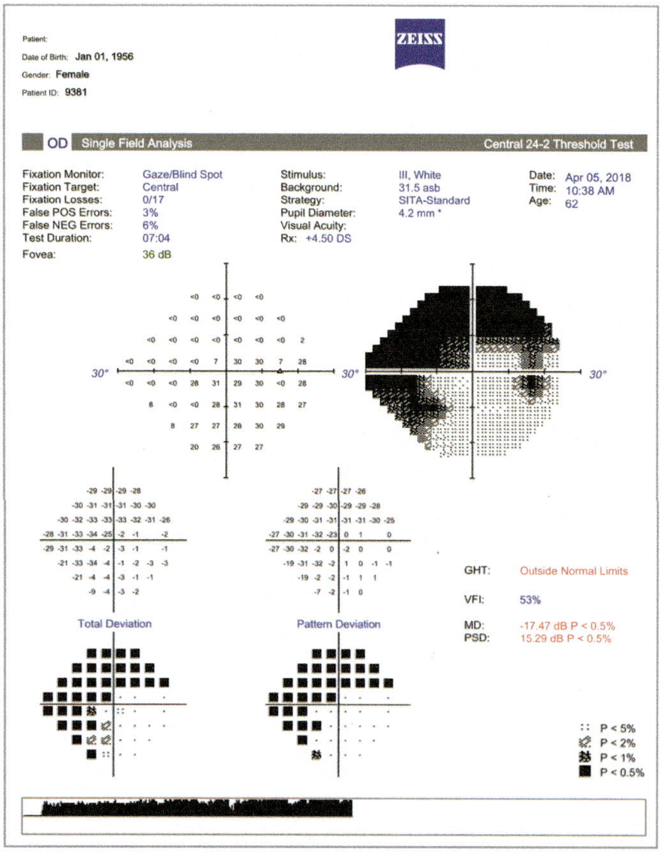

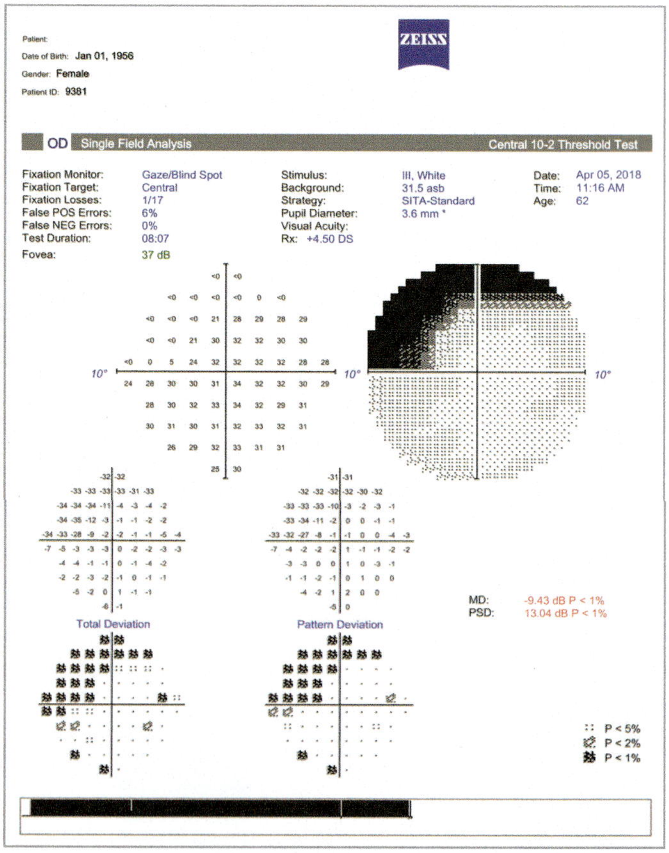

FL 0/17; FP 3%; FN 6%
Fovea 36 dB; GHT-ONL; VFI 53%
MD -17.47 dB P < 0.5%; PSD 15.29 dB P < 0.5%

FL 1/17; FP 6%; FN 0%
Fovea 37 dB
MD -9.43 dB P < 1%; PSD 13.04 dB P < 1%

Case 11 RE

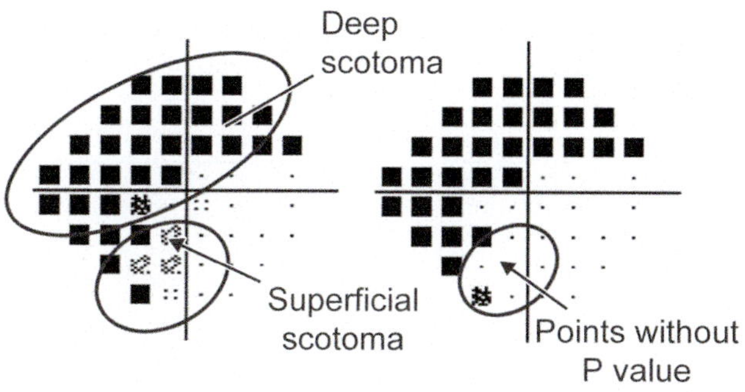

Probability plots

Location and extent of the field defect: Biarcuate scotoma located in the nasal half of the field and extending into upper temporal quadrant. More than 90% of the points in the scotoma are represented by black squares (P < 0.5%). During the conversion of TDNP to pattern deviation numerical plots (PDNP) the superficial scotomas in the TDPP became nonsignificant in the PDPP. From this we know the direction of progression. The direction of progression is towards lower nasal quadrant and also towards fixation.

Conversion of total deviation plots to pattern deviation plots

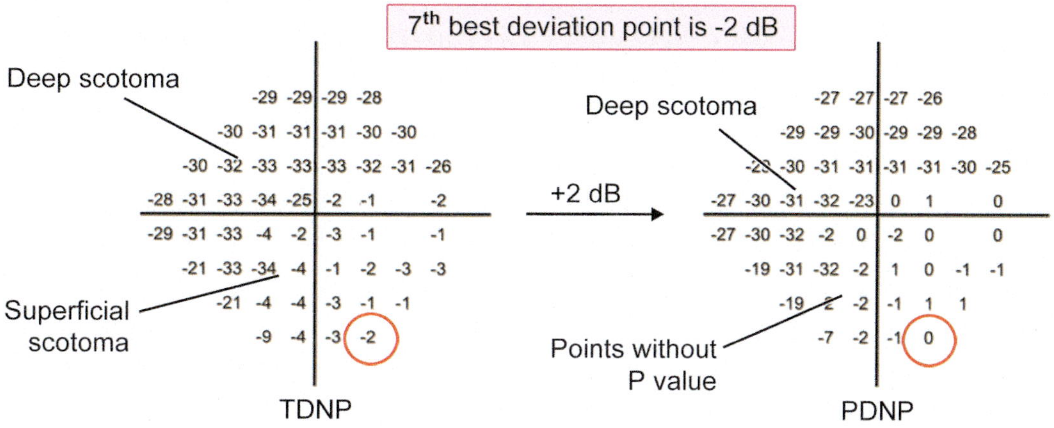

Depth of the field defect (TDNP): The loss of sensitivity at most of the points in both upper and lower arcuate scotomas is around 30 dB and MD index is -17.47 dB P < 0.5%, the 7th best deviation point is -2 dB. So by adding +2 dB to all the deviation values in the TDNP, it could not change P < 0.5% of the most of the points during the conversion of TDNP to PDNP. This is the reason why both the probability plots are looking almost similar.

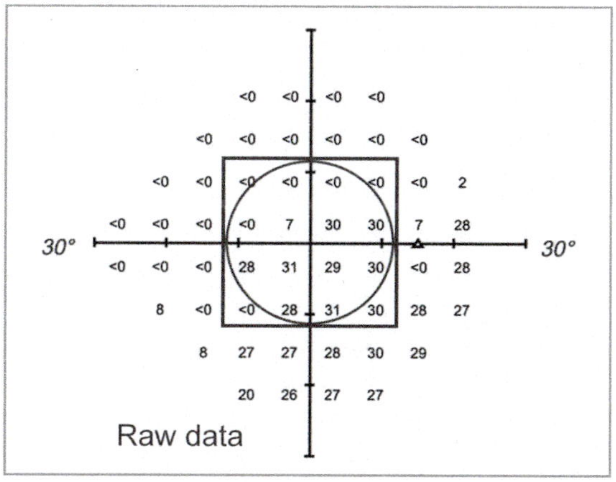

Raw data: There are three absolute scotomas among the 16 points in the 10° circle area. So it is an absolute indication to repeat the test with 10-2 point pattern.

Case 11 RE (10-2)

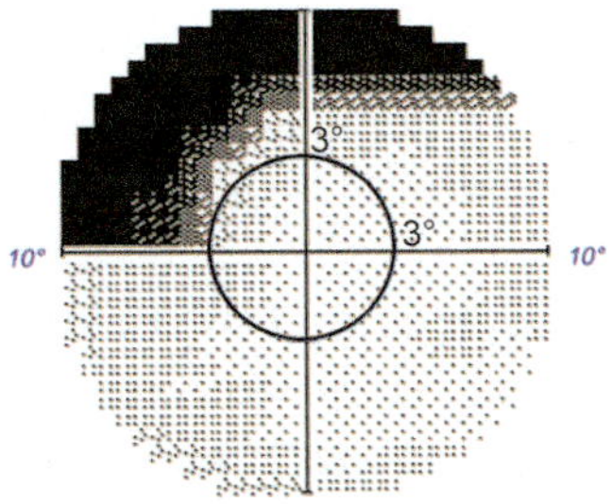

Grey scale

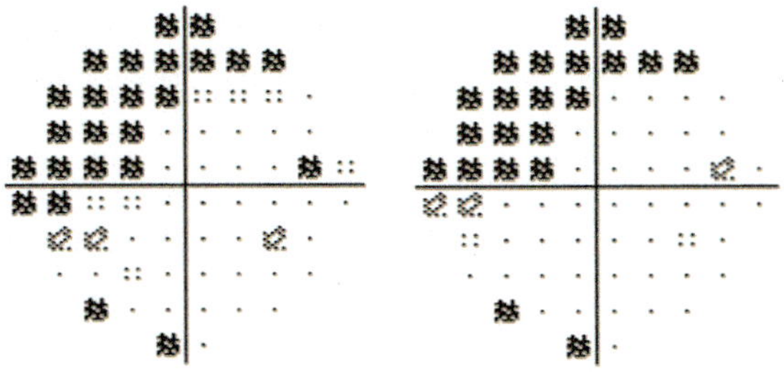

Probability plots

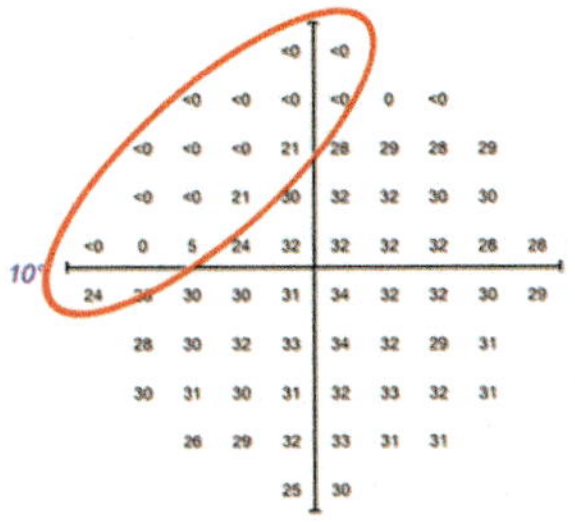

Raw data

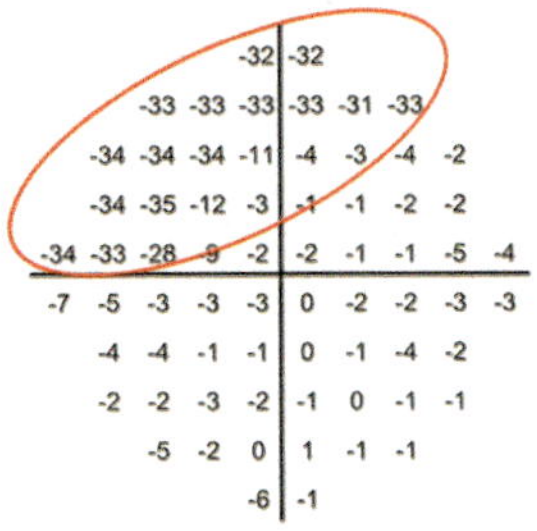

TDNP

MD -9.43 dB P < 1%
PSD 13.04 dB P < 1%

Raw data, the grey scale and TDNP are important components. In the 10-2 SFA printout, most of the points in the field defect are absolute scotomas. The field defect started outside 10° circle almost progressed into 3° circle in the upper nasal quadrant. The macular program area is not involved **MD 10-2 -9.43 dB P < 1%.** Though 95% points are absolute scotomas in the field defect, since the MD index is the average of the deviation values of all 68 points of 10-2 point pattern, the MD index value is **-9.43 dB P< 1%**. The 3° circle area around fixation is not involved. That is one good sign.

> Raw data—Most of the points in the localized scotoma are absolute scotomas. When the field defect is having absolute scotomas and progressing towards fixation, we should aim for low target IOP.

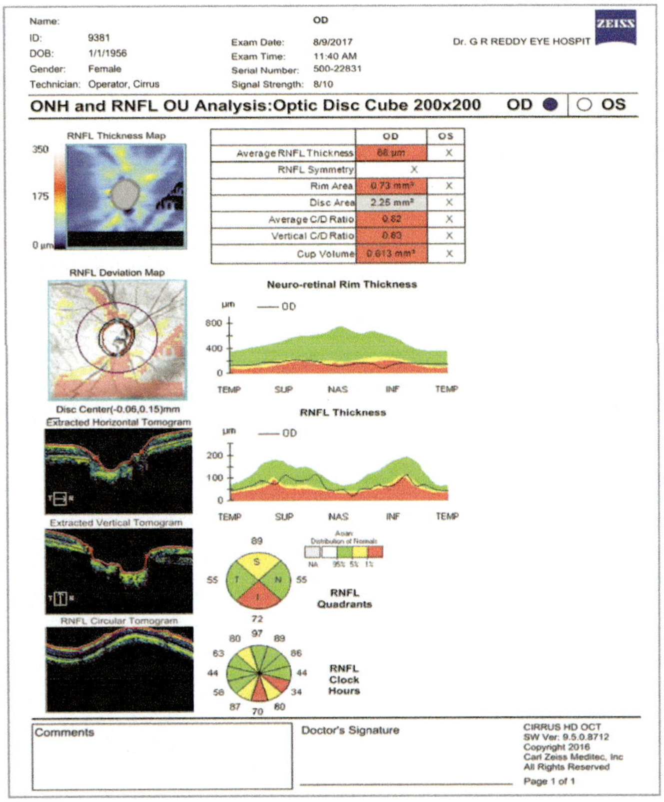

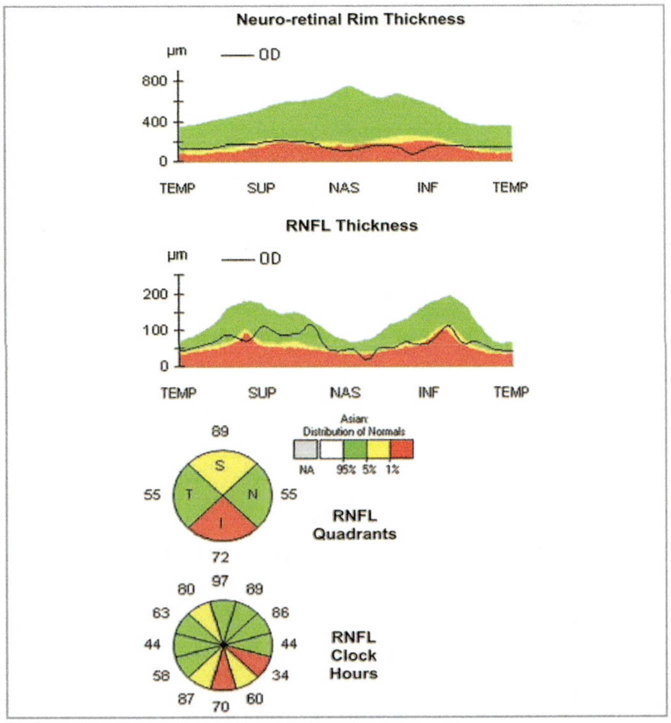

> OCT is correlating to the fundus and visual fields.

Case 11 RE

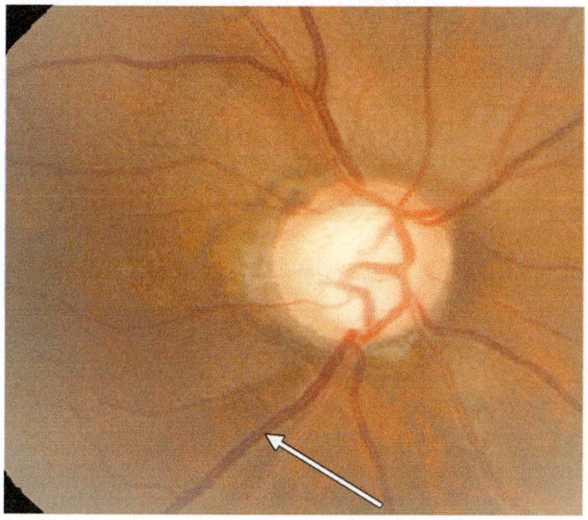

Case 11 LE

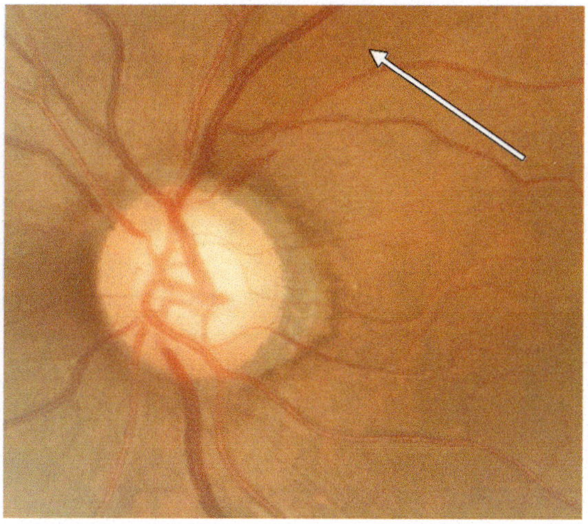

RNFL defect in both the eyes.

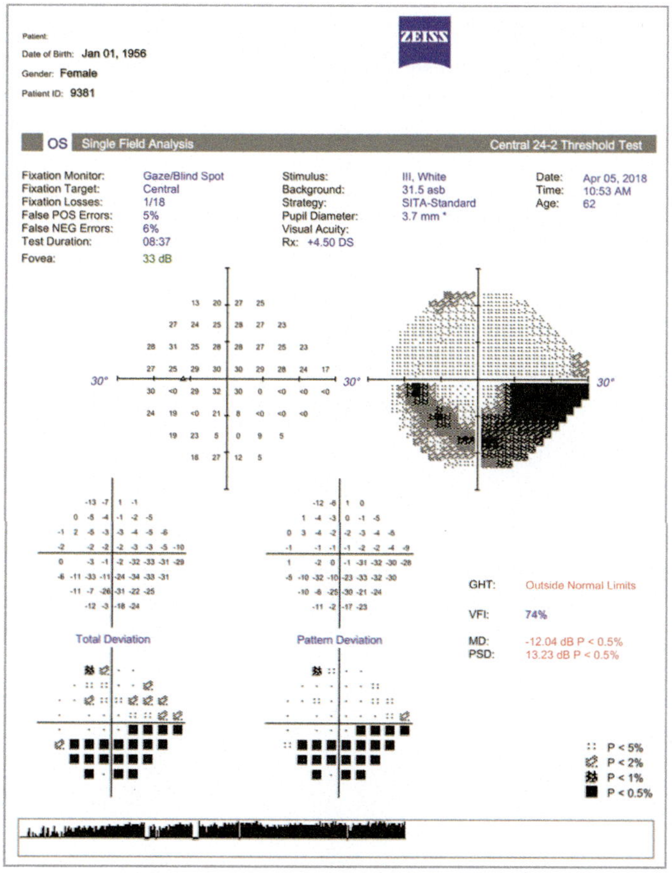

FL 1/18; FP 5%; FN 6%
Fovea 33 dB; GHT-ONL; VFI 74%
MD -12.04 dB P < 0.5%; PSD 13.23 dB P < 0.5%

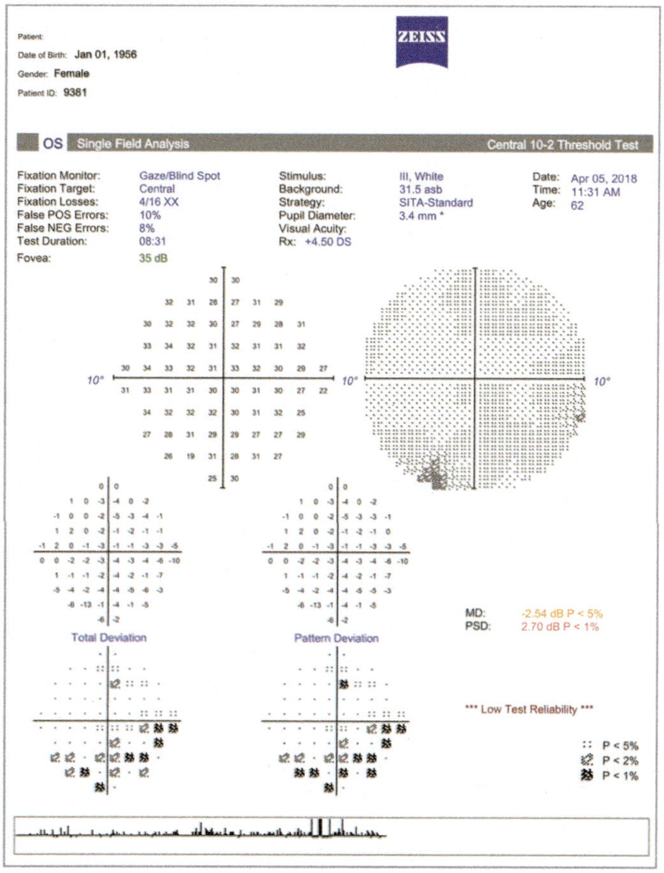

FL 4/16 XX; FP 10%; FN 8%
Fovea 35 dB
MD -2.54 dB P < 5%; PSD 2.70 dB P < 1%

Case 11 LE 24-2

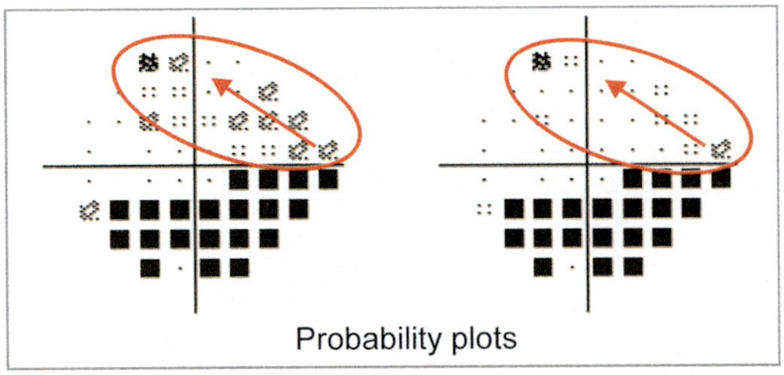

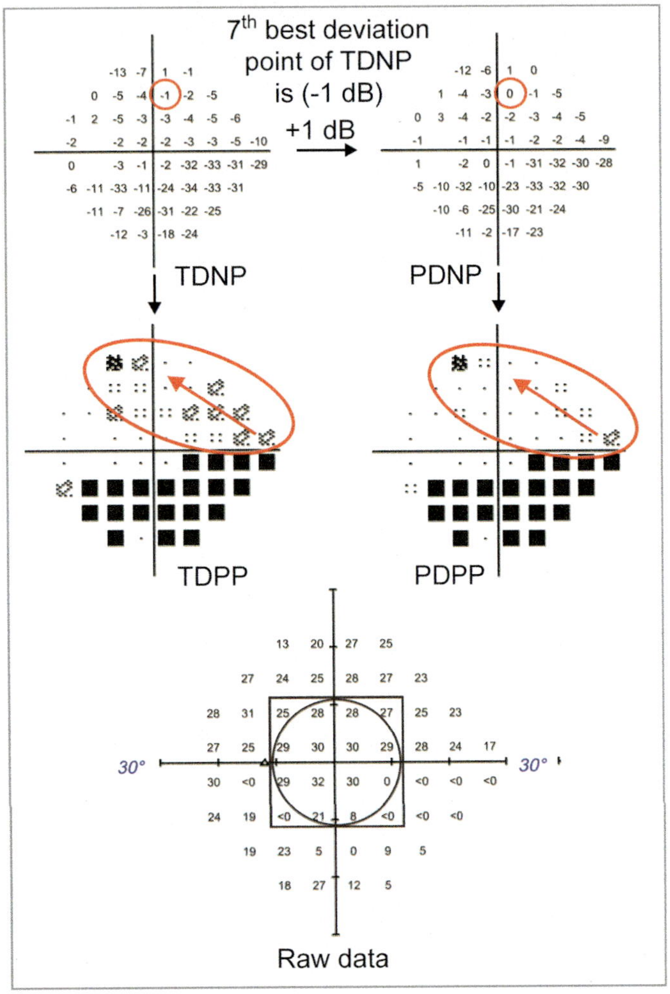

Location and extent of the field defect (Probability plots): Biarcuate field defect in the nasal half of the field in which all the points in the lower arcuate scotoma are represented by black squares P < 0.5% (deep scotomas) and the points in the upper arcuate scotoma are represented by P < 2% (superficial scotomas).

Conversion of TDNP to PDNP: 7th best deviation point of TDNP is (-1 dB). So +1 dB is added to all the points to convert TDNP to PDNP. The deviation values of the newly formed deviation plot (PDNP) will be same as TDNP as +1 dB is added to all the deviation values of TDNP. So, TDNP and PDNP deviation values will be similar. This is the reason why the probability plots look similar in most of the localized field defects.

Depth of the scotoma: The loss of sensitivity at most of the points in the lower arcuate scotomas is around 30 dB and MD index is -12.04 dB P < 0.5%. Because the MD index is the average of all points of TDNP, it is not a true index to represent the depth of a localized field defect. The value of MD index is always less than the actual depth of a localized field defect.

Raw data: About 50% of the points in the lower arcuate scotomas are absolute scotomas and the loss of sensitivity of the remaining points is also very severe. When the presenting IOP is causing absolute scotoma we should aim for low target IOP.

Indication for 10-2 point pattern: There is one absolute scotoma at one point which is 9° from the vertical axis and 3° from the horizontal axis in the lower nasal quadrant. An absolute scotomas in the 10° circle area is an indication to repeat the test with 10-2 point pattern.

Case 11 LE 10-2

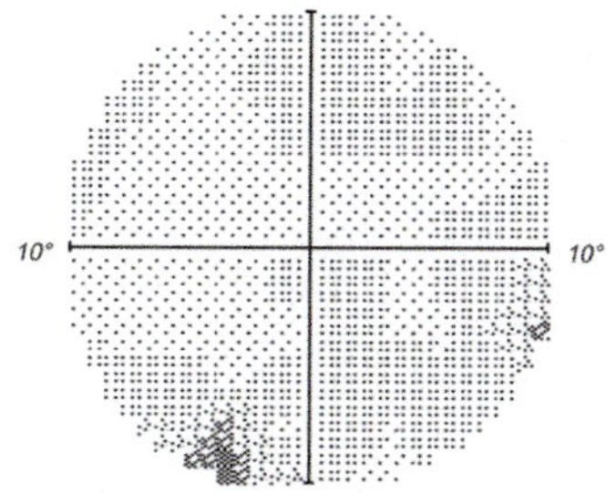

Grey scale

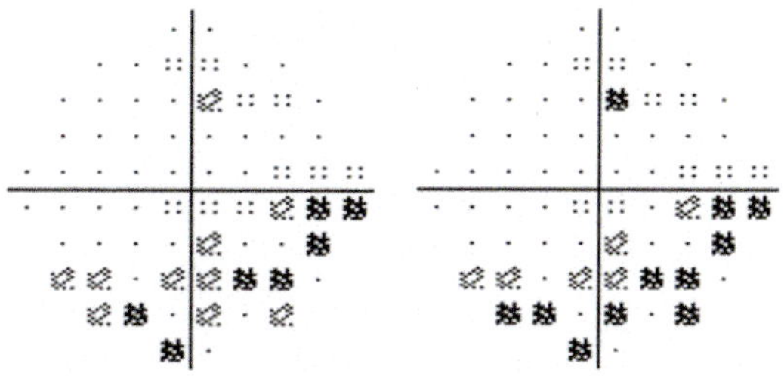

Probability plots

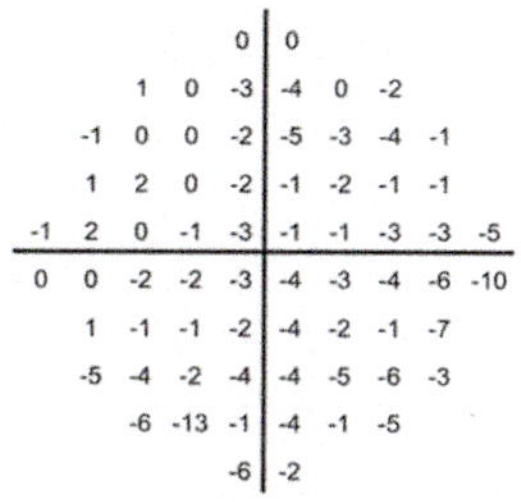

TDNP

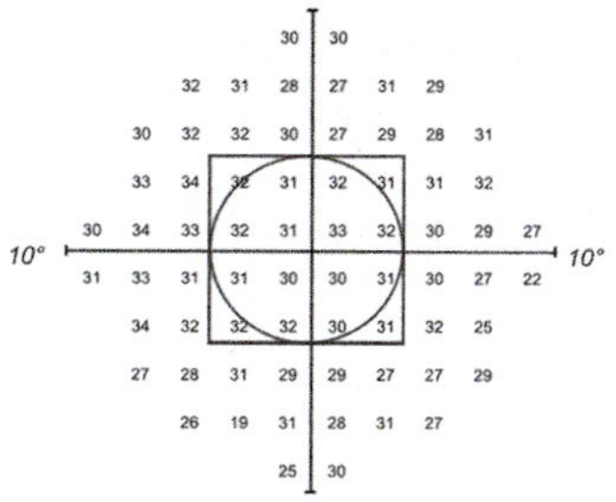

Raw data

24-2 MD -12.04 dB P < 0.5%
PSD 13.23 dB P < 0.5%

10-2 MD -2.54 dB P <5%
PSD 2.70 dB P < 1%

Fixation losses 4/18
Unreliable field

The sensitivities of the points in the 10° circle area of 10-2 point pattern are good and the **MD -2.54 dB P < 5%**

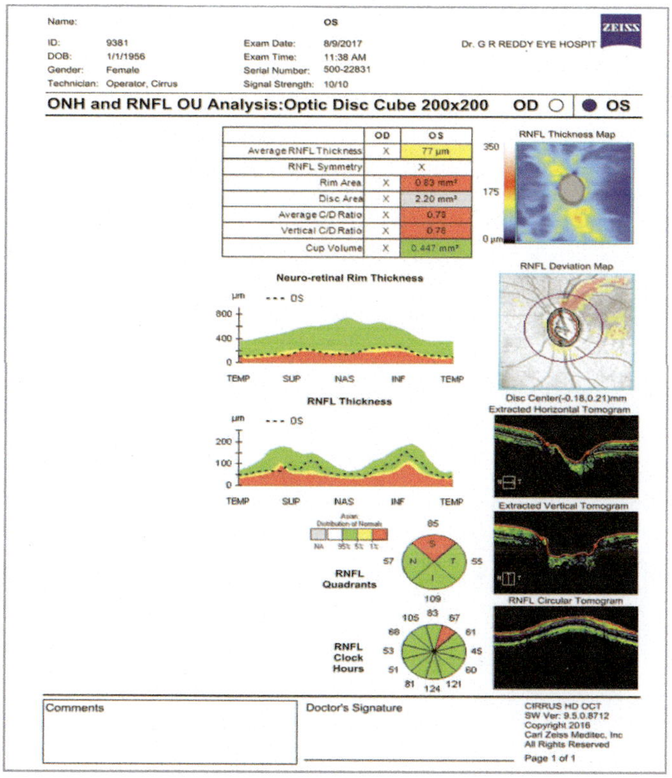

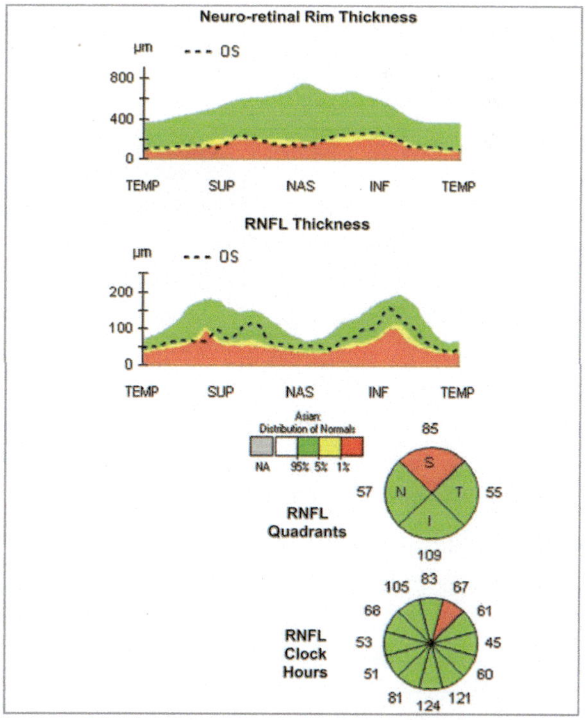

OCT is correlating to the fundus and visual fields.

Case 12 RE **Case 12 LE**

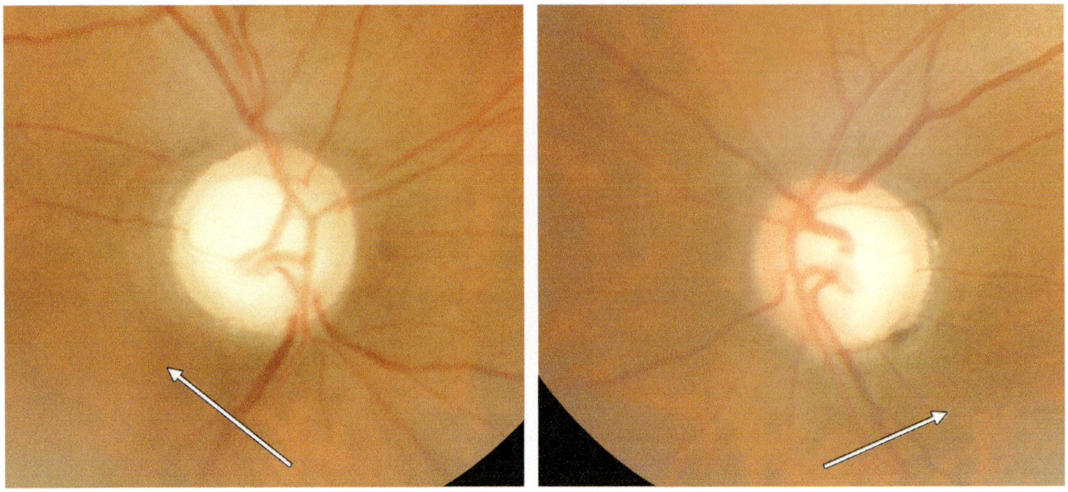

Advanced glaucomatous disc with RNFL defect in both the eyes.

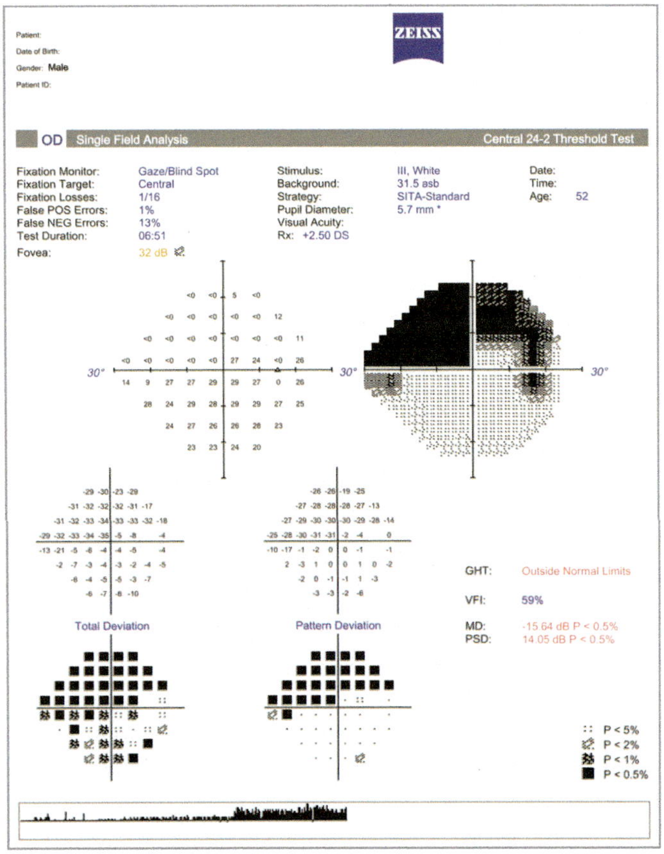

FL 1/16; FP 1%; FN 13%

Fovea 32 dB; GHT-ONL; VFI 59%

MD -15.64 dB P < 0.5%; PSD 14.05 dB P < 0.5%

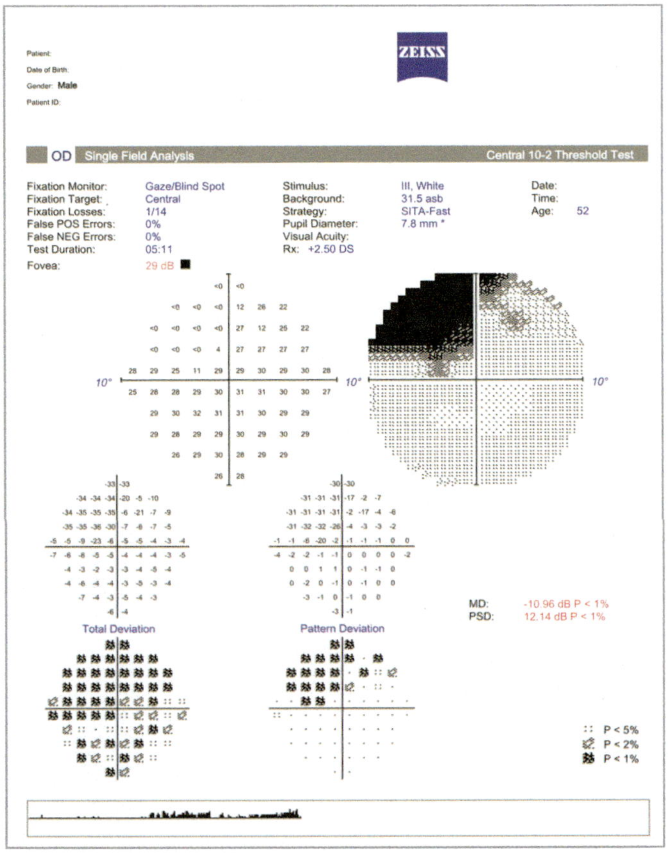

FL 1/14; FN 0%; FP 0%

Fovea 29 dB

MD -10.96 dB P <1%; PSD 12.14 dB P < 1%

Case 12 RE 24-2

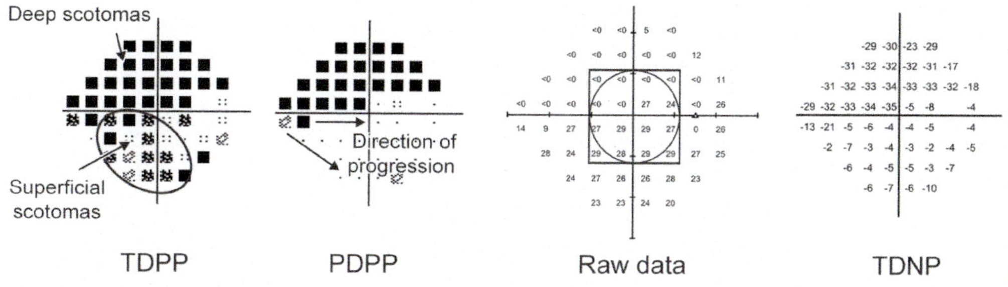

Location and extent of the field defect: TDPP is showing almost generalized depression with deep scotomas in the upper half of the field and superficial scotomas in the lower half of the field. So from the probability plot it is evident that the disease process started in the upper half of the field and progressed towards lower half of the field. The direction of progression is towards fixation and also downwards towards the lower nasal quadrants.

Depth of the field defect: The loss of sensitivity is around 30 dB at most of the points in the upper half of the field defect and around 5 dB at most of the points in the lower half of the field defect. The MD index is -15.64 dB P < 0.5%.

Raw data: Most of the points in the upper half of the field defect are absolute scotomas. There are 6 absolute scotomas among the 16 points in the 10° circle area. So, it is an absolute indication to repeat the test with 10-2 point pattern.

Case 12 RE 10-2

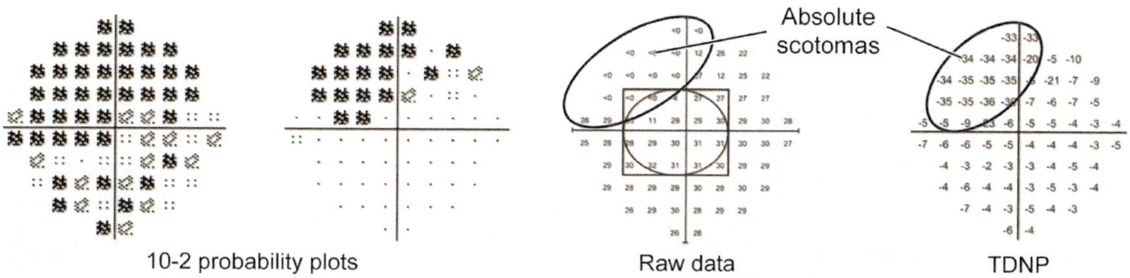

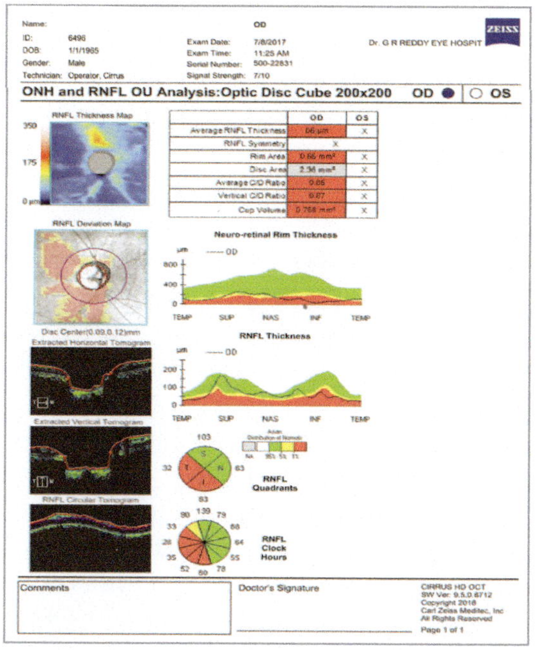

In 10-2 printout concentrate on grey scale, raw data, total deviation numerical plot and MD index. **Raw data—Absolute scotomas in the upper nasal quadrant in the 10° circle area. MD -10.96 dB P < 1%.**

MD -10.96 dB P < 1%
PSD 12.14 dB P < 1%

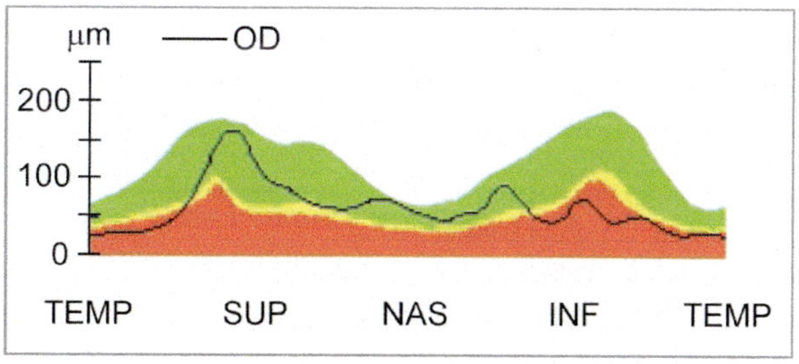

OCT is correlating to the fundus and visual fields.

Case 12 RE **Case 12 LE**

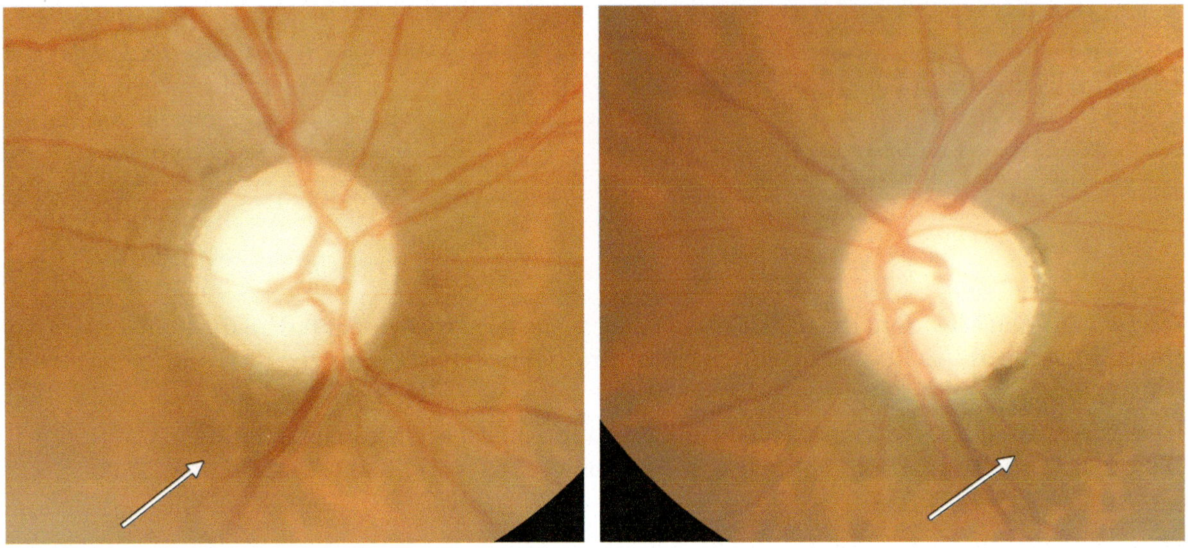

Advanced glaucomatous disc with RNFL defects in both the eyes.

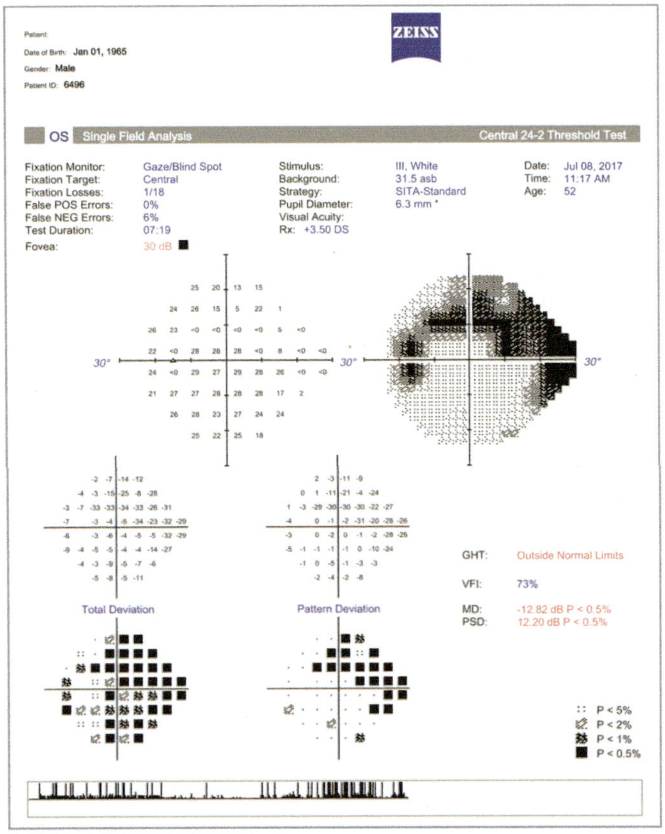

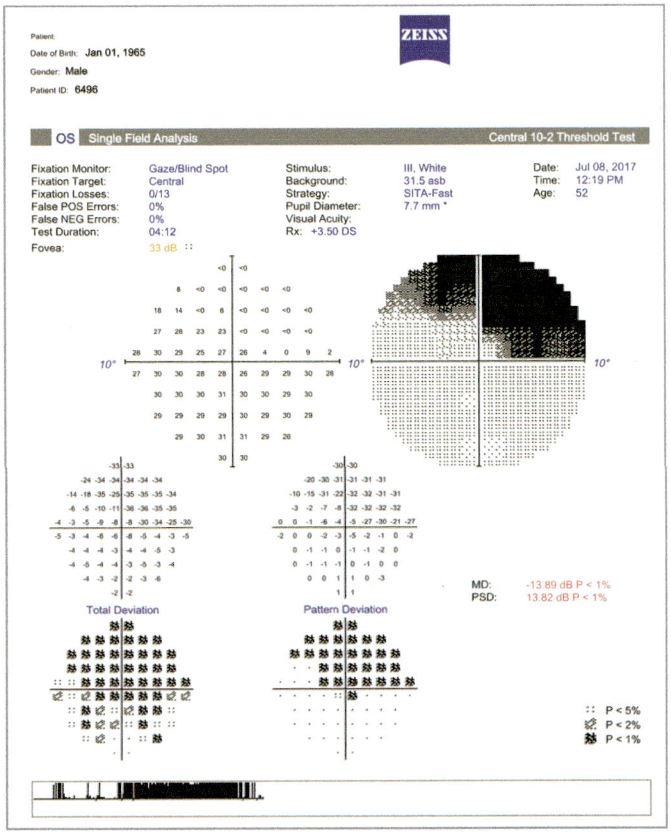

FL 1/18; FP 0%; FN 6%
Fovea 30 dB; GHT-ONL; VFI 73%
MD -12.82 dB P < 0.5%; PSD -12.20 dB P < 0.5%

FL 0/13; FP 0%; FN 0%
Fovea 33 dB
MD -13.89 dB P < 1%; PSD 13.82 dB P < 1%

Case 12 LE -24-2

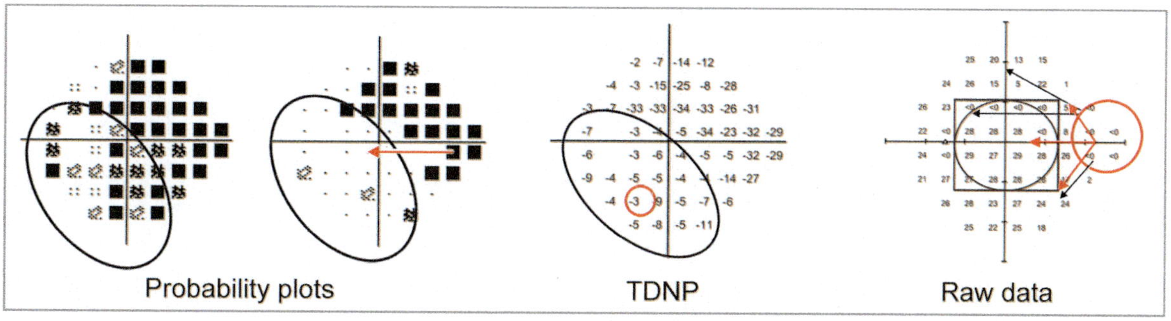

Location and extent of the field defect: TDPP is showing field defect in the nasal half of the field and extending to temporal quadrants. During the conversion of TDNP to PDNP the superficial scotomas in the TDPP become nonsignificant and the deep scotomas are highlighted in the PDPP. From this, we know the direction of progression. The direction of progression is towards lower nasal quadrant and also towards fixation.

Raw data: As shown in the Figure, the points in the red circle area all the points are absolute scotomas. Actually, the disease process started as nasal step and progressed mainly upwards and five points in the 10° circle area are also absolute scotomas.

Indication for 10-2 point pattern: There are five absolute scotomas among the 16 points in the 10° circle area. So, it is an absolute indication to repeat the test with 10-2 point pattern.

Case 12 LE 10-2

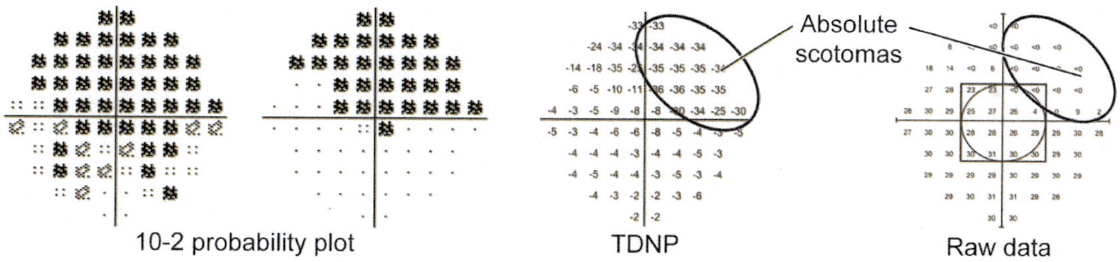

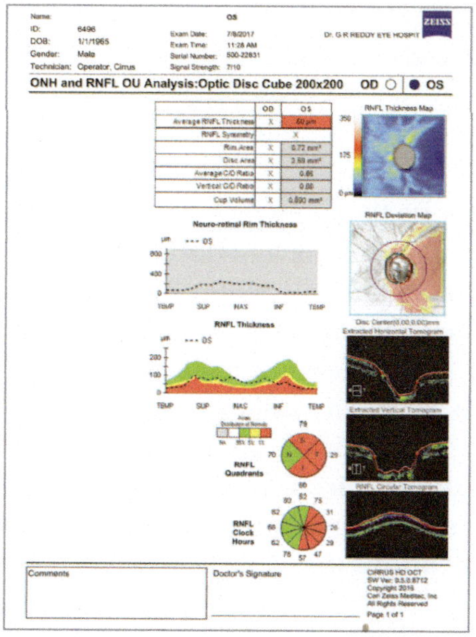

In 10-2 printout concentrate on grey scale, raw data, total deviation numerical plot and MD index.

Raw data: Absolute scotomas in the upper nasal quadrant in the 10° circle area.

MD -13.89 dB P < 1

VFI is not present in 10-2 program.

OCT is correlating with the fundus and visual fields.

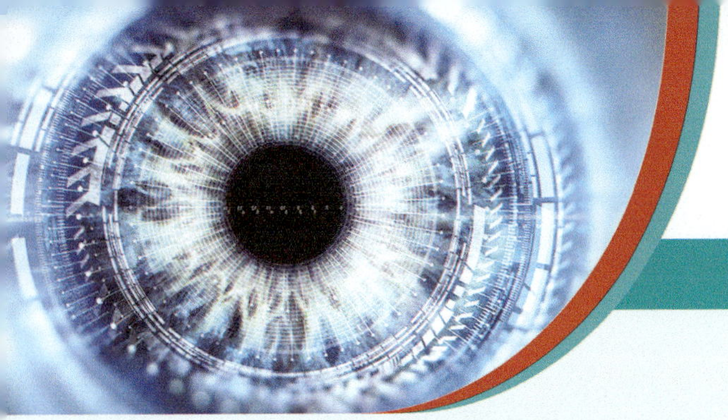

Interpretation of Single Field Analysis Printouts of Type 2 Primary Open-angle Glaucoma

TYPE 2 POAG: FIELD DEFECT DOMINANT WITHIN 10° CIRCLE AREA

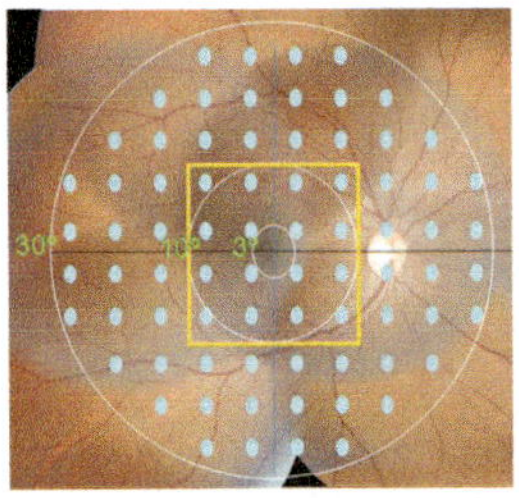

30-2 point pattern

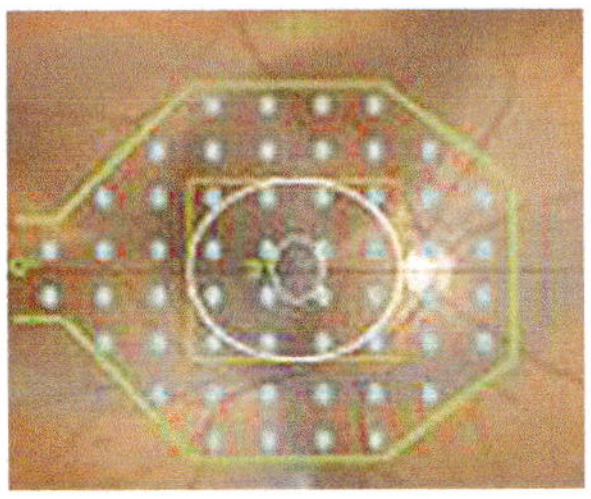

24-2 point pattern

Step 1: In glaucoma suspect or in established glaucoma always select 30-2 or 24-2 point pattern, 30-2 or 24-2 SFA printouts which are the base line printouts for a glaucoma patient.

Step 2: To know whether we have to repeat the test with 10-2 point pattern.

We normally ask for 10-2 point pattern field test when the field defect is extending into 10° area in 30-2 or 24-2. But in Type 2 glaucomas (glaucomas starting within 10° circle area) single field analysis (SFA) printouts of 24-2 or 30-2 will have few scotomas and some times they may look almost normal. In such cases we should able to repeat the test with 10-2 point pattern to pickup glaucoma at an early stage. For that, we should know how to evaluate the 10° circle area of 30-2 or 24-2 printouts.

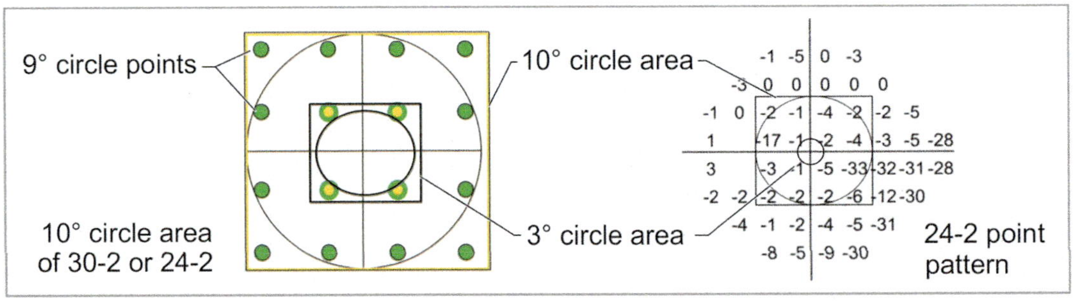

There are 16 points in the 10° circle area of 30-2 or 24-2 point patterns. Basically they are divided into two groups as 3° circle points and 9°circle points. The 3° circle points are 4 in number and the 9°circle points are 12 in number. We should concentrate on these 16 points in probability plots, grey scale, total deviation numerical plot (TDNP), and raw data. Loss of sensitivity first affects probability plots. Loss of sensitivity more than 6 dB to 7 dB will be represented by a black square ($P < 0.5\%$). As the measured sensitivity of these points will be around 30 dB even after 8–10 dB loss of sensitivity 30 dB sensitivity will have good shade in the grey scale. So minimal loss of sensitivity will not affect the 10° circle area in the grey scale. **Even one black square in the probability plots with or without black shade in the 10° circle area in the grey scale is an indication to repeat the test with 10-2 point pattern. An absolute scotoma in the raw data or, loss of sensitivity more than 30 dB among these 16 points are definite indications to repeat the test with 10-2 point pattern**.

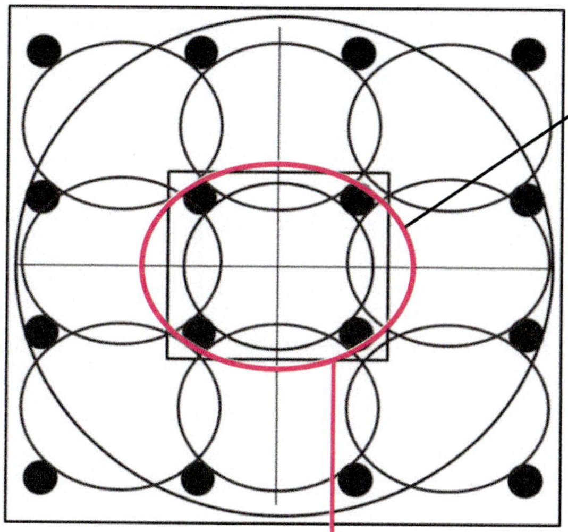

10° circle area of 24-2 point or 30-2 point patterns

Bare areas in 30-2 or 24-2 are filled with 64 points in 10-2 point pattern. The inner 4 points of 30-2 or 24-2 are included in 10-2 point pattern. All the remaining 12 outer set points of 10° circle **area of 24-2 point or 30-2** are not included in 10-2 point pattern. The total number of points in 10-2 point pattern are 68 (64+4). The inner set 4 points belong to 3° circle area of 30-2 or 24-2 will be tested in both 30-2 or 24-2 and 10-2 point patterns tests.

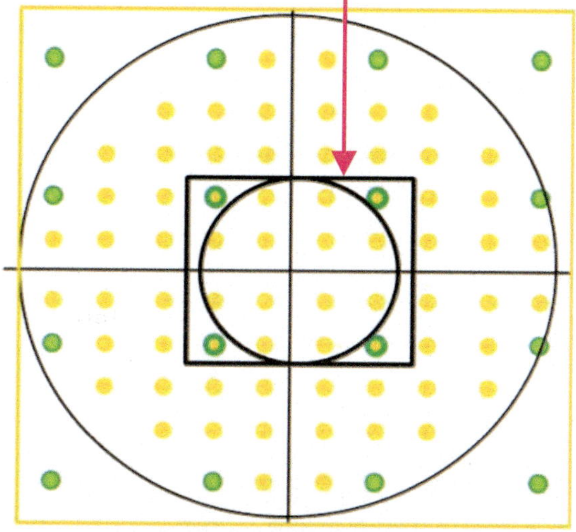

10° circle area (8° points)

The 3° circle bare area around fixation of 30-2 or 24-2 is filled with 12 points in the 10-2 point pattern. The inner set 4 points belonging to 3° circle are present both in 30-2 or 24-2 and 10-2 point pattern. The 3° circle area of 10-2 will have 16 points (12+4) in **10-2 point pattern.**

The total number of points in the 10° circle area are 80 (68 points of 10-2 + 12 outer set points of 30-2 or 24-2).

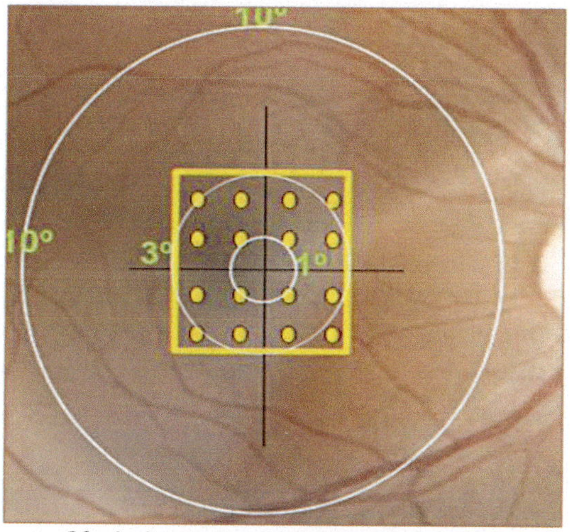

3° circle area of 10-2 point pattern
(macular program)

The 3° circle area of 10-2 point pattern contains 16 points. Basically they are divided into two groups as 1° circle points and 3° circle points. The 1° circle points are 4 in number and the 3° circle points are 12 in number. These 16 points form the macular program. In advanced cases of glaucoma, we advice macular program tests with stimulus size III or V to assess foveal status.

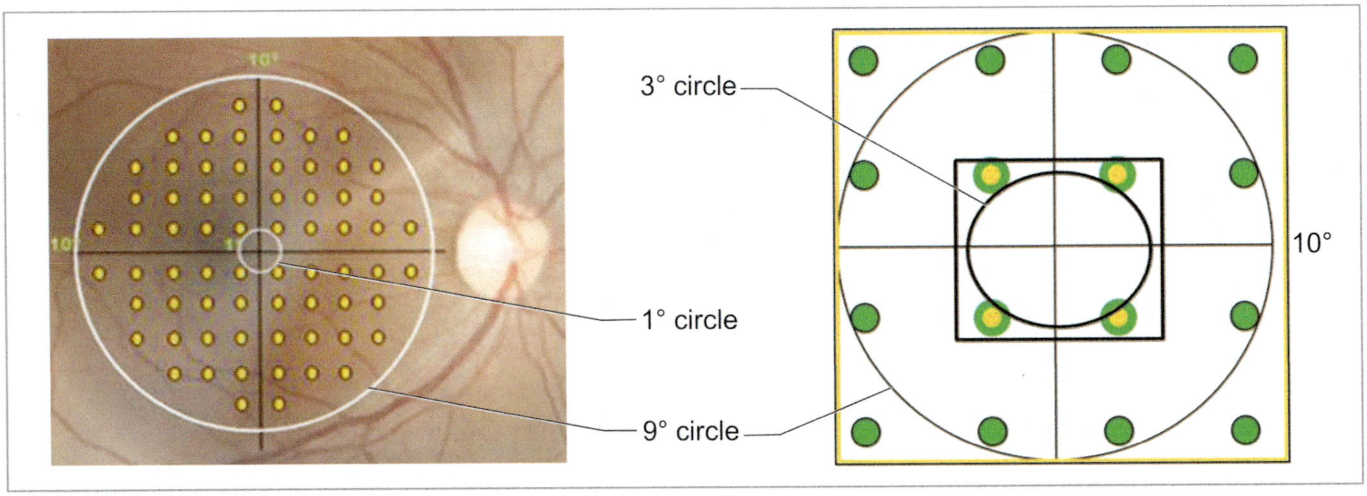

The 3° circle area of 10-2 contains 16 points in the 3° circle area. So we are testing up to fixation in 10-2 point patterns. Foveal split depends on the sensitivity of the 16 points in the 3° circle area.

The 3° circle area of 30-2 or 24-2 contains 4 points and within 3° circle there are no points. We are not testing up to fixation in 30-2 or 24-2 point patterns. So we should not comment on foveal split from 30-2 or 24-2 point patterns.

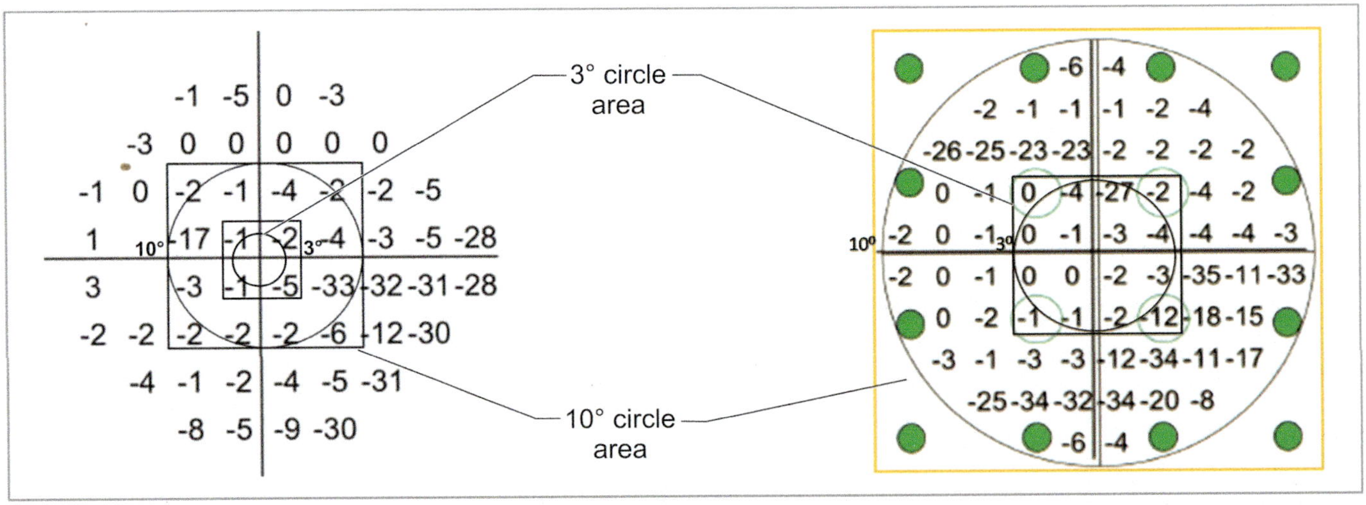

There is a huge untested area (bare area) in the 10° circle area in the 30-2 or 24 -2 point patterns. This untested area is now filled with points in 10-2 point pattern. The outer set of 12 points of 10° circular area of 24-2 or 30-2 are not included in 10-2 point pattern. The inner 4 points of 30-2 or 24-2 are included in the 10-2 point pattern.

Indications to Repeat the Test with 10-2

We will study a case belonging to type 2 open angle glaucoma (field defect dominant within 10° circle). Though the case was picked at an early stage, target intraocular pressure (IOP) could not be achieved and hence (glaucoma field defect) progressed. We will study the probability plots, grey scale, TDNP and raw data in 24-2 SFA printouts to know the indications to repeat the test with 10-2 point pattern.

2014—24-2

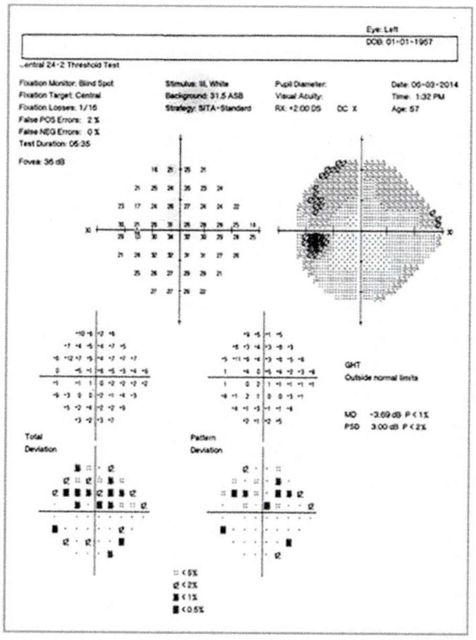

2017—24-2

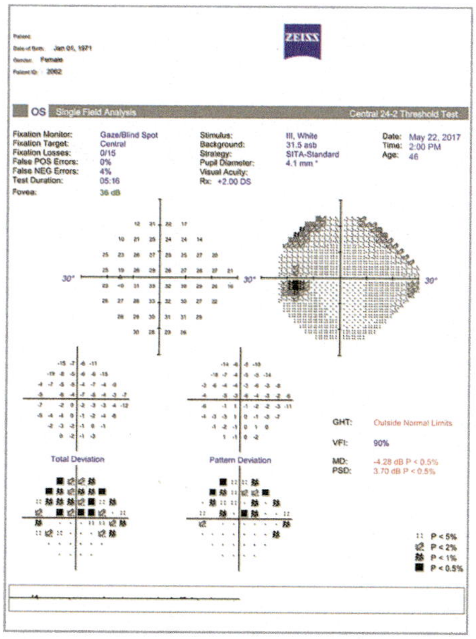

2018—24-2

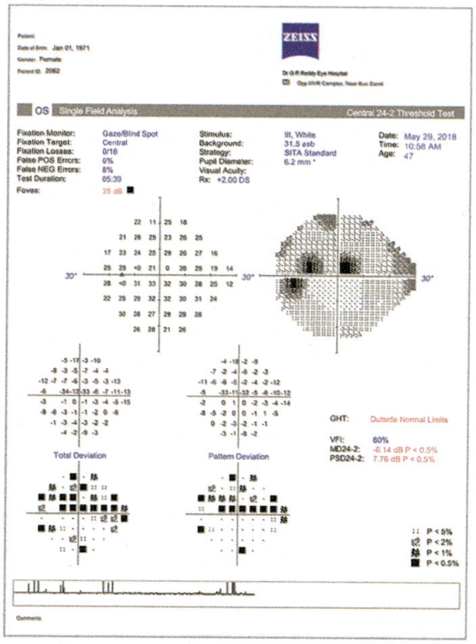

2014—10-2

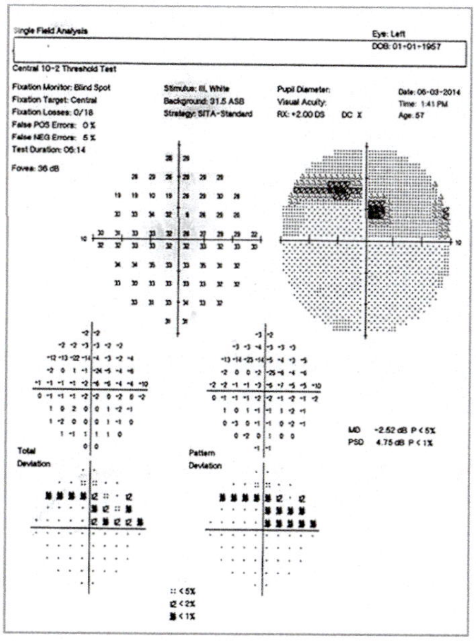

2017—10-2

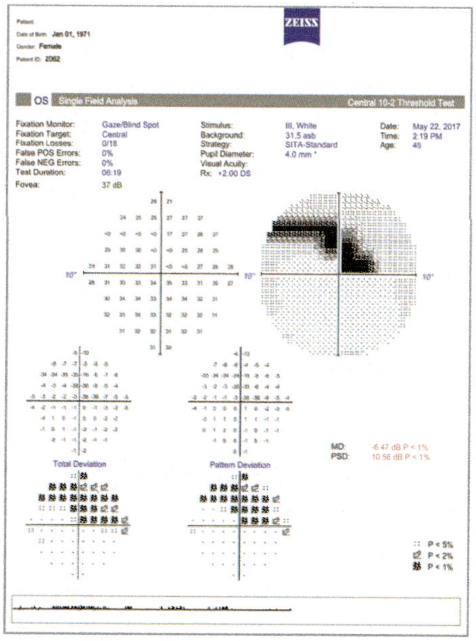

2018—10-2

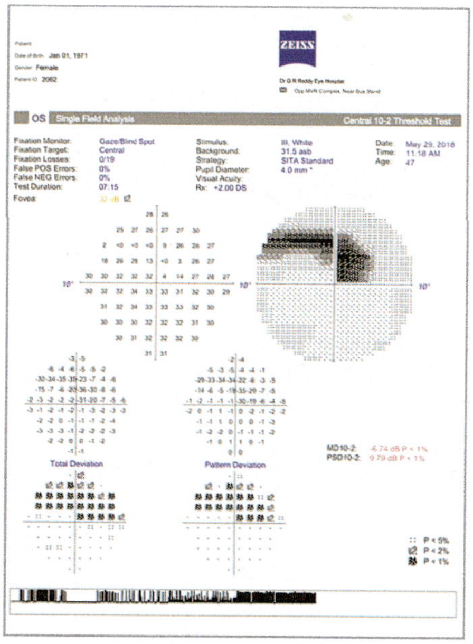

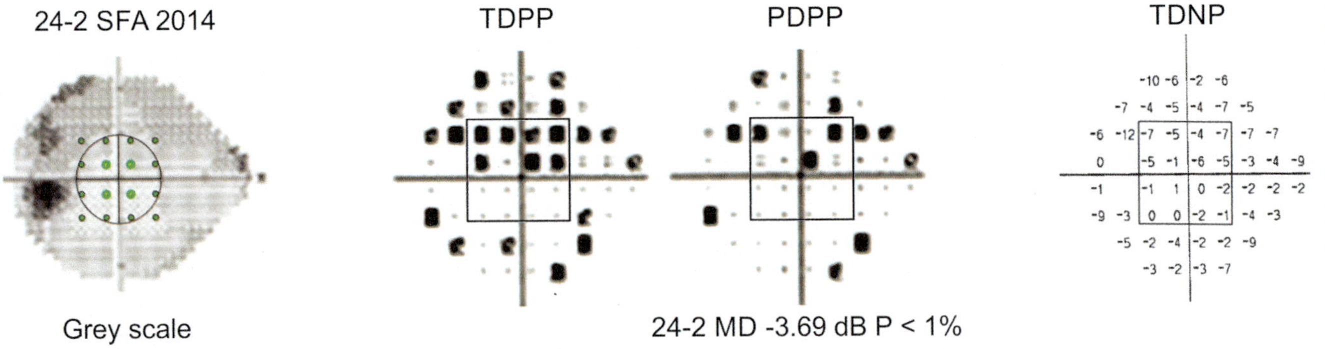

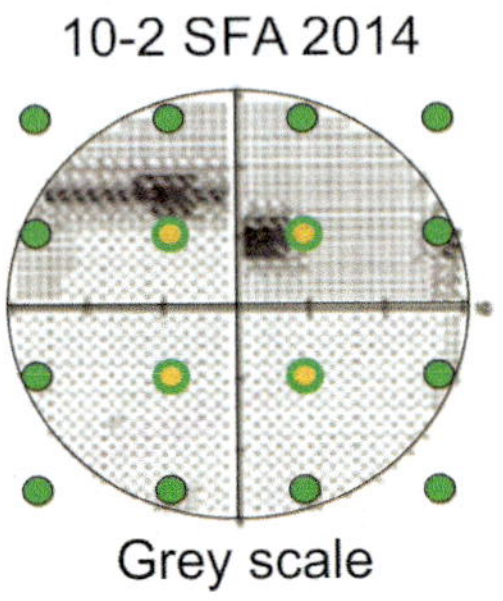

Concentrate on the 10° circle area in grey scale, pattern deviation probability plot (PDPP), TDNP, (raw data) to know whether we should repeat the test with 10-2 point pattern or not. In this SFA printout, there is no indication either from grey scale or TDNP (Raw data) for the repetition of the test with 10-2 point pattern. Out of the 16 points, 3 scotomas which have significant P value (black squares) are highlighted in PDPP. In this SFA printout total deviation probability plot (TDPP) and PDPP are giving clue for the repetition of the test with 10-2 point pattern.

> Localized scotoma which is present in the bare area of 30-2 or 24-2 is seen in 10-2 SFA 2014.

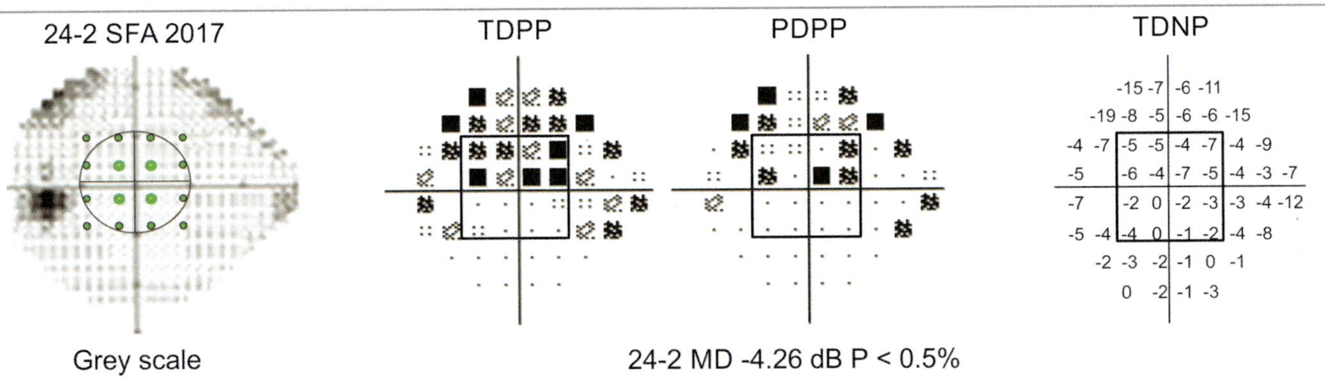

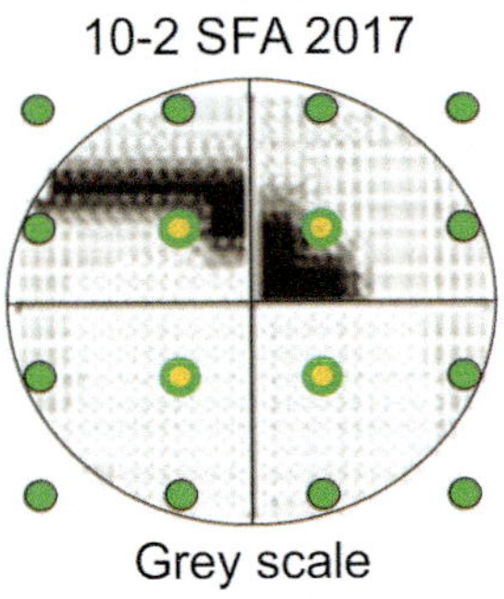

Even in 2017 SFA printout, there are no indications either from grey scale or TDNP (raw data) for the repetition of the test with 10-2 point pattern. But in PDPP, out of the 16 points, 4 points have significant P value (black squares). **In this SFA printout, TDPP and PDPP are giving the clue that the field defect is progressing and need for the repetition of the test with 10-2 point pattern.**

> 2017—10-2 SFA. The localized scotoma which is progressing in the bare area of 30-2 or 24-2 is seen in 10-2 SFA 2017.

24-2 SFA 2018

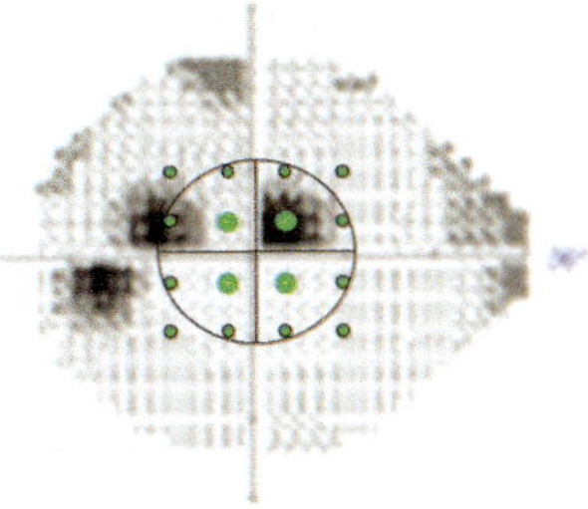

Grey scale

TDPP

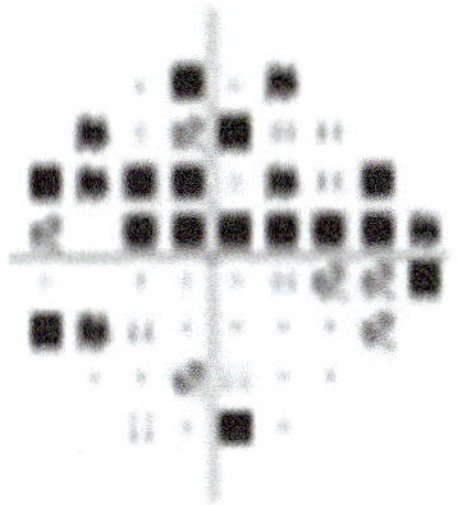

PDPP

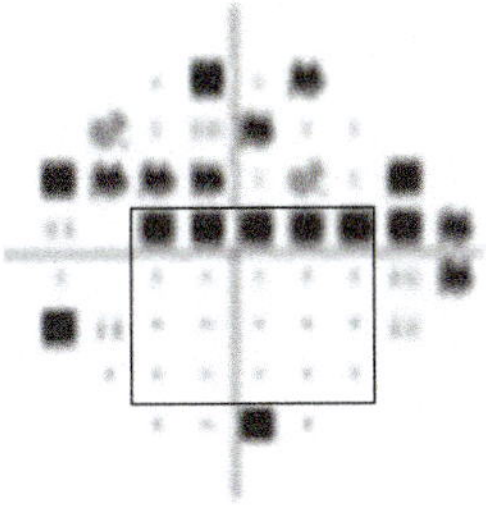

MD -6.14 dB P < 0.5%

TDNP

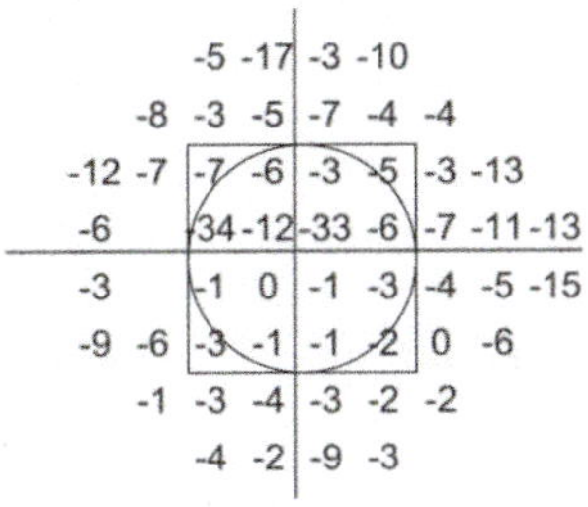

10-2 SFA 2018

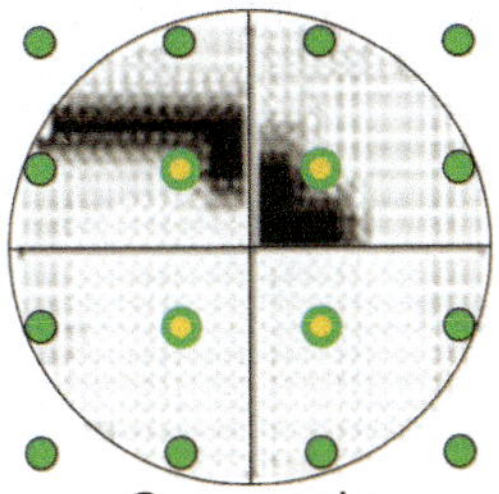

Grey scale

In 2018 SFA printout, there are clues in grey scale and TDNP (Raw data) for the repetition of the test with 10-2 point pattern. In TDPP and PDPP significant P value points (black squares) are increased from 3 to 6 indicating that the field defect is progressing and the need to change the target IOP to still more lower levels or we have to go for surgery.

2018 24-2 SFA—Along with probability plots grey scale and TDNP (raw data) are giving indications to repeat the test with 10-2 point pattern.

24-2 SFA printout	*Probability plots*	*Grey scale*	*TDNP and Raw data*
2014 24-2 SFA printout	3 black squares in the 10° circle area	No clue from grey scale	No severe loss in the 10° circle area
2017 24-2 SFA printout	Number of black squares increased in the 10° circle area	No clue from grey scale	No severe loss in the 10° circle area
2018 24-2 SFA printout	Number of black squares increased in the 10° circle area	Black shade appeared in the 10° circle area	Two points showed severe loss in the 10° circle area

Glaucomas starting within 10° circle area will have major field defect within 10° circle area and few scotomas outside 10° circle area. The major field defect in the 10° circle area may not be appreciated well in 24-2 SFA printout. We will study 24-2 SFA printouts of glaucomas started in 10° circle area to know the indications in 24-2 SFA printout to repeat the test with 10-2 point pattern to pickup type 2 and type 3 glaucomas at an early stage.

When we suspect glaucoma, first we ask 30-2 or 24-2 point pattern visual field test. Then we should look for indications to repeat the test with 10-2 point pattern or not.

We will study 24-2 SFA printouts of type 2 and type 3 glaucoma.

Example 1

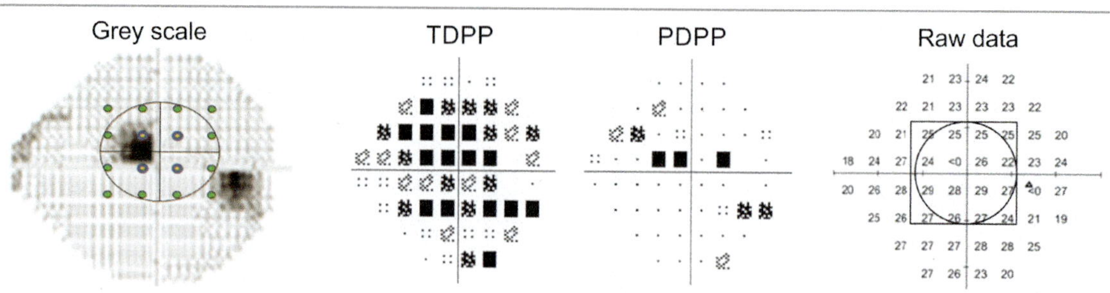

Dark shade in the upper nasal quadrant close to fixation within the 10° circle area in the grey scale and 3 black squares in the 10° circle area of PDPP are giving indications to repeat the test 10-2 point pattern.

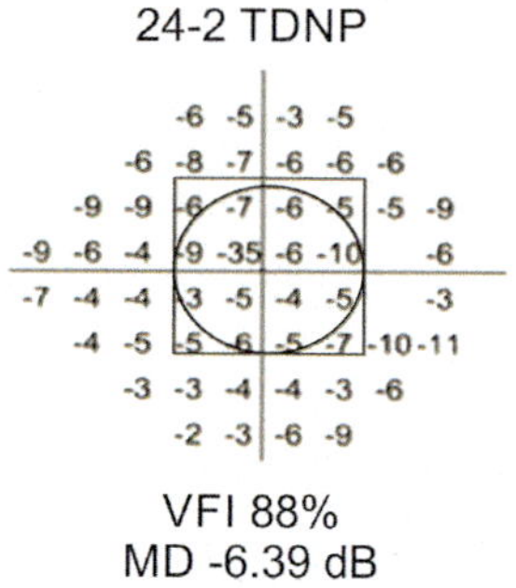

TDNP—First 4 worst deviation points in the 10° circle area: -35 dB, -10 dB, -9 dB, -7 dB.
Raw data—First 4 worst sensitivity points in the 10° circle area: <0 dB, 22 dB, 24 dB, 25 dB.
The sensitivities of the remaining 12 points are better than the sensitivities of these points.

In this example, probability plots, grey scale and TDNP (raw data) are giving indications to repeat the test with 10-2 point pattern

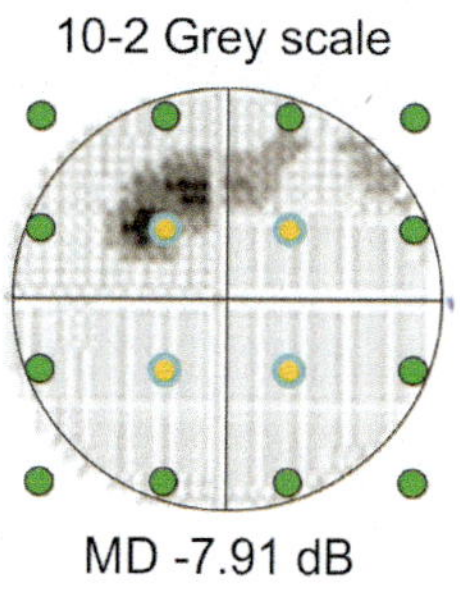

Example 2

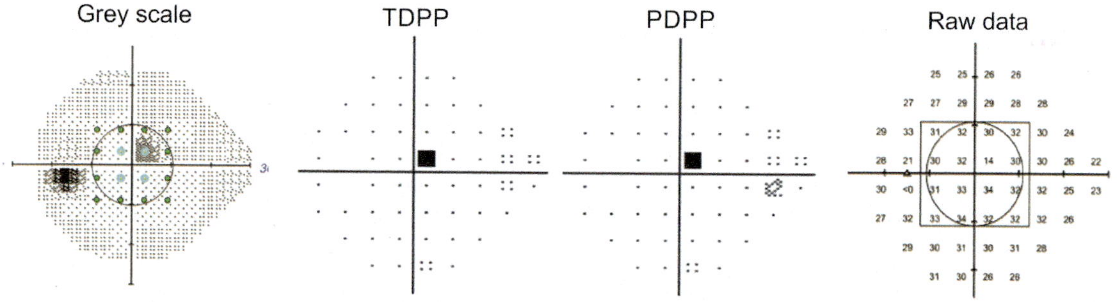

Grey scale—Dark shade in the upper nasal quadrant close to fixation within the 10° circle area.
Probability plots—One point in the 10° circle area of probability plots is represented by black square.

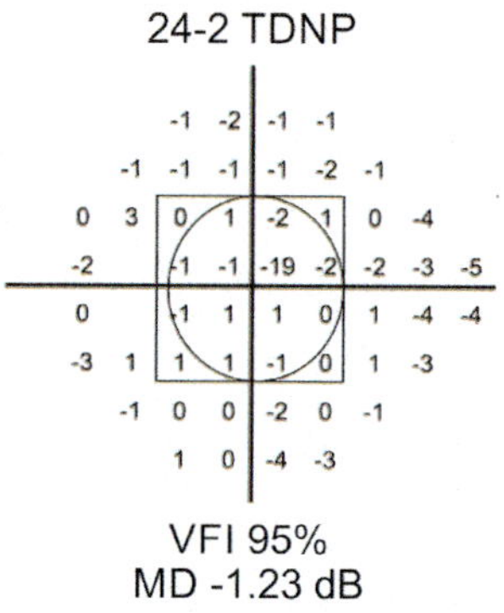

TDNP—First 4 worst deviation points in the 10° circle area: -19 dB, -2 dB, -2 dB, -1 dB.
Raw data: First 4 worst sensitivity points in the 10° circle area: 14 dB, 30 dB, 30 dB, 30 dB.
The sensitivities of the remaining 12 points are better than the sensitivities of these points.

In this example, probability plots, grey scale and TDNP (raw data) are giving indications to repeat the test with 10-2 point pattern.

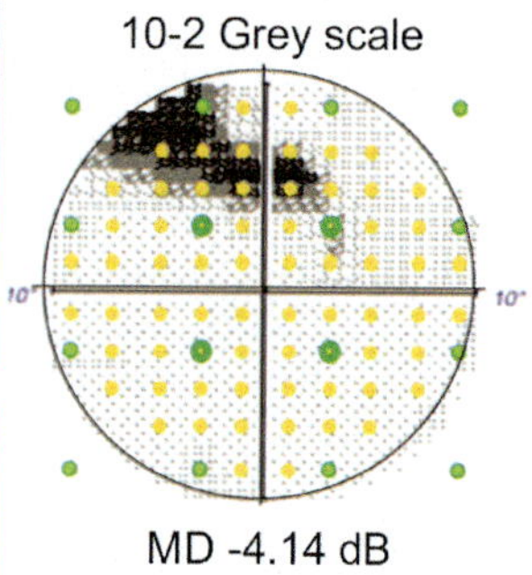

Example 3

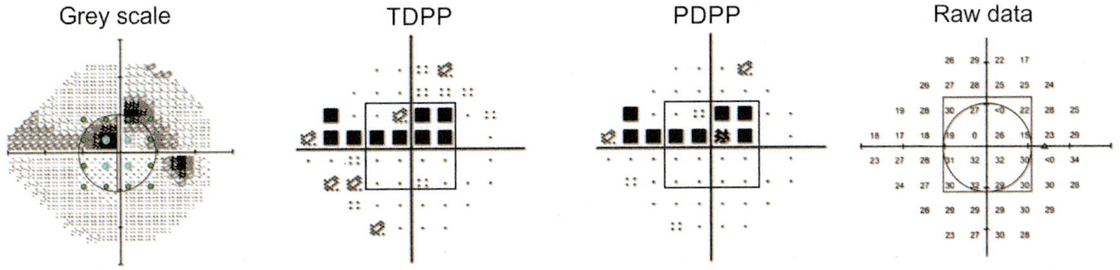

Grey scale—Dark shade in the upper nasal quadrant close to fixation within the 10° circle area.

Probability plots—Six points in the 10° circle area of probability plots is represented by black square.

24-2 TDNP

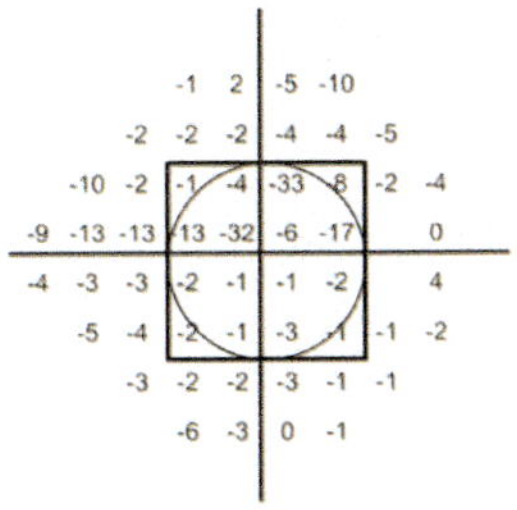

MD -5.23 dB
VFI 84%

TDNP—First 4 worst deviation points in the 10° circle area: -33 dB,-32 dB,-17 dB,-13 dB.
Raw data—First 4 worst sensitivity points in the 10° circle area: < 0 dB, < 0 dB, 19 dB, 19 dB.
The sensitivities of the remaining 12 points are better than the sensitivities of these points.

In this example, probability plots, grey scale and TDNP (raw data) are giving indications to repeat the test with 10-2 point pattern.

10-2 Grey scale

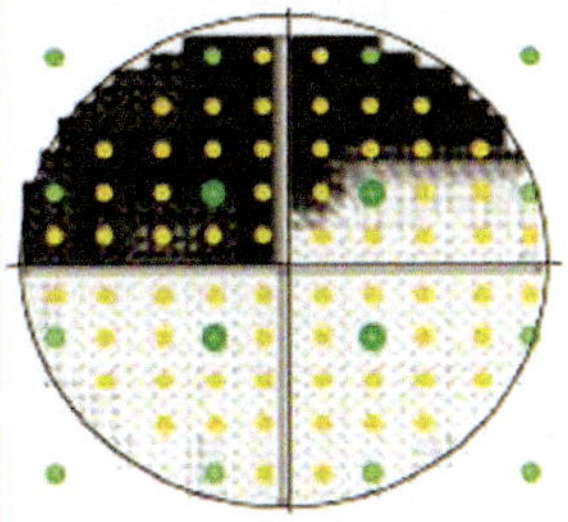

MD -12.84 dB
No VFI index

Example 4

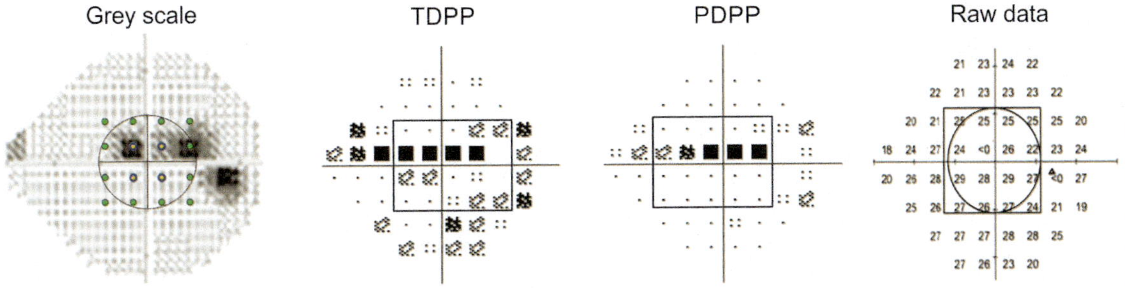

Grey scale—Dark shade in the upper half of the field close to fixation within the 10° circle area.

Probability plots—Four points in the 10° circle area of probability plots is represented by black square.

24-2 TDNP

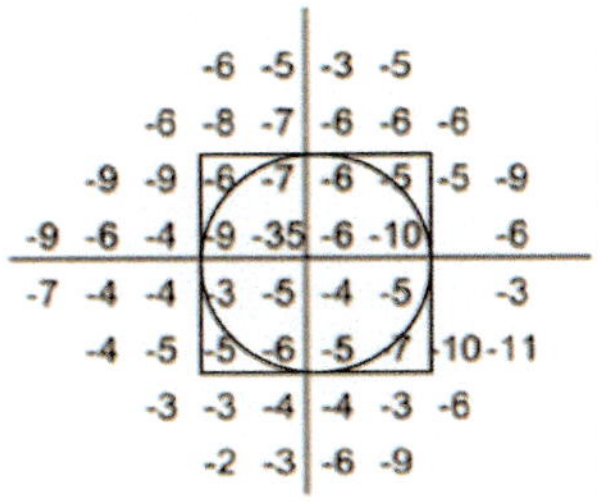

MD -4.62 dB
VFI 87%

TDNP—First 4 worst deviation points in the 10° circle area: -35 dB, -10 dB, -9 dB, -7 dB.
Raw data—First 4 worst sensitivity points in the 10° circle area: < 0 dB, 22 dB, 22 dB, 24 dB.
The sensitivities of the remaining 12 points are better than the sensitivities of these points.

In this example, probability plots, grey scale and TDNP (raw data) are giving indications to repeat the test with 10-2 point pattern.

10-2 Grey scale

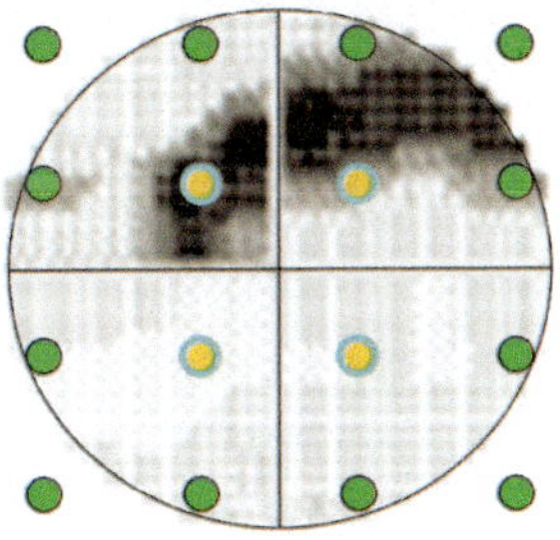

MD -8.29 dB

Example 5

Grey scale | TDPP | PDPP | Raw data

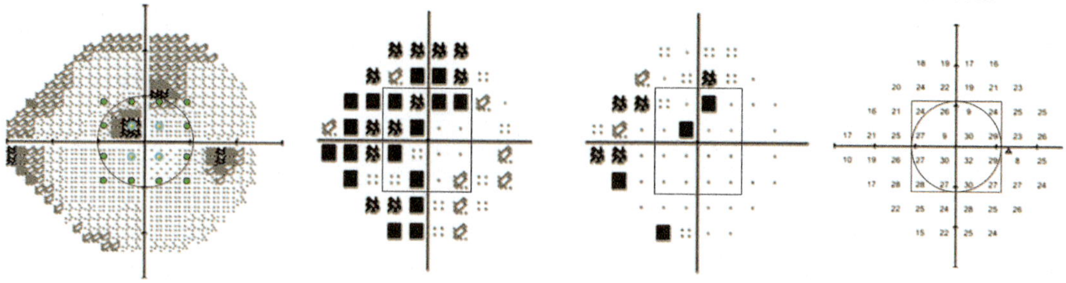

Grey scale—Dark shade in the upper nasal quadrant close to fixation within the 10° circle area.

Probability plots—Two deep scotomas in generalized depression in the 10° circle area are highlighted in the PDPP.

24-2 TDNP

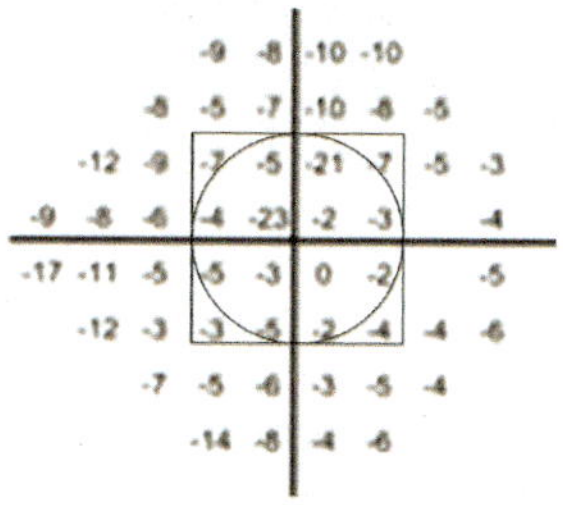

VFI 86%
MD -6.46 dB

TDNP—First 4 worst deviation points in the 10° circle area: -23 dB, -21 dB, -7 dB, -5 dB.
Raw data—First 4 worst sensitivity points in the 10° circle area: 9 dB, 9 dB, 24 dB, 24 dB.
The sensitivities of the remaining 12 points are better than the sensitivities of these points.

In this example, probability plots, grey scale and TDNP (raw data) are giving indications to repeat the test with 10-2 point pattern

10-2 Grey scale

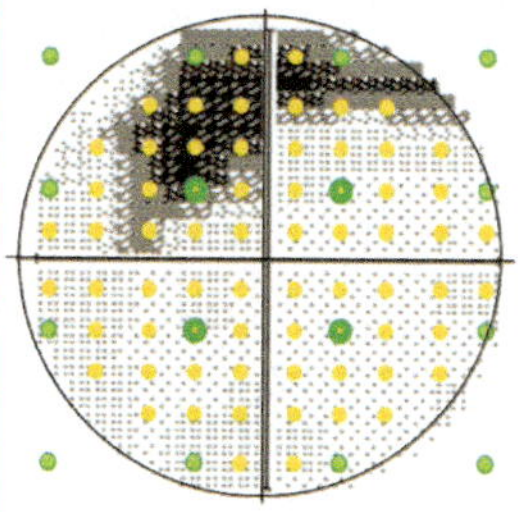

MD -7.20 dB

Example 6

Grey scale | TDPP | PDPP | Raw data

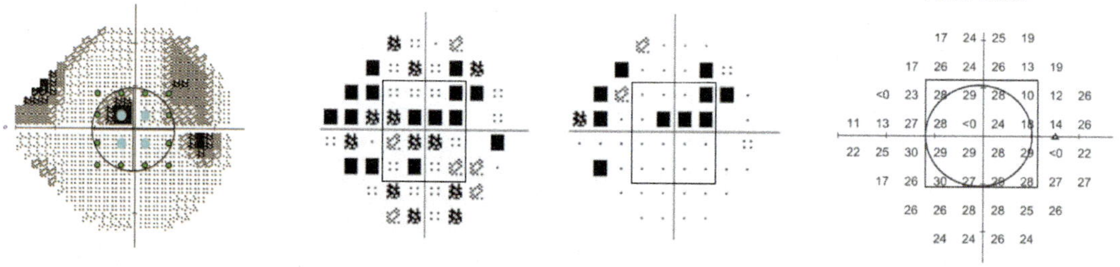

Grey scale—Dark shade in the upper nasal quadrant close to fixation within the 10° circle area.

Probability plots—Four deep scotomas in generalized depression in the 10° circle area are highlighted in the PDPP.

24-2 TDNP

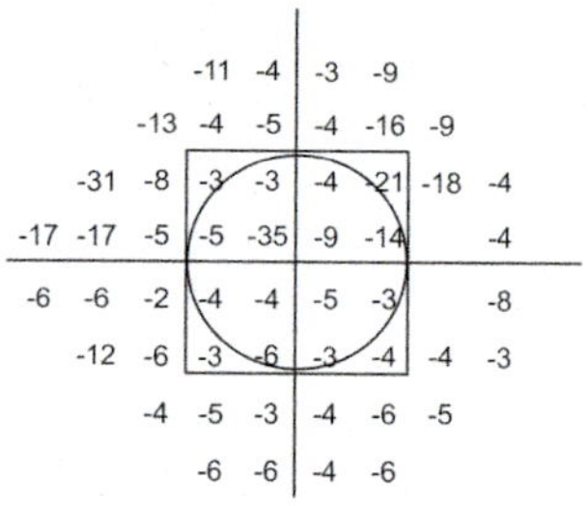

VFI 83%
MD -7.42 dB

TDNP—First 4 worst deviation points in the 10° circle area: -35 dB, -21 dB, -14 dB, -9 dB.
Raw data—First 4 worst sensitivity points in the 10° circle area: < 0 dB, 10 dB, 18 dB, 24 dB.
The sensitivities of the remaining 12 points are better than the sensitivities of these points.

In this example, probability plots, grey scale and TDNP (raw data) are giving indications to repeat the test with 10-2 point pattern.

10-2 Grey scale

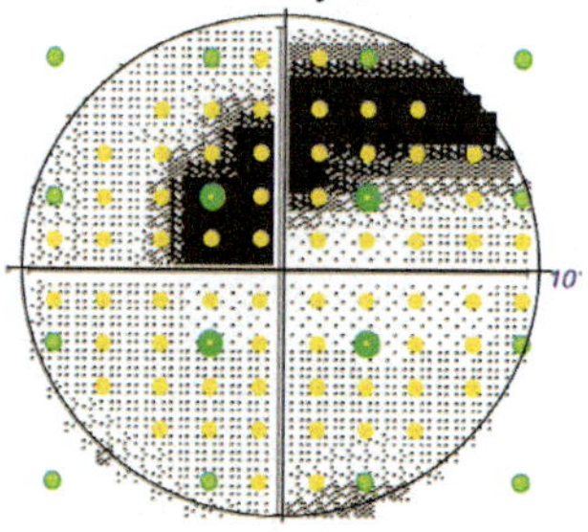

MD -10.85 dB

Case 13 RE

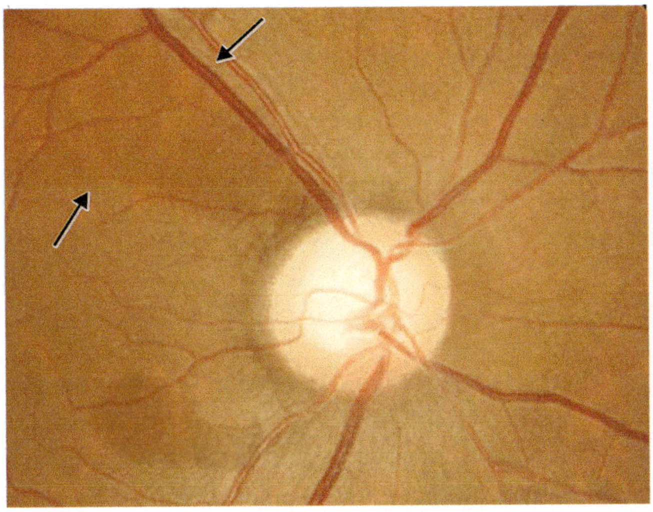

Case 13 LE

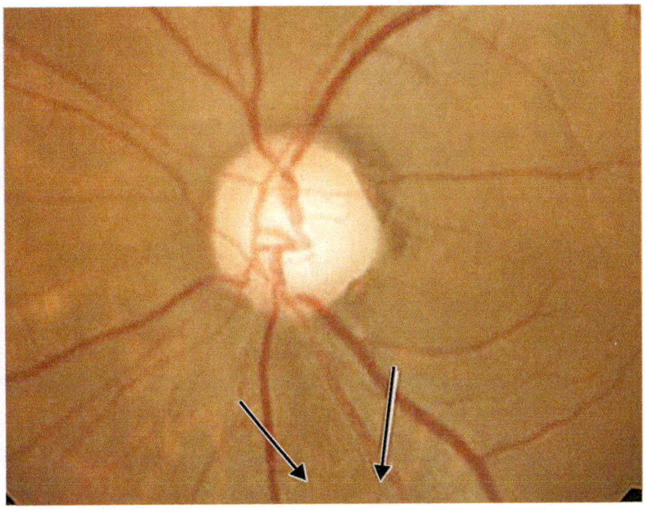

RNFL defect present in both the eyes.

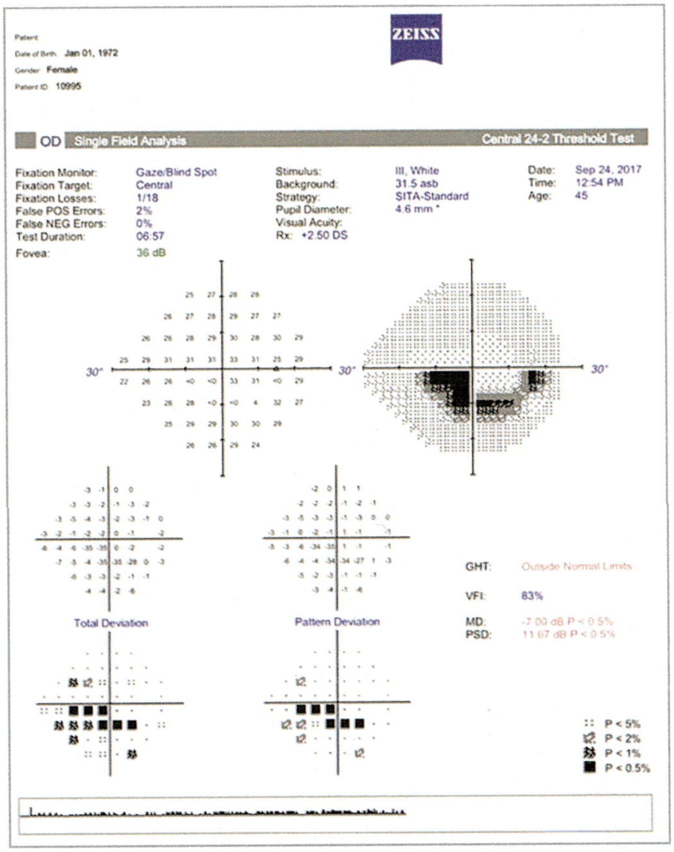

FL 1/18; FP 2%; FN 0%
Fovea 36 dB; GHT-ONL; VFI 83%
MD -7.00 dB P < 0.5%; PSD 11.67 dB P < 0.5%

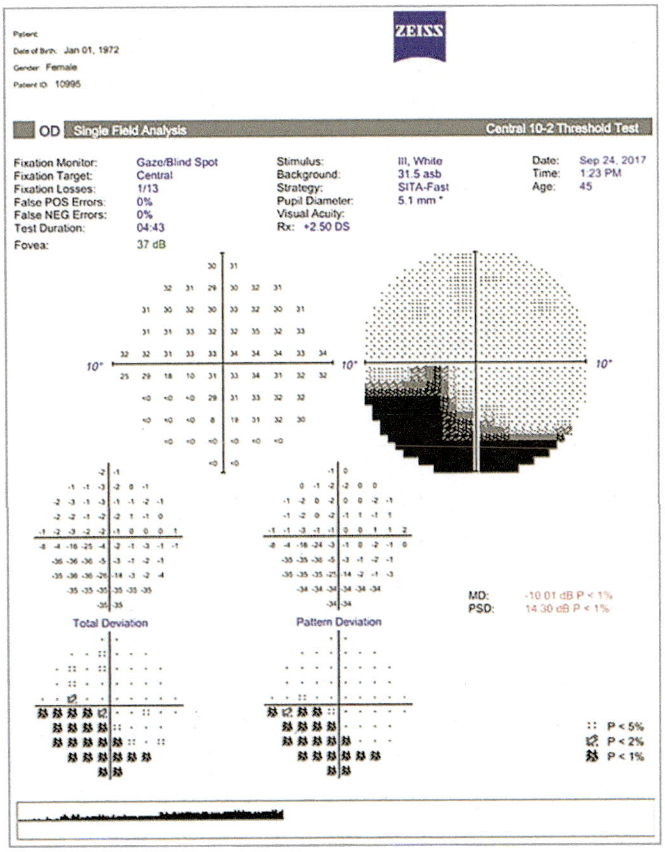

FL 1/13; FP 0%; FN 0%
Fovea 37 dB
MD -10.01 dB P < 1%; PSD 14.30 dB P < 1%

Case 13 RE

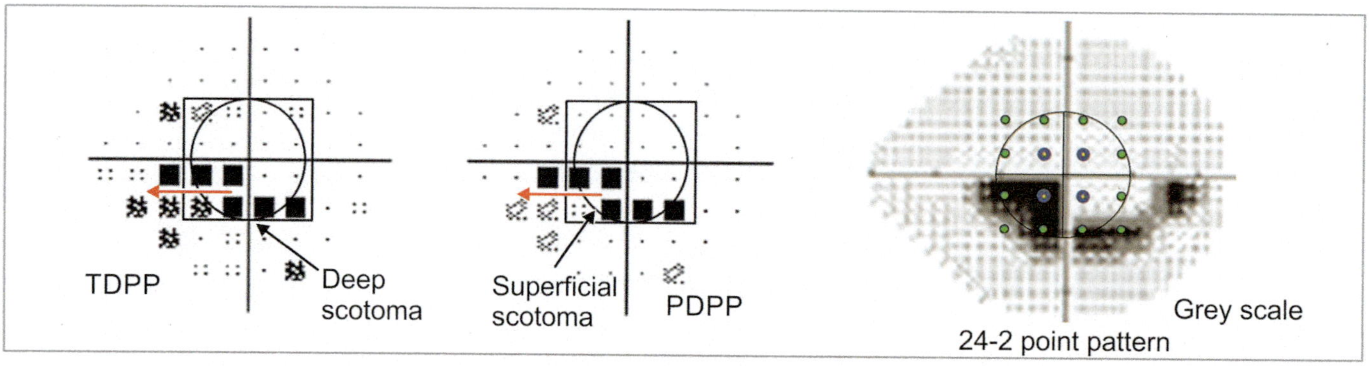

Location and extent of the field defect (Probability plot)—Field defect mainly located in the lower nasal quadrant in the 10° circle area and most of the points are represented by black squares. Normally the deep scotomas retain the P < 0.5% and the superficial scotomas change their P values either to P < 2% or to P < 5%. During the conversion of total deviation plots to pattern deviation plots, the scotomas (P < 1%) of the TDPP will be changed to either to P < 2% or P < 5% in the PDPP. From the probability plots it is evident that the disease process started in the 10° circle and is progressing away from fixation.

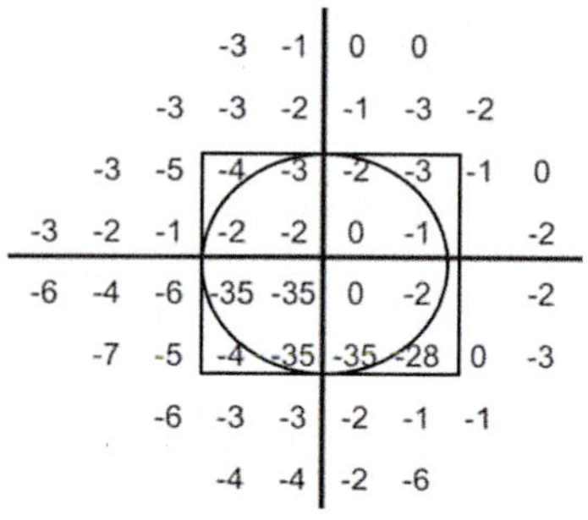

TDNP

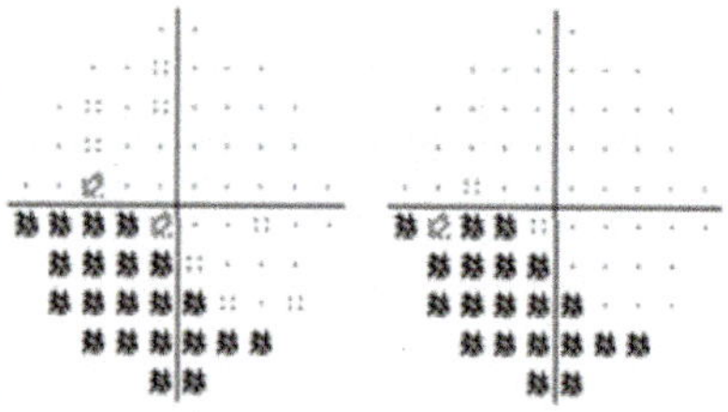

10-2 Probability plots

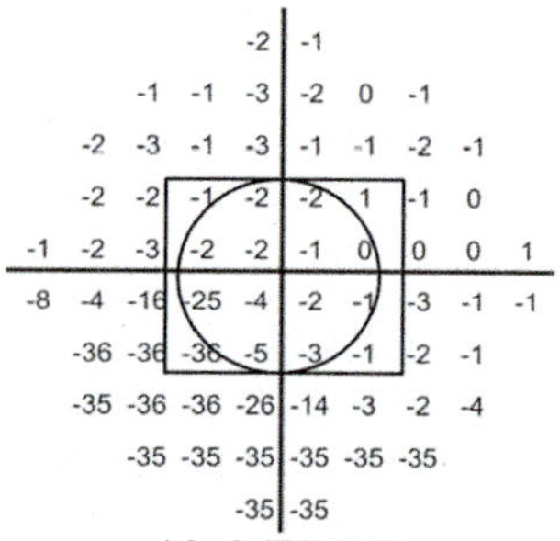

10-2 TDNP

Depth of the field defect (TDNP)—The loss of sensitivity is -35 dB at 4 points in the 10° circle area. All these 4 points are absolute scotomas. **MD -7.00 dB P < 0.5%.** Since the loss of sensitivity of the points in the 10° circle area is very severe, we should repeat the test with 10-2 point pattern.

24-2 MD -7.00 dB P < 0.5%

PSD 11. 67 dB P < 0.5%

VFI 83%

10-2 MD -10.01 dB P < 1%

10-2 PSD 14.30 dB P < 1%

The field defect started within 3° circle and progressed away from fixation and towards the lower nasal quadrant. Almost all the points in the field defect are absolute scotomas.

Normally we expect the 24-2 MD index will be higher than the 10-2 MD index. Since the field defect started within 10° circle area 10-2 MD index is higher than the 24-2 MD index.

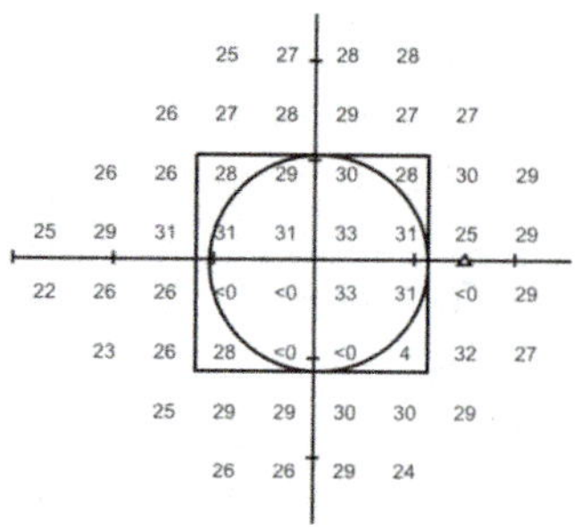

Raw data

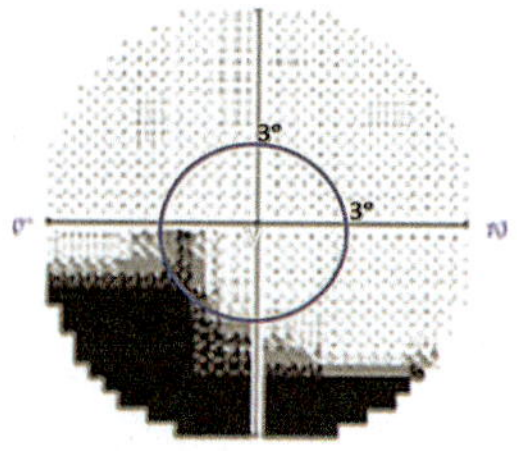

10-2 Grey scale

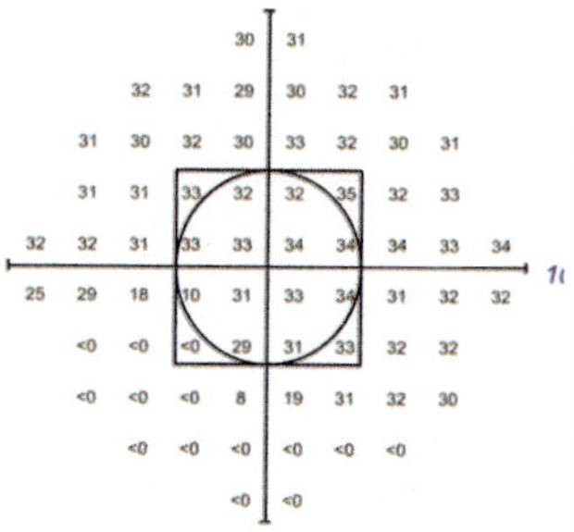

10-2 Raw data

Normally glaucoma progression will be analyzed on the basis of either MD index or VFI index (guided progression analysis-GPA). The most important point to note is VFI is not calculated in 10-2 printouts. So for glaucomas starting within 10° circle (Type 2 glaucomas), glaucoma progression will be analysed only on the basis of change in MD index. To assess progression we should repeat the test both with 24-2 and 10-2 point patterns.

Case 13 LE

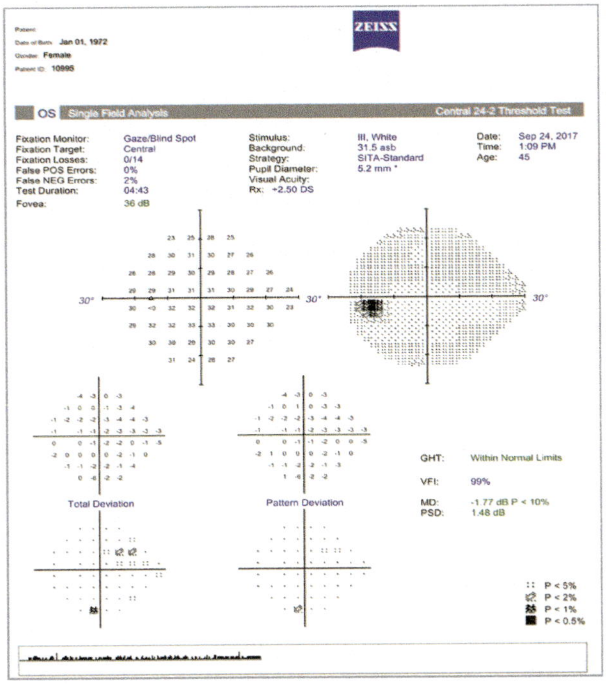

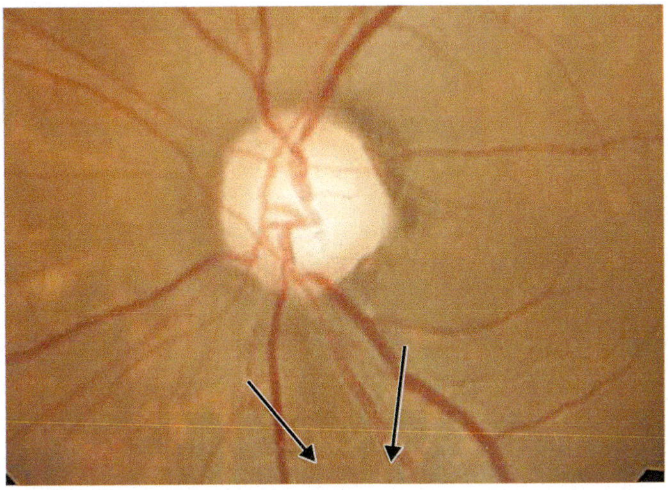

FL 0/14; FP 0%; FN 2%
Fovea 36 dB

GHT-WNL
VFI 99%
MD -1.77 dB P < 10%
PSD 1.48 dB

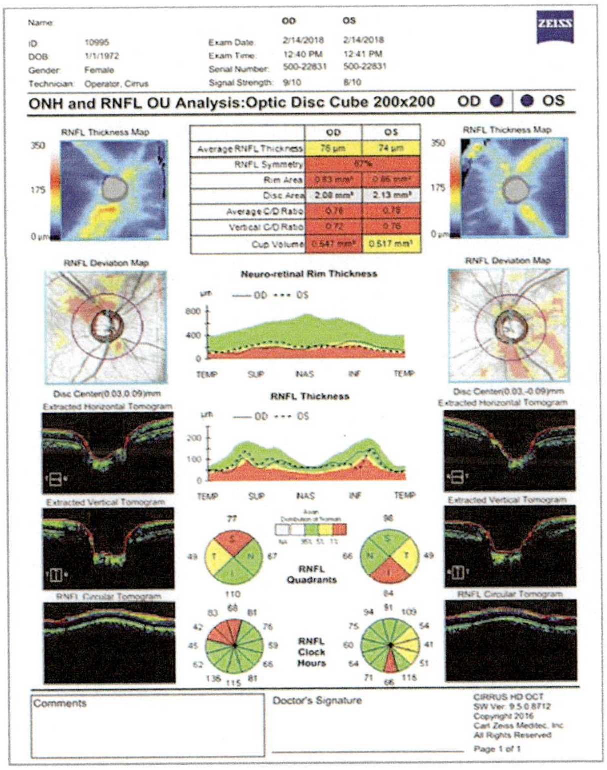

The fundus is showing RNFL defect and it is appreciated in the OCT. But the field defect is not appreciated in the 24-2 SFA printout. Always note the direction of RNFL defect. In this case RNFL defect is directed towards periphery. In such situations, the field defect will be located outside 30° circle and it will not be picked up by 24-2 or 30-2 point patterns. This is the most important take home message from this case.

Case 14 RE **Case 14 LE**

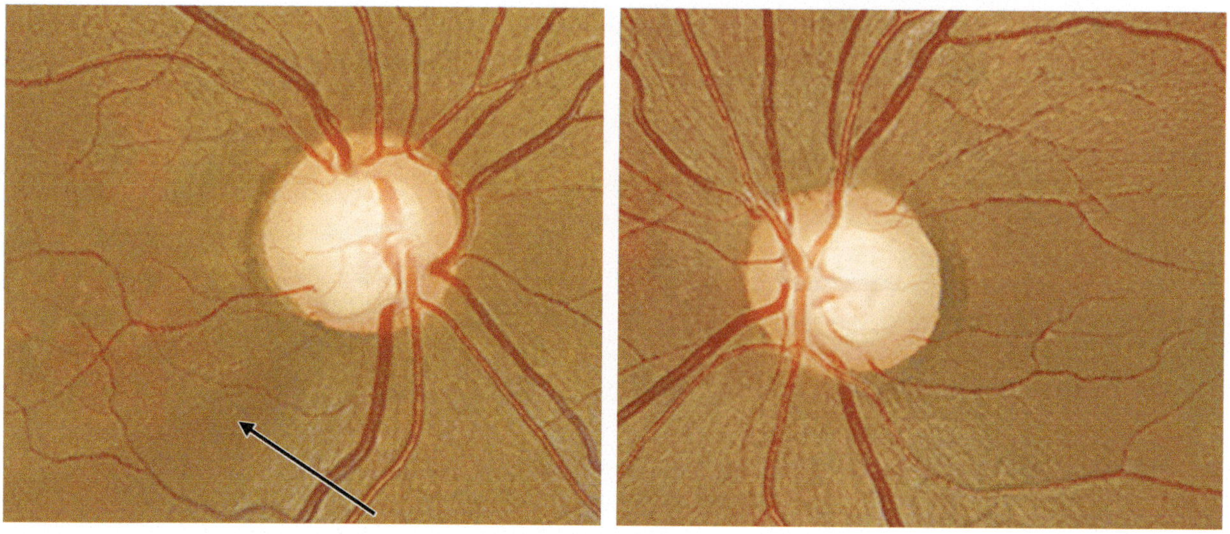

RNFL defect in the right eye.

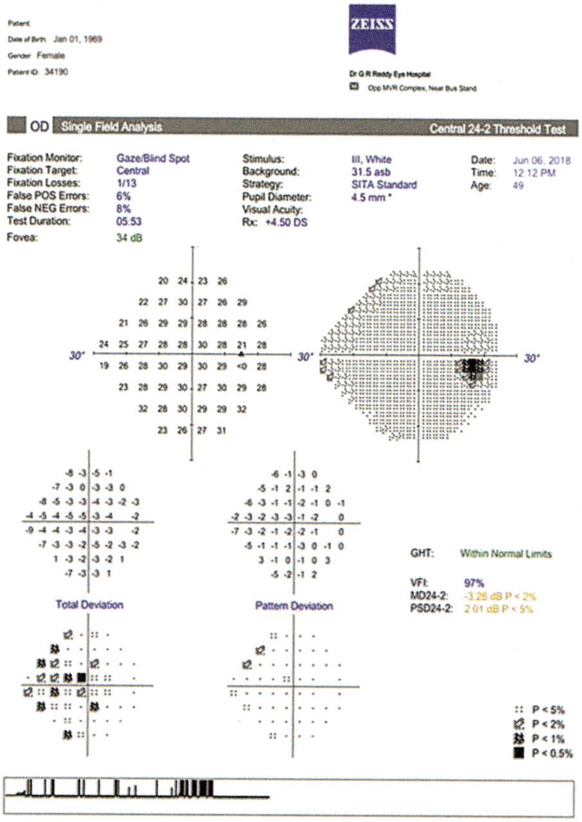

FL 1/13; FP 6%; FN 8%
Fovea 34 dB; GHT-WNL; VFI 97%
MD -3.28 dB P < 2%; PSD 2.01 dB P < 5%

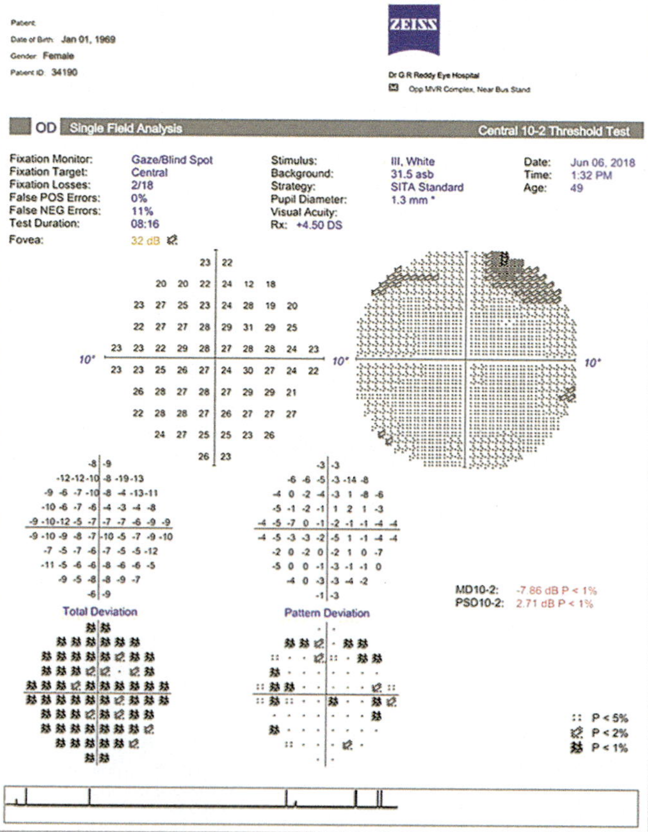

FL 2/18; FP 0%; FN 11%
Fovea 32 dB
MD -7.86 dB P < 1%; PSD 2.71 dB P < 1%

Case 14 RE

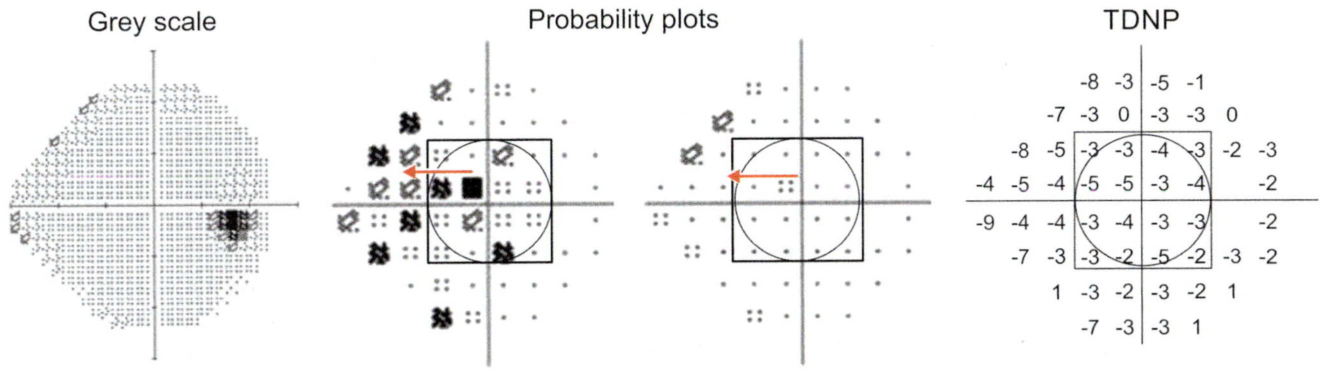

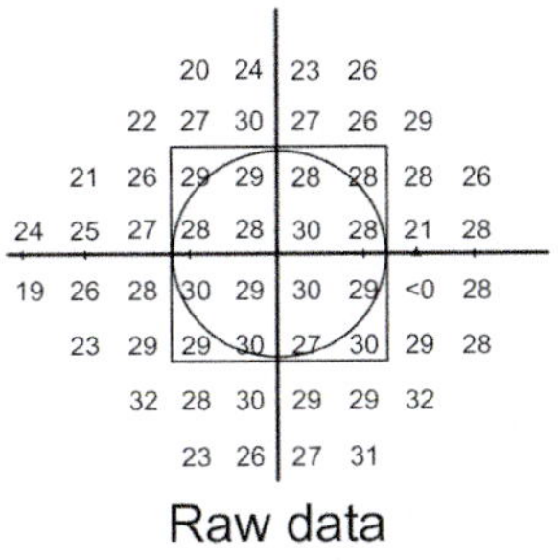

Location and extent of the field defect (Probability plot)—Field defect is mainly located in the upper nasal quadrant in the 10° circle area and one point is represented by black squares in TDPP.

GHT-WNL, VFI 97%, MD -3.28 dB P < 2%, PSD 2.01 dB P < 5%, IOP is 20 mm Hg and RNFL defect is present.

The only indication to repeat the test with 10-2 point pattern is a black square in the 10° circle area. 5 dB loss of sensitivity in the 10° area will not be appreciated in the grey scale, but it will be better appreciated in the probability plots. Actually the disease started within 10° circle area and is progressing away from fixation.

Case 14 RE (10-2)

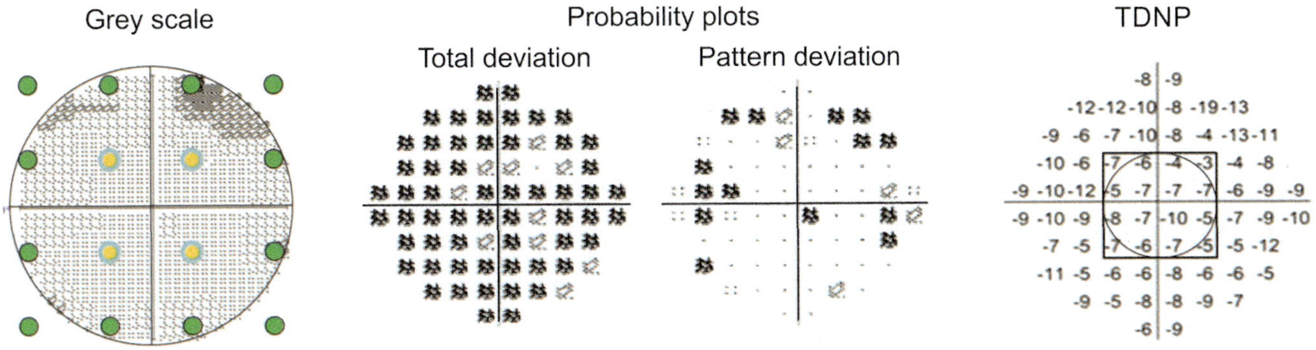

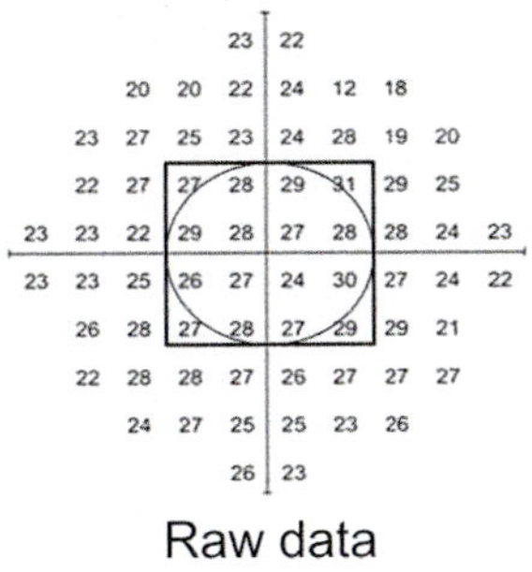

Note that the MD index in 10-2 point pattern is -7. 86 dB P < 1% and MD index in 24-2 point pattern is -3.28 dB P < 1%. Because the disease started within 10° circle area MD index is more in 10-2 point pattern.

In Type 2 and Type 3 glaucomas, we require both 30-2 or 24-2 and 10-2 point pattern SFA printouts as base line printouts for progression analysis. We have to analyse progression by change in MD index. We can not assess progression dependent on VFI index as it is not present in 10-2 printouts.

Case 14 LE

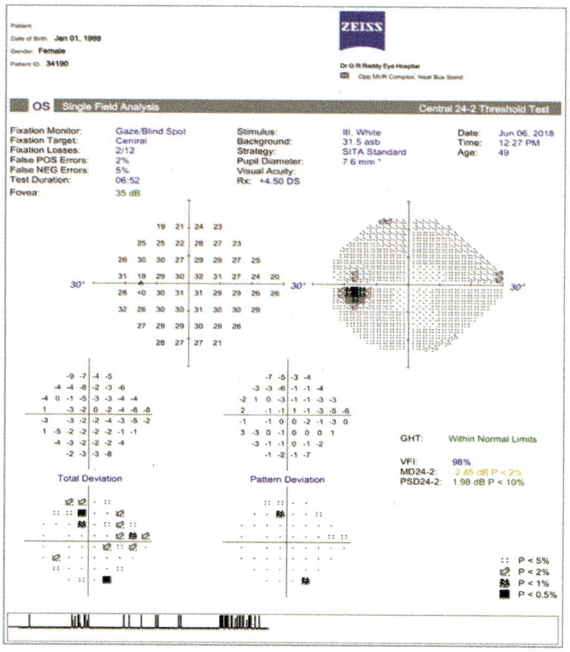

FL 2/12
FP 2%
FN 5%
Fovea 35 dB
GHT-WNL
VFI 98%
MD -2.85 dB P <2%
PSD 1.98 dB P <10%

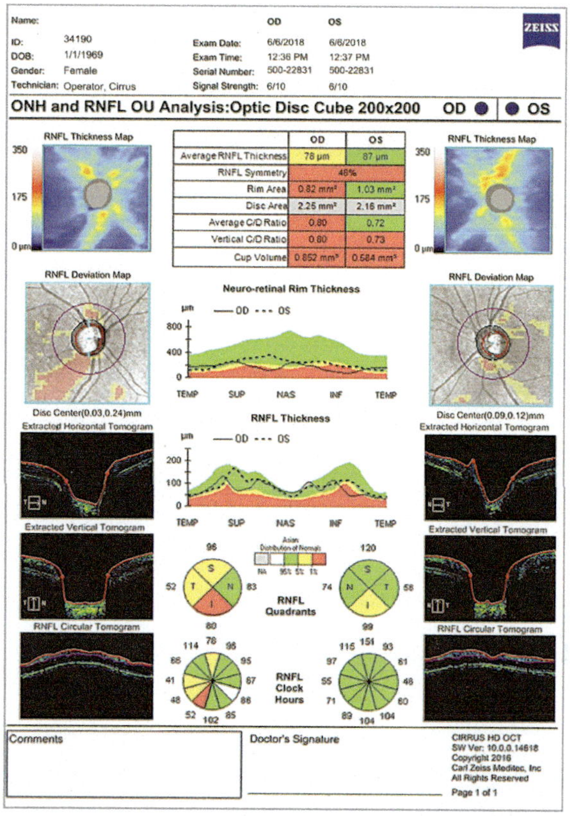

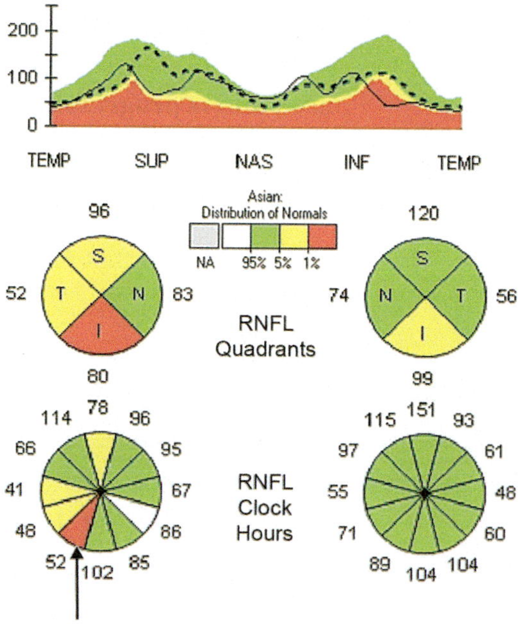

Thinning between 7 and 9 clock hours in the OCT in right eye gives clue to repeat the test with 10-2 point patterns

Right eye (RE): Fundus (RNFL defect) and OCT are correlating to one another. We get the most important information from OCT clock hour map, that is, the direction of the RNFL defect. This information helps us to select a proper point pattern. If maculopapillary fibers are involved, the thinning will be shown between 7 and 9 clock hours in the OCT in right eye. This information gives us a clue to select 10-2 point pattern.

Case 15 RE | **Case 15 LE**

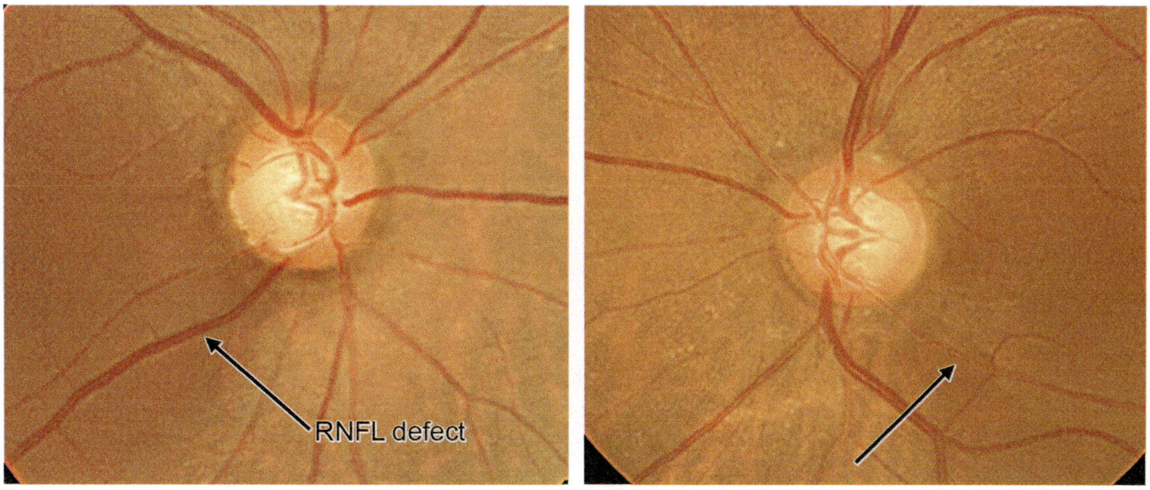

RNFL defect in both the eyes.

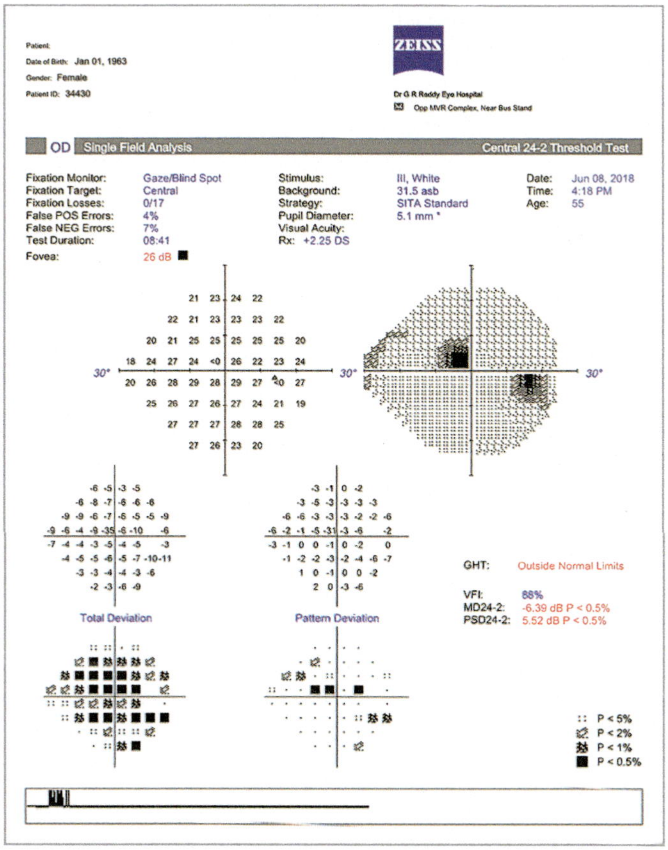

FL 0/17; FP 4%; FN 7%
Fovea 26 dB; GHT-ONL; VFI 88%
MD -6.39 dB P < 0.5%; PSD 5.52 dB P < 0.5%

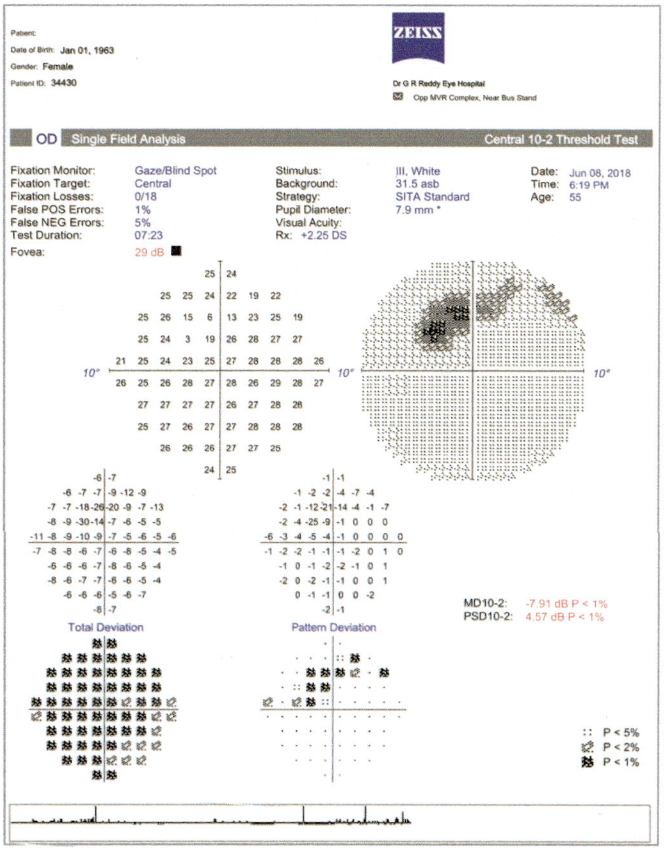

FL 0/18; FP 1%; FN 5%
Fovea 29 dB
MD -7.91 dB; P < 1%; PSD 4.57 dB; P < 1%

Case 15 RE

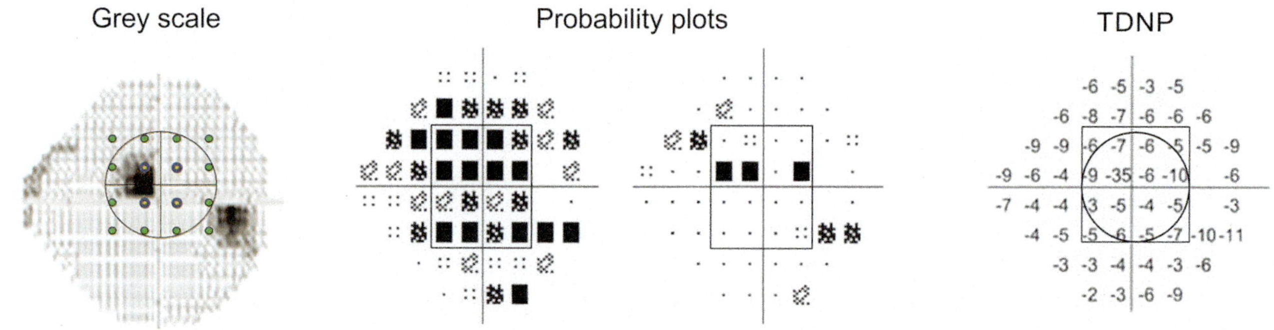

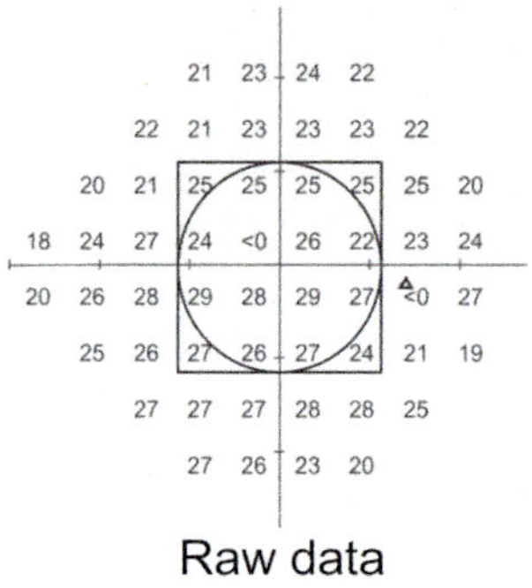

The grey scale and PDPP show a localized scotoma in the upper nasal quadrant within the 10° circle area and the raw data is showing an absolute scotoma at 3° point in the upper nasal quadrant. These are the indications to repeat the test with 10-2 point pattern.

GHT ONL, VFI 88%, MD -6.39 dB P < 0. 5%, PSD 5.52 dB P < 0.5%.

The outer 12 points in the 10° circle area of 30-2 or 24-2 are not included in 10-2 point pattern and hence, the sensitivities of these points will not be seen in the raw data of 10-2 point pattern. The inner 4 points on the 3° circle are tested in both 30-2 and 10-2 point patterns.

Case 15 10-2 RE

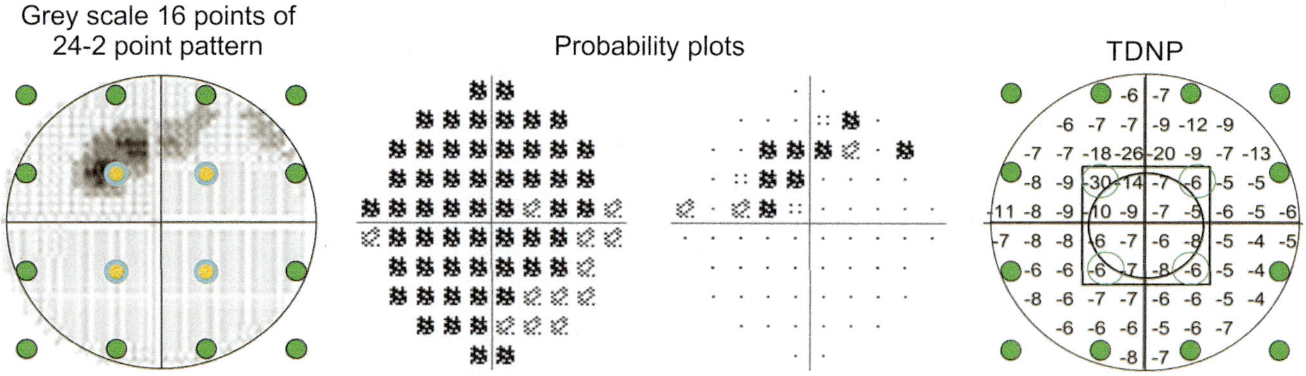

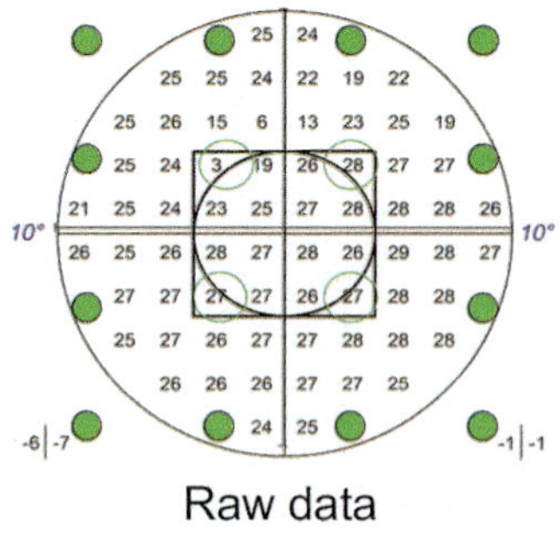

The localized scotoma is progressing towards upper temporal quadrant and travelling between the 3° and 9° points. This is the reason why the scotoma is not appreciated in 24-2 grey scale. Note that the **MD index of 10-2 point pattern is -7.91 dB P < 1%** and MD index in 24-2 point pattern is -6.39 dB P < 0.5%. Because the disease started within 10° circle area, MD index is more 10-2 point pattern.

Target IOP—Since the field defect is close to fixation we should aim for low target IOP. Since most of the cases of the type 2 glaucomas are normotensive glaucomas, avoid beta blockers.

Case 15 LE

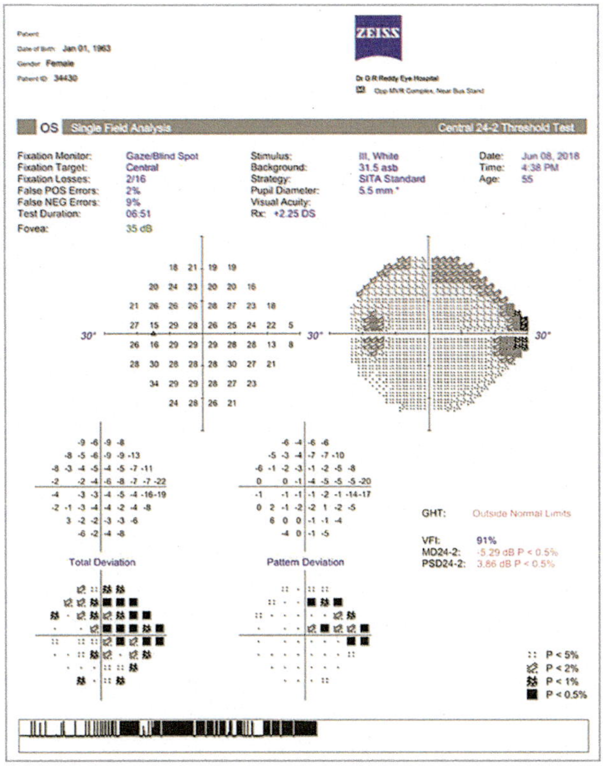

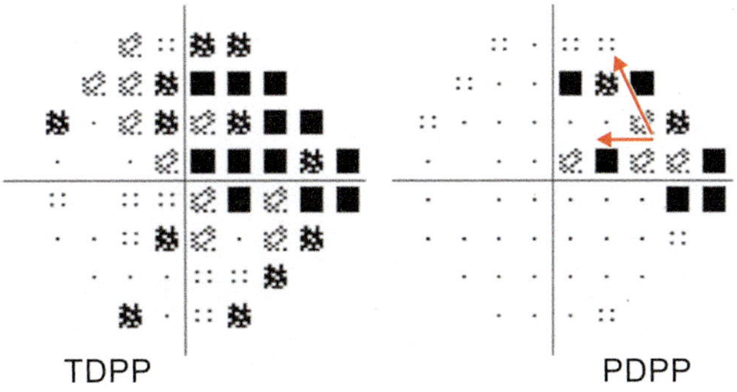

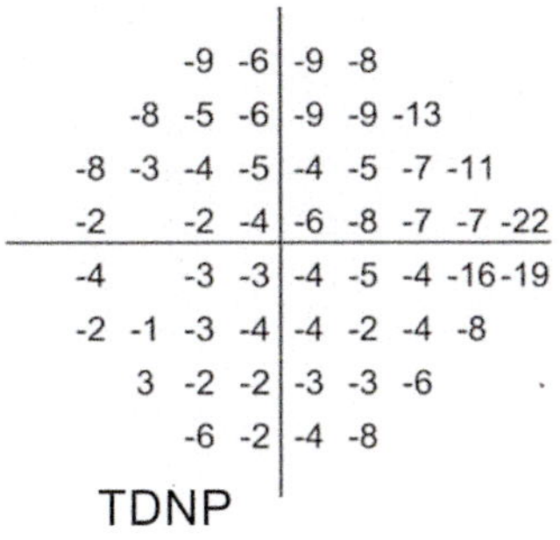

VFI 91%
MD -5.29 dB
P < 0.5%

In the LE, glaucoma started outside 10° circle and the direction of progression is towards fixation.

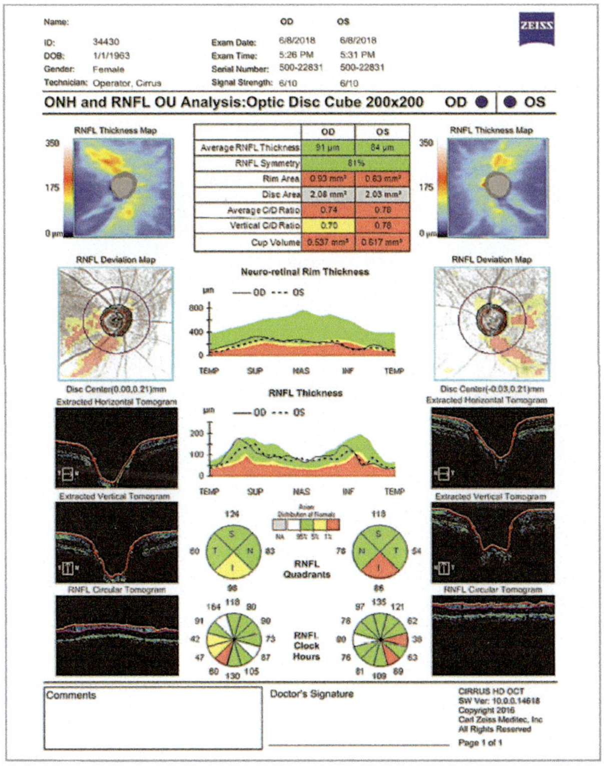

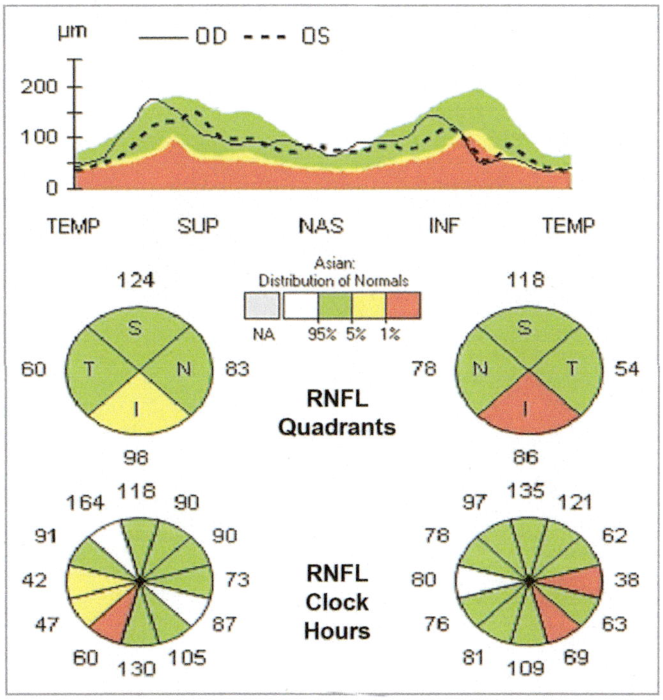

Thinning between 7 and 9 clock hours in the OCT in right eye gives clue to repeat the fields test with 10-2 point pattern.

Case 16 RE **Case 16 LE**

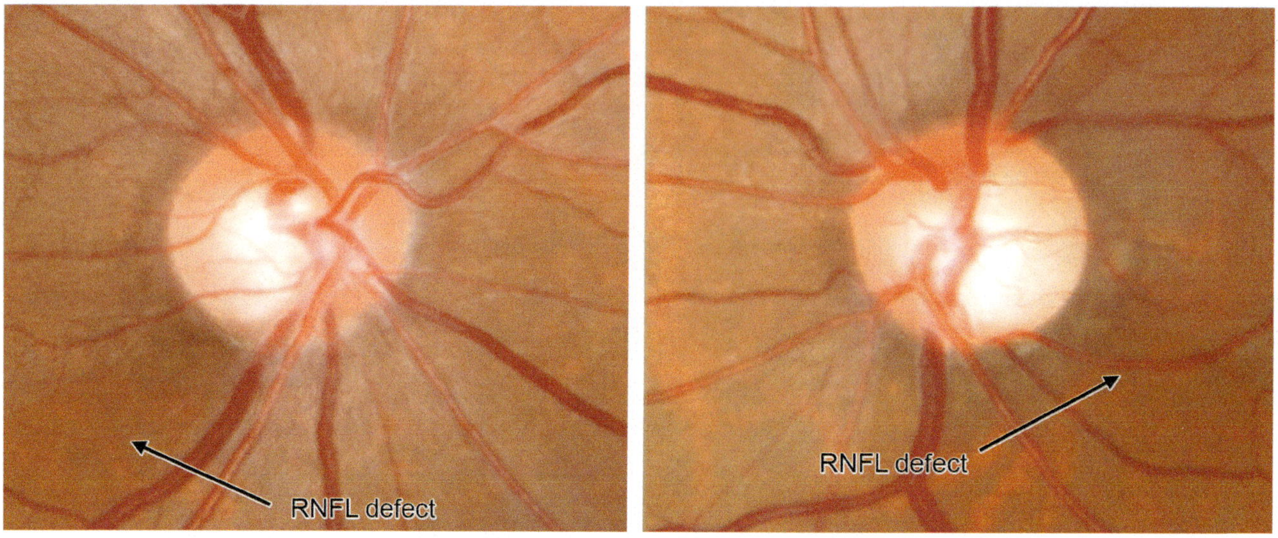

RNFL defect in both the eyes.

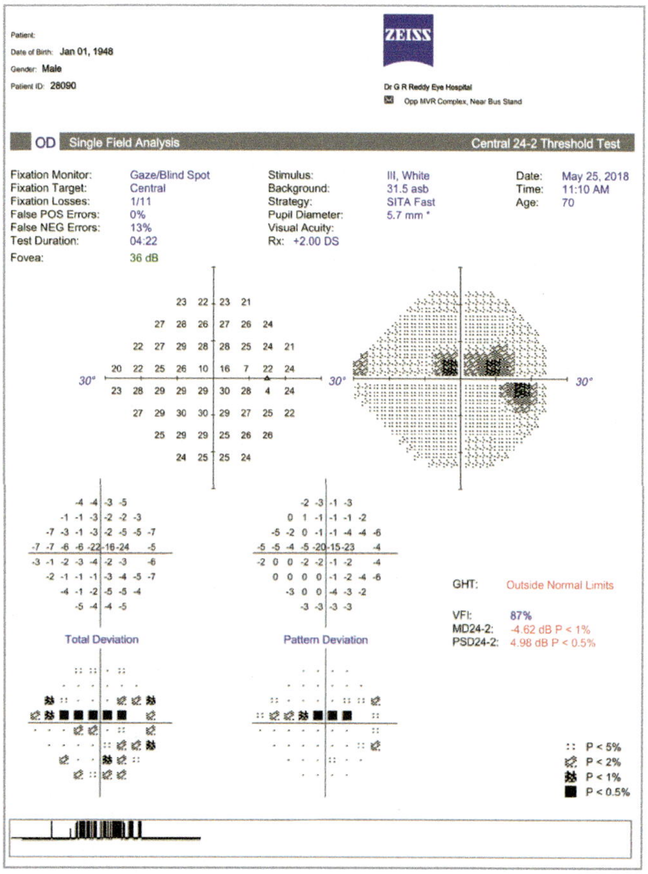

FL 1/11; FP 0%; FN 13%
Fovea 36 dB; GHT-ONL; VFI 87%
MD -4.62 dB P < 1%; PSD 4.98 dB P < 0.5%

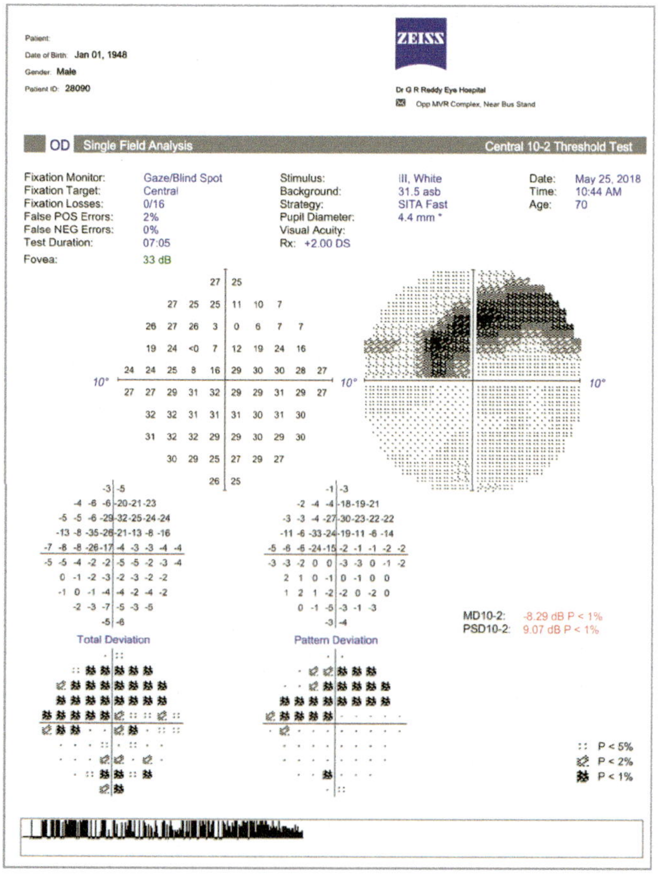

FL 0/16; FP 2%; FN 0%
Fovea 33 dB
MD -8.29 dB P < 1%; PSD 9.07 dB P < 1%

Case 16 RE

Grey scale

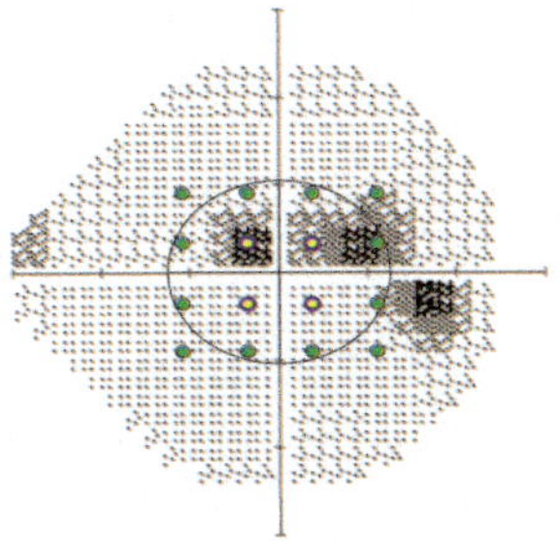

Probability plots

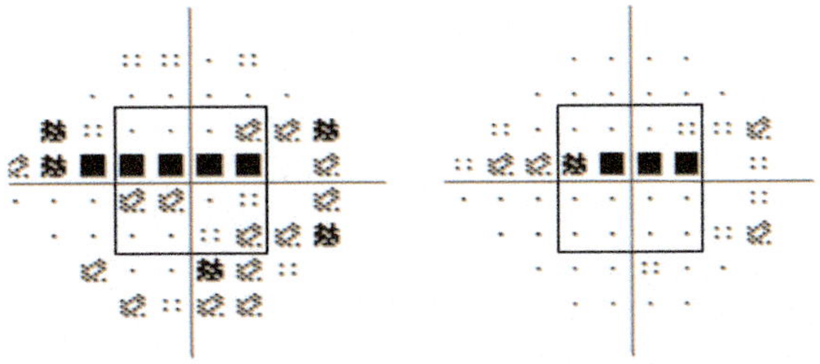

TDNP

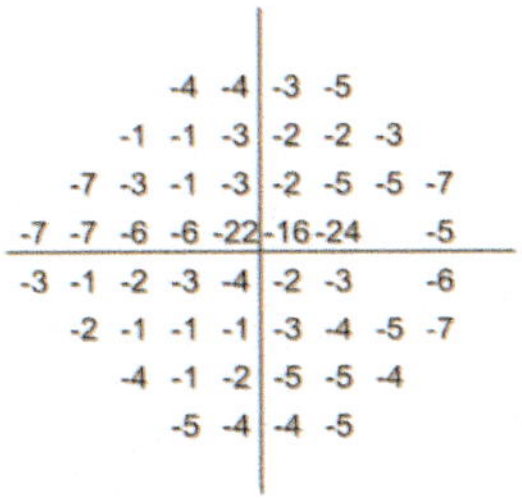

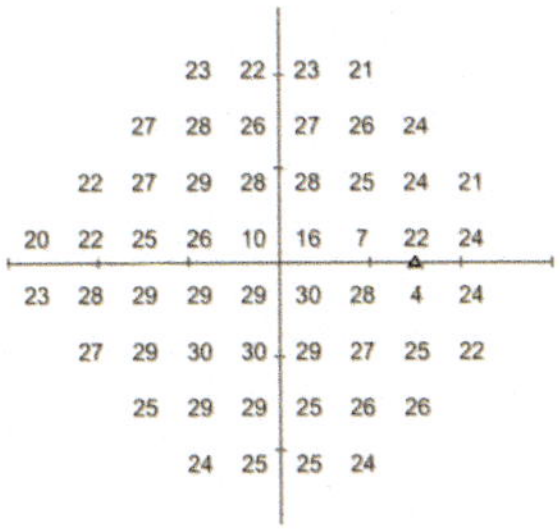

Raw data

The grey scale and probability plots are showing localized scotoma in the upper nasal and temporal quadrants within the 10° circle area.

The loss of sensitivity at 2 points of 3° circle is severe. We have to repeat the test with 10-2 point pattern.

VFI 87%

24-2 MD -4. 62 dB P <1%

Case 16 RE

Point pattern (Grey scale)

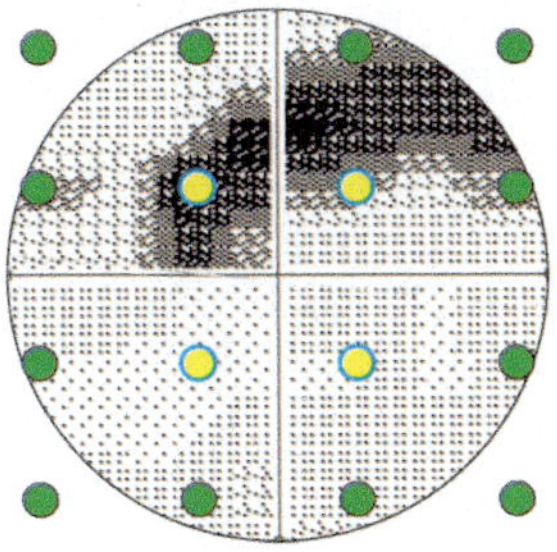

Probability plots

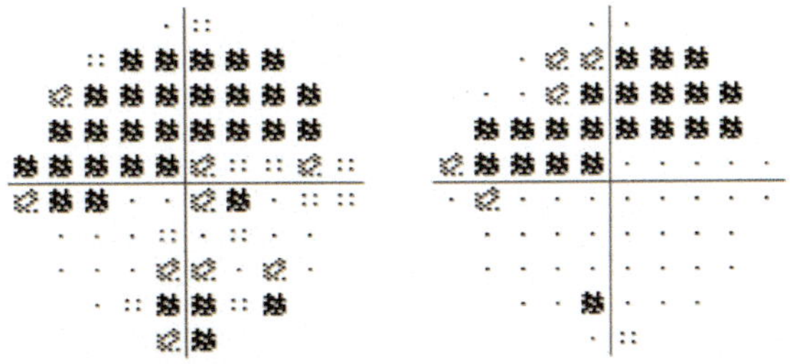

TDNP

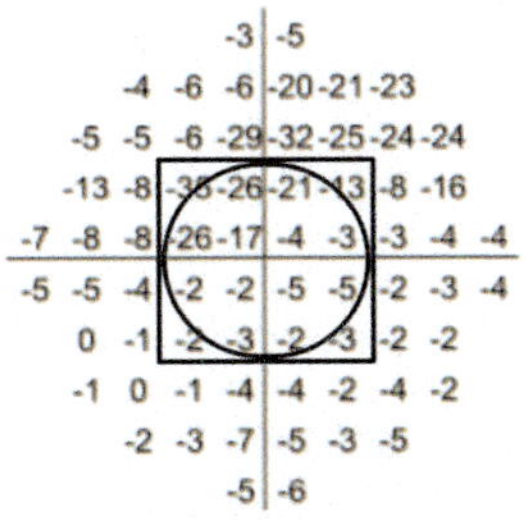

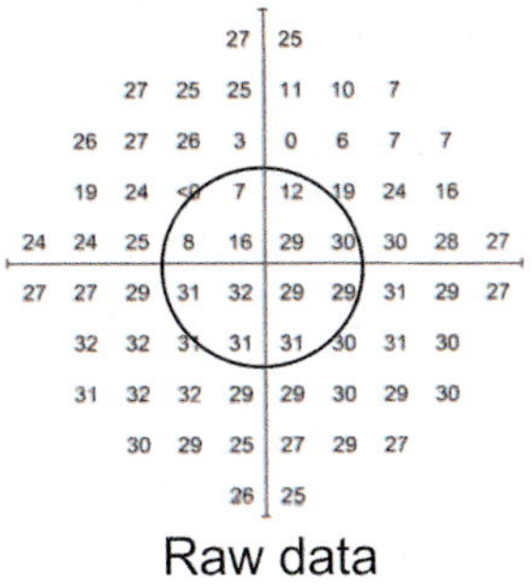

Raw data

The localized scotoma is progressing towards upper temporal quadrant and involving the 3° and 9° points in 24-2 point pattern. This is the reason why the scotoma is appreciated in 24-2.

Note that the MD index in 10-2 point pattern is -8.29 dB P < 1% and MD index in 24-2 point pattern is -4.62 dB P < 1%. This is the reason why we should not grade glaucomas on the basis of MD index values.

Because the disease started within 10° circle area MD index is more 10-2 point pattern. In follow-up tests we should have both 24-2 and 10-2 SFA printouts to assess progression.

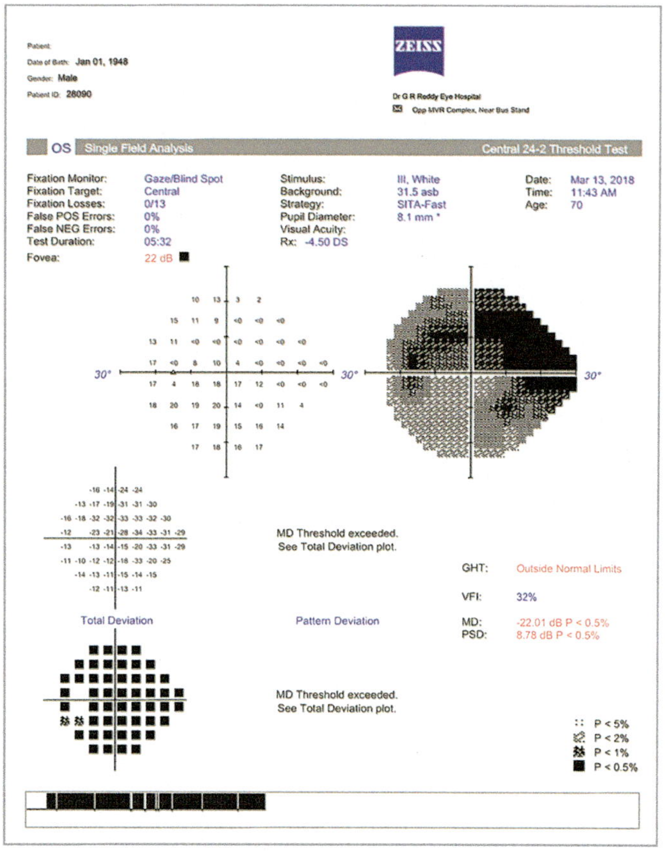

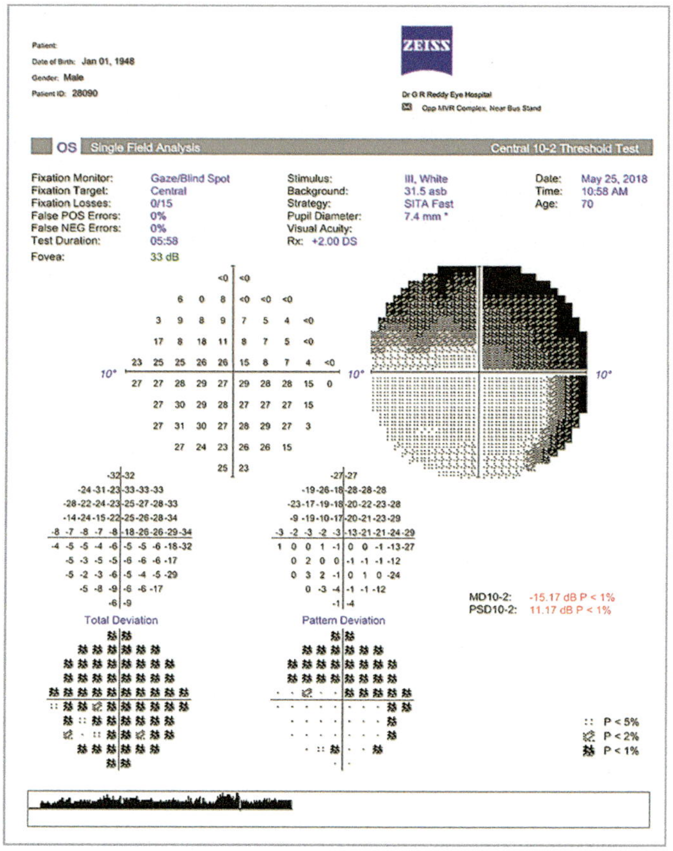

VFI 32%
MD -22.01 dB P < 0.5%; PSD 8.78 dB P < 0.5%

FL 0/15; FP 0%; FN 0%; Fovea 33 dB
MD -15.17 dB P < 1%; PSD 11.17 dB P < 0.5%

Case 16 LE

Grey scale

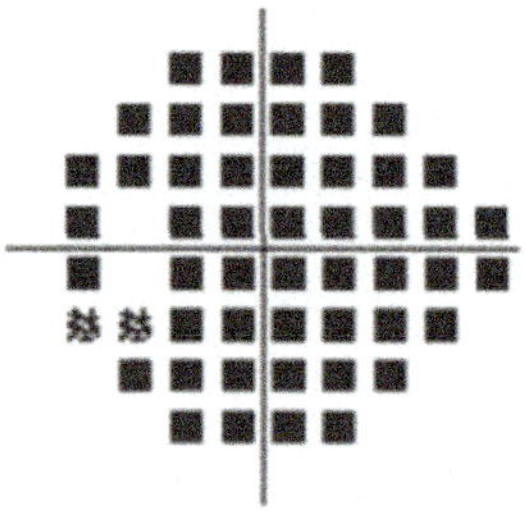

MD threshold exceeded
See total deviation plot

Probability plots

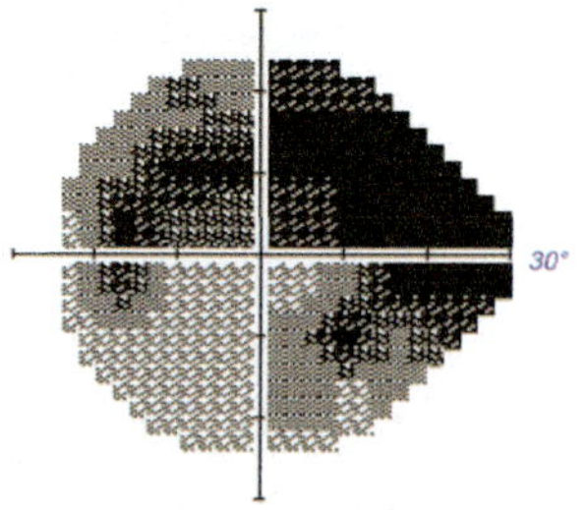

TDNP

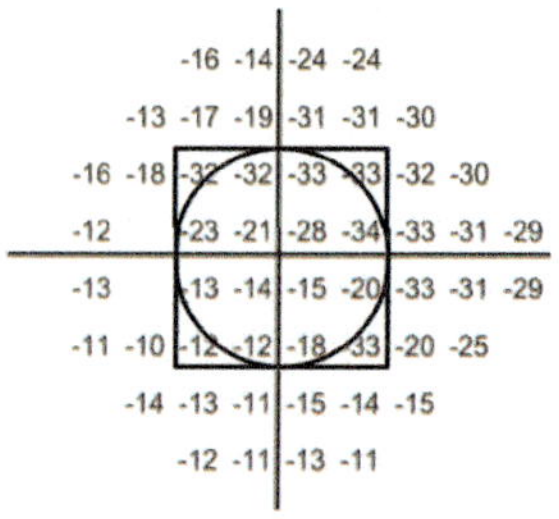

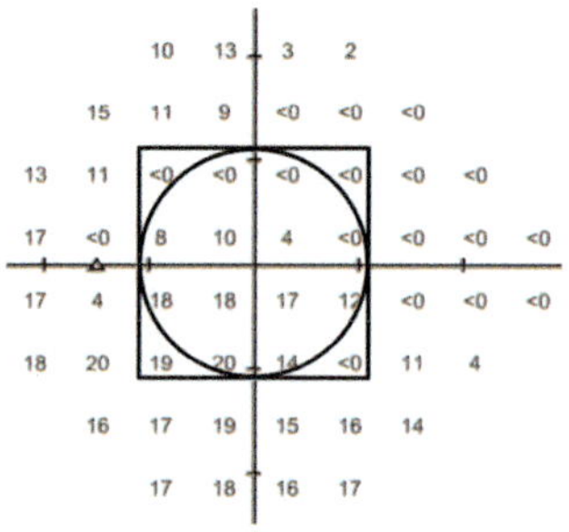

Raw data

One important point, one should learn from this case, is that both eyes need not have the same type of glaucoma. The left eye is having type 1 glaucoma in which glaucoma started outside 10° circle and progressed towards 10° circle area. We repeat the test with 10-2 point pattern to know the extent of the residual field. Right eye is having type 2 glaucoma in which glaucoma started inside 10° circle and progressed to periphery. We repeat the test with 10-2 point pattern to know the exact extent, depth of the field defect.

Case 16 10-2 LE

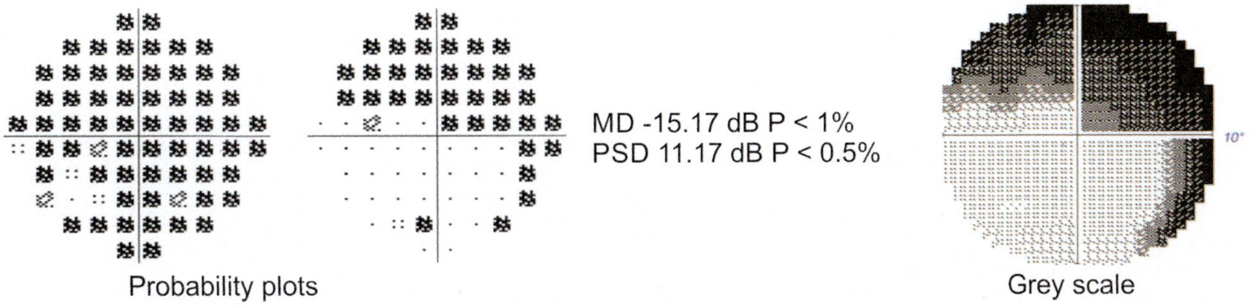

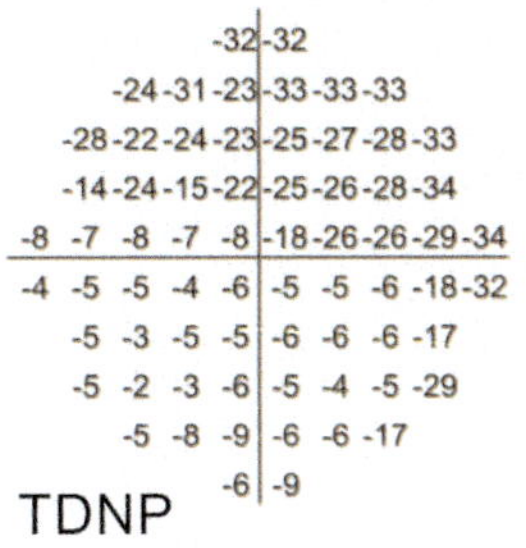

In this case the sensitivities of the 16 points within 3° circle area are good. There is no foveal split. By seeing the grey scale and probability plots we should not come to conclusion regarding the foveal split. Raw data is the final base to comment on foveal split.

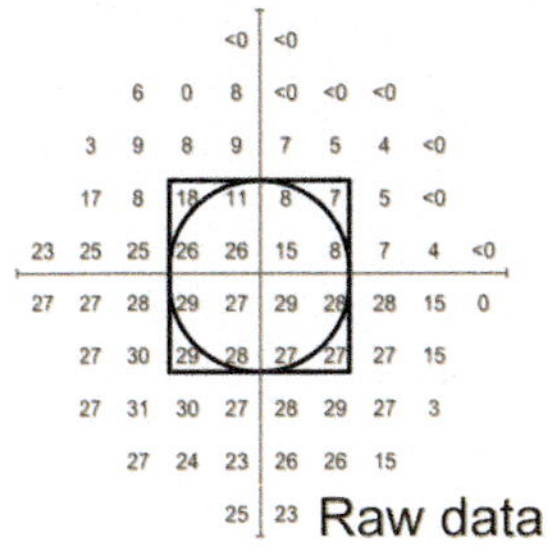

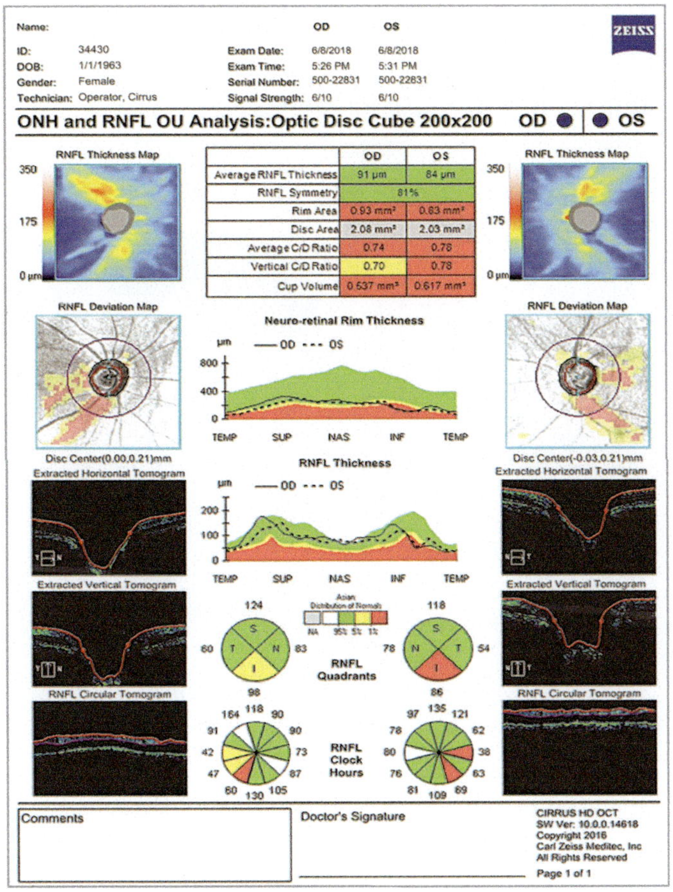

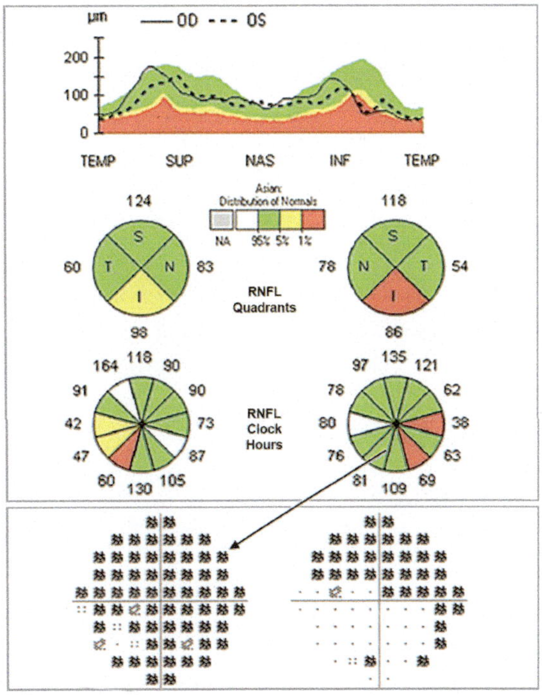

The relative scotoma in the field is represented by red color in OCT and RNFL defect need not represent absolute scotoma. We saw many cases in which RNFL defect is representing a relative scotomas. Absolute scotomas are not required to produce RNFL defect.

Case 17 RE

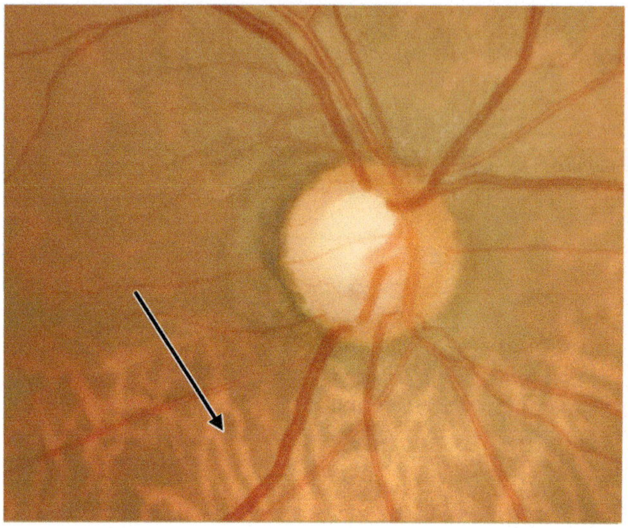

Case 17 LE

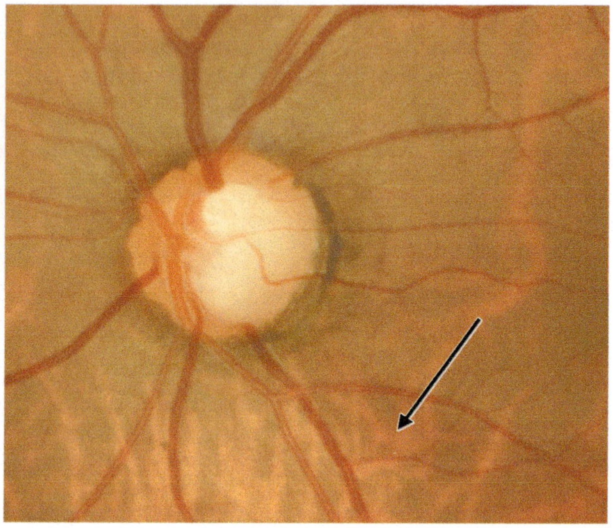

RNFL defect in both the eyes.

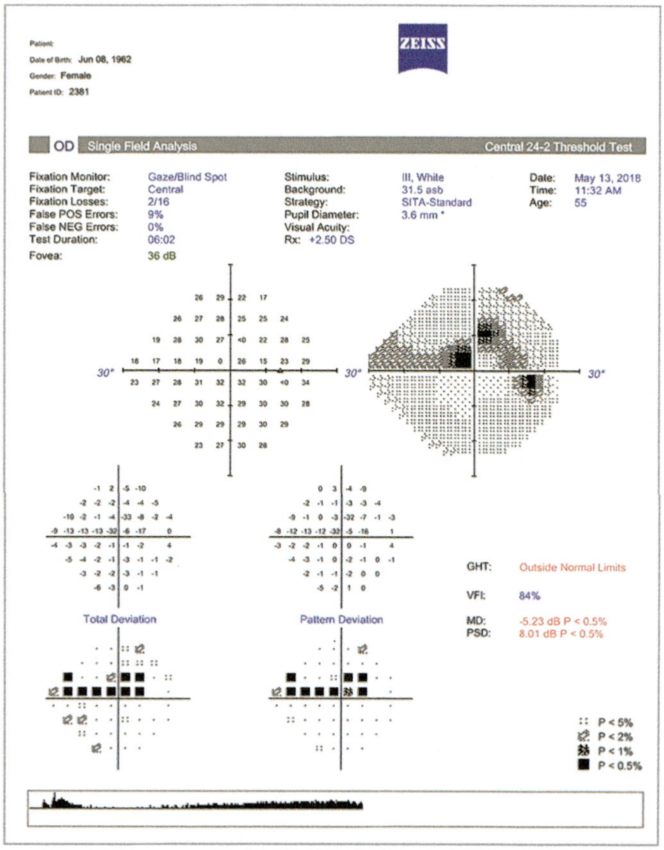

FL 2/16; FP 9%; FN 0%
Fovea 36 dB; GHT-ONL; VFI 84%
MD -5.23 dB P < 0.5%; PSD 8.01 dB P < 0.5%

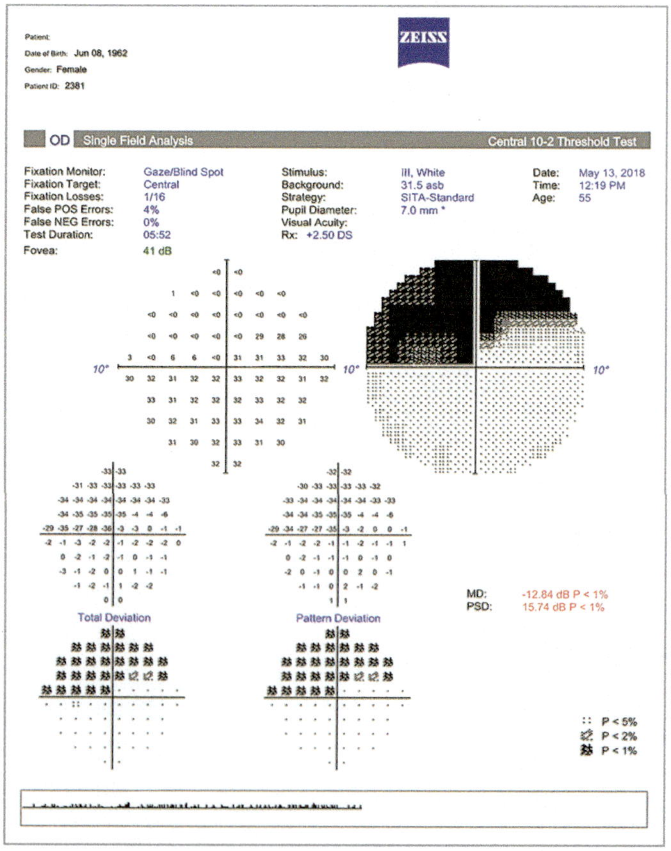

FL 1/16; FP 4%; FN 0%
Fovea 41 dB
MD -12.84 dB P < 1%; PSD 15.74 dB P < 1%

Case 17 RE

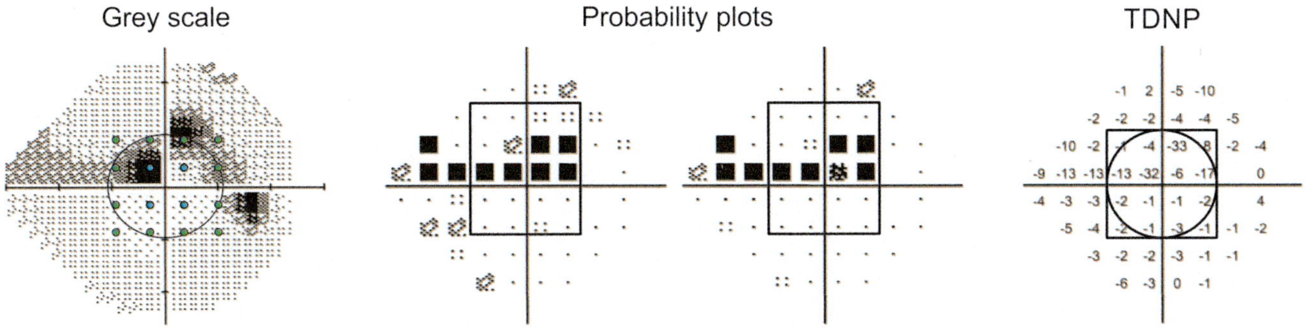

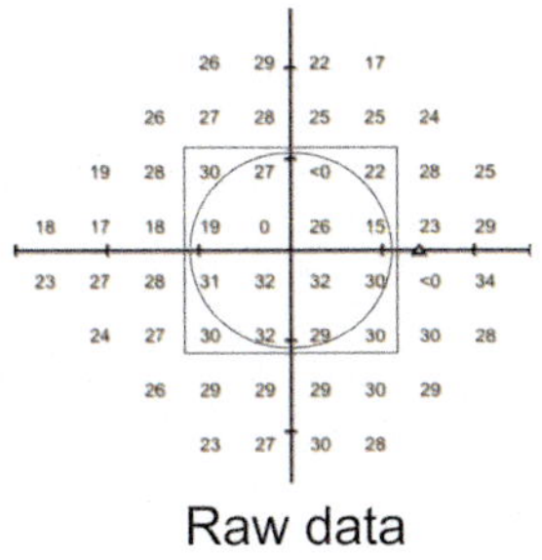

VFI 84%
MD -5.23 dB P < 0.5%

The grey scale and probability plots are showing localized scotoma in the upper nasal and temporal quadrants within the 10° circle area.

The loss of sensitivity started within the 10° circle area and is progressing along the horizontal axis in the upper nasal quadrant. An absolute scotoma on 3° nasal point is an indication to repeat the test with 10-2 point pattern.

Case 17 10-2 RE

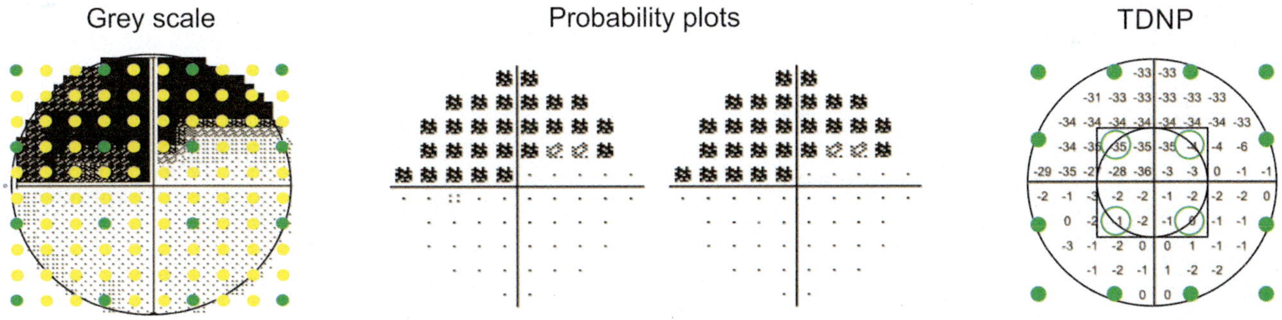

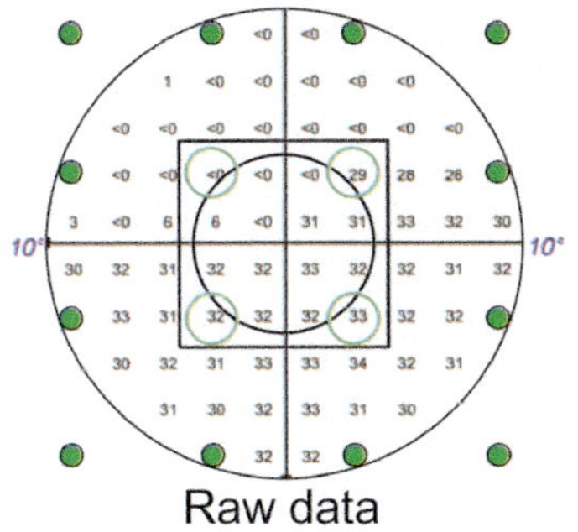

10-2 MD -12.84 dB P < 1%
24-2 MD -5.23 dB P < 0.5%

Note that the MD index in 10-2 point pattern is -12.84 dB P < 1% and MD index in 24-2 point pattern is -5. 23 dB P < 0. 5%. Because the disease started within 10° circle area MD index is more in 10-2 point pattern.

There are more than 10 absolute scotomas in the 10-2 printout.

From this case one should learn the importance of knowing when to repeat the test with 10-2 point pattern. We know the extent, depth and foveal status in 10-2 printout. This information is important to set target IOP to arrest progression. In this case, the role of 24-2 printout is to give an indication to repeat the test with 10-2 point pattern.

Case 17 24-2 LE

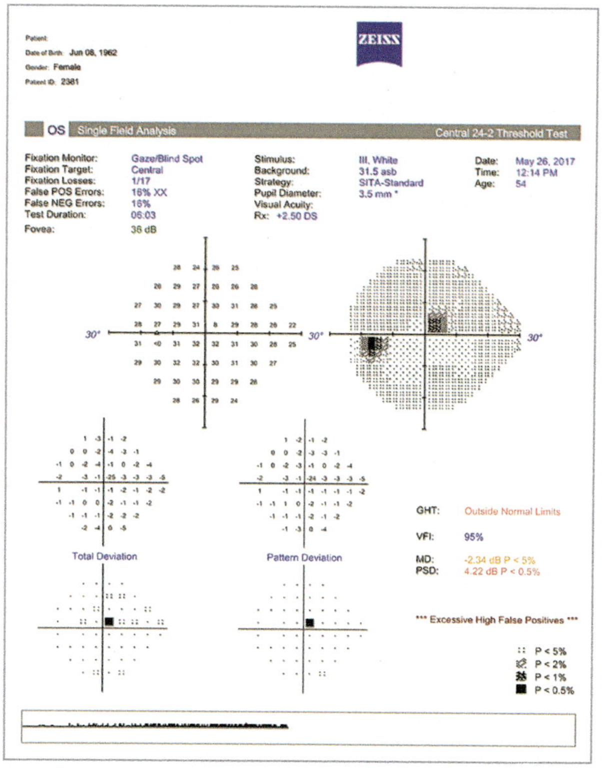

FL 1/17; FL 16% XX; FN 16%
Fovea 36 dB; GHT-ONL; VFI 95%
MD -2.34 dB P < 0.5%; PSD 4.22 dB P < 0.5%

Case 17 10-2 LE

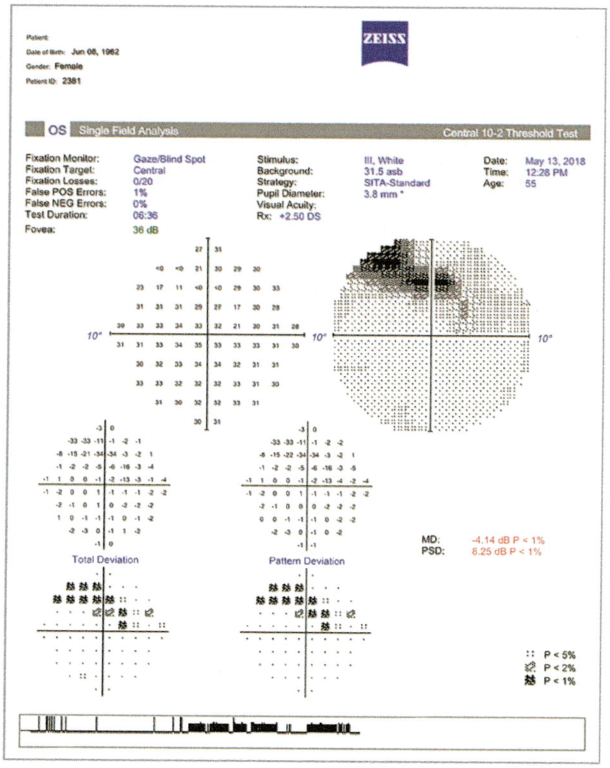

FL 0/20; FP 1%; FN 0%
Fovea 36 dB
MD -4.14 dB P < 1%; PSD 8.25 dB P < 1%

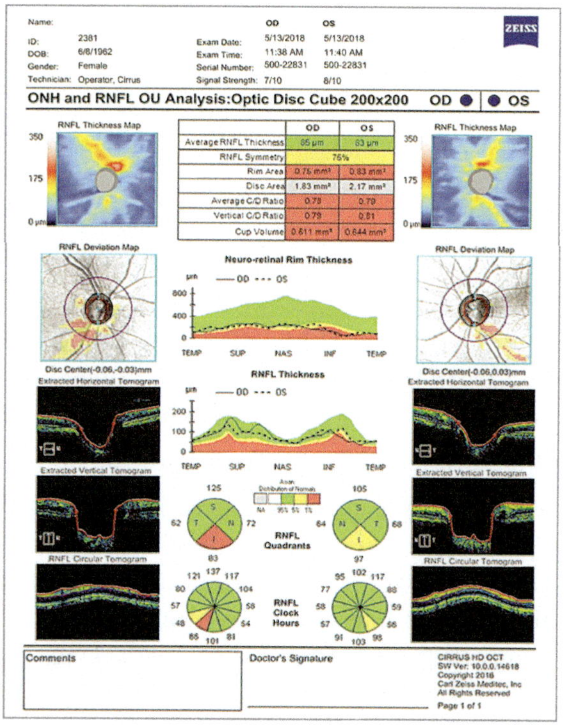

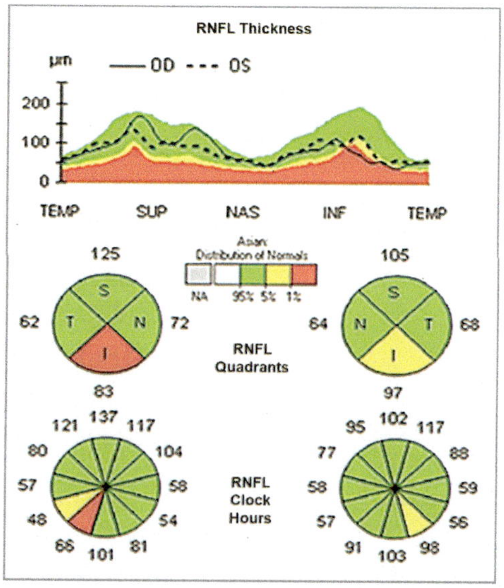

In this case LE OCT is normal. But the ganglion cell damage was picked up in fields. From this case we should learn that it is not always true to say that OCT picks up ganglion cell damage earlier than white on white perimetry.

Case 17 24-2 LE

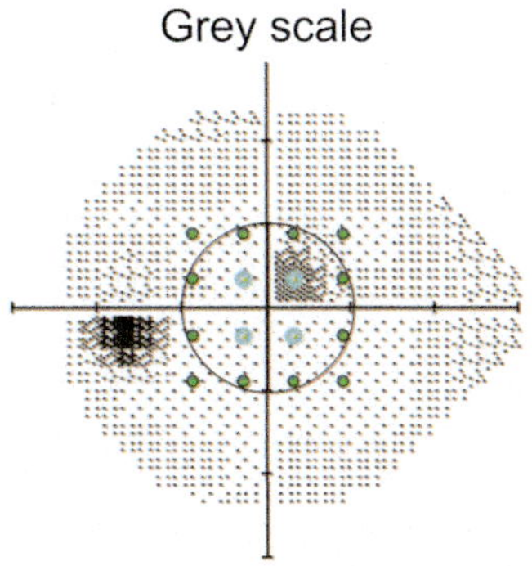

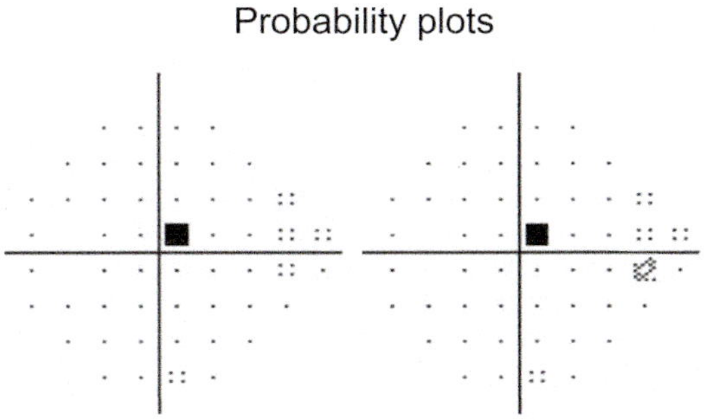

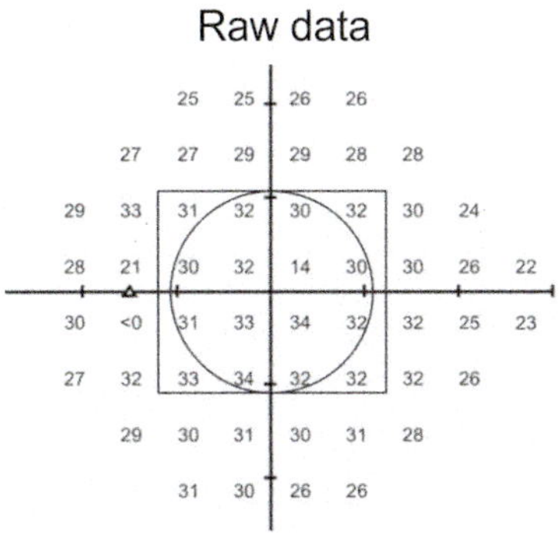

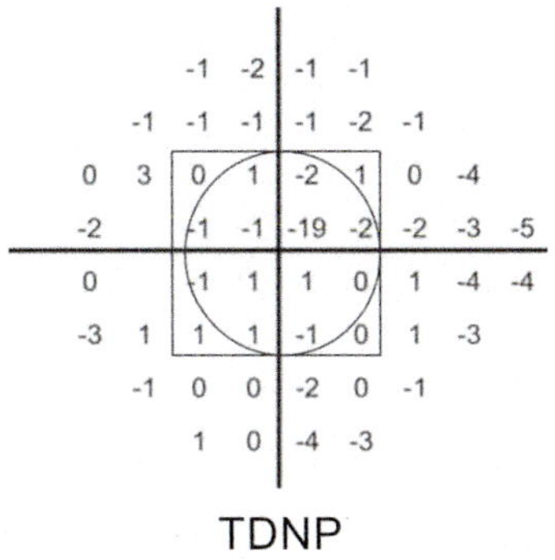

The grey scale and probability plots are showing localized scotoma in the upper nasal quadrants within the 10° circle area. **The loss of sensitivity** at 3° point in the upper nasal quadrant is 19 dB and the sensitivity of the remaining 15 points is very good.

If the loss of sensitivity is severe even at one point, we should repeat the test 10-2 point pattern.

Case 17 10-2 LE

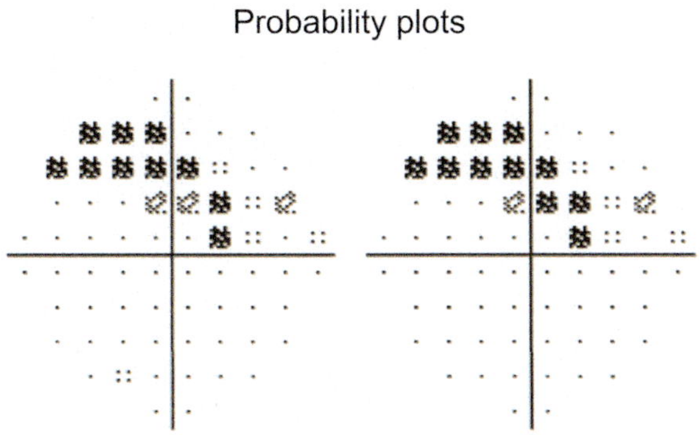

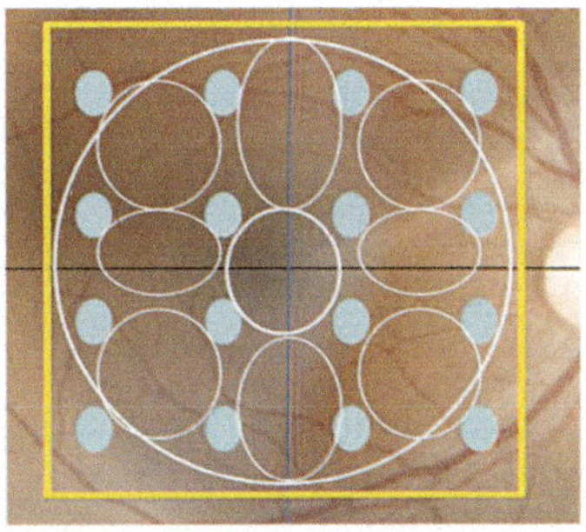

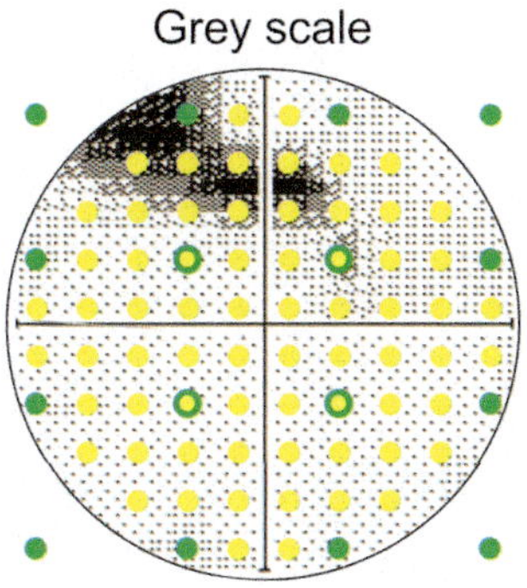

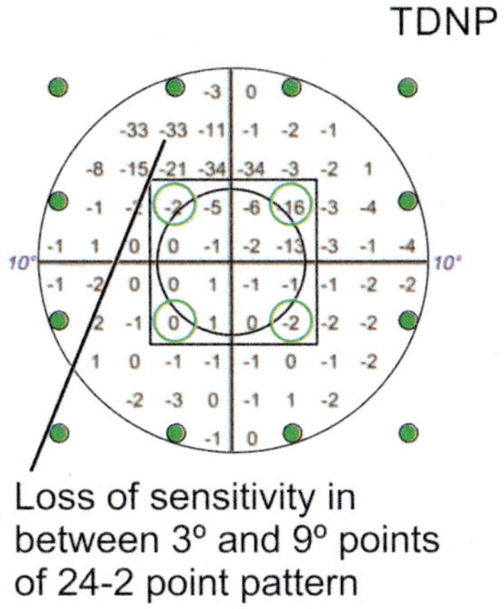

There is a huge untested area within 10° circle area of 24-2 point pattern. The field defect involving the area in between the points will be picked up in the 10-2 point pattern. If we suspect glaucoma, we should do the field test either with 30-2 or 24-2 point pattern. Even if the loss of sensitivity is significant even at one point among the 16 points in the 10°circle area, we should repeat the test 10-2 point pattern.

Note that the MD index in 10-2 point pattern is -4.14 dB P < 1% and MD index in 24–2 point pattern is -1. 23 dB. Because the disease started within 10° circle area MD index is more in 10-2 point pattern.

Case 18 RE **Case 18 LE**

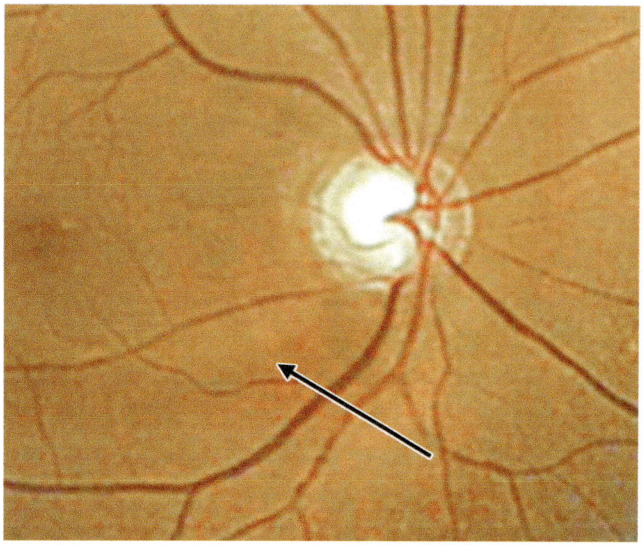

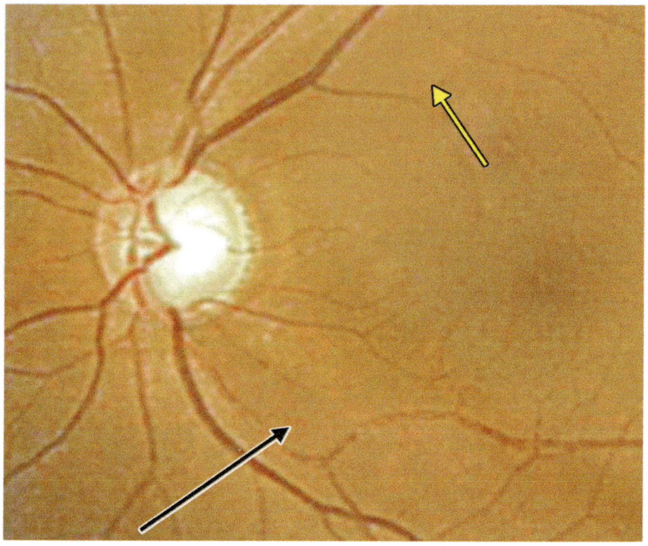

RNFL defects in both the eyes.

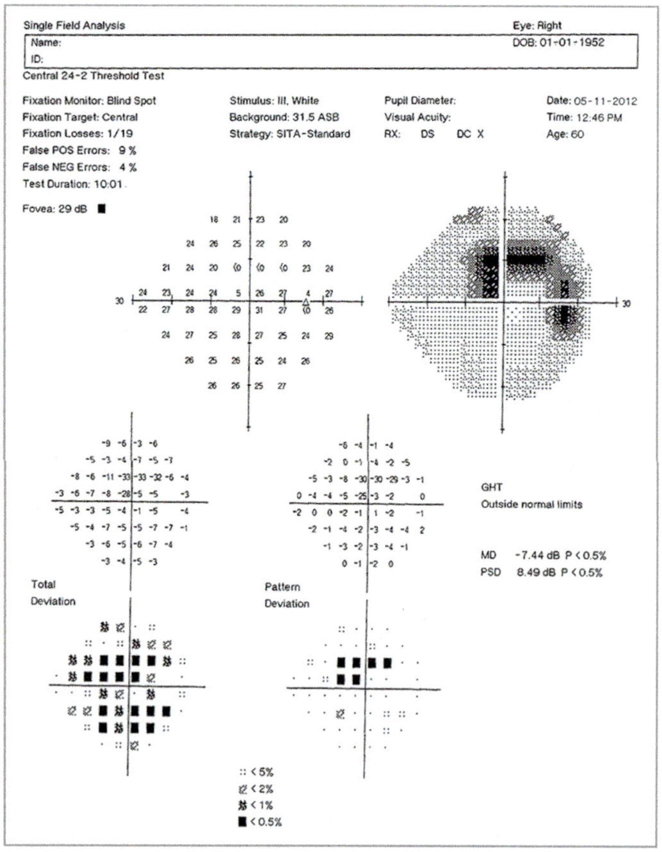

FL 1/19; FP 9%; FN 4%
Fovea 29 dB
MD -7.44 dB P < 0.5%; PSD 8.49 dB P < 0.5%

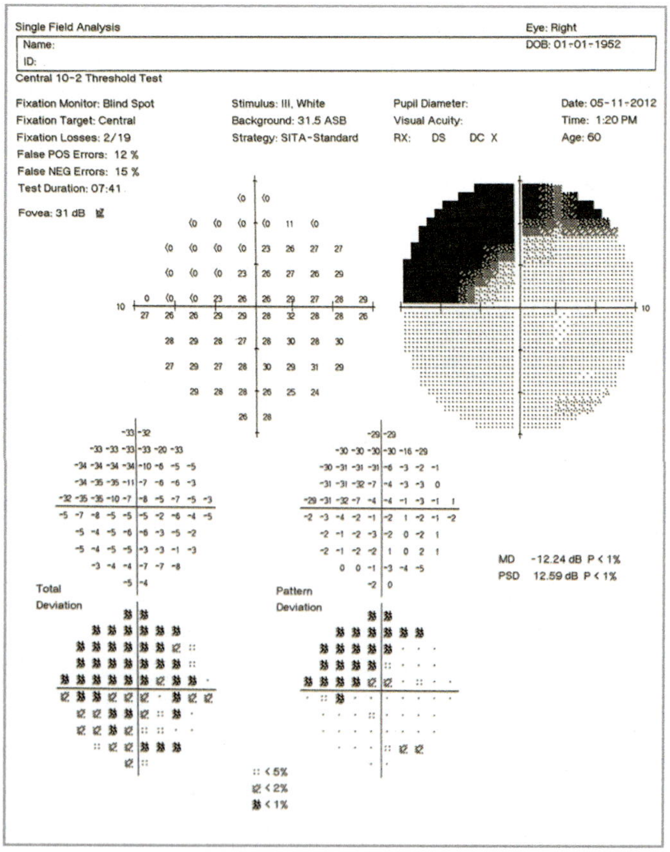

FL 2/19; FP 12%; FN 15%
Fovea 31 dB
MD -12.24 dB P < 1%; PSD 12.59 dB P < 1%

Case 18 RE

Grey scale

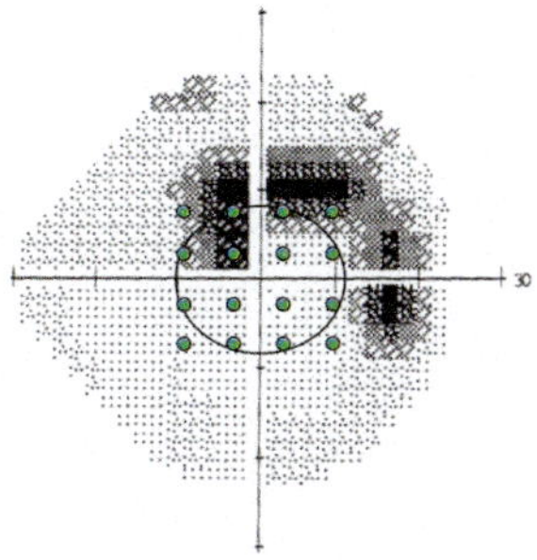

Probability plots

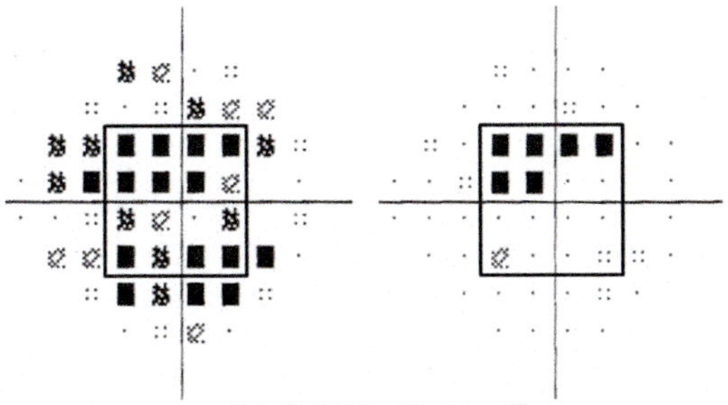

Raw data

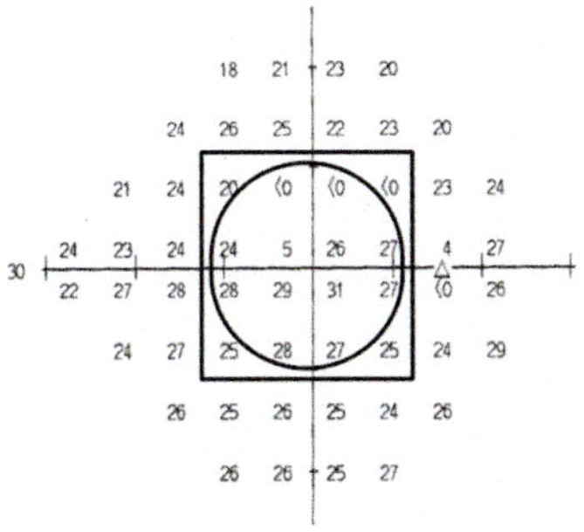

24-2 MD -7.44 dB

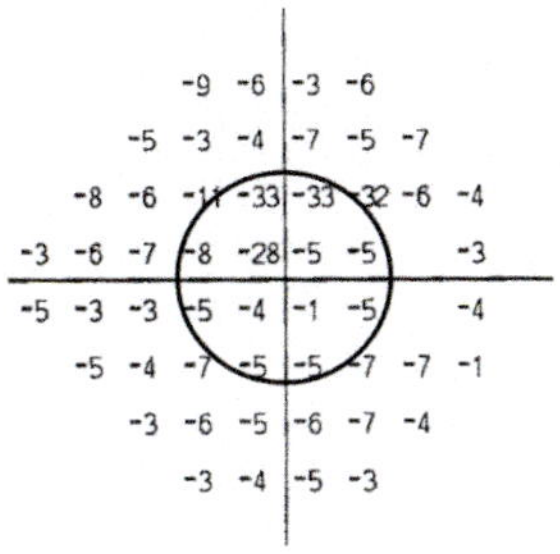

TDNP

The grey scale and probability plots are showing localized scotoma in the upper nasal quadrants within the 10° circle area. **The PDPP is showing black squares at 6 points within the 10° circle area. So we should repeat the test with 10-2 point pattern.**

TDNP—First 4 worst deviation points in the 10° circle area: -33 dB, -33 dB, -28 dB, -8 dB.

Raw data—First 4 worst sensitivity points in the 10° circle area are: 0 dB, 0 dB, 0 dB, 5 dB.

The sensitivities of the remaining 12 points are better than the sensitivities of these points.

Case 18 10-2 RE

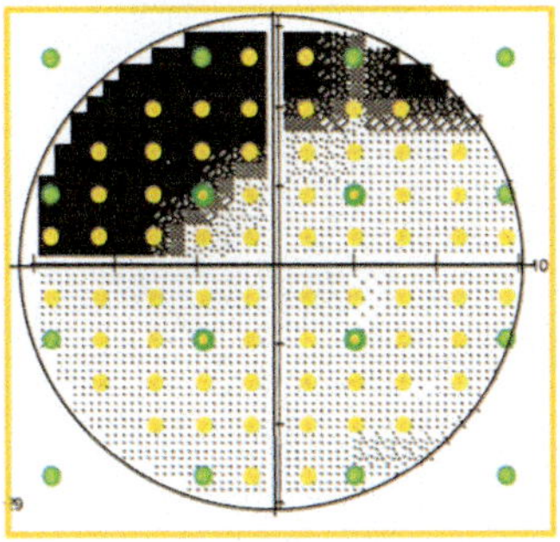

Grey scale

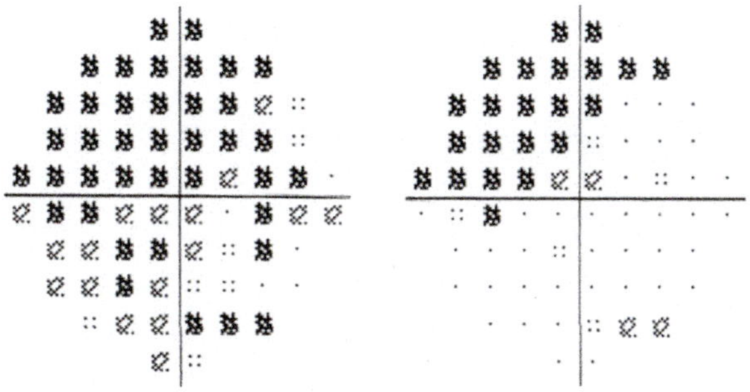

Probability plots

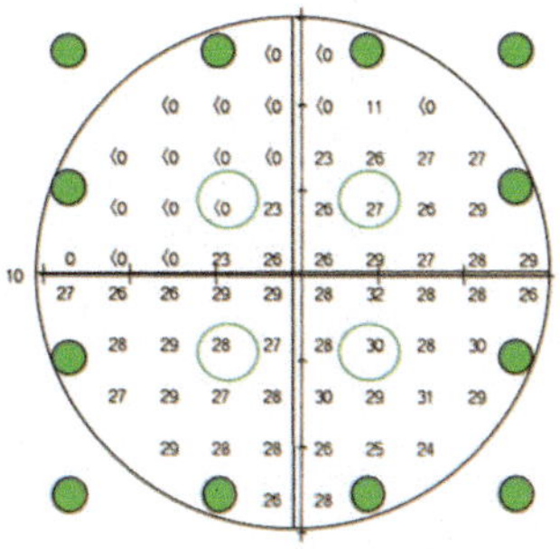

Raw data

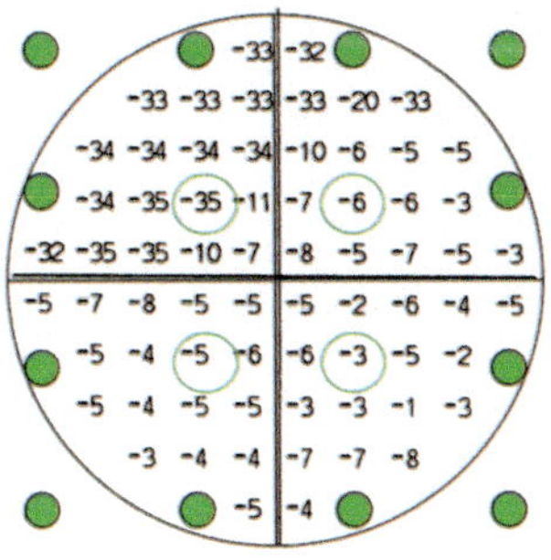

TDNP

Note that the MD index in 10-2 point pattern is -12.24 dB P < 1% and MD index in 24-2 point pattern is -7.44 dB P < 0.5%. Because the disease started within 10° circle area and almost all the points in the upper nasal quadrant are absolute scotomas, MD index is more in 10-2 point pattern.

From this case one should learn the importance of knowing when to repeat the test with 10-2 point pattern. We know the extent, depth and foveal status of the field defect in 10-2 printout. This information is important to set target IOP to arrest progression. In this case the role of 24-2 printout is to give an indication to repeat the test with 10-2 point pattern.

Case 18 RE **Case 18 LE**

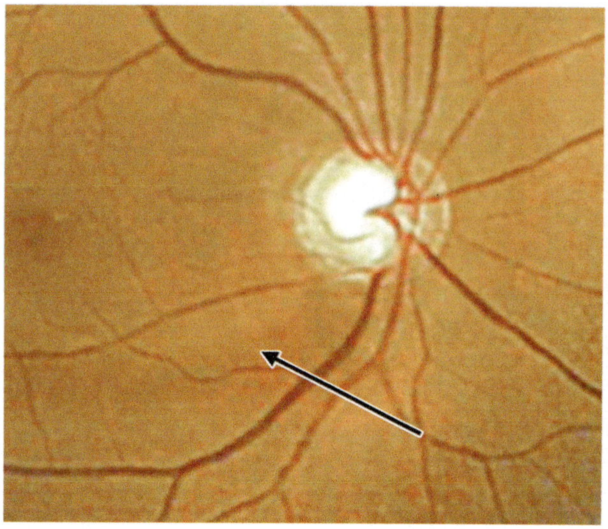

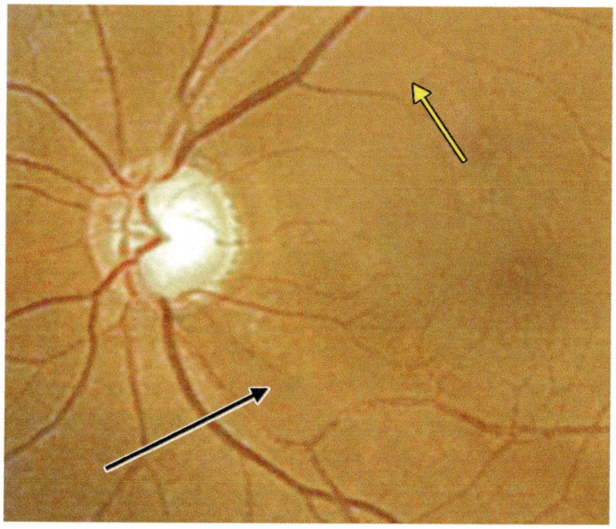

RNFL defects in both the eyes.

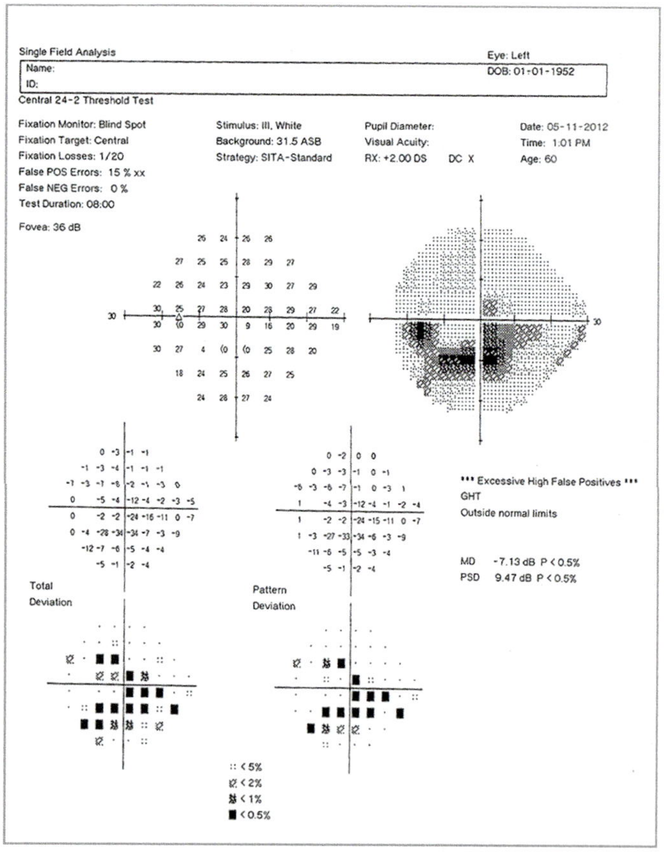

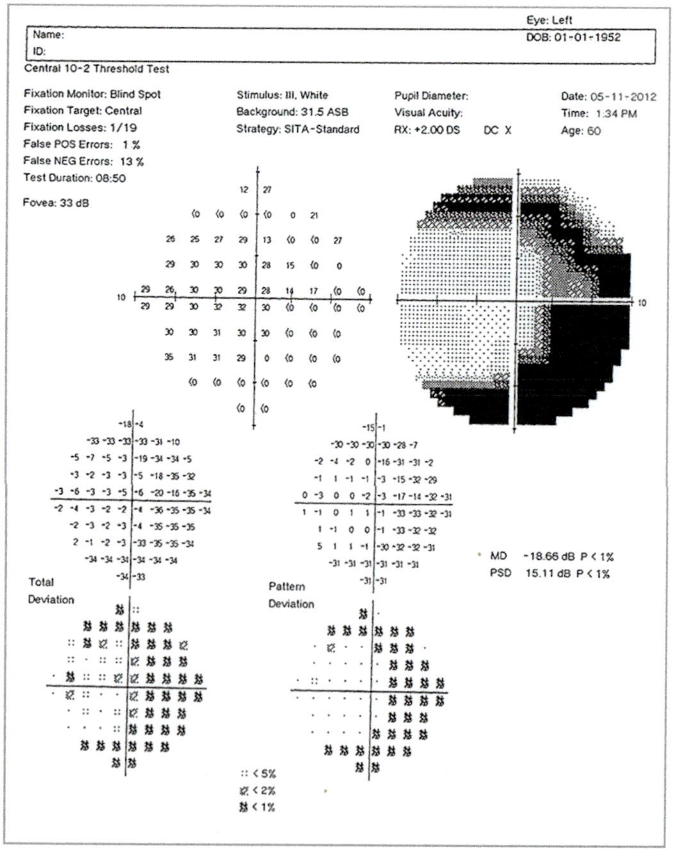

FL 1/20; FP 15% XX; FN 0%
Fovea 36 dB; GHT-ONL
MD -7.13 dB P < 0.5%; PSD 9.47 dB P < 0.5%

FL 1/19; FP 1%; FN 13%
Fovea 33 dB
MD -18.66 dB P < 1%; PSD 15.11 dB P < 1%

Case 18 RE

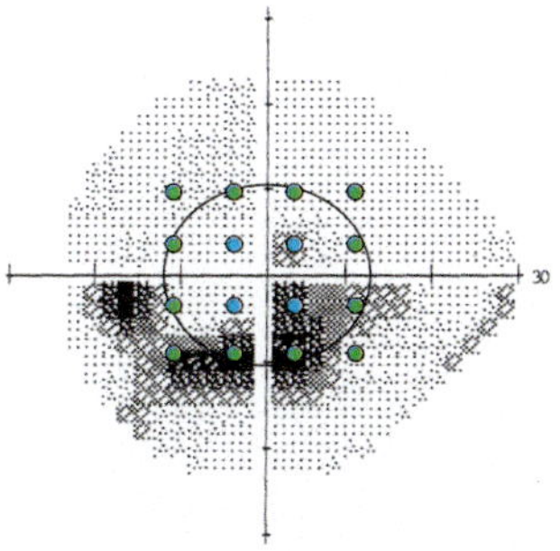

Grey scale

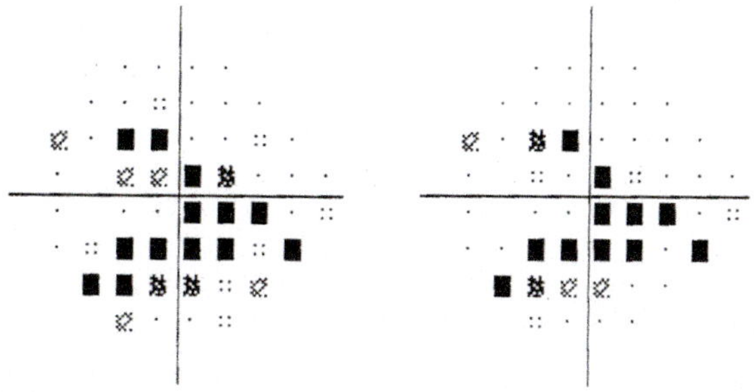

Probability plots

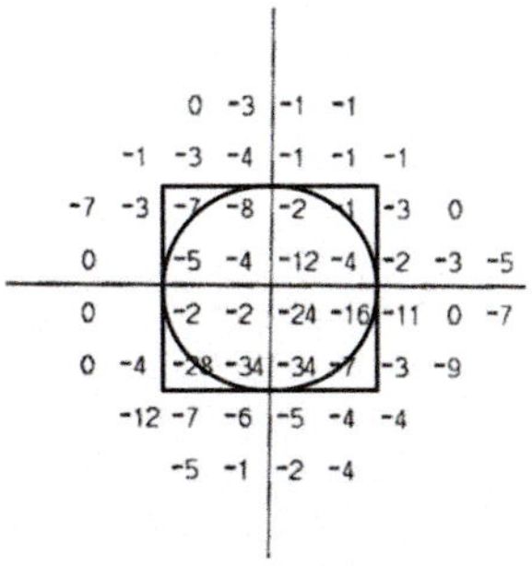

TDNP

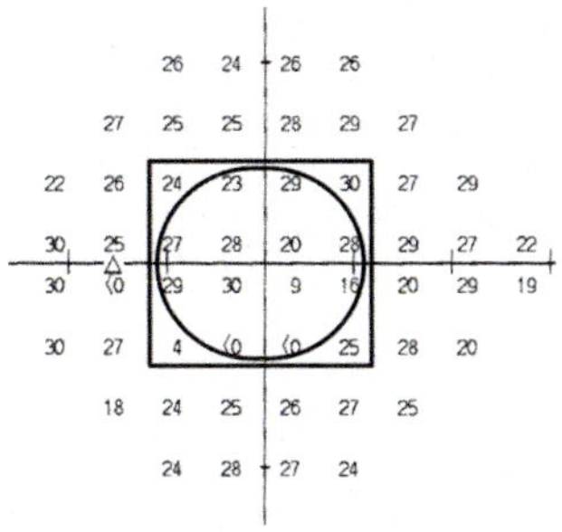

Raw data

The dark shade in the lower nasal quadrant extended up to fixation. The probability plots are showing biarcuate scotoma within the 10° circle area. All the points in the localized scotoma are almost represented by black squares. We should repeat the test with 10-2 point pattern.

The points with loss of sensitivity less than 6 dB within the 10° circle area will have sensitivity around 30 dB. The points with 30 dB sensitivity will be given good shade in the grey scale. So the field defects with loss of sensitivity around 5 dB will not be appreciated in the grey scale. But the points with loss of sensitivity around 6 dB will be well appreciated in the probability plots, but will not be appreciated in the grey scale.

Case 18 10-2 LE

Grey scale

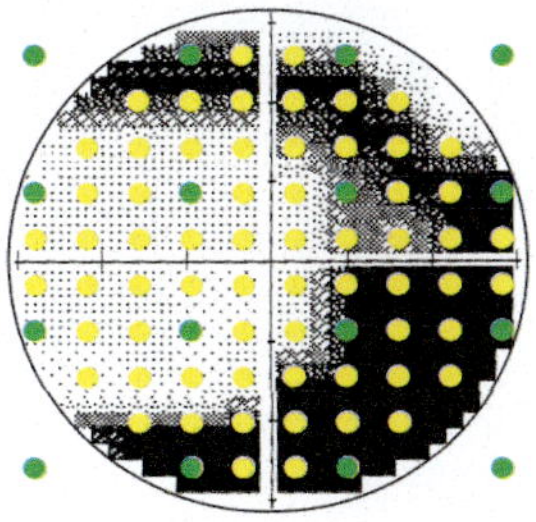

Probability plots

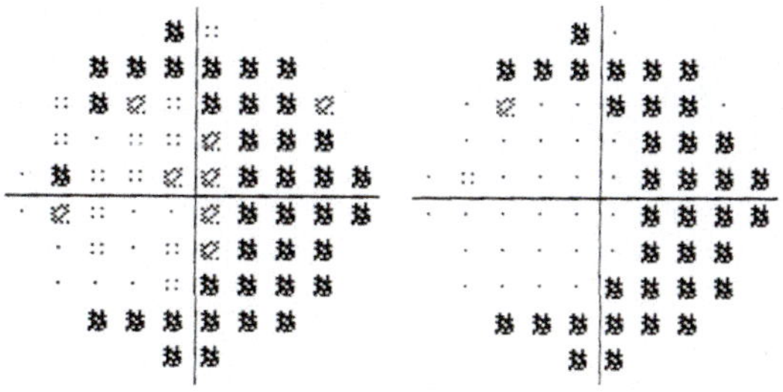

TDNP

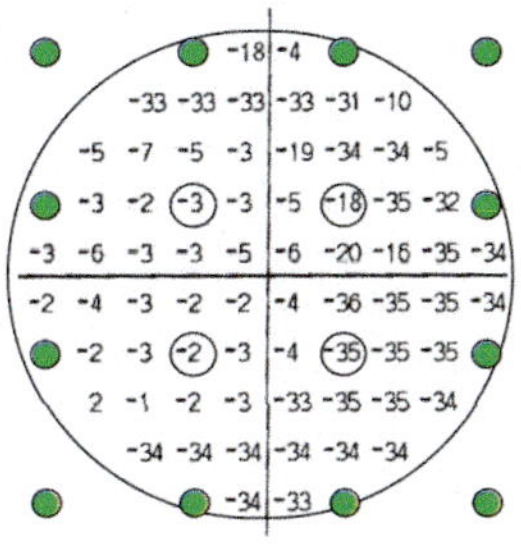

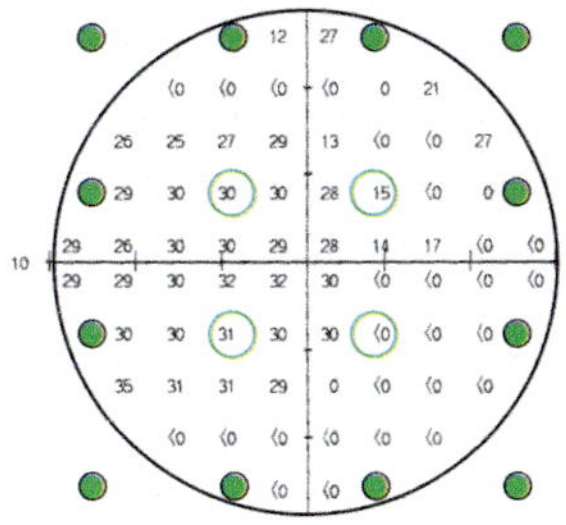

Raw data

The 10-2 probability plots are showing biarcuate scotoma and extending into 3° circle which is not a good sign. Because the upper arcuate scotomas are progressing in between 3° and 9° points, they are not appreciated in 24-2 grey scale.

Note that the MD index in 10-2 point pattern is -18.66 dB P < 1% and MD index in 24-2 point pattern is -7.13 P < 0. 5% dB. Because the disease started within 10° circle area MD index is more in 10-2 point pattern.

Case 19 RE **Case 19 LE**

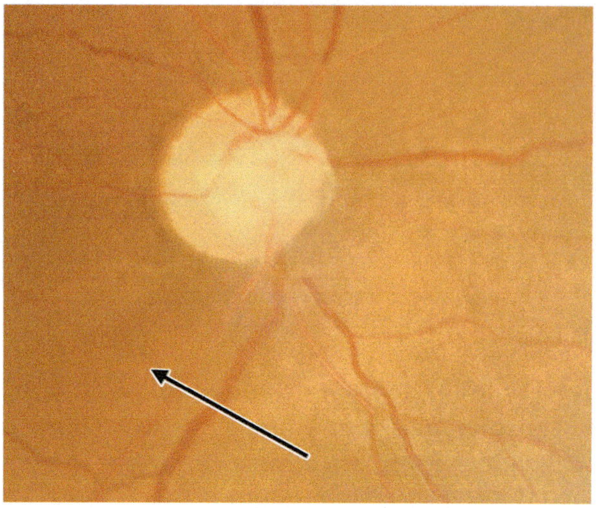

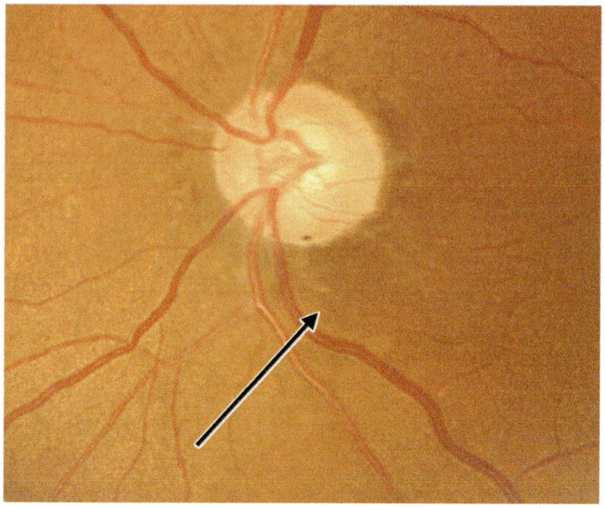

RNFL defects in both the eyes.

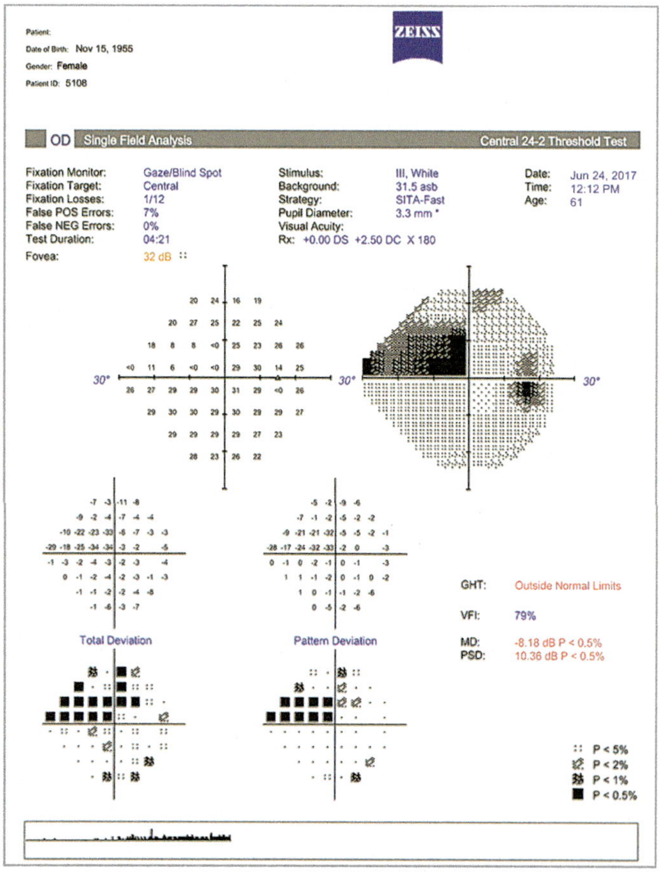

FL 1/12; FP 7%; FN 0%
Fovea 32 dB; VFI 79%
MD -8.18 dB P < 0.5%; PSD 10.36 dB P < 0.5%

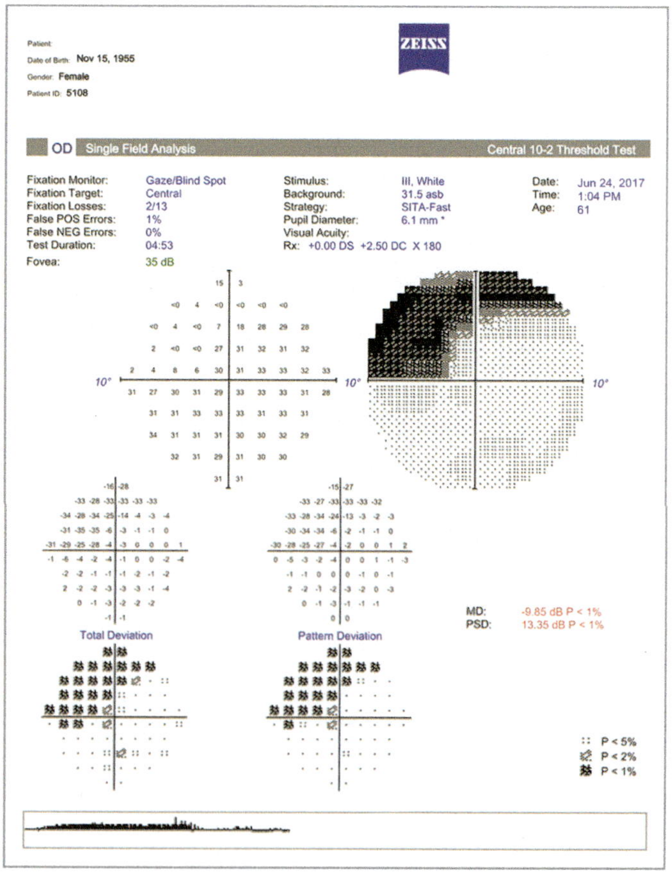

FL 2/13; FP 1%; FN 0%
Fovea 35 dB
MD -9.85 dB P < 1%; PSD 13.35 dB P < 1%

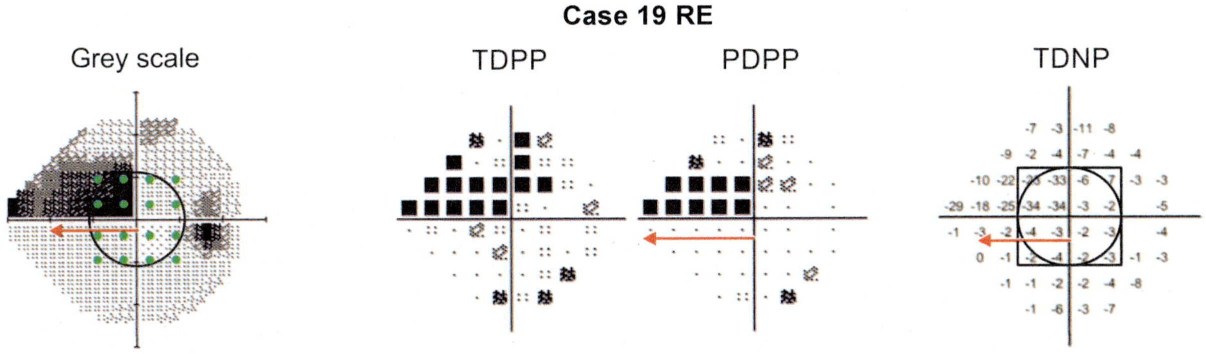

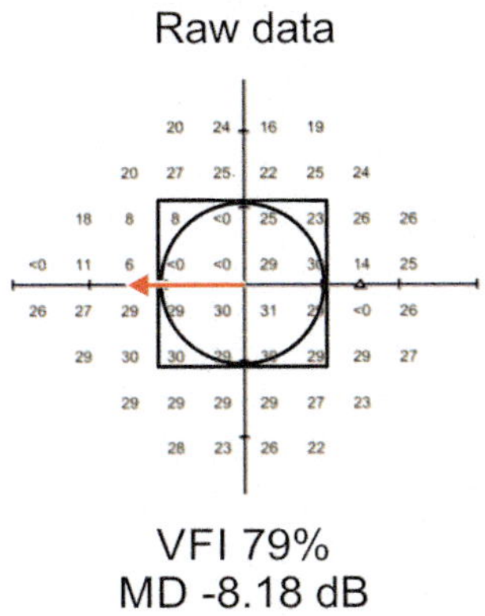

Location and extent of the field defect—probability plot. The most important point in this case is to identify the absolute scotomas within the 10° circle and one among the three is on the 3° circle point. It indicates glaucoma started close to fixation and is progressing outwards.

To know the exact extent and depth of the field defect we should repeat the test with 10-2 point pattern.

Identification of type 2 glaucomas is very important.

The 24-2 VFI misguides the treatment approach in type 2 glaucomas.

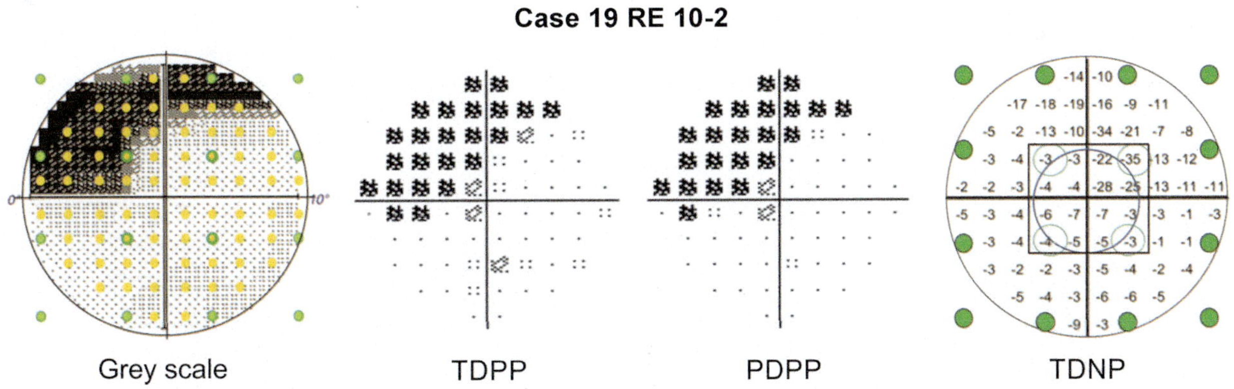

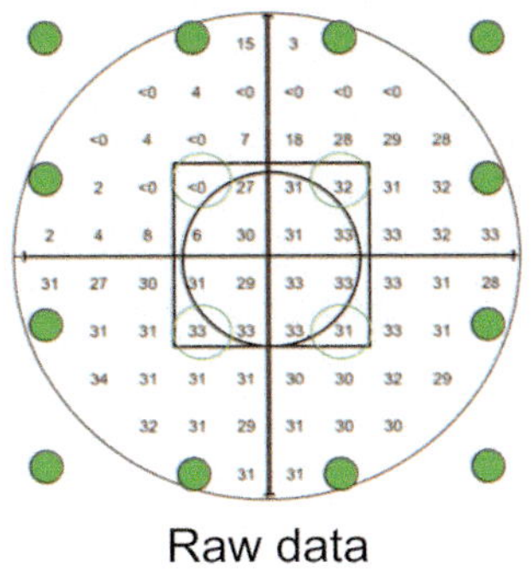

As the field defect is progressing between 3° and 9° points, the field defect is not well-appreciated in the upper temporal area within the 10° circle area of 24-2 grey scale.

In type 2 glaucomas 10-2 MD index (-9. 85 dB) will be always more than 24-2 MD index (-8.18 dB).

The 24-2 VFI 79% misguides the treatment approach in type 2 glaucomas as VFI is not calculated in 10-2 SFA printouts.

Low target IOP must be aimed for and, if needed, antiglaucoma surgical approach is indicated in type 2 and type 3 glaucomas.

Case 19 LE 10-2

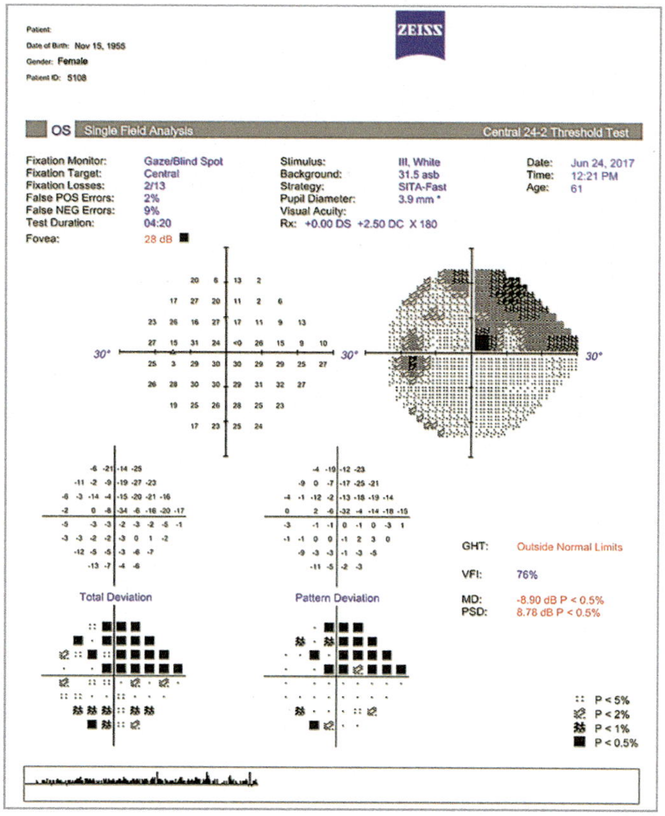

FL 2/13; FP 2%; FN 9%; Fovea 28 dB
GHT-ONL; VFI 76%
MD -8.90 dB P < 0.5%; PSD 8.78 dB P < 0.5%

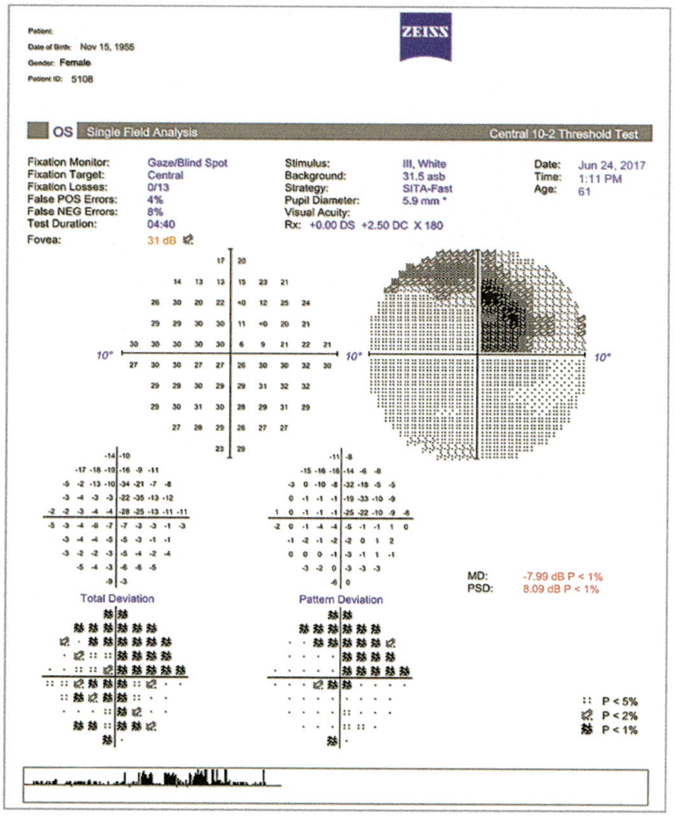

FL 0/13; FP 4%; FN 8%
Fovea 31 dB
MD -7.99 dB P < 1%; PSD 8.09 dB P < 1%

Case 19 LE

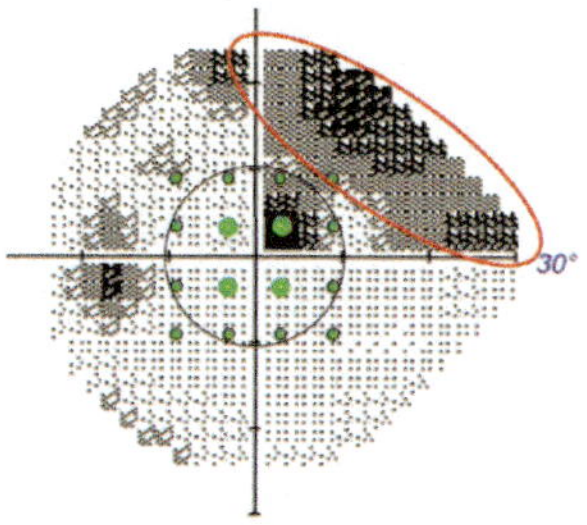

Grey scale

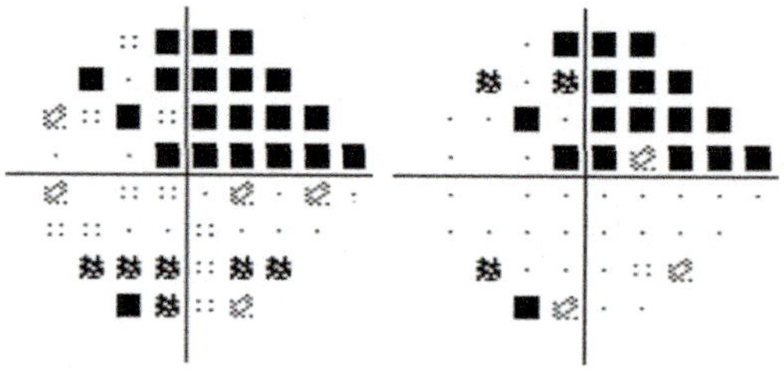

Probability plots

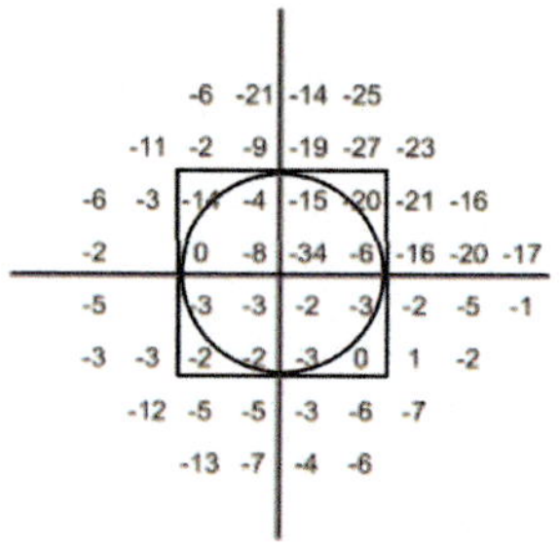

TDNP

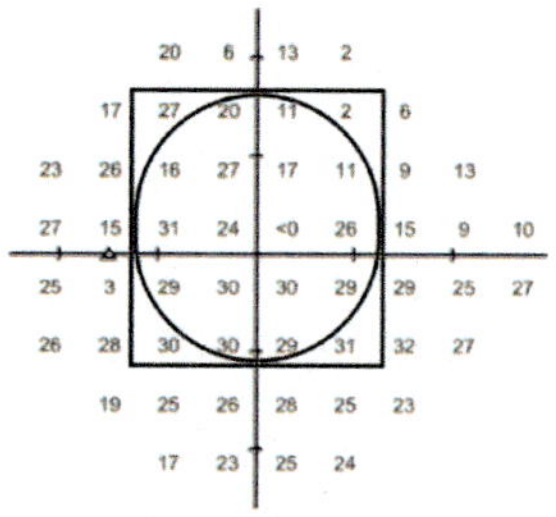

Raw data

From the grey scale, TDNP and raw data, it is clearly evident that glaucomatous damage started both within 10° circle area and outside 10° circle area.

VFI 76%

MD -8. 90 dB P < 0. 5%

Absolute scotoma in the 10° circle area is an indication to repeat the test with 10-2 point pattern.

Case 19 10-2 LE

Grey scale | Probability plots | TDNP

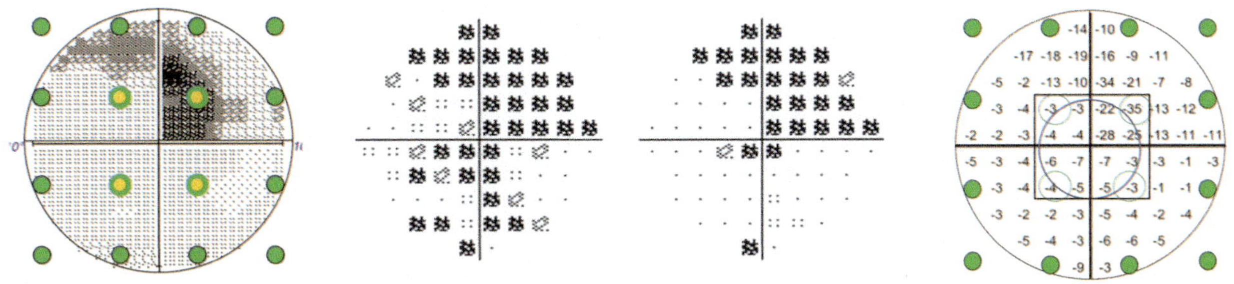

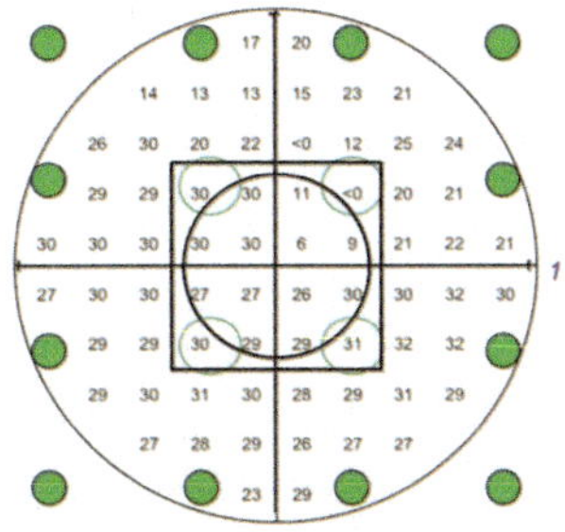

Raw data

As the field defect is progressing between 3° and 9° points the field defect is not well-appreciated in the upper temporal area within the 10° circle area of 24-2 grey scale.

Note that the MD index in 10-2 point pattern is **-7. 99** dB P < 1% and MD index in 24-2 point pattern is -8. 90 dB P < 0. 5%. Because the disease started both within and outside 10° circle area the MD index can be more either in 24-2 point pattern or 10-2 point pattern.

In type 2 and type 3 glaucomas we should aim at low target IOP and if needed antiglaucoma surgical approach is indicated.

Case 19 RE/LE

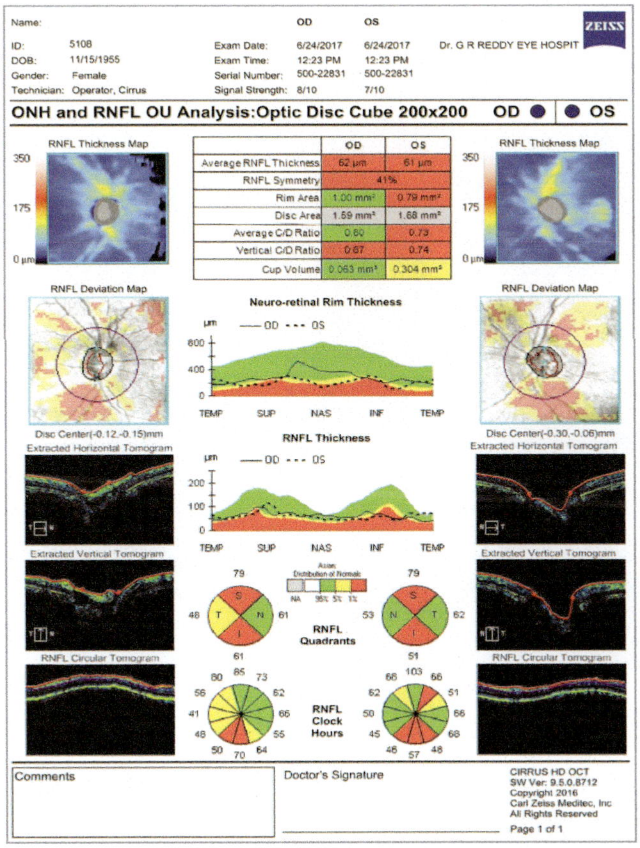

The most important point to remember is in type 2 glaucomas (field defect starts within 10° circle) and type 3 glaucomas (type 2 glaucomas associated with field defects outside 10° circle) better to avoid beta blockers. Most of the type 2 glaucomas are mostly normotensive glaucomas. So treat type 2 glaucoma as NTG.

OCT is correlating with fundus and field defects

CHAPTER

8

Interpretation of Single Field Analysis Printouts of Type 3 Primary Open-angle Glaucoma

TYPE 3 POAG—ISOLATED FIELD DEFECTS WITHIN AND OUTSIDE 10° CIRCLE AREA

I am presenting six cases of **clinically suspected or established** Type 3 glaucoma (Isolated **field defects within and outside 10° circle**). As in Type 2, most of the cases of Type 3 have definite clinical signs from the fundus as definite notch, retinal nerve fiber layer (RNFL) defect and intraocular pressure (IOP) is high in most of the cases. Whether it is a case of glaucoma suspect or established case of glaucoma we must have 30-2 or 24-2 point pattern printouts as they are base line print-outs. Now we should know how to evaluate the 10° circle area of 30-2 or 24-2 printouts to know whether we should repeat the test with 10-2 point pattern to pick up these group of cases at an early stage. Direction of RNFL defect is very important. The direction of RNFL defect towards macula is an indication is repeat the test with 10-2 point pattern. Optical coherence tomography (OCT) shows RNFL thinning between 6-7° clock position in right eye and 6-5° clock position in left eye in Type 2 and Type 3 glaucomas.

Case 20 RNFL defect in both the eyes.

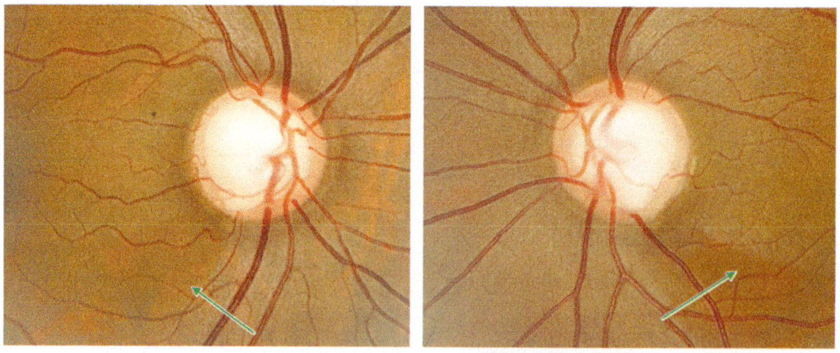

Case 21 RNFL defect in both the eyes.

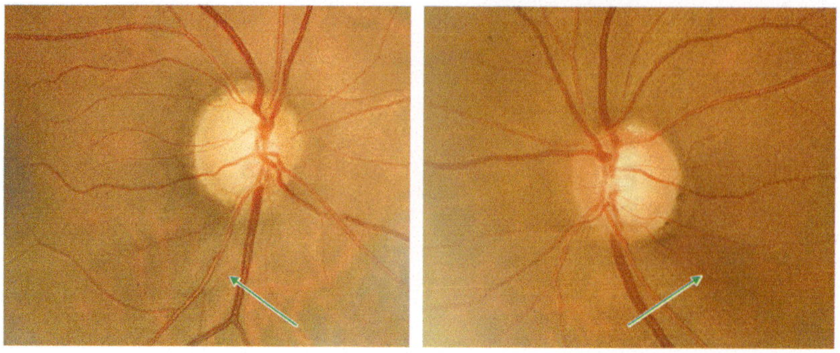

Case 22 RNFL defect in left eye.

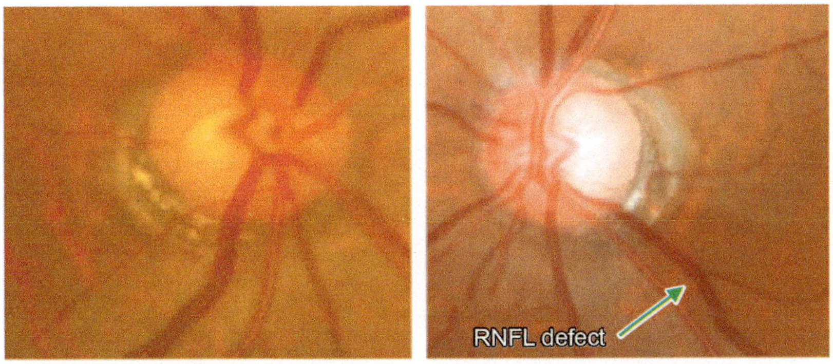

Case 23 RNFL defect in both the eyes.

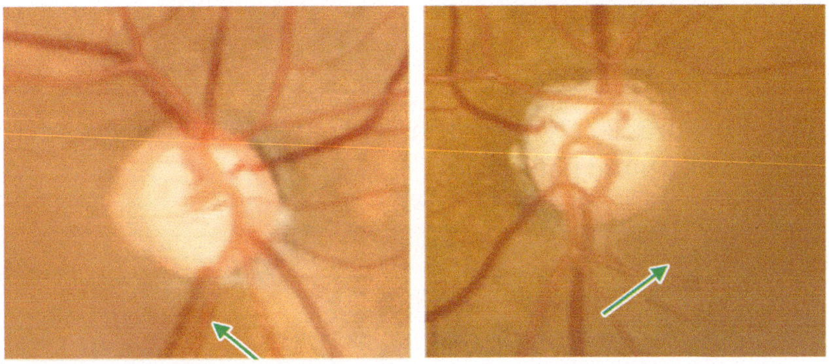

Case 24 RNFL defect in both the eyes.

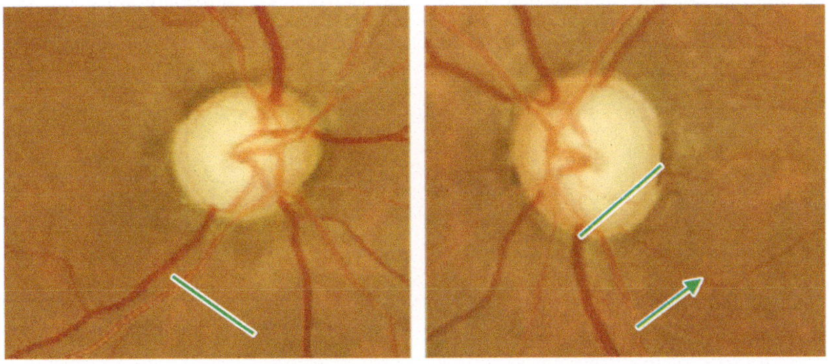

Case 25 RNFL defect in left eye.

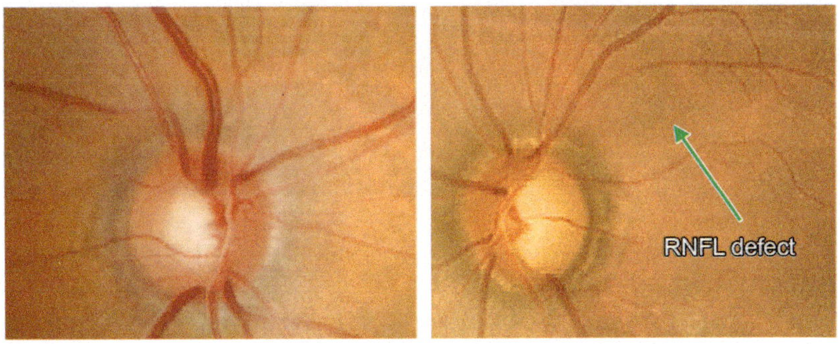

Case 20 RE

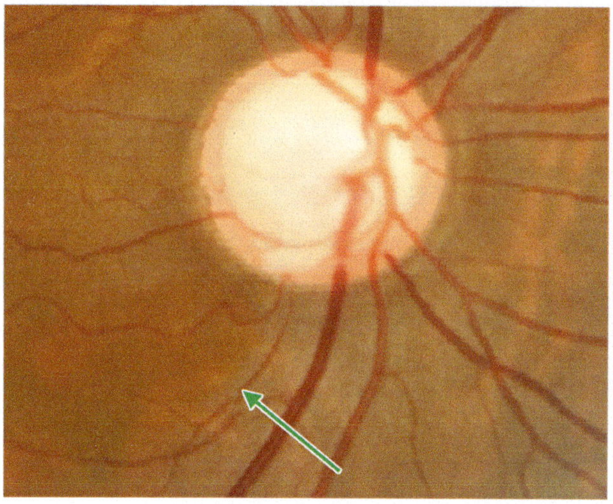

Case 20 LE

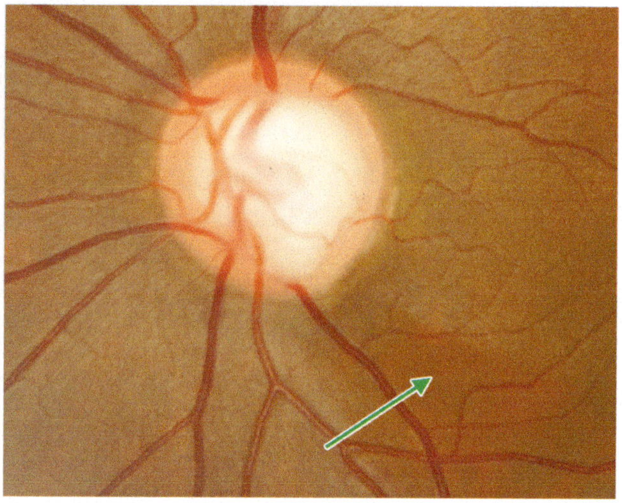

Note that the direction of RNFL defect is towards macula. If RNFL defect is directed towards macula, always repeat the test with 10-2 point pattern.

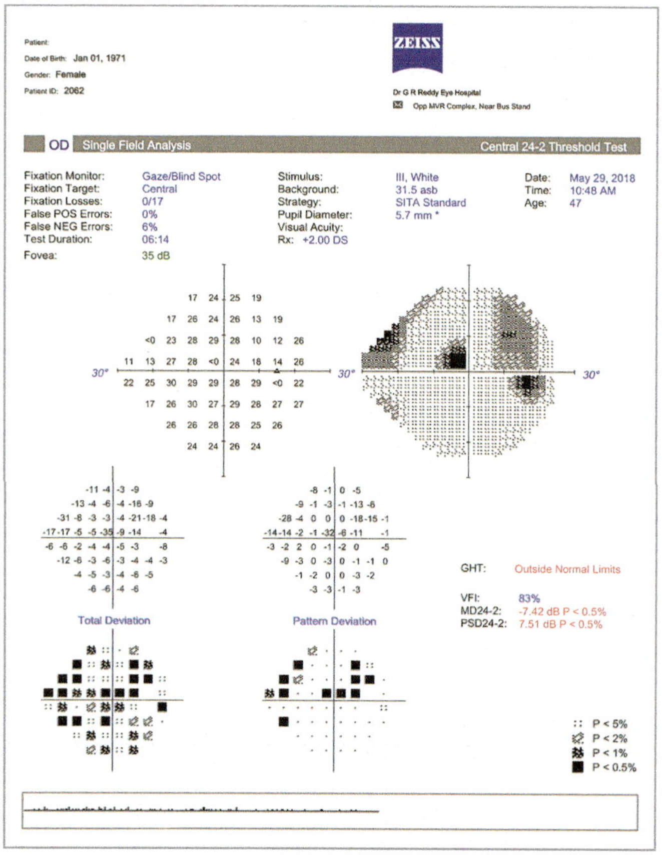

FL 0/17; FP 0%; FN 6%
Fovea 35 dB; GHTONL; VFI 83%
MD -7.42 dB P < 0.5%; PSD 7.51 dB P < 0.5%

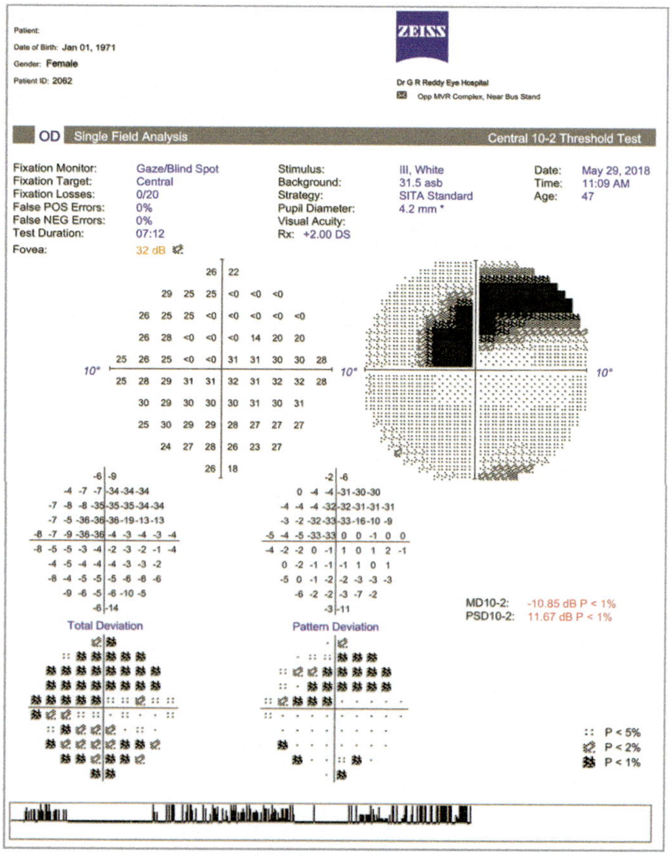

FL 0/20; FP 0%; FN 0%
Fovea 32 dB
MD -10.85 dB P < 1%; PSD 11.67 dB P < 1%

Case 20 RE

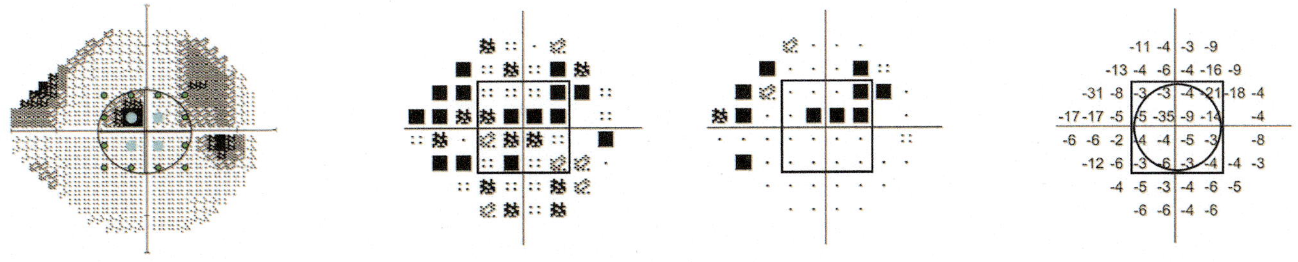

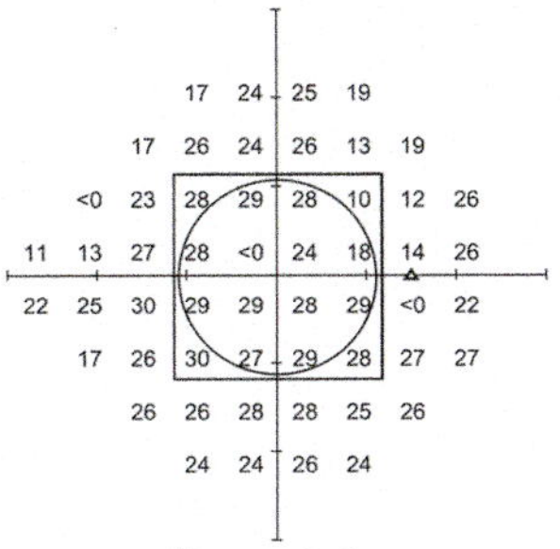

The multifocal origin of glaucoma is clearly evident from the grey scale and the probability plots. The most striking feature in this raw data is that the sensitivity of the 3° point in the upper nasal quadrant is 0 dB (Absolute scotoma). It indicates that the glaucoma started within 10° circle. Probability plots, grey scale and raw data (TDNP) are giving indications to repeat the test with 10-2 point pattern.

24-2 MD index is -7.42 dB. We should not grade glaucomas on the basis of MD index alone. Identification of the type of glaucoma is important. For that one should know how to evaluate the 24-2 or 30-2 printouts to know when to repeat the test with 10-2 point pattern.

Case 20 RE 10-2

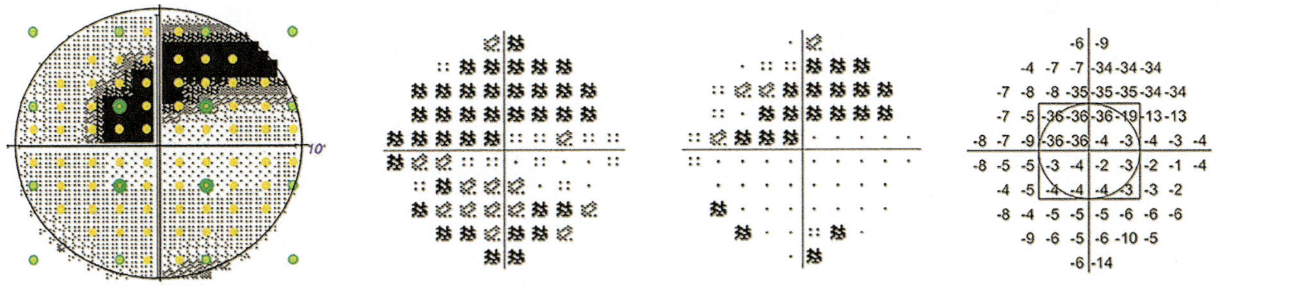

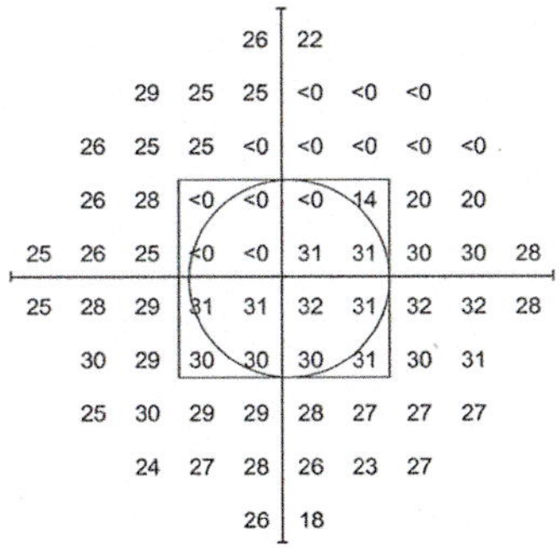

Location and progression of the field defect—The probability plots are showing biarcuate scotoma in the total deviation probability plot and the deep upper arcuate scotoma is highlighted in the pattern deviation probability plot (PDPP). Most of the points in the field defect are absolute scotomas. Since the scotoma is located in between 3° and 9° points they are not appreciated in the 24-2 grey scale.

Comment on 24-2 visual field index (VFI)—In the Type 2 and Type 3 glaucomas we should not consider VFI value. Unfortunately VFI is not calculated in 10-2 point pattern printouts. This a case of glaucoma with **24-2 MD index -7.42 dB** and with foveal split. The approach of management of glaucoma changes when it is associated with foveal split. So we should not grade glaucomas on the basis of MD index alone.

In this case the treatment of glaucoma must be aggressive.

Case 20 LE

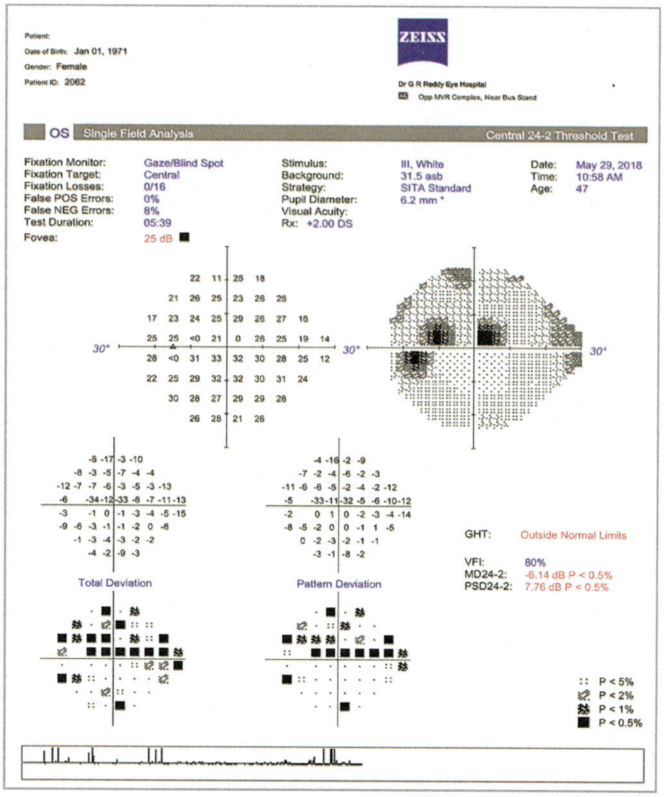

FL 0/16; FP 0%; FN 8%
Fovea 25 dB; VFI 80%
MD -6.14 dB P < 0.5%; PSD 7.76 dB P < 0.5%

Case 20 LE 10-2

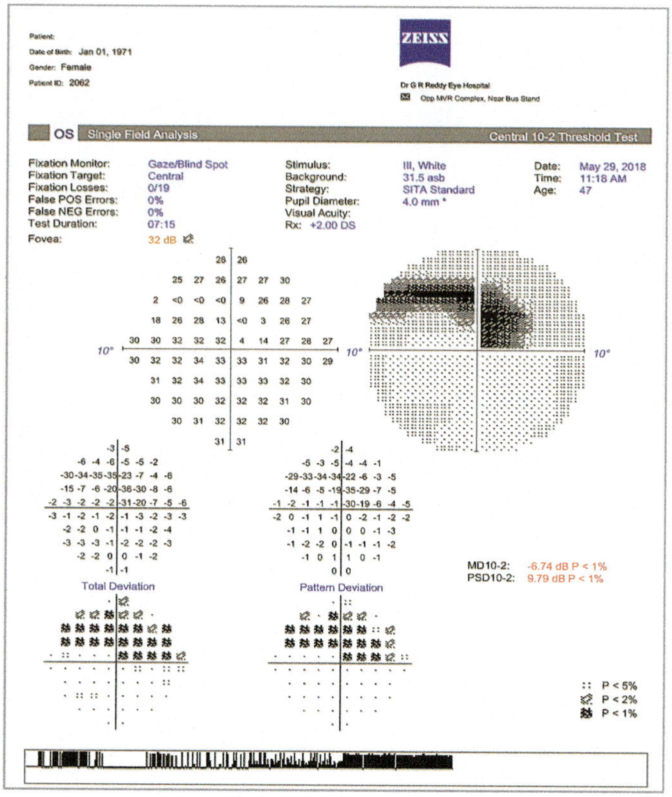

FL 0/19; FP 0%; FN 0%
Fovea 32 dB
MD -6.74 dB P < 1%; PSD 9.79 dB P < 1%

Case 20 LE

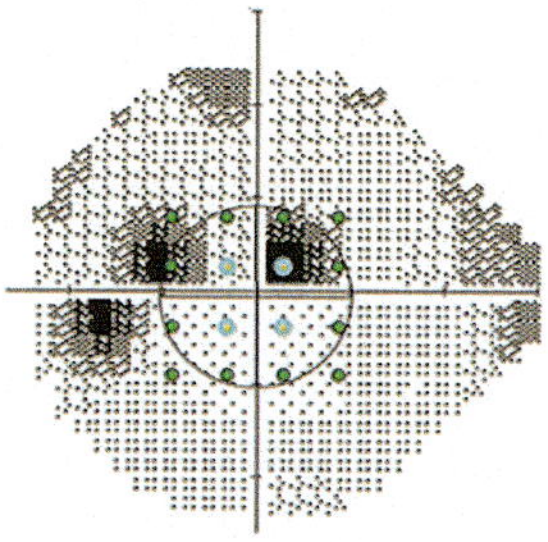

Grey scale

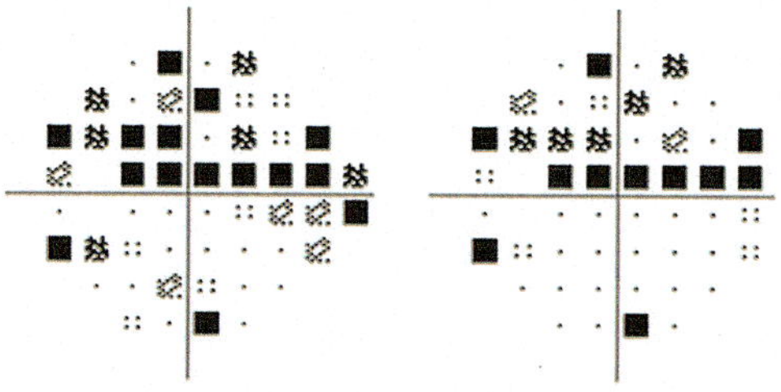

Probability plots

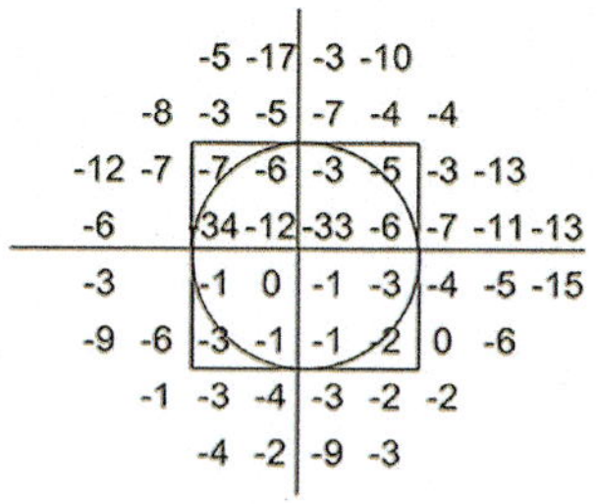

TDNP

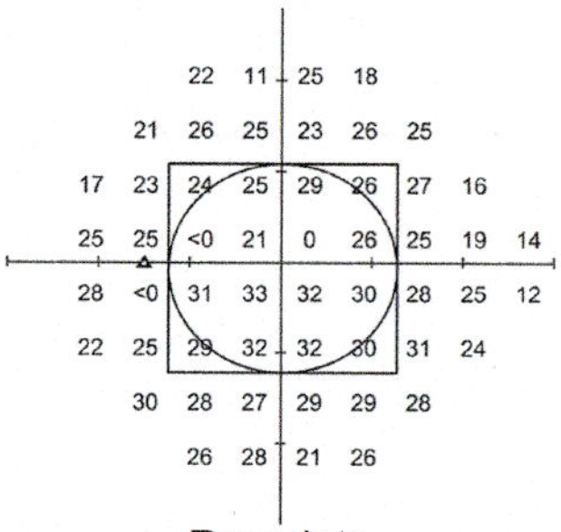

Raw data

Identification of location of field defect—Grey scale is giving clues that there is ganglion cell damage within 10° circle and outside 10° degree circle.

Probability plots—In this case, it is clearly evident from the probability plots that glaucoma started close to fixation.

RAW DATA—Out of 16 points in the 10° circle area, there are two absolute scotomas. The most striking feature in this raw data is that the sensitivity of the 3° point in the upper nasal quadrant is 0 dB (Absolute scotoma). Probability plots, grey scale and raw data (TDNP) are giving indications to repeat the test with 10-2 point pattern.

Case 20 LE 10-2

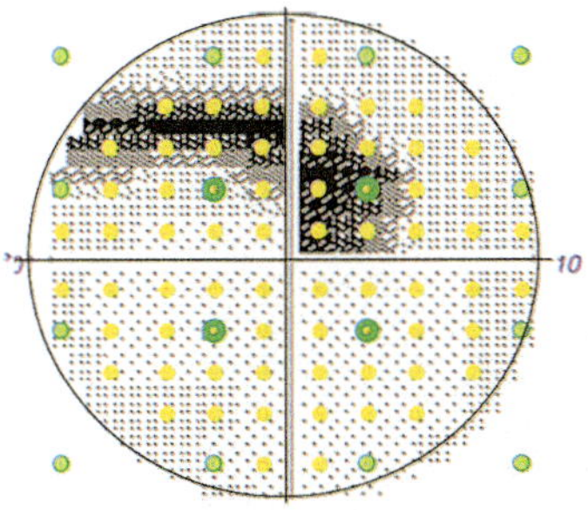

Grey scale

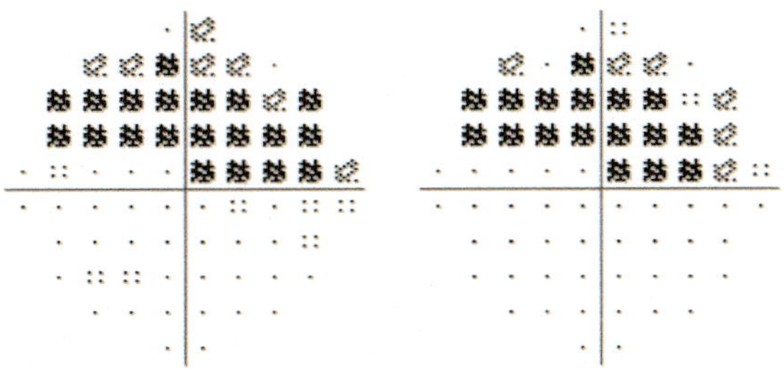

Probability plots

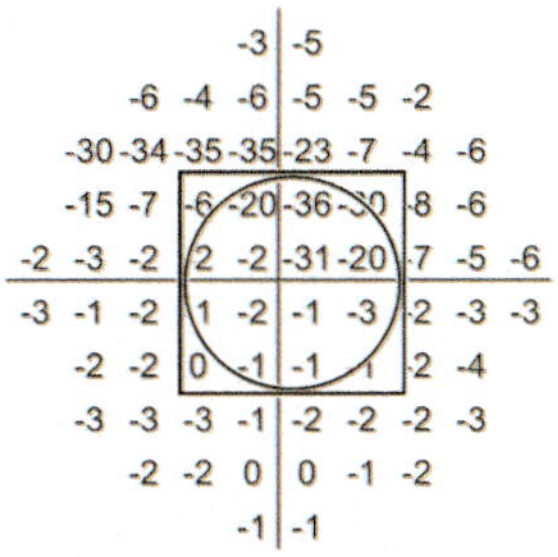

TDNP

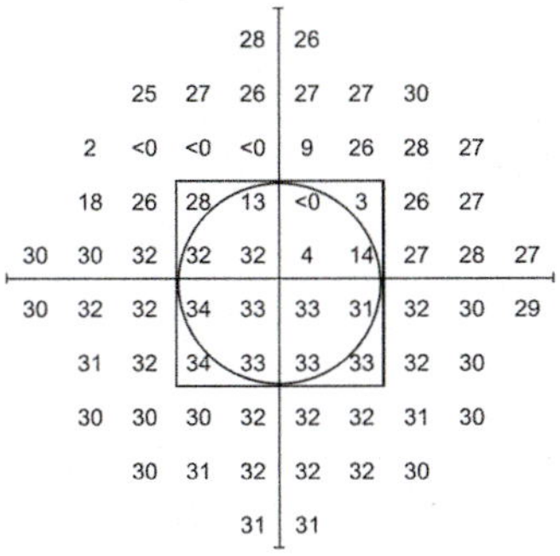

Raw data

The most important point in this printout is that glaucoma started within the 3° circle in the upper nasal quadrant.

3 points have severe loss of sensitivity in the upper nasal quadrant within 3° circle. One point is absolute scotoma and the two remaining points have the sensitivity around 5 dB.

Note that the extent of the scotoma is better appreciated in the probability plots and depth is better appreciated in the grey scale. The 24-2 VFI is 88% and no VFI in 10-2 program.

In the category of glaucomas starting within 10° circle 24-2 VFI value gives wrong impression about the visual status. We have to plan for very low target IOP till we plan for surgery.

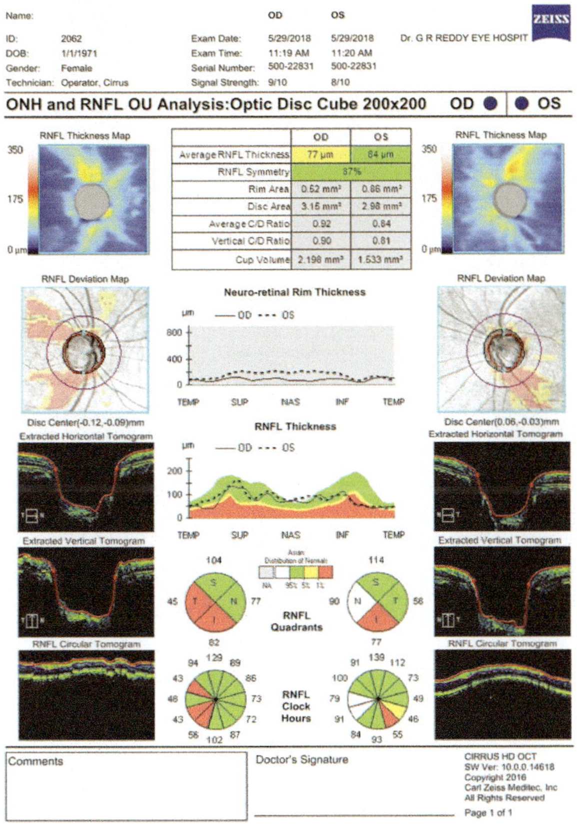

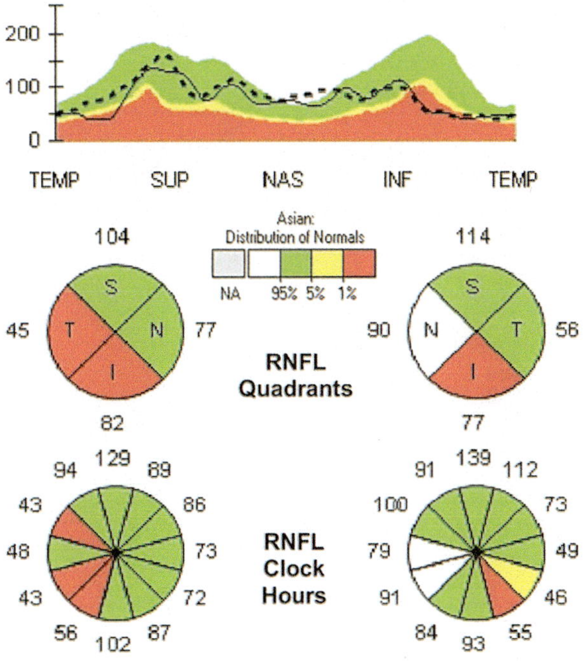

In the left eye OCT mappings are not proportionate to the field defect.

Case 21 RE

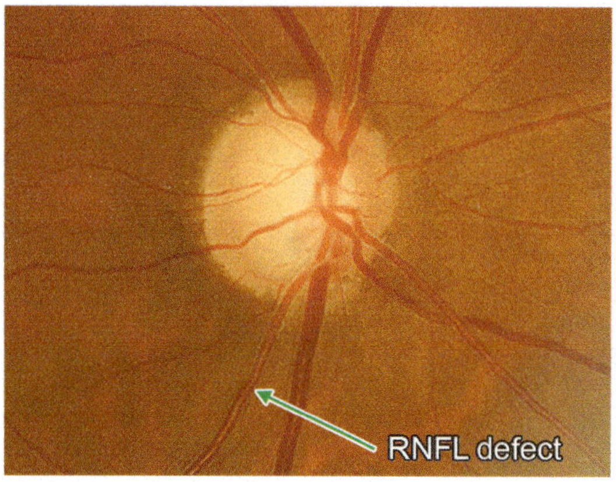

Case 21 LE

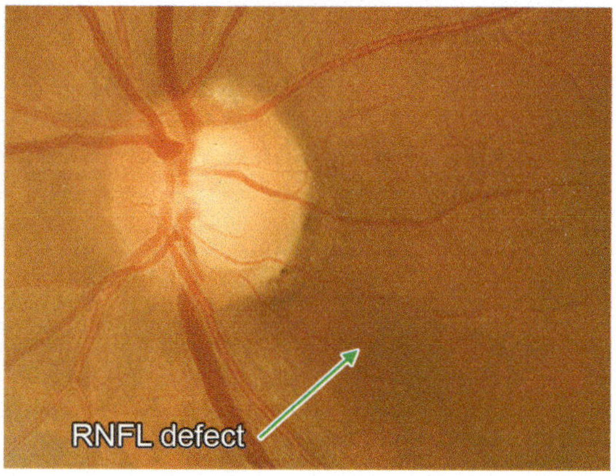

In this case, glaucoma is suspected on the basis of increased IOP and RNFL defect in both the eyes and the visual fields confirmed the diagnosis.

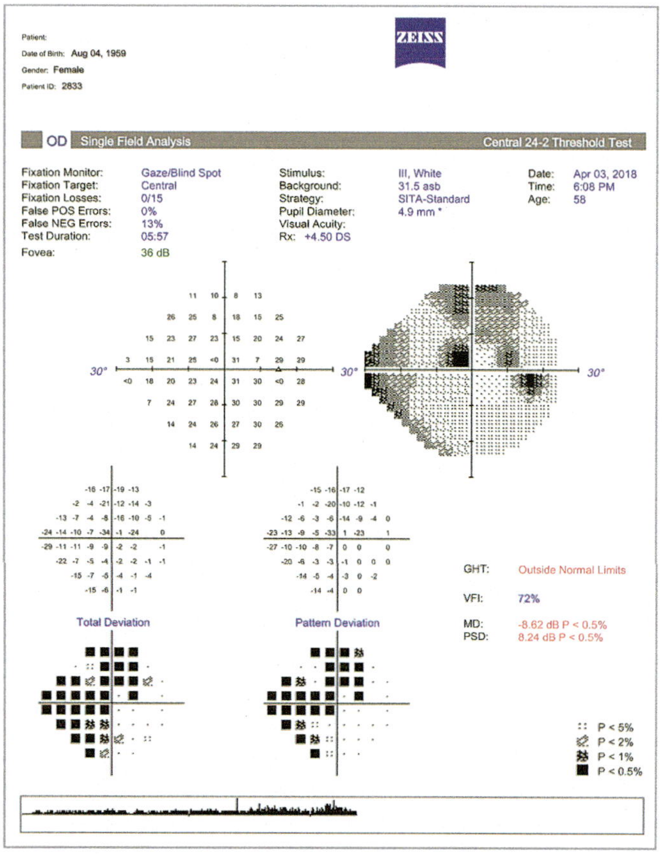

FL 0/15; FP 0%; FN 13%
Fovea 36 dB; VFI 72%
MD -8.62 dB P < 0.5%; PSD 8.24 dB P < 0.5%

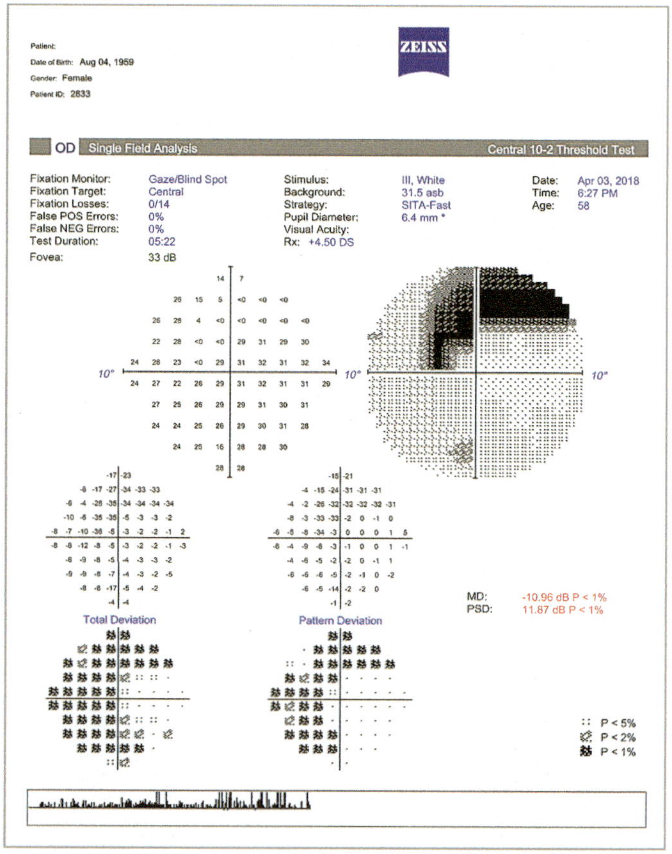

FL 0/14; FP 0%; FN 0%
Fovea 33 dB
MD -10.96 dB P < 1%; PSD 11.87dB P < 1%

Case 21 RE

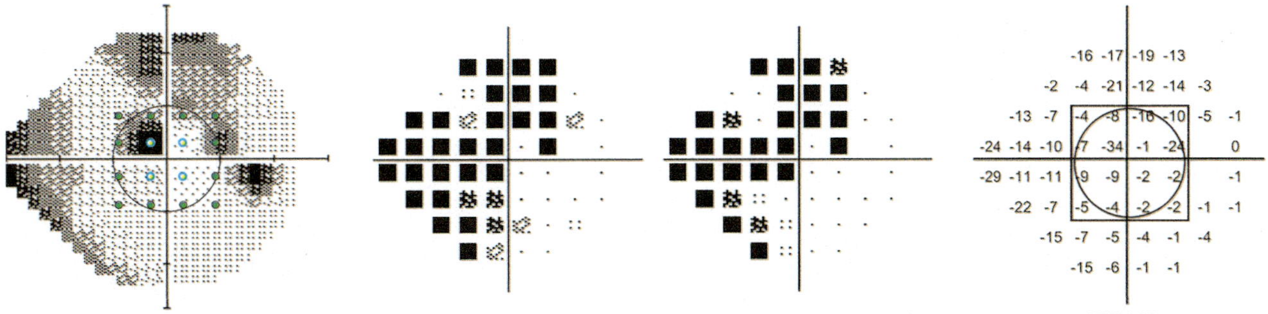

Grey scale | Probability plots | TDNP

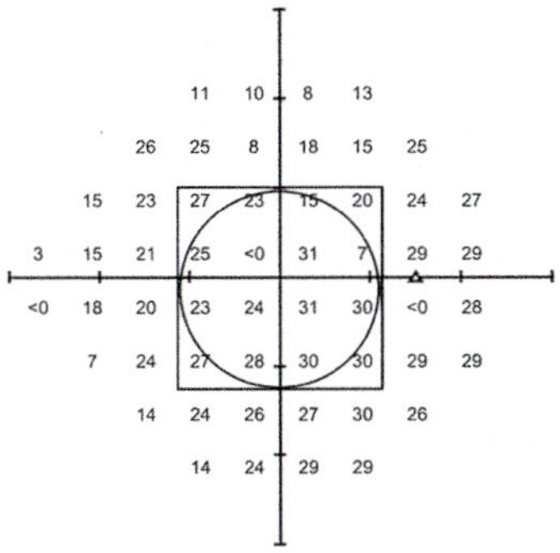

Raw data

Identification of location of field defect—Grey scale is giving clues that ganglion cell damage started within 10° circle and outside 10° degree circle. In this case from the probability plots alone it is not possible to identify the multicentric origin of glaucoma.

RAW DATA—Out of 16 points in the 10° circle area 3° upper nasal point is absolute scotoma. This tells glaucoma started close to fixation. So we have to repeat the test with 10-2 point pattern. There are two separate localized field defects outside 10° circle area.

Case 21 RE 10-2

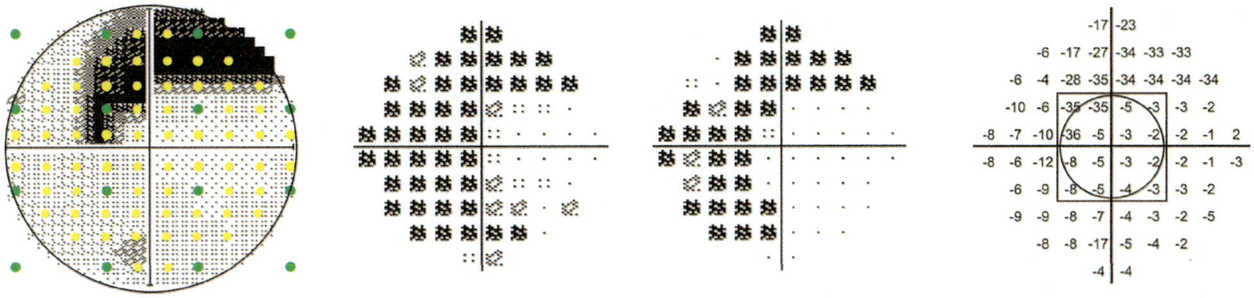

Grey scale | Probability plots | TDNP

Case 19 RE 10-2

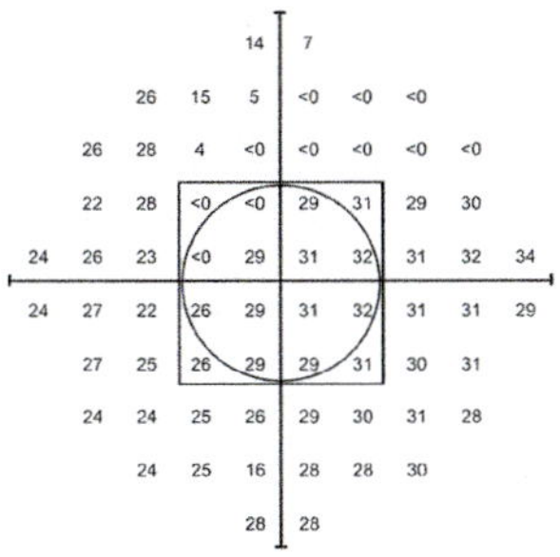

Raw data

10-2 Probability plots are showing biarcuate scotoma involving the nasal half of the field. The sensitivity of most of the points in the lower nasal quadrant is around 25-30 dB and have good shade in the grey scale. Minimal loss of sensitivity will not be appreciated in the grey scale. But the points with 8 dB loss will be represented by significant P value symbol in the probability plots. The value of VFI in 24-2 is 72%. VFI index is not given for 10-2 point program. The 10-2 MD is -10.96 dB and 24-2 MD is -8.62 dB. The field defect extended in to 3° circle, and we have to set very low target IOP or plan for surgery.

Case 21 LE

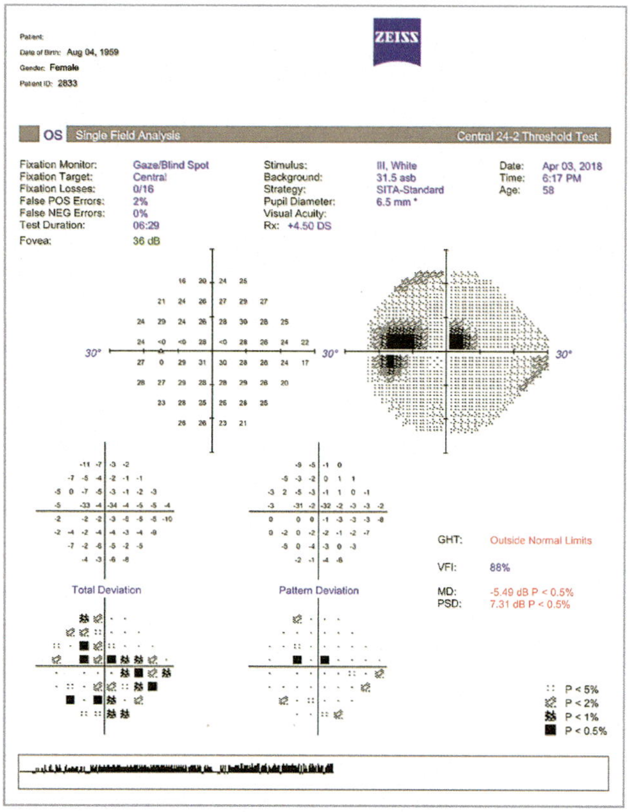

FL 0/16; FP 2%; FN 0%
Fovea 36 dB; VFI 88%
MD -5.49 dB P < 0.5%; PSD 7.31 dB P < 0.5%

Case 21 LE 10-2

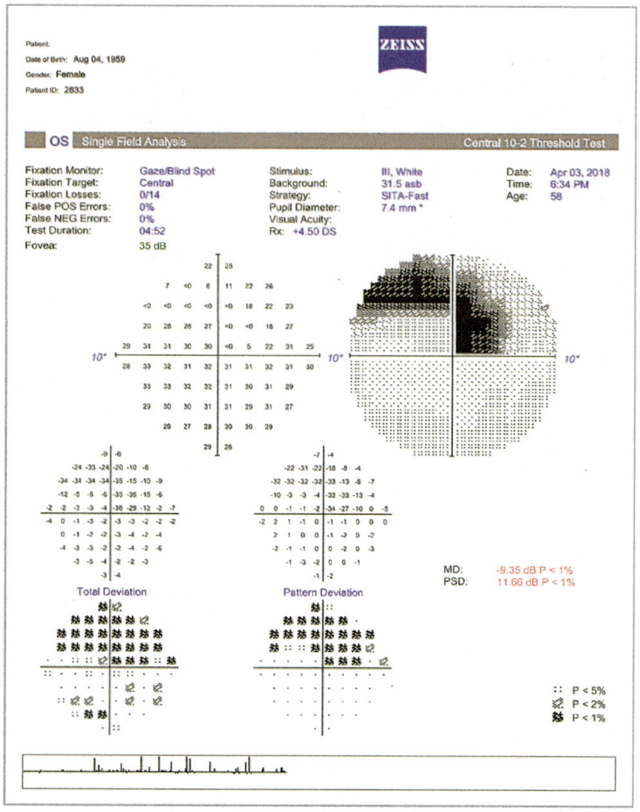

FL 0/14; FP 0%; FN 0%
Fovea 35 dB
MD -9.35 dB P < 1%; PSD 11.66 dB P < 1%

Case 21 LE 24-2

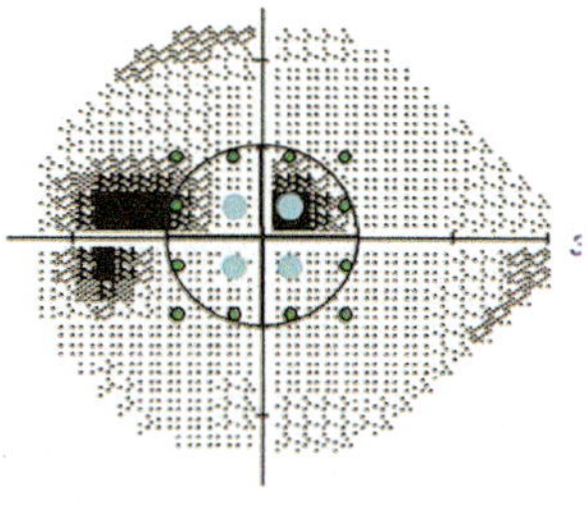

Grey scale

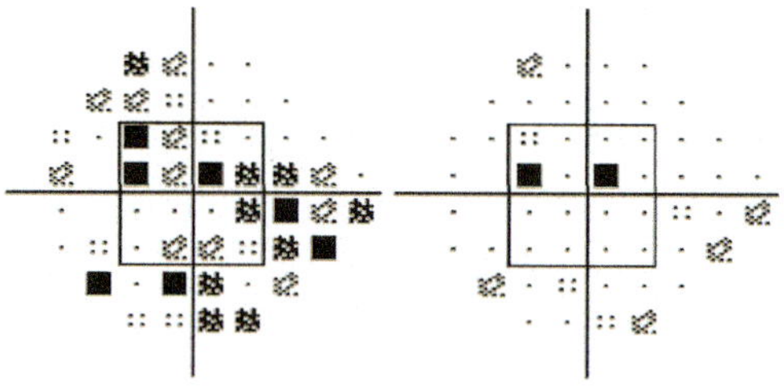

Probability plots

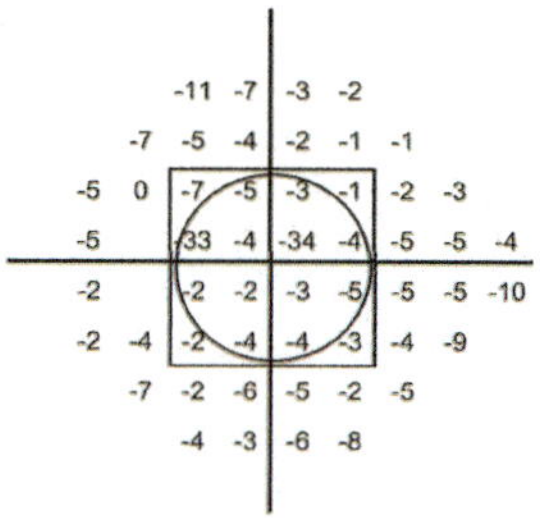

TDNP

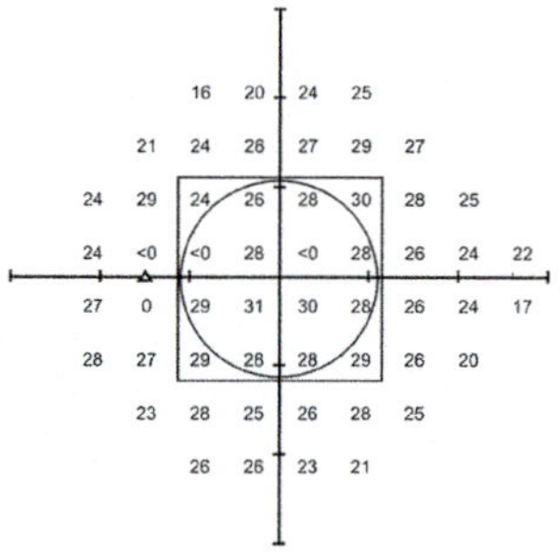

Raw data LE

Identification of location of field defect—Grey scale is giving clues that ganglion cell damage started within 10° circle and outside 10° degree circle.

Probability plots—In this case, it is clearly evident from the probability plots that glaucoma started close to fixation.

RAW DATA—Out of 16 points in the 10° circle area, there are two absolute scotomas. This tells glaucoma started close to fixation.

Probability plots, grey scale and raw data (TDNP) are giving indications to repeat the test with 10-2 point pattern.

CASE 21 LE 10-2

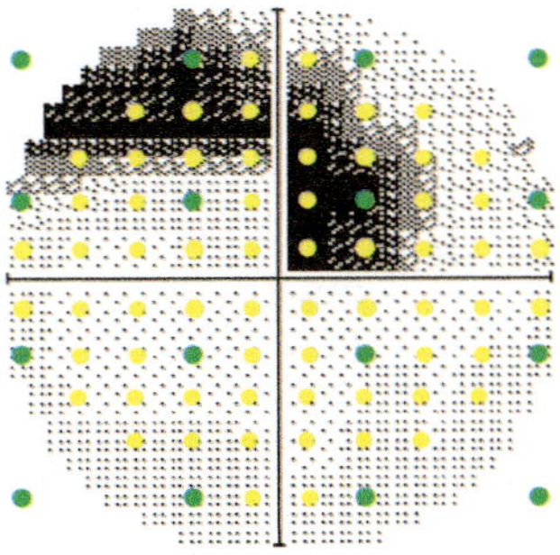

Grey scale

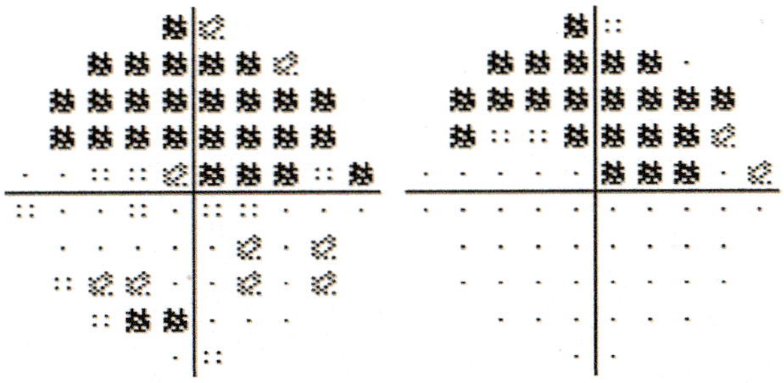

Probability plots

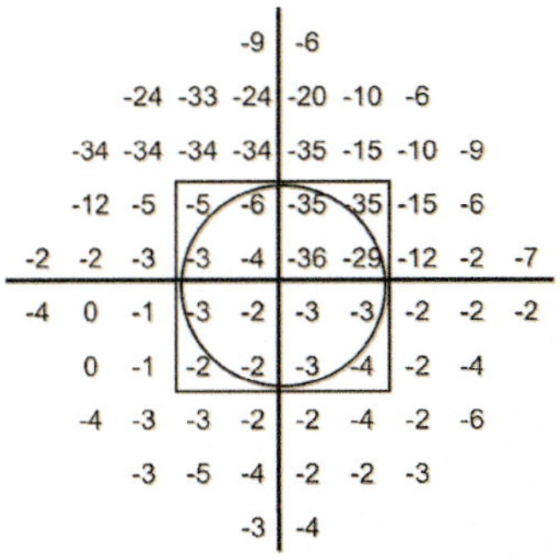

TDNP

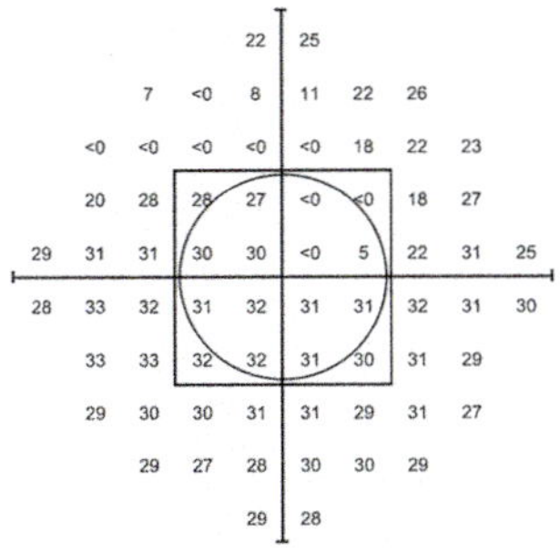

Raw data

The most important point in this printout is glaucoma started within the 3° circle in the upper nasal quadrant. 3 points are absolute scotomas in the nasal quadrant within 3° circle and the remaining point's sensitivity is 5 dB.

Note that the extent of the scotoma is better appreciated in the probability plots and depth is better appreciated in the grey scale. The 24-2 VFI is 88% and no VFI in 10-2 program.

In the category of glaucomas starting within 10° circle 24-2 VFI value gives wrong impression about the visual status. We have to maintain very low target IOP till we plan for surgery.

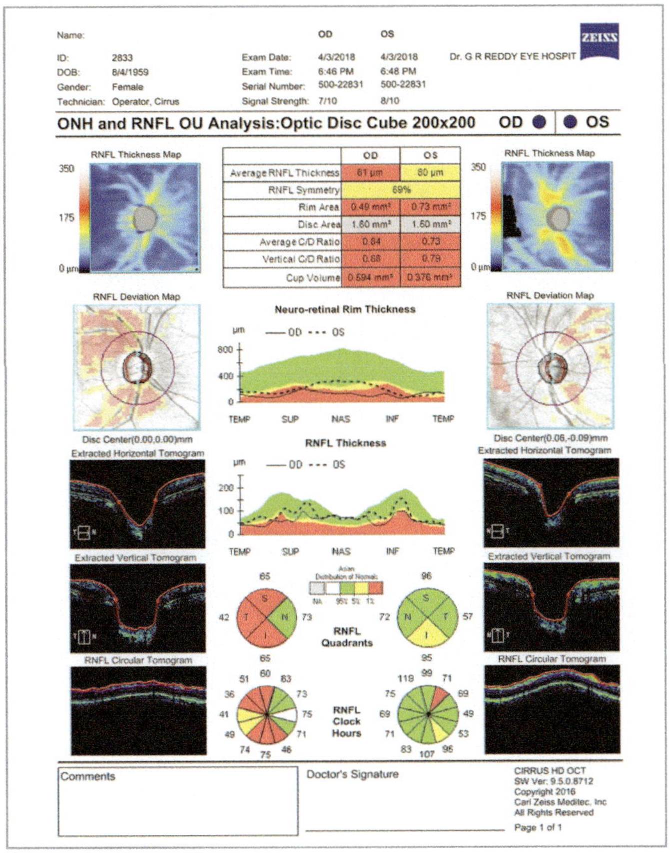

Thinning between 7 and 9° clock hours in the OCT gives clue to repeat the fields test with 10-2 point pattern.

By seeing the OCT we can not assess the depth and location of the field defect exactly.

Case 22 RE

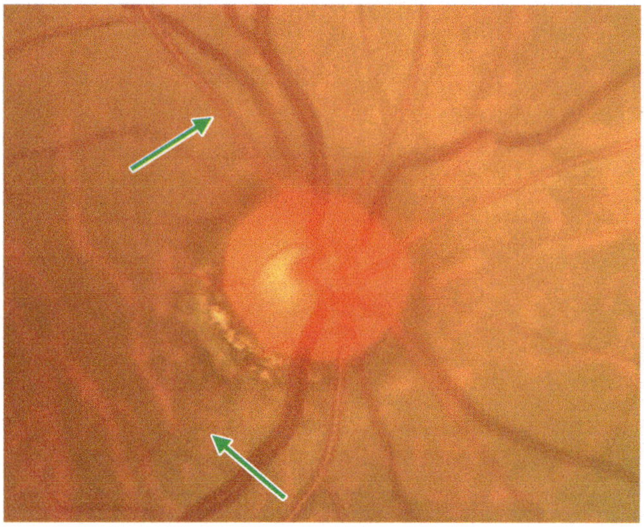

Case 22 LE

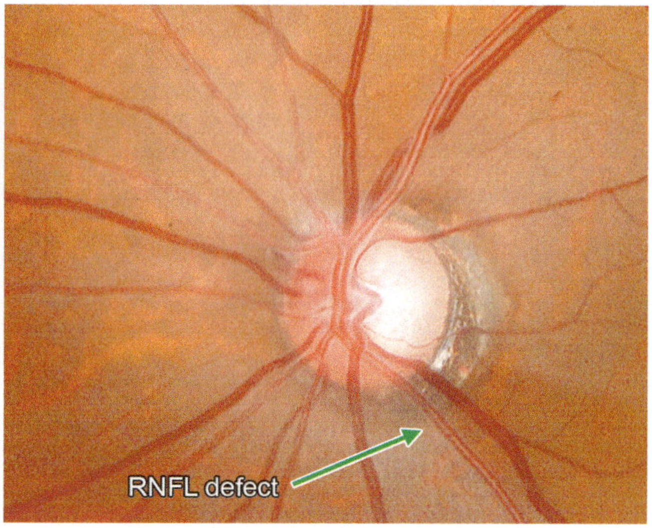

LE RNFL defect present.

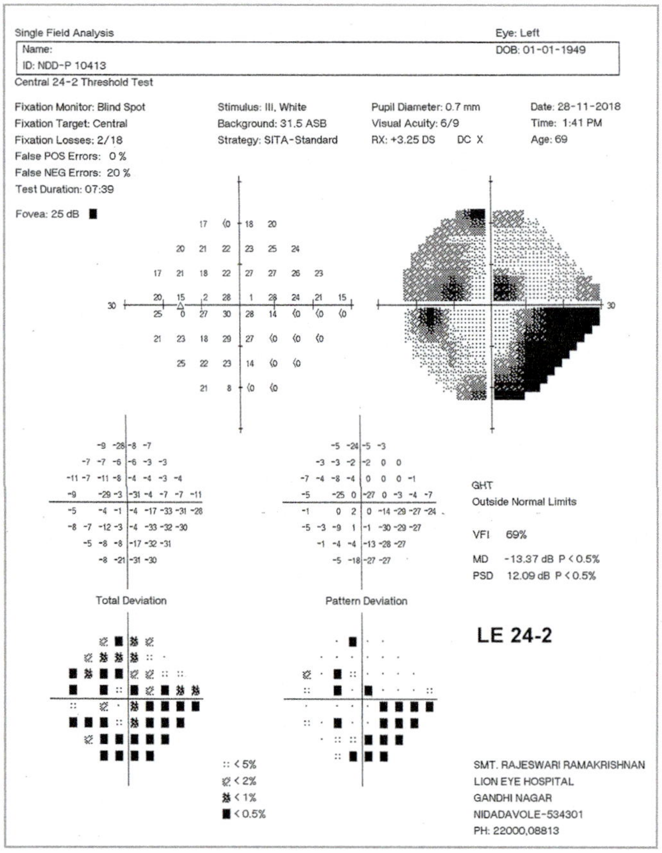

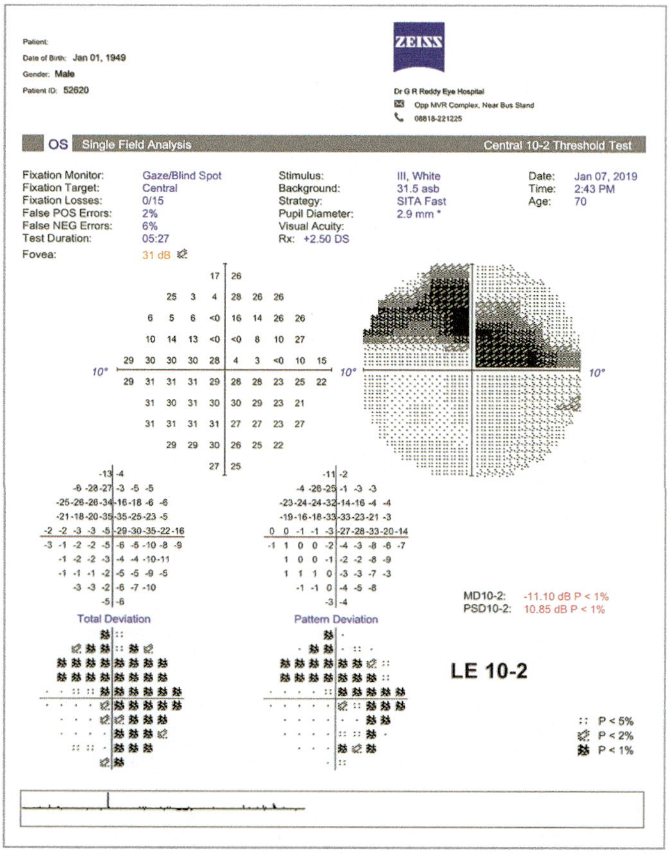

FL 2/18; FP 0%; FN 20%
Fovea 25 dB; VFI 69%
MD -13.37 dB P < 0.5%; PSD 12.09 dB P < 0.5%

FL 0/15; FP 2%; FN 6%
Fovea 31 dB
MD -11.10 dB P < 1%; PSD 10.85 dB P < 1%

Case 22 LE

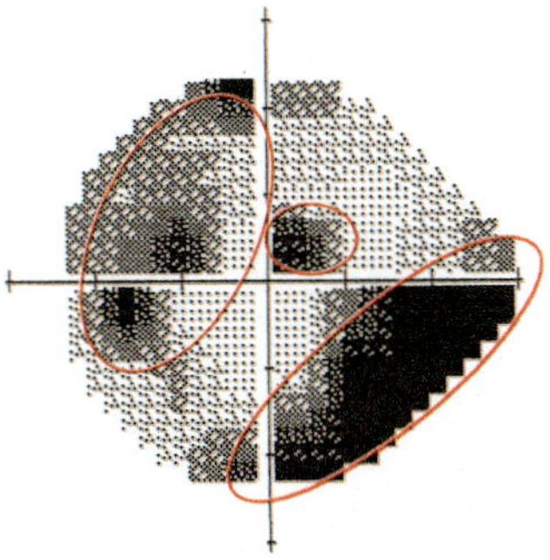

Grey scale

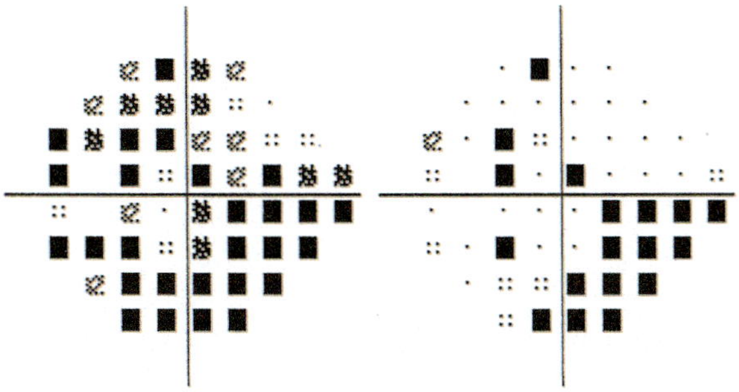

Probability plots

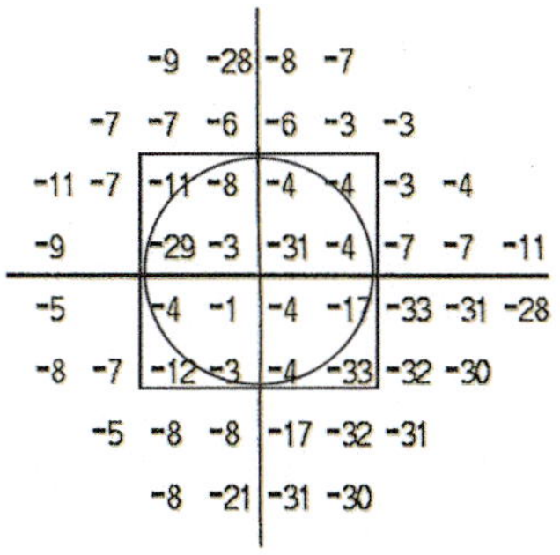

TDNP

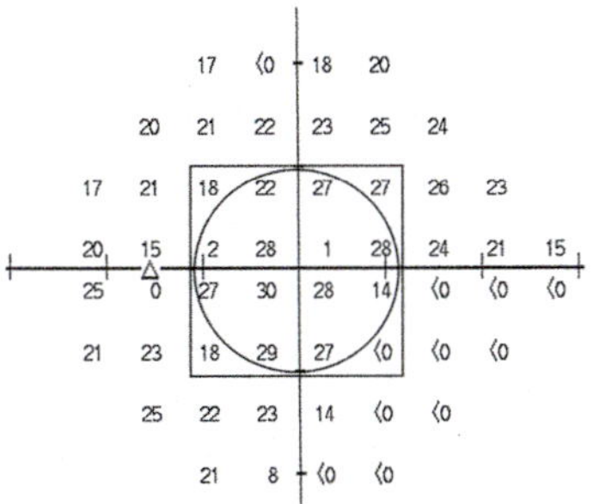

Raw data

In this printout the multifocal origin of glaucoma is better appreciated in the grey scale than in the probability plots. Lower arcuate scotoma is seen in the nasal quadrant.

RAW DATA—Out of 16 points in the 10° circle area two are almost absolute scotoma in the lower nasal quadrant. Localized absolute lower arcuate scotoma in the nasal quadrant.

24-2 VFI is 69% VFI is not calculated in 10-2 program. So, the most important point to remember is that the progression of the glaucoma starting in 10° circle can not be analyzed on the basis of change in VFI. So progression analysis for glaucomas starting in 10° circle will be calculated on the basis of change in MD index.

Case 22 LE 10-2

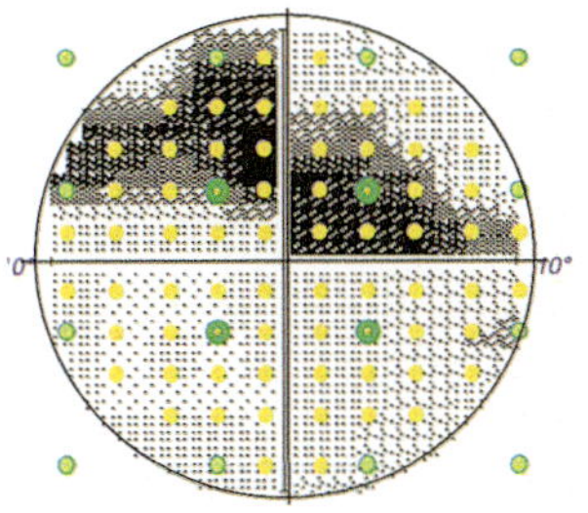

Grey scale

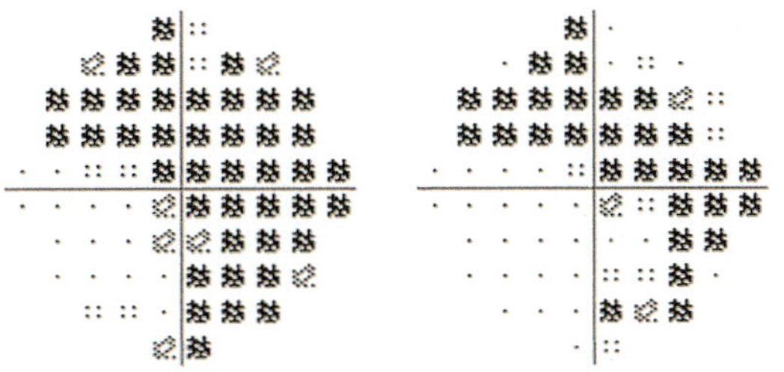

Probability plots

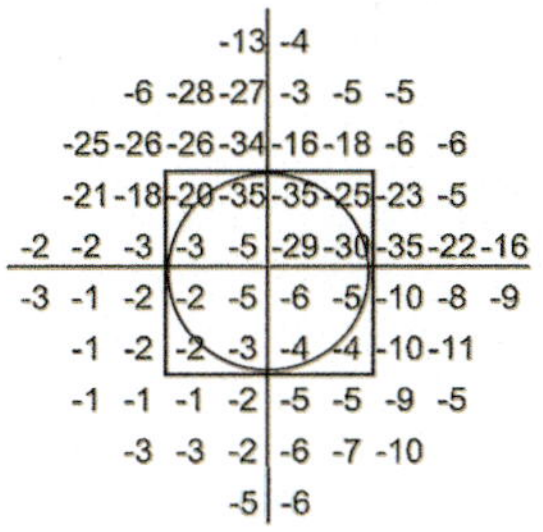

TDNP

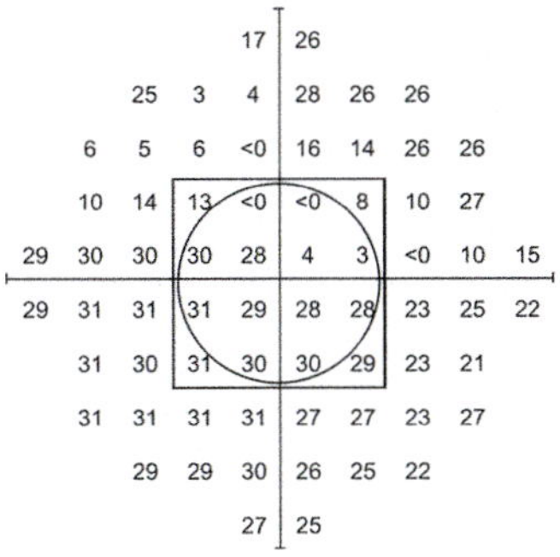

Raw data

Note that the extent of the 3 black squares in the 10° circle area in 24-2 program will be better appreciated in 10-2 program. The loss of sensitivity 4 dB to 11dB in the lower nasal quadrant is better appreciated in the probability plots than in the grey scale. We always concentrate on the 16 points in the 10° circle area in 24-2 point pattern to know whether we should repeat the test with 10-2 point pattern or not and again we concentrate on the 16 points in the 3° circle area in 10-2 point pattern to find out about foveal status.

In this case, the field defect has extended into 3° circle area **we have to maintain very low IOP till we plan for surgery.**

Case 22 RE

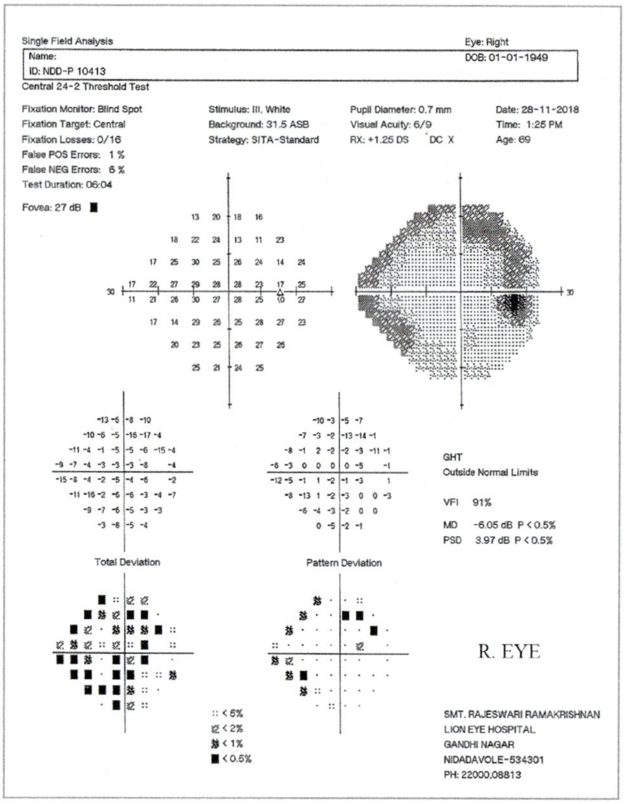

Fixation losses	**0/16**
False POS Errors	**1%**
False NEG Errors	**6%**
Fovea	**27 dB**

GHT Outside Normal Limits
VFI 91%
MD -6.05 dB P < 0.5%
PSD 3.97 dB P < 0.5%

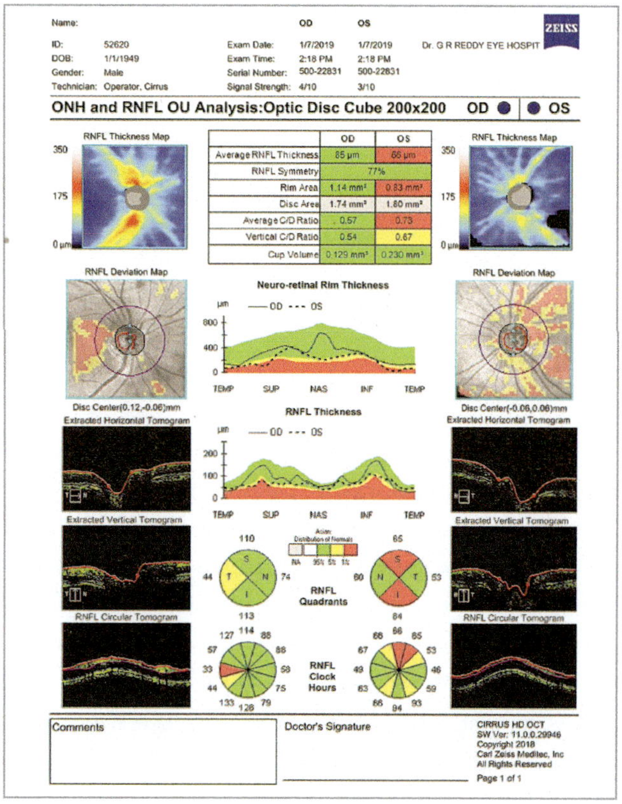

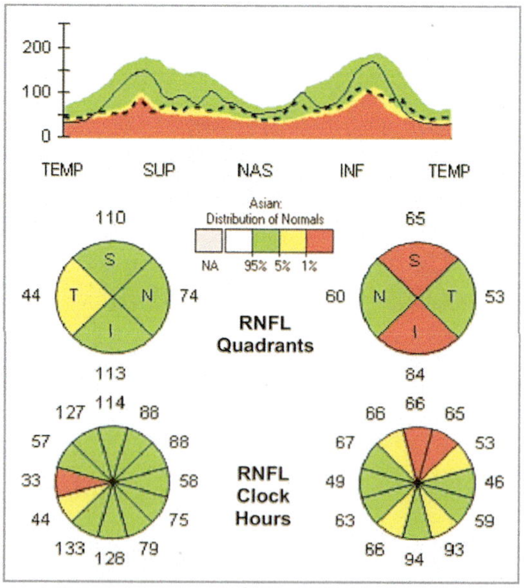

Visual fields and OCT are not correlating with each other. The huge field defect in the 10° circle area (L.EYE) is not shown in OCT clock hour map.

Case 23 RE

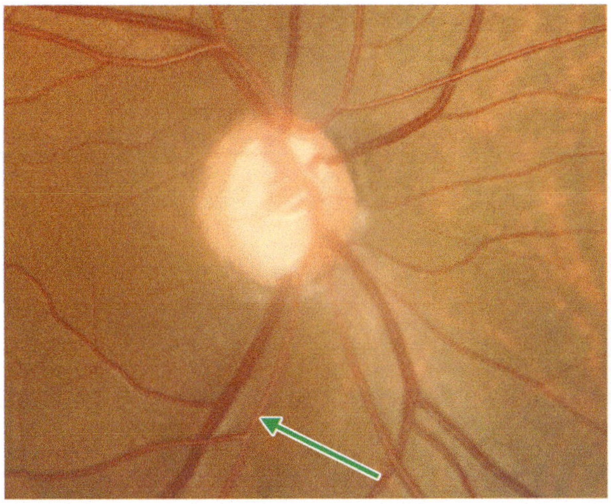

Case 23 LE

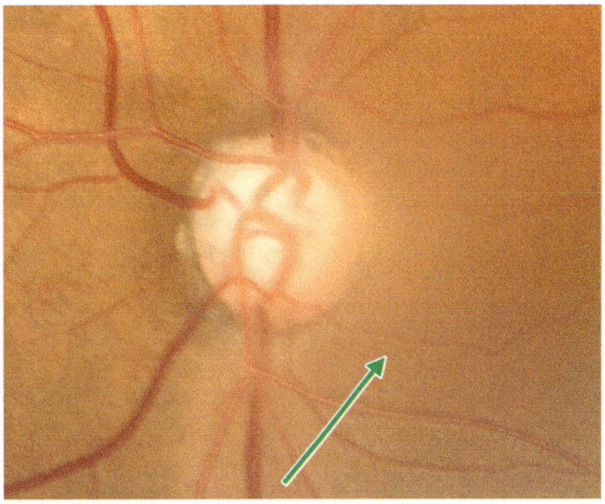

RNFL defect present in both the eyes.

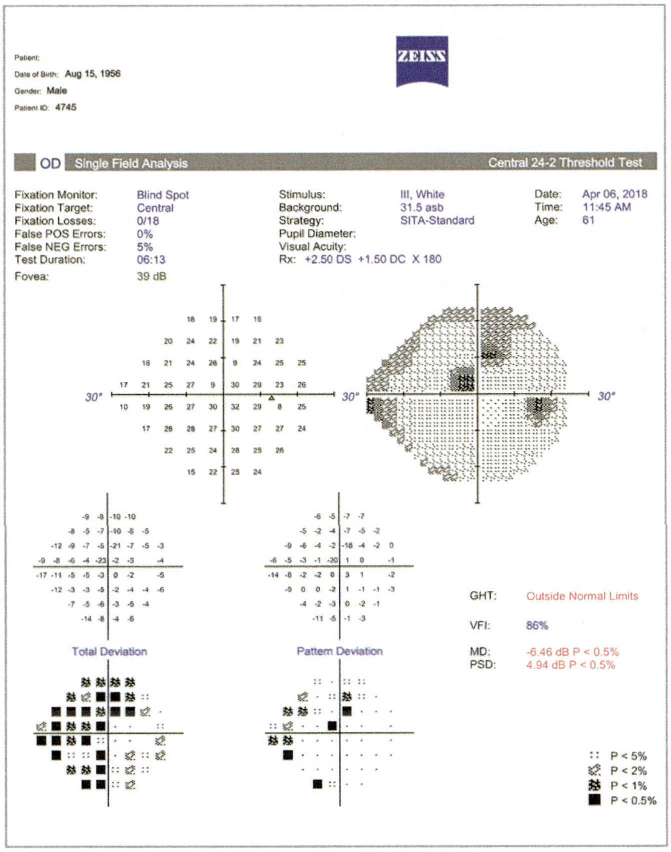

FL 0/18; FP 0%; FN 5%
Fovea 39 dB; VFI 86%
24-2 MD -6.46 dB

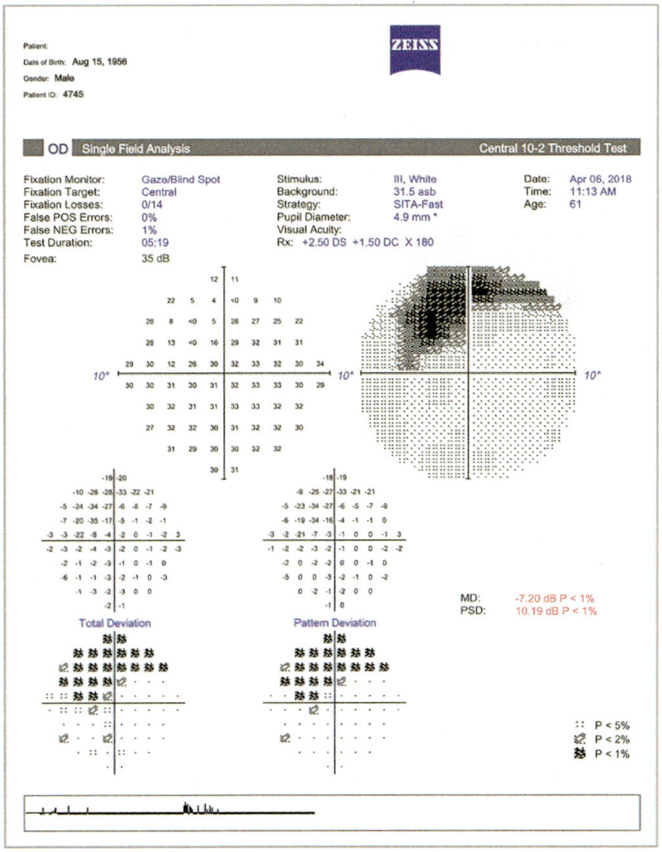

FL 0/14; FP 0%; FN 1%
Fovea 35 dB
10-2 MD -7.20 dB

Case 23 RE

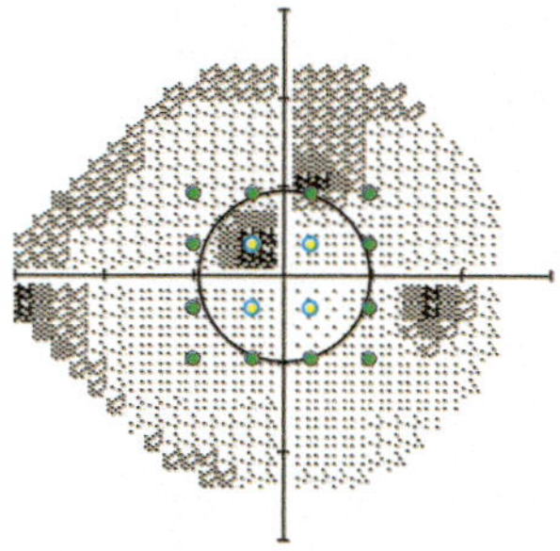

Grey scale

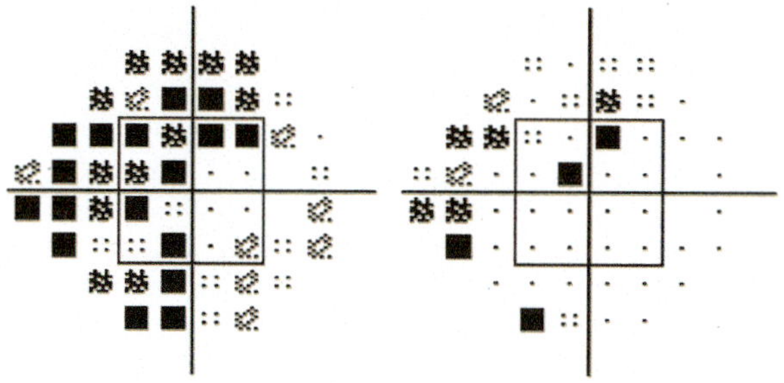

Probability plots

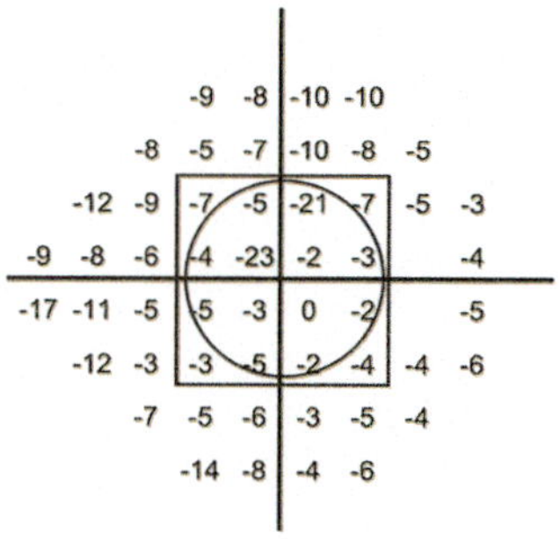

TDNP

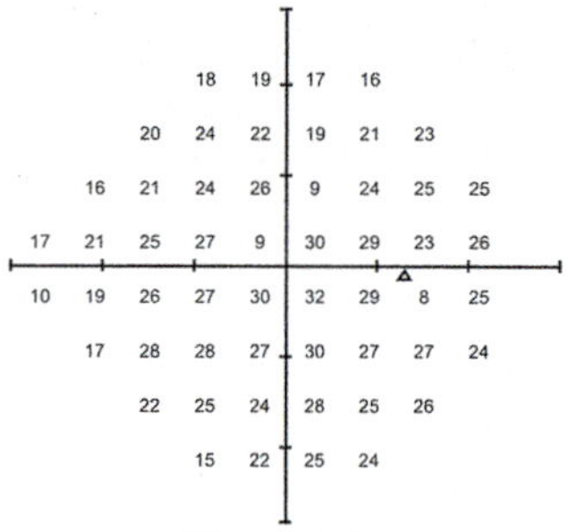

Raw data

Location of the field defect—The presence of the field defect in and outside the 10° circle is clearly evident from the grey scale and the probability plots in this printout. The sensitivity of the 3° circle point in the upper nasal quadrant is 9 dB, (-23 dB in TDNP)

Probability plots, grey scale and raw data (TDNP) are giving indications to repeat the test with 10-2 point pattern.

VFI 86%
24-2 MD index is -6.46 dB

Case 23 RE 10-2

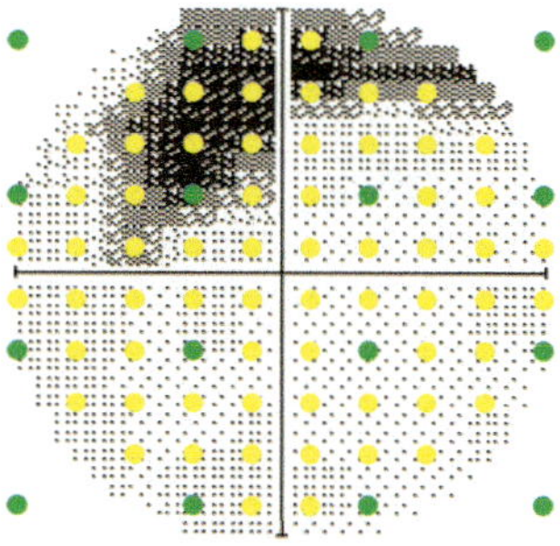

Grey scale

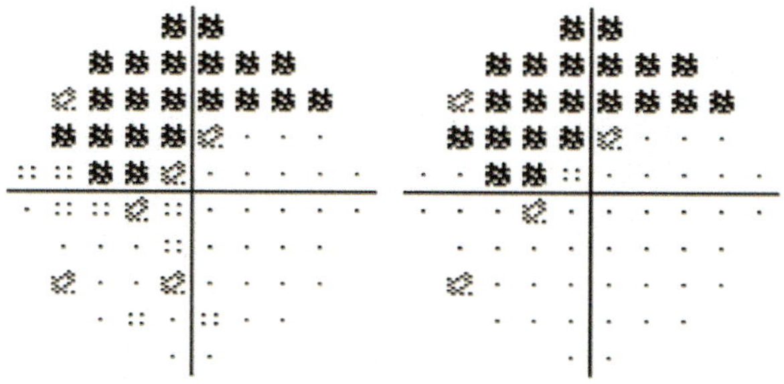

Probability plots

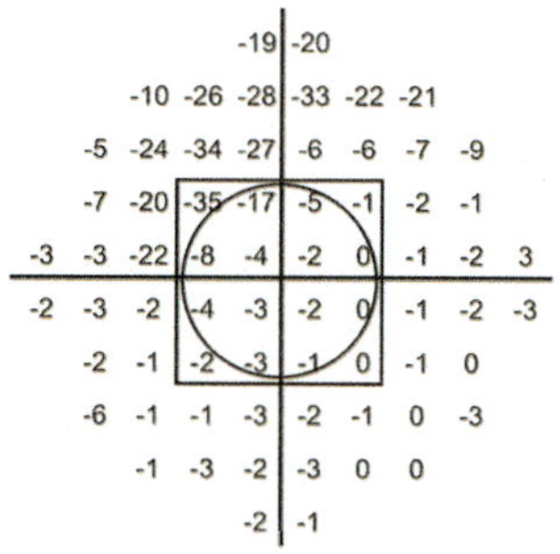

TDNP

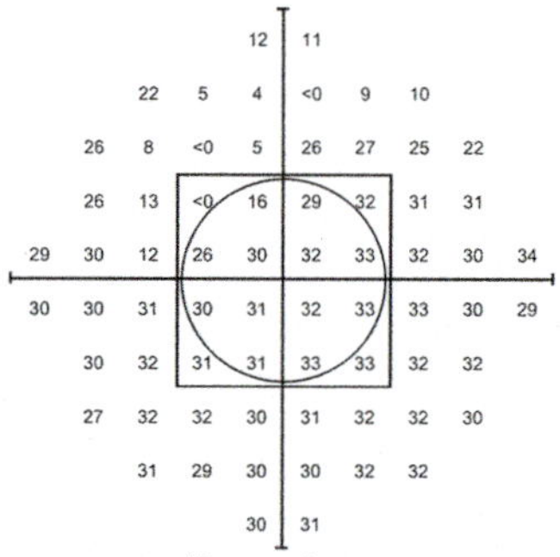

Raw data

Location of the field defect—Upper arcuate scotoma in the nasal quadrant progressing between 3° and 9° points towards temporal quadrant. The field defect is extended to the 3° circle in the upper nasal quadrant. This is a bad prognostic sign. **24-2 MD index is -6.46 dB 10-2 MD index is -7.20 dB No VFI in 10-2 printouts.**

So for glaucoma progression we have to depend on change in MD index since the field defect extended to the 3° circle we have to set very low target IOP or plan for antiglaucoma surgery at the earliest.

Case 23 LE

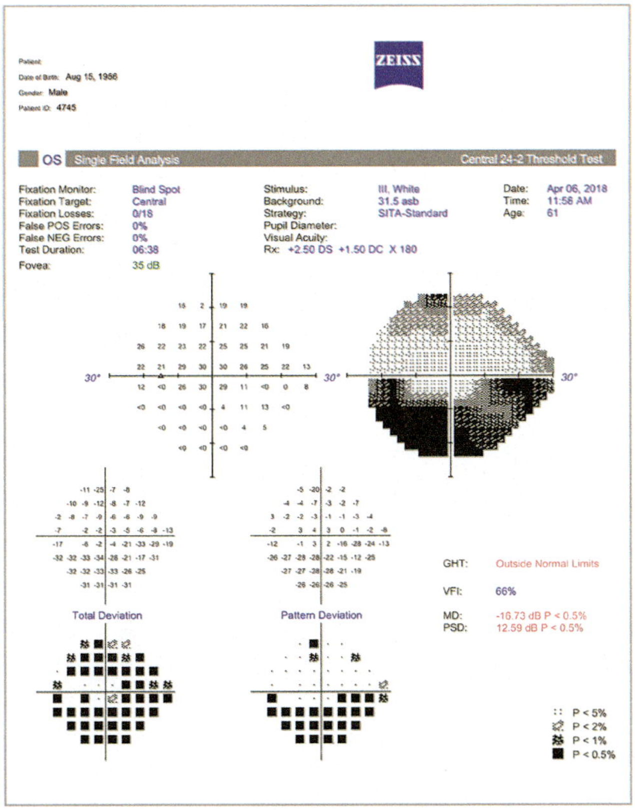

FL 0/18; FP 0%; FN 0%
Fovea 35 dB; VFI 66%
MD -16.73 dB P < 0.5%

Case 23 LE 10-2

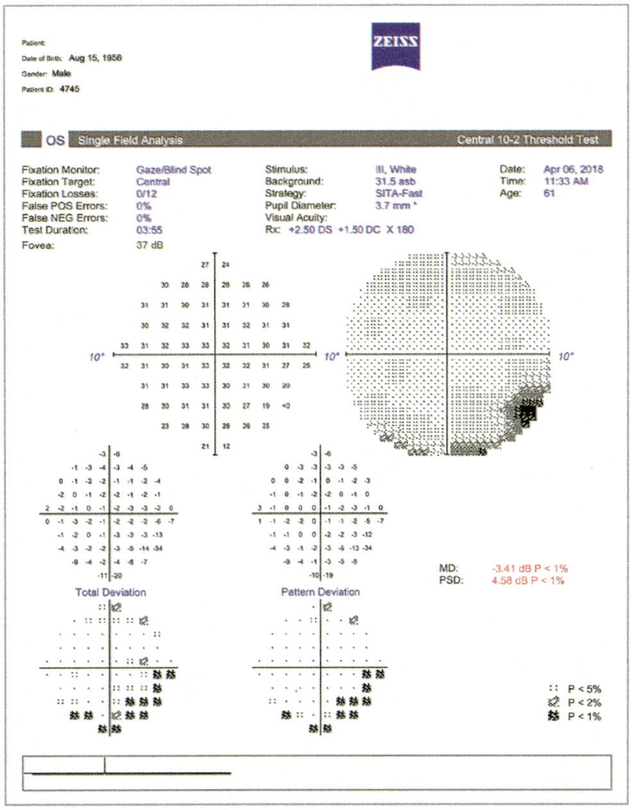

FL 0/12; FP 0%; FN 0%
Fovea 37 dB
MD -3.41 dB P < 1%

Case 23 LE

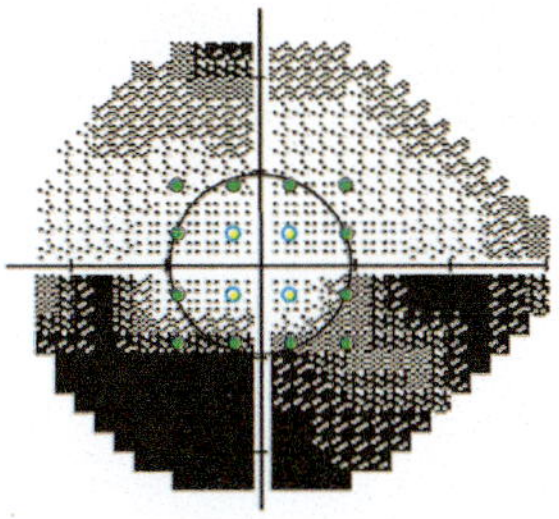

Grey scale

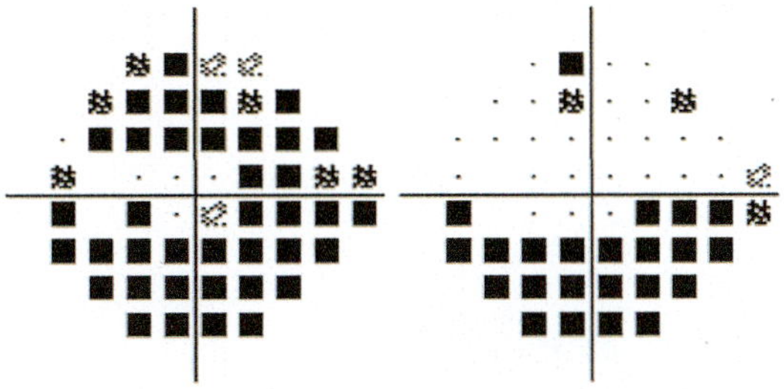

Probability plots

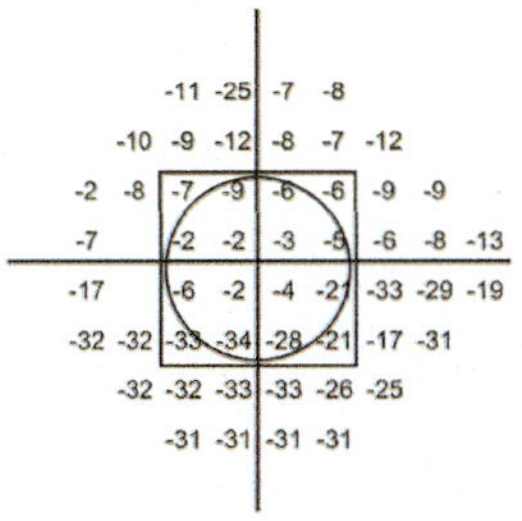

TDNP

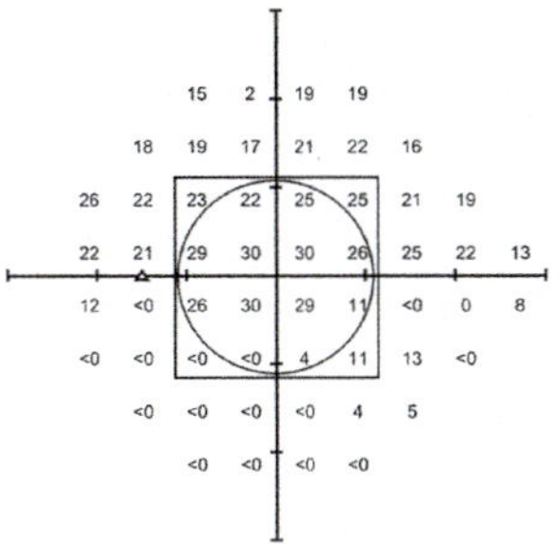

Raw data

Location of the field defect—In this patient glaucoma started outside 10° circle and progressed toward fixation. Glaucoma started in the lower temporal quadrant (All black squares absolute scotomas in this quadrant). The generalized depression in TDPP is caused by glaucoma only as there is no cataract in this patient and the foveal sensitivity is 37 dB. Deep scotomas are highlighted in PDPP and field defect is progressing towards upper quadrant.

VFI 66%; MD -16.73 dB; PSD 12.59 dB

Case 23 LE 10-2

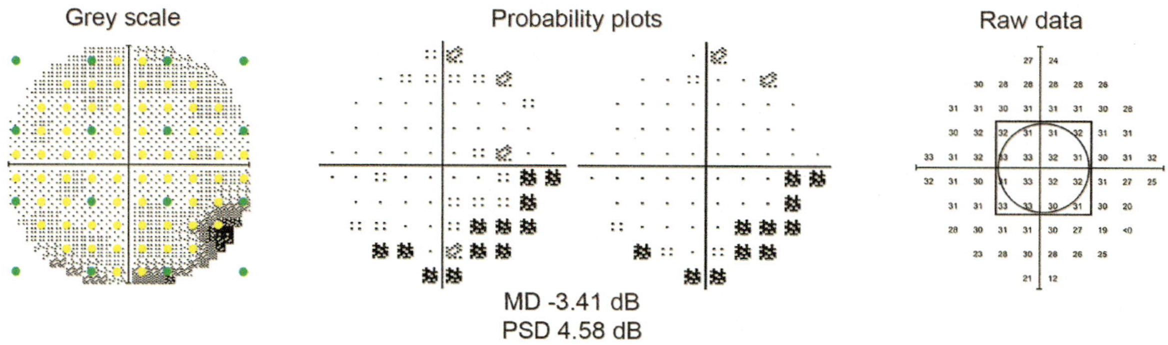

Primary open-angle glaucomas can be divided into 3 types on the basis of location of the field defect

Type-1: Field defect dominant outside 10° circle area.

Type-2: Field defect dominant inside 10° circle area.

Type-3: Field defect dominant in and outside 10° circle area.

Before we start treating a case of glaucoma, we should know the type of glaucoma we are dealing with. In this case right eye is having type 2 primary open-angle glaucoma (POAG) and left eye is having type 1 POAG.

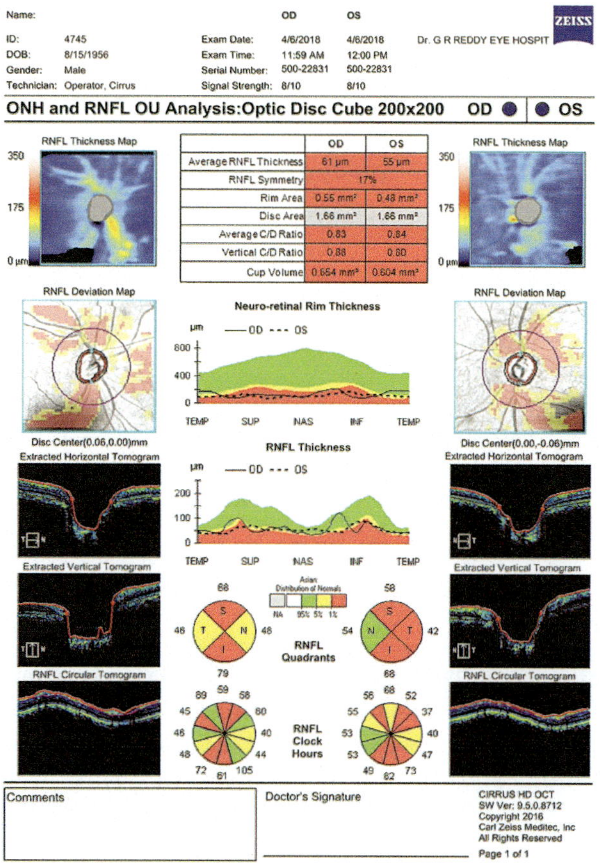

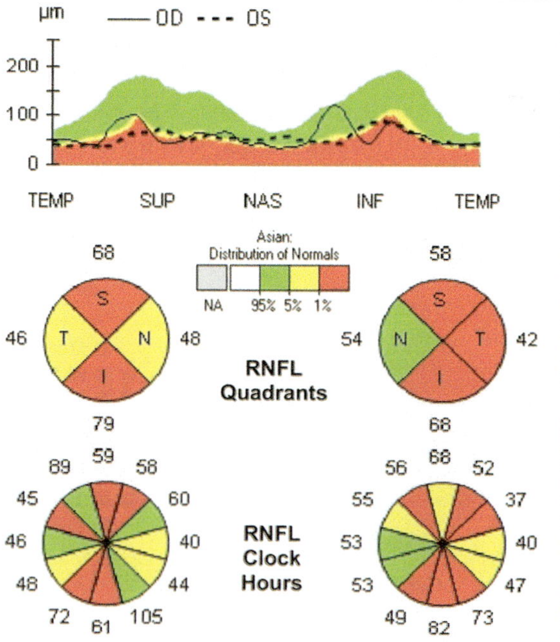

OCT mappings are correlating with fundus findings and field defects.

Case 24 RE

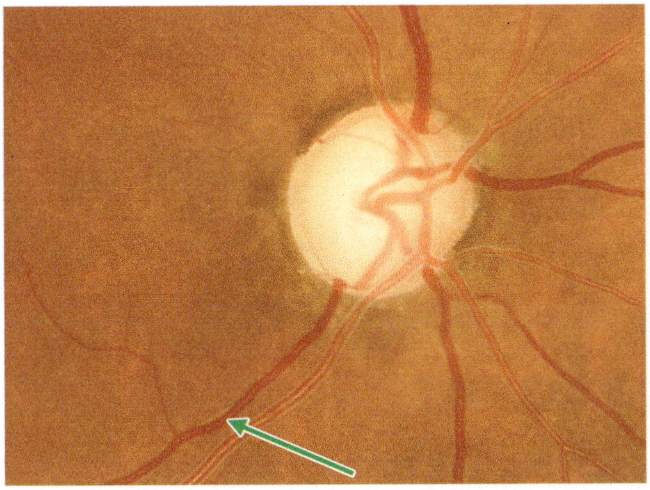

Case 24 LE

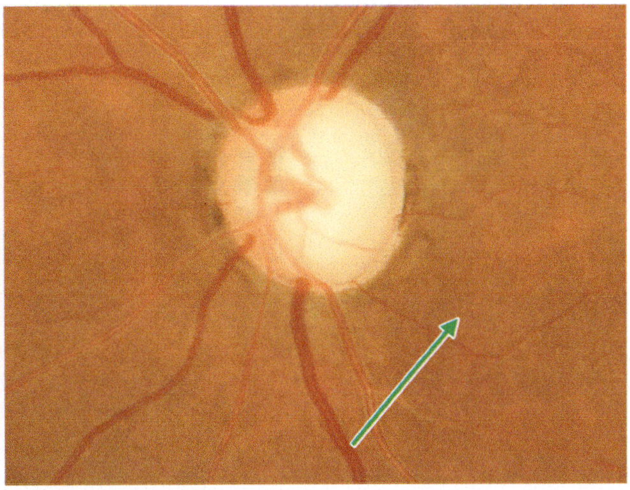

RNFL defect present in both the eyes.

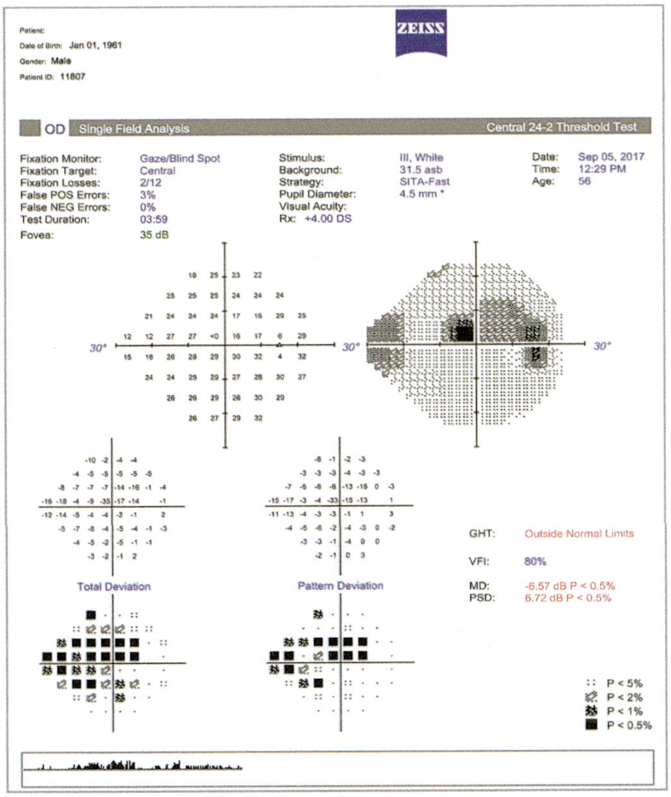

FL 2/12; FP 3%; FN 0%
Fovea 35 dB; VFI 80%
MD -6.57 dB

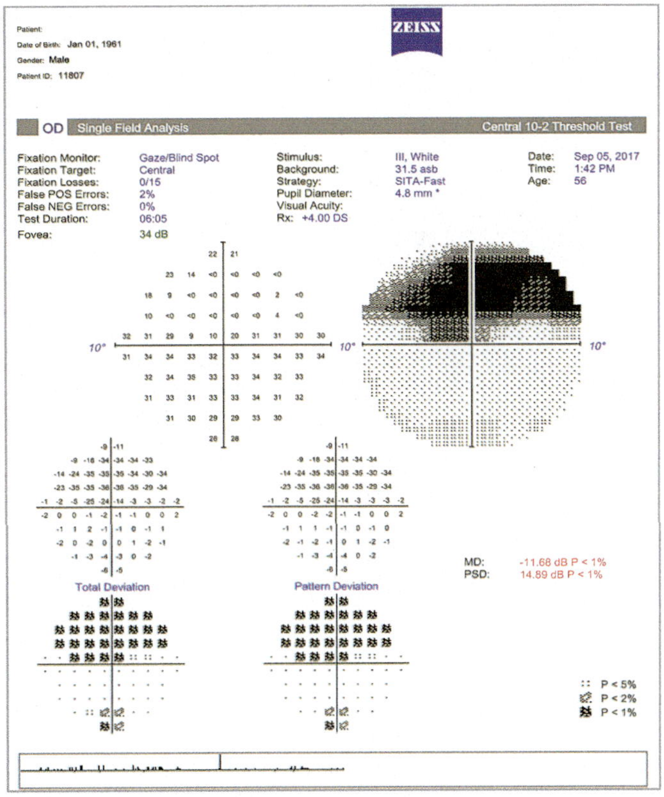

FL 0/15; FP 2%; FN 0%
Fovea 34 dB
MD -11.68 dB

Case 24 RE

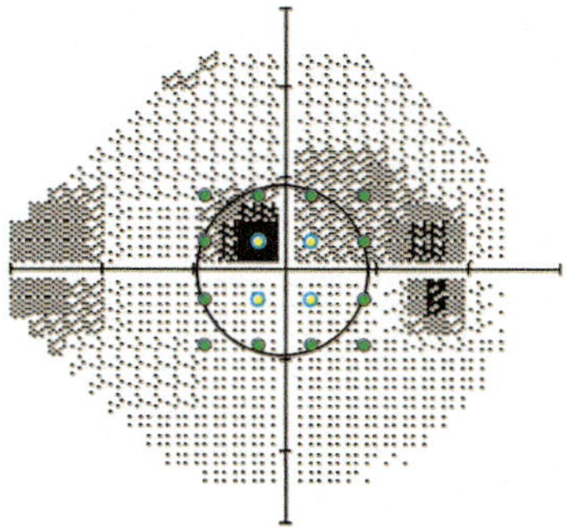

Grey scale

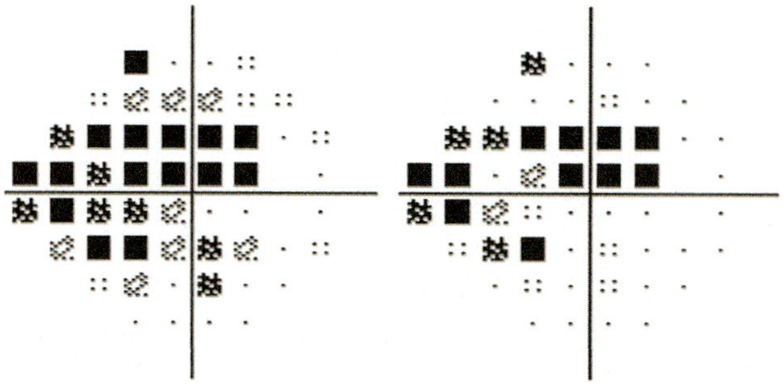

Probability plots

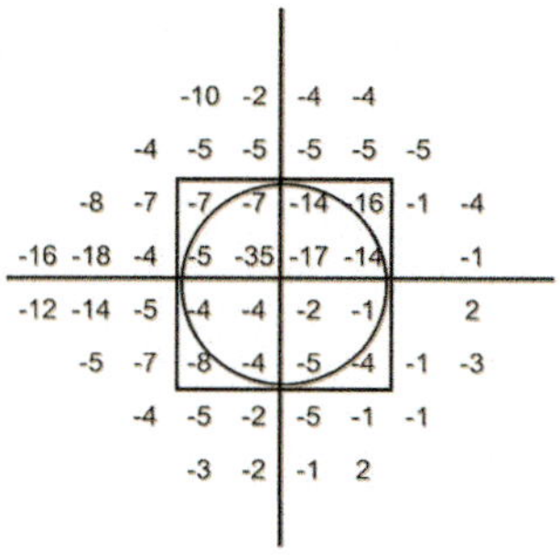

TDNP

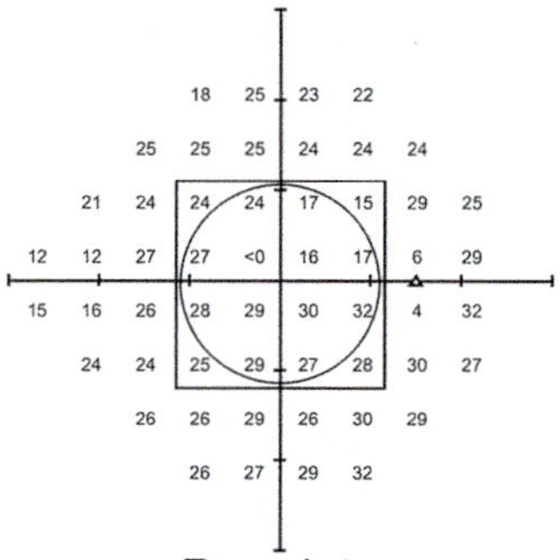

Raw data

Location of the field defect. The presence of the field defect in and outside 10° circle is clearly evident from the grey scale. The 3° point in the upper nasal quadrant is an absolute scotoma. The field defect extending into 3° circle which is a bad prognostic sign and is an indication to repeat the test with 10-2 point pattern.

MD -6.57 dB; VFI 80%

Case 24 RE 10-2

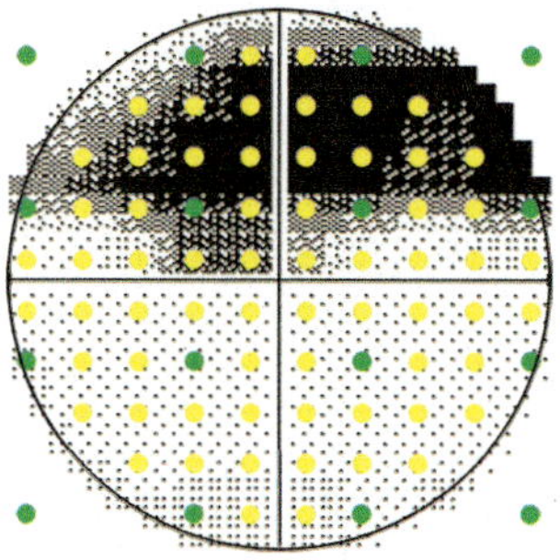

Grey scale

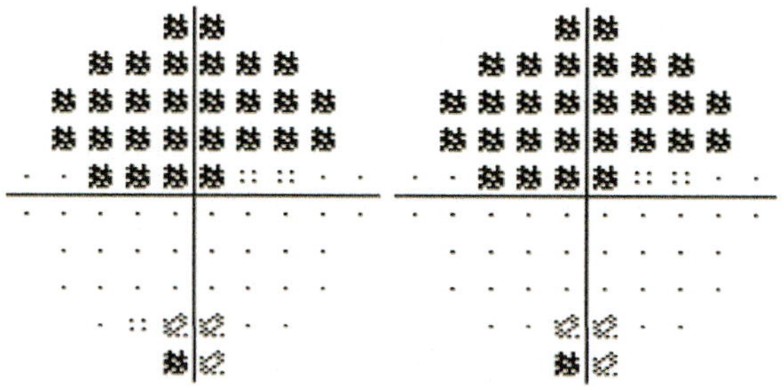

Probability plots

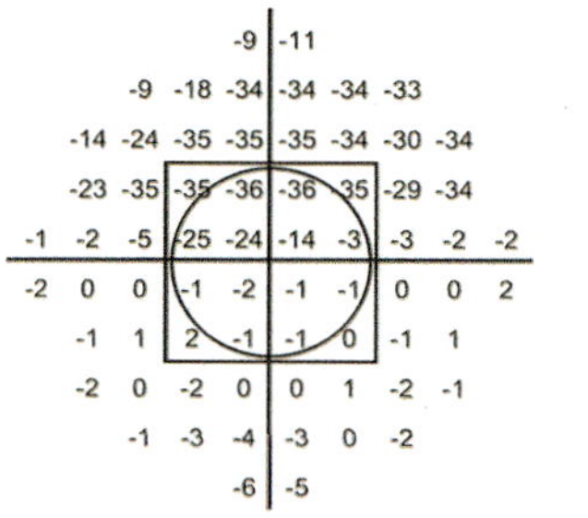

TDNP

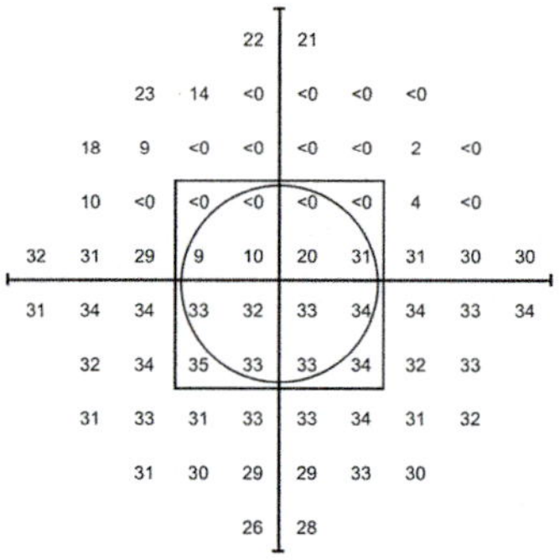

Raw data

The field defect started within 10° circle and progressed towards fixation and also towards upper temporal quadrant. Most of the points in the field defect in between the 3° and 9° points are not appreciated in the 24-2 SFA printout. 24-2 VFI will not carry any value when glaucoma's starting within 10° circle.

24-2 **MD -6.57 dB and 10-2 MD index -11.68 dB.**

Till surgery is planned, very low target IOP must be maintained.

Case 24 LE

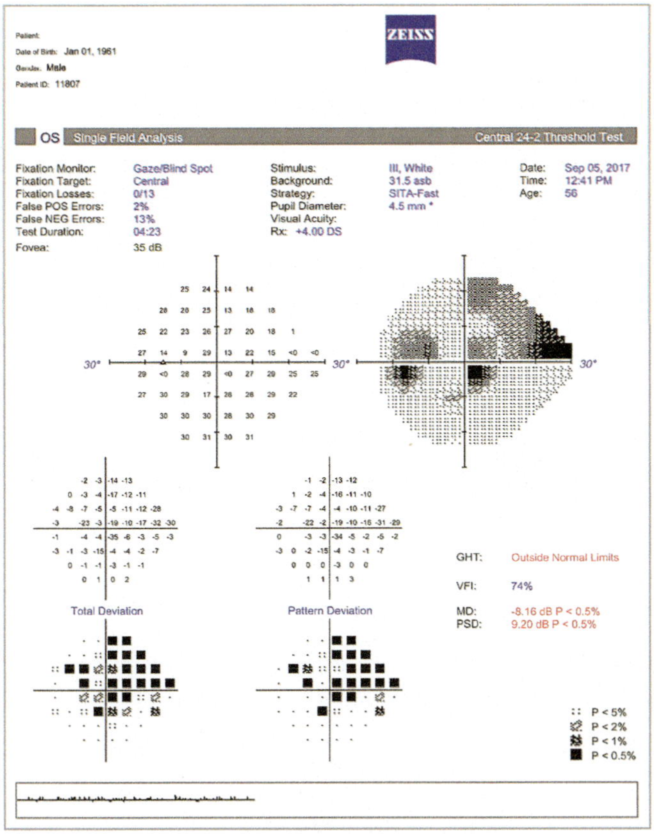

FL 0/13; FP 2%; FN 13%
Fovea 35 dB; VFI is 74%
24-2 MD -8.16 dB

Case 24 LE 10-2

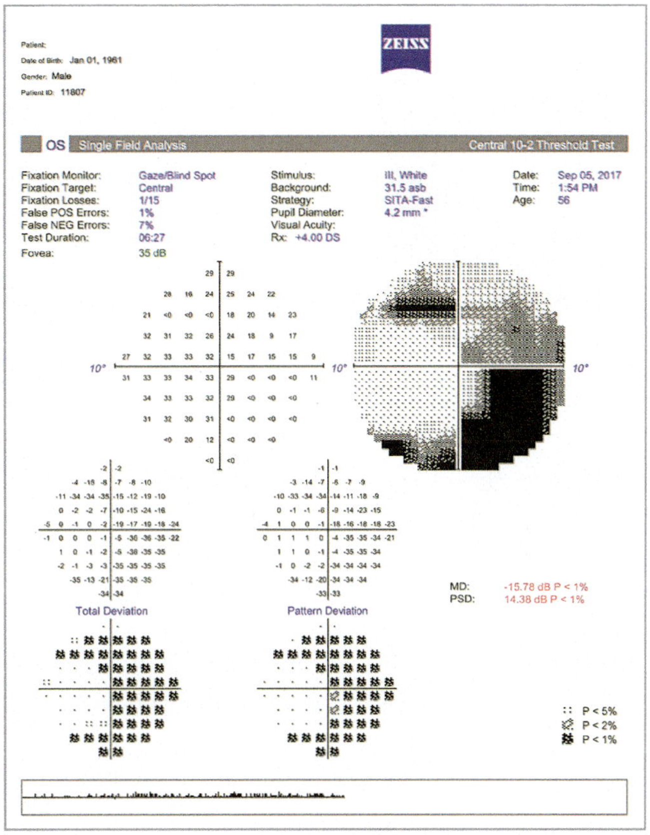

FL 1/15; FP 1%; FN 7%
Fovea 35 dB
10-2 MD -15.78 dB

Case 24 LE

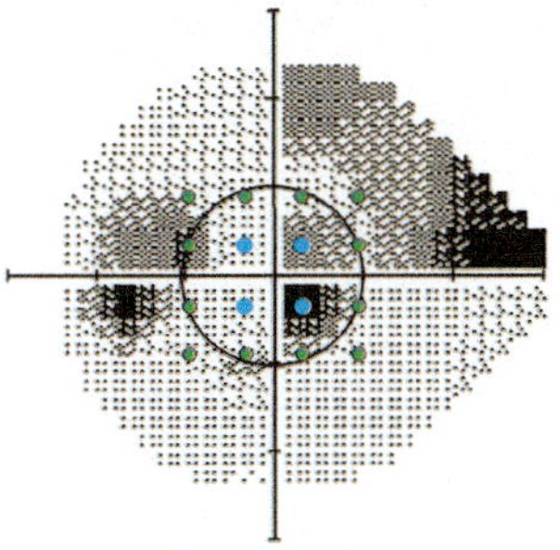

Grey scale

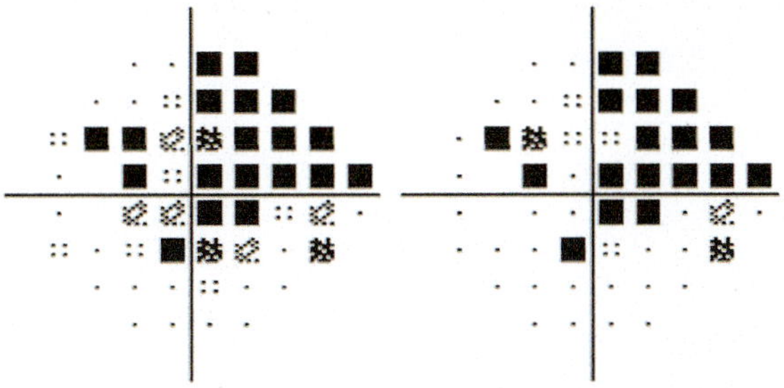

Probability plots

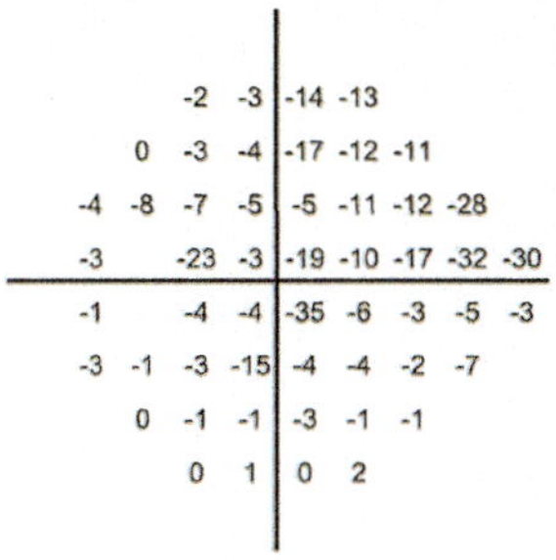

TDNP

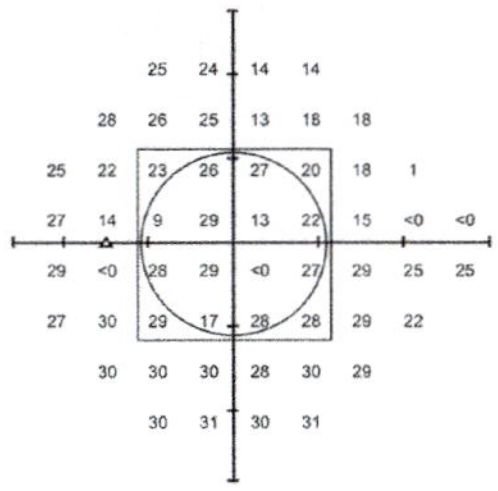

Raw data

The presence of the field defects in and outside 10° circle is clearly evident from the grey scale. The 3° point in the lower nasal quadrant is absolute scotoma and the sensitivities of the remaining points are good and again there a localized scotoma in the upper nasal quadrant outside the 10° circle.

VFI 74%
24-2 MD index -8.16 dB

Case 24 LE 10-2

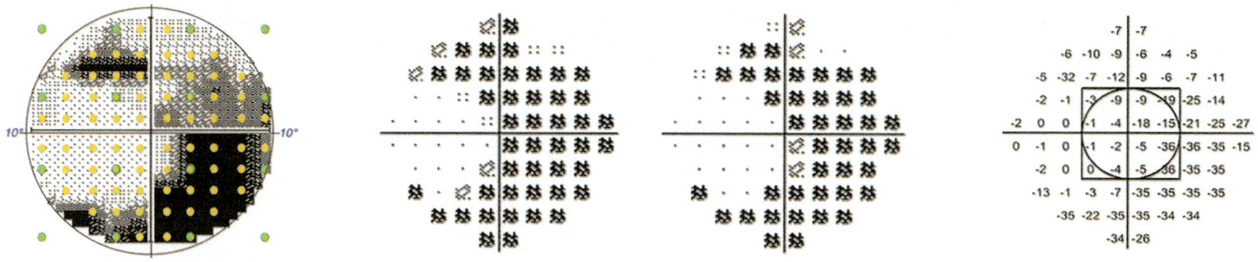

Grey scale Probability plots TDNP

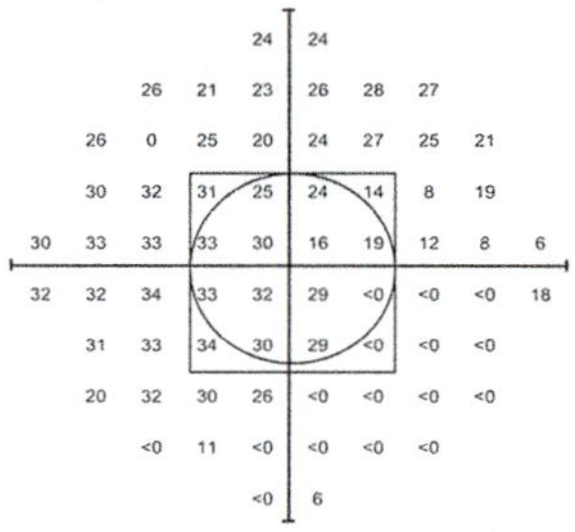

Raw data

At the beginning the field defect started with in the 10° circle in the lower nasal quadrant. It progressed towards fixation and upwards into upper nasal quadrant. The bi arcuate pattern field defect is better appreciated in the probability plots than the grey scale.

1. **10-2 MD index is -15.78 dB**
2. **24-2 MD index is -8.16 dB**
3. **24-2 VFI is 74% and VFI is not calculated in 10-2.**

> In a case of glaucoma the most important point is know the type of glaucoma we are dealing with. For that, in every 24-2 SFA, we should see the sensitivity of the 16 points in the 10° circle to decide whether we should repeat the test with 10-2 point pattern or not.

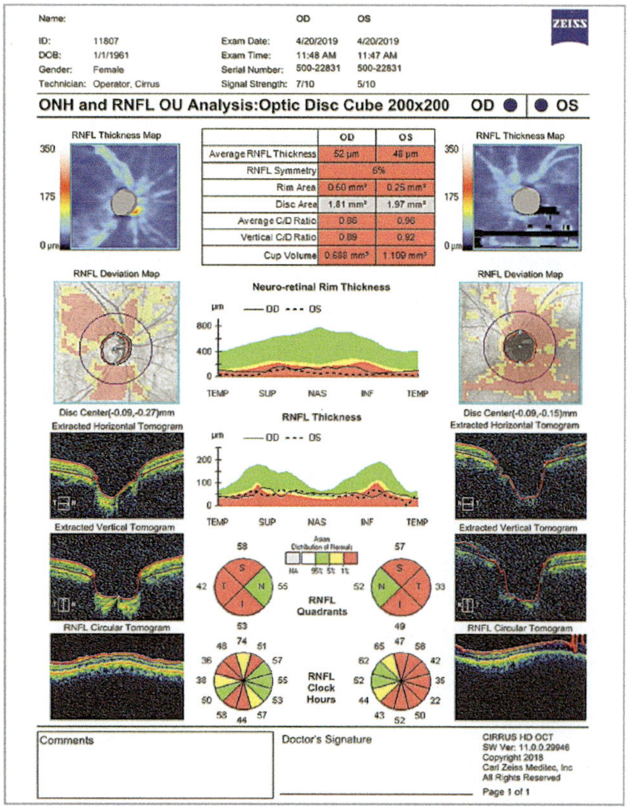

In advanced cases of glaucoma, there is no role of OCT.

Case 25 RE

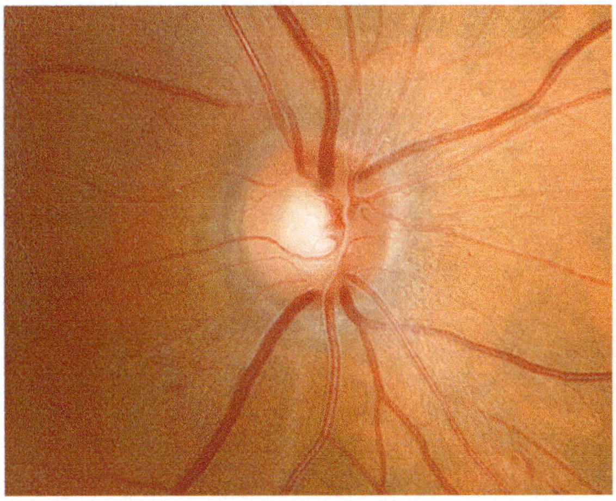

Case 25 LE

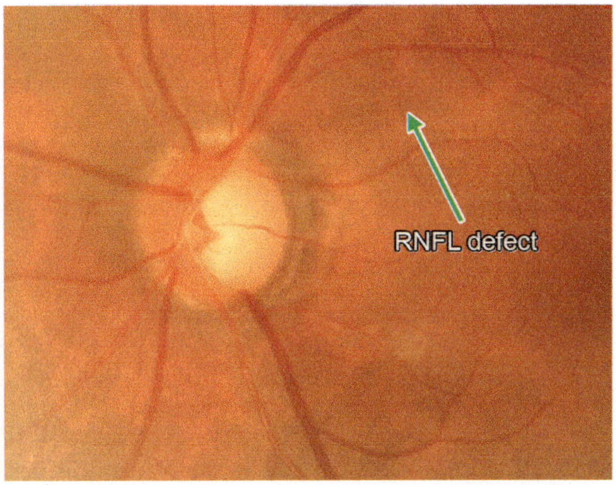

This case has been under my care for antiglaucoma treatment since 2004. Aimed target IOP 15 mm Hg was perfectly achieved and the 24-2 visual fields were stable since then. In 2018, the patient complained that he was not comfortable while reading even with best N.V. correction. That made me ask for 10-2 printout. To my surprise there was a huge scotoma in between the 3° and 9° points in LE 24-2 printout. This is the reason why the scotoma was not appreciated in the 24-2 grey scale.

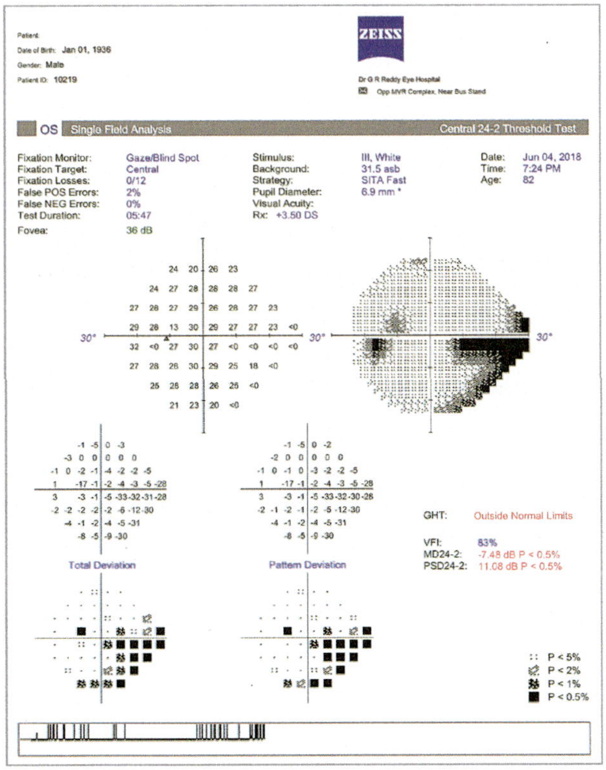

FL 0/12; FP 2%; FN 0%
Fovea 36 dB; VFI 83%
MD -7.48 dB P < 0.5%; PSD 11.08 dB P < 0.5%

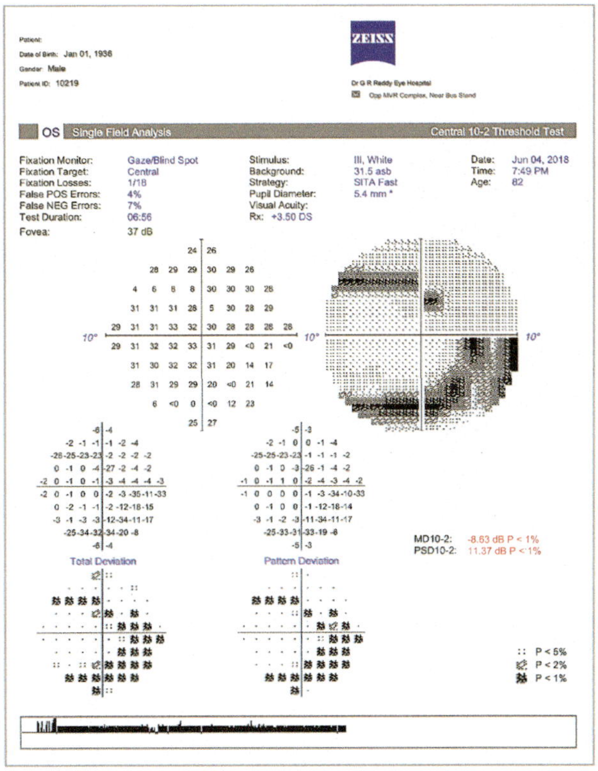

FL 1/18; FP 4%; FN 7%
Fovea 37 dB
MD -8.63 dB P < 1%; PSD 11.37 dB P < 1%

Case 25 LE

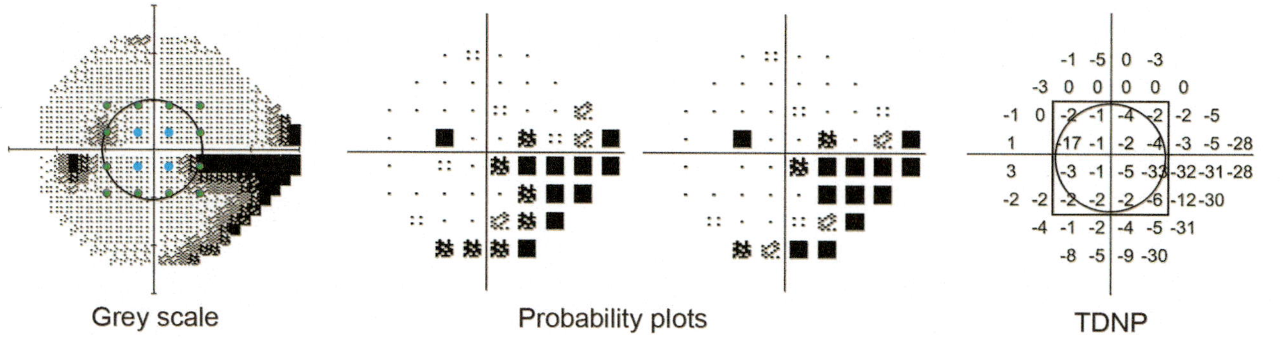

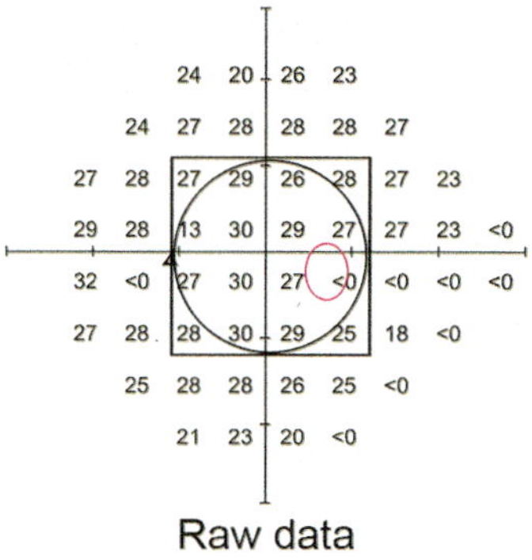

The grey scale and the probability plots are showing arcuate scotoma in the lower nasal quadrant. Within 10° circle there one absolute scotoma as shown in the raw data. If there is an absolute scotoma among the 16 points in the 10° circle we have to repeat the test with 10-2 point pattern.

VFI 83%

MD -7.48 dB P< 0.5%

Case 25 LE 10-2

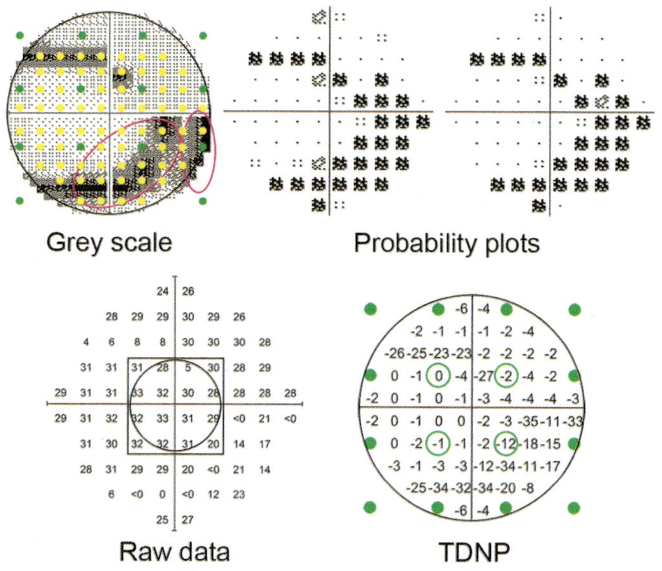

Biarcuate scotoma is well appreciated in the probability plots than in the grey scale. The lower arcuate scotoma in 24-2 is appearing like a single scotoma. But from the grey scale, it is clearly evident that they are two isolated scotomas. Because the scotoma is passing in between 3° and 9° points, (bare area of 24-2 point pattern) the scotoma is not appreciated in 24-2 grey scale.

In this case we have to assess progression analysis in both 24-2 printout and 10-2 printout. In this case I missed glaucoma progression within 10° area. I do not know when this scotoma started.

MD -8.63 dB P < 1% VFI is not calculated in 10-2.

Identification of type of POAG is very important. Then only we will have both 24-2 and 10-2 base line printouts instead of having only 24-2 SFA printout alone. This case belongs to type 3 glaucoma (Isolated scotomas present in and outside 10° circle).

Case 25 RE

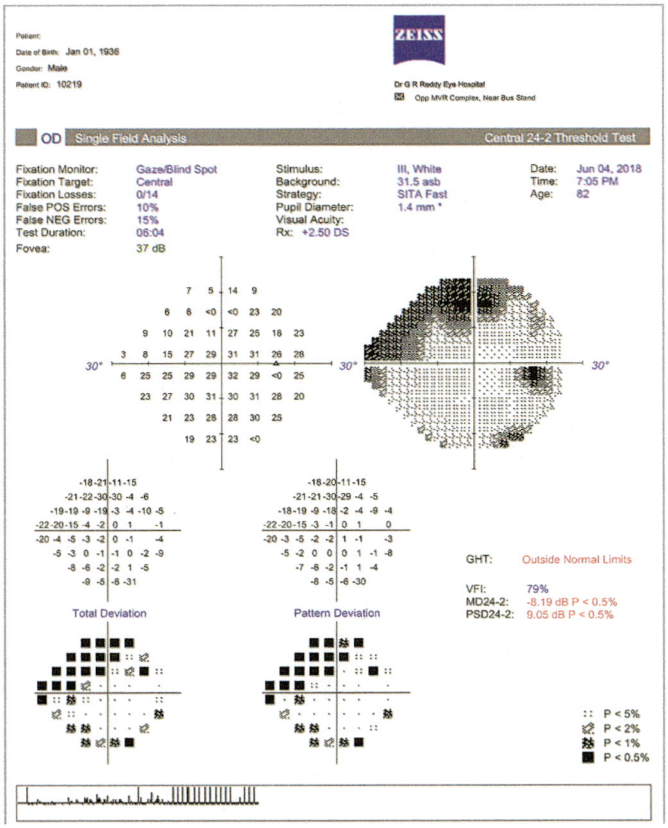

FL 0/14
FP 10%
FN 15%
Fovea 37 dB
VFI 79%
MD -8.19 dB P < 0.5%
PSD 9.05 dB P < 0.5%

Case 25 RE

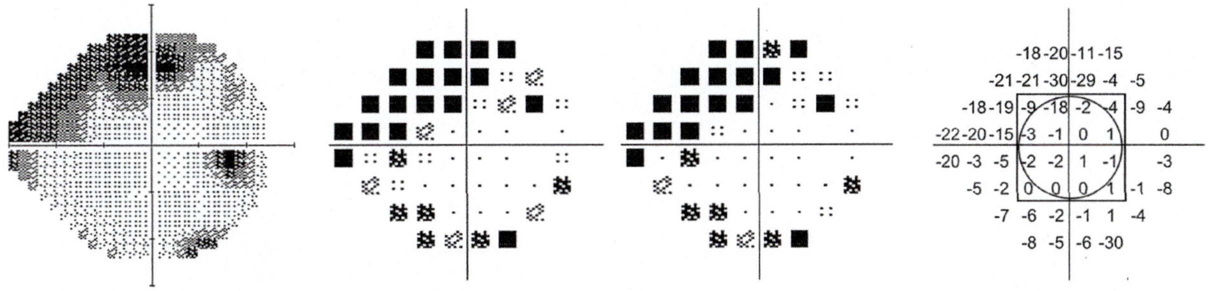

Grey scale Probability plots TDNP

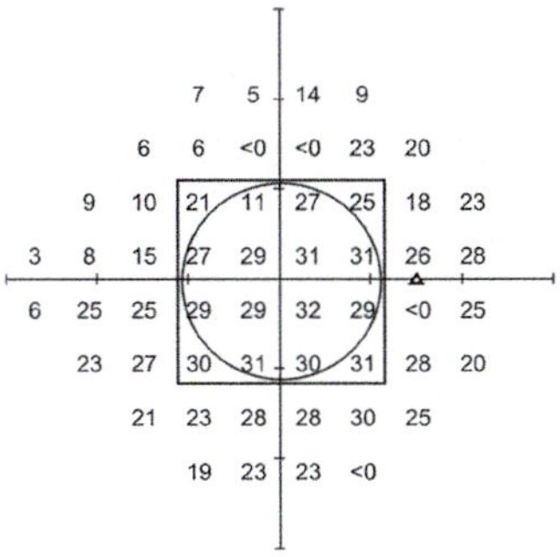

Raw data

The most important take home message from this case is that both eyes need not to have the same type of glaucoma. In this case, right eye is having type 1 glaucoma and left eye is having Type 3 glaucoma. So, the target IOP in both the eyes need not be the same. In left eye we should aim for low target IOP and in right eye the target IOP need not be as low as left eye.

Case 25 RE

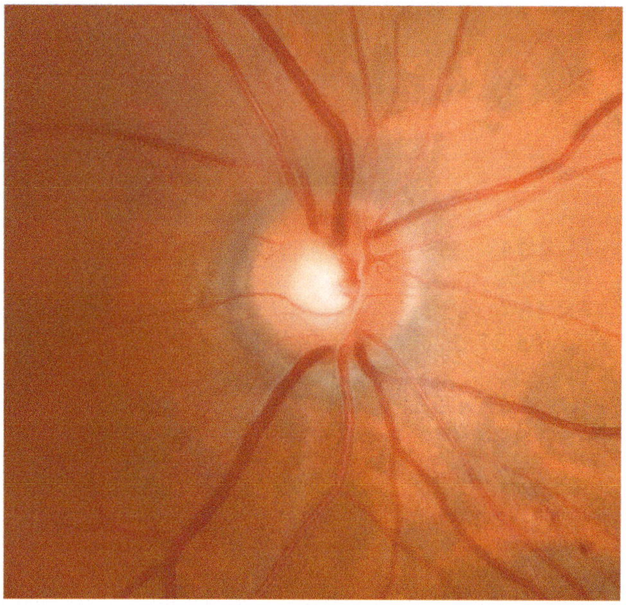

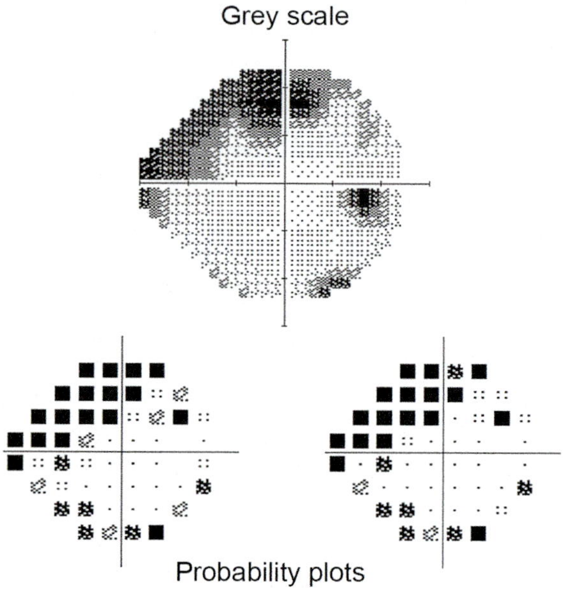

RNFL clock hour map is showing RNFL thinning at 6° clock. Usually 6° clock RNFL thinning represents peripheral field defect.

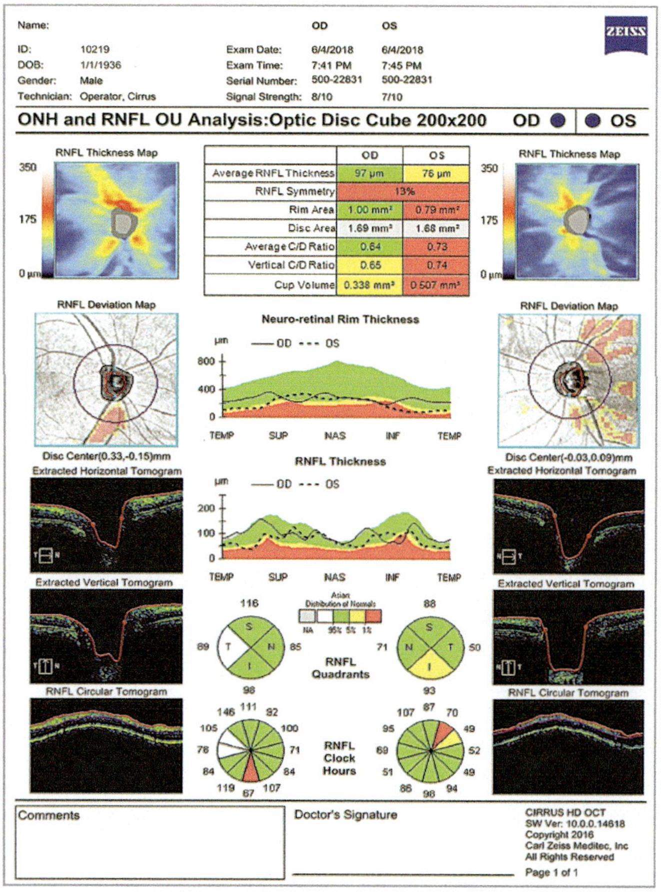

Case 25 LE

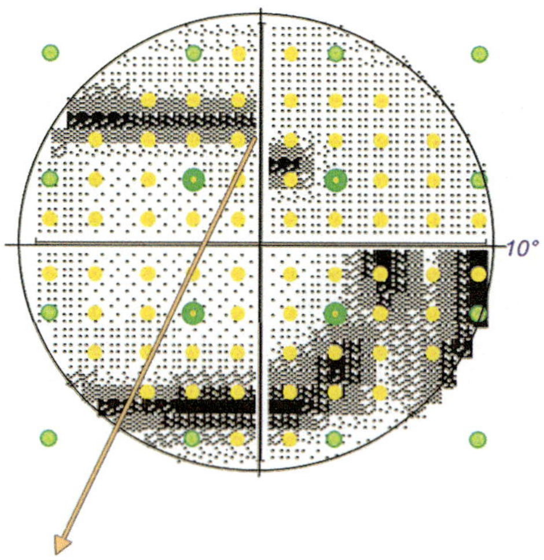

This field defect is not picked up by OCT.
OCT CAN NEVER REPLACE PERIMETRY.
The location, extent, depth will not be known exactly in OCT.

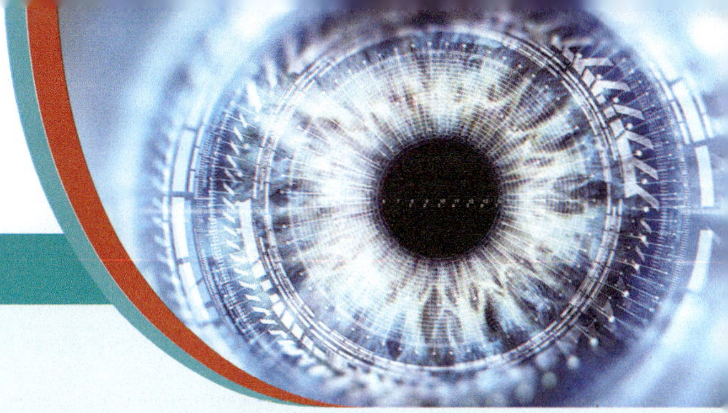

CHAPTER

9

Interpretation of Single Field Analysis Printouts of Cataract Associated with Glaucoma

Interpretation of visual fields when glaucoma is associated with cataract.

Perimetry plays a major role to diagnose glaucoma when it is associated with cataract, and to set target intraocular pressure (IOP) in established case of glaucoma **with cataract.**

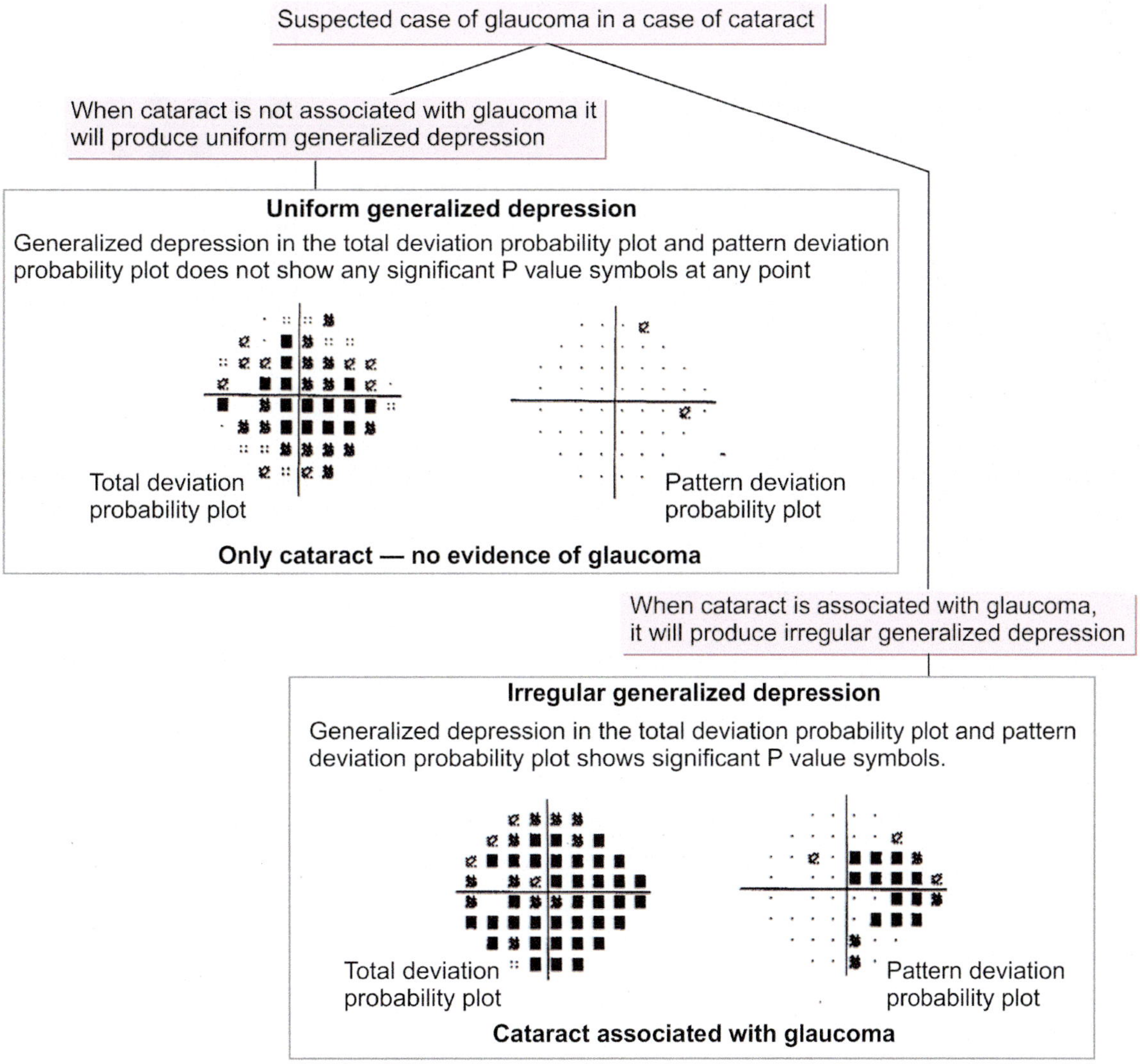

INTERPRETATION OF SFA PRINTOUT: A CASE OF GLAUCOMA SUSPECT WITH CATARACT

When we suspect glaucoma in a case of cataract, it is very important to have good understanding in interpreting probability plots to diagnose glaucoma. We apply Anderson's criteria to pattern deviation probability plot to label whether the field defect is due to glaucoma or not. Cataract associated with glaucoma, will produce irregular generalized depression. In irregular generalized depression the total deviation probability plot (TDPP) shows generalized depression and the localized field defect (deep scotoma) in generalized depression will be highlighted in pattern deviation probability plot (PDPP). Glaucoma will be diagnosed by the location and pattern of the localized field defect in PDPP. Depending on the location, extent and depth of the field defect the target IOP will be set.

Anderson's criteria to diagnose glaucoma in a case of cataract.

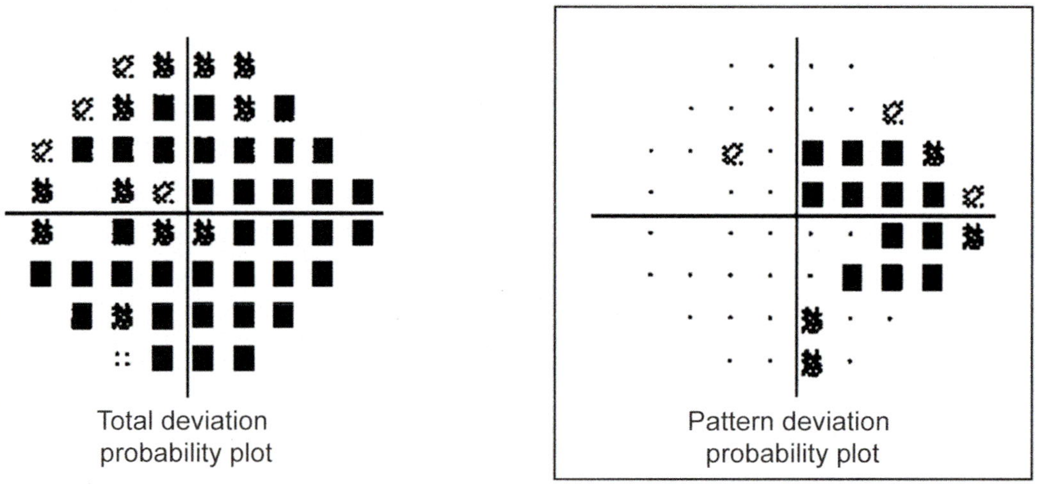

Pattern deviation probability plot—Anderson's criteria can be applied either to the TDPP in a localized scotoma and PDPP in generalized field defect. When **cataract is associated with glaucoma,** the total deviation probability plot shows generalized field defect due to cataract. So, concentrate on pattern deviation probability plot and apply Anderson's criteria to pattern deviation probability plot.

Estimation of depth of the field defect caused by glaucoma in a case of cataract.

Glaucoma with cataract will cause irregular generalized depression (generalized depression in the total deviation probability plot and localized field defect or defects in the pattern deviation probability plot). Normally generalized depression in the total deviation probability plot is due to cataract or improperly corrected near vision during the test or due to glaucoma itself or due to combinations of the above said causes. To estimate the depth of the field defect caused by glaucoma with cataract, we have to eliminate the uniform generalized depression caused by cataract. Always note the dB value of the 7th best deviation point of total deviation numerical plot, from which we can estimate how much generalized depression is eliminated from the total deviation numerical plot (TDNP). If the value of the 7th best deviation point is not high, the pattern deviation plots give us the depth of the localized field loss caused by glaucoma. So concentrate on pattern deviation numerical plot (PDNP) to know the depth and the extent of the localized field defect caused by glaucoma. In advanced cases of glaucoma, there will be some effect of glaucoma on total deviation plots. If the value of the 7th best deviation point is high, some depth of generalized depression due to glaucoma is also eliminated from the TDNP during its conversion to PDNP. See the value of loss of foveal sensitivity. Usually the foveal sensitivity will not be affected during the initial stage of glaucoma. If the loss of foveal sensitivity and the dB value of the 7th best deviation point of TDNP are approximately equal, pattern deviation numerical plot gives the correct picture regarding the depth and extent of the field defect caused by glaucoma. If the dB value of the 7th best deviation point of TDNP is very high when compared to loss of foveal sensitivity, it indicates some part of generalized depression in the total deviation plot is due to glaucoma and pattern deviation plot does not give the correct picture regarding the depth of glaucomatous field defect.

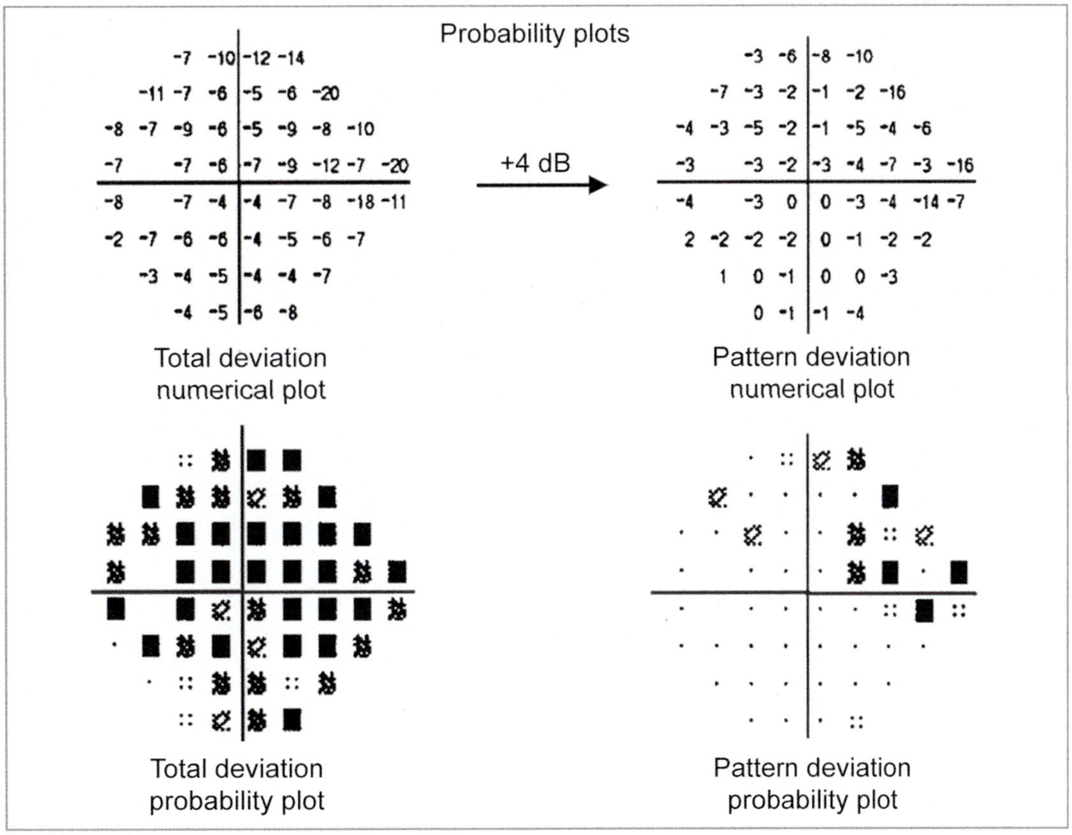

In this example, the 7th best deviation point of TDNP is -4 dB. The sensitivity at each point in TDNP is elevated by 4 dB to form the PDNP. The uniform generalized depression caused by cataract is eliminated from TDNP to form the pattern deviation plots. So the pattern deviation plots give us the depth and extent of field loss caused by glaucoma. **The most important point to be noted is whenever the elevation of each point's sensitivity of TDNP is not high (4 dB) as in this example, we can take the depth of the localized field defect of PDNP as the total indicator of glaucomatous nerve damage.** If the elevation of each point's sensitivity of TDNP is high, one should not depend on pattern deviation plot alone to assess the depth of the field defect caused by glaucoma. In such situations the generalized field defect in the total deviation plot is partly due to glaucoma and partly due to cataract. When an advanced case of glaucoma is associated with cataract, the 7th best deviation point will be very high and the entire generalized depression caused by cataract and generalized depression caused by glaucoma will be excluded from the total deviation plot to form the pattern deviation plot. So in cases of cataract associated with advanced glaucoma, very deep localized scotomas of glaucoma will be highlighted in the pattern deviation plots.

To assess the depth of the field defect caused by glaucoma, associated with cataract, the 7th best point of TDNP and foveal sensitivity are very important to evaluate the pattern deviation numerical plot.

Estimation of depth of the field defect caused by glaucoma when associated with cataract

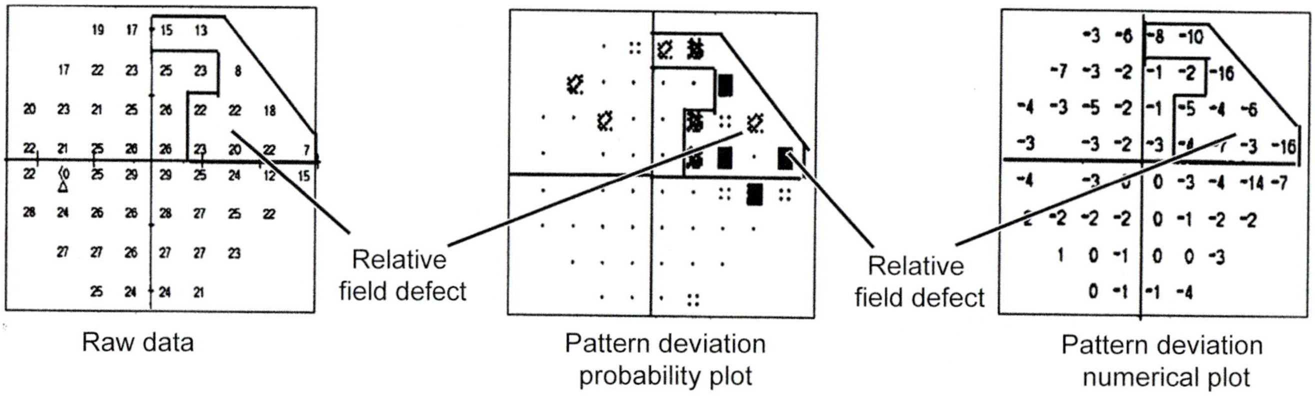

The depth of the field defect due to glaucoma (early glaucoma) will be known from the pattern deviation numerical plot especially when the 7th best deviation value is not high

The target IOP will be determined according to the extent and the depth of the field defect (from the pattern deviation numerical plot). See the raw data to know whether the black square is representing absolute scotoma or not and also to know the foveal status. In this case the nerve damage is not severe. So we need not keep the IOP at very low level. See the MD index (-7.02 dB P < 0.5%) to know the average loss of sensitivity which includes the average loss of sensitivity due to cataract also.

Case 26 RE Glaucoma suspect in a case of cataract

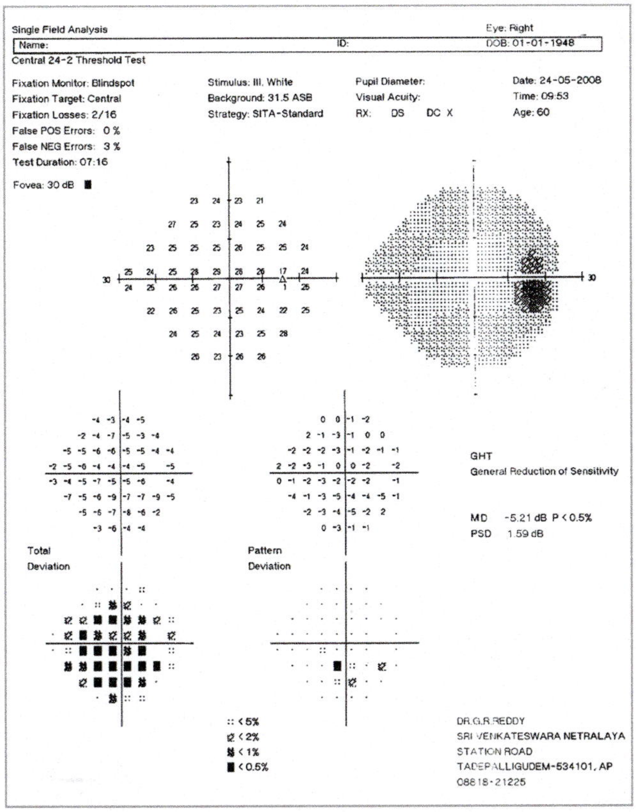

24-2 SITA Standard
FL 2/16; FP 0%; FN 3%
PSD 1.59 dB
MD -5.21 dB P < 0.5%
Foveal sensitivity 30 dB
7th best deviation point of TDNP -4 dB

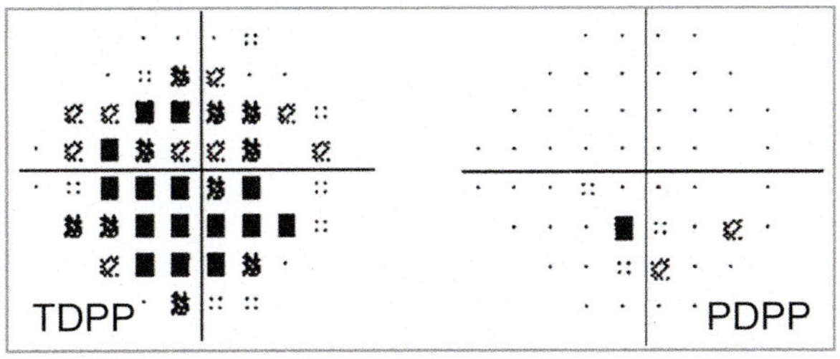

Generalized depression in TDPP and normal PDPP is a feature of uniform generalized field defect. The other features of uniform generalized depression are uniform shade in grey scale, normal PDPP, low PSD and the 7th best deviation point's dB value and MD index are almost same.

We know cataract causes uniform generalized depression and cataract with glaucoma causes irregular generalized depression. So there is no evidence of glaucoma in this case.

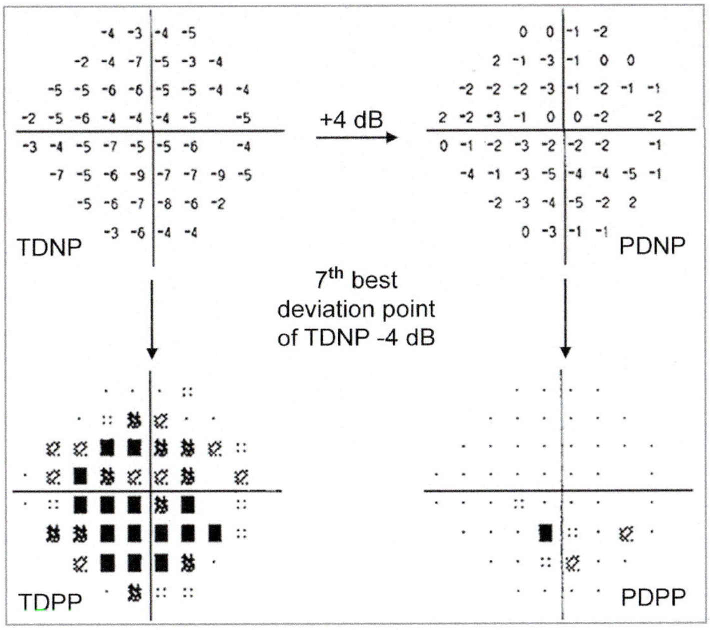

TDNP is converted to PDNP by elevating each point's sensitivity of TDNP by 4 dB, the deviation values of PDNP came to normal range and are varying mostly from -2 dB deviation to -4 dB deviation. The sensitivity of most of the points of PDNP are within the normal range and hence are not represented by any significant P value symbol in the PDPP and thus a normal pattern deviation probability plot is seen.

Case 26 LE Glaucoma suspect in a case of cataract

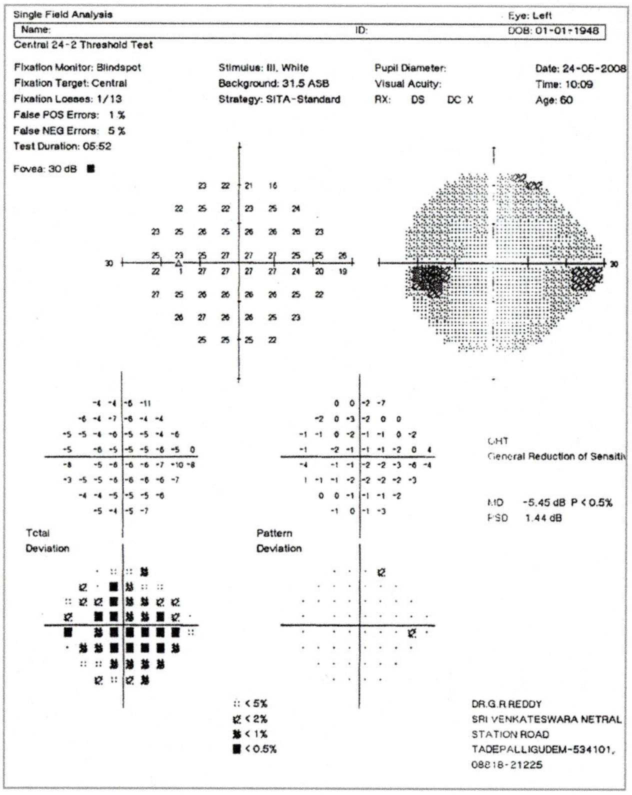

24-2 SITA Standard
FL 1/13; FP 1%; FN 5%

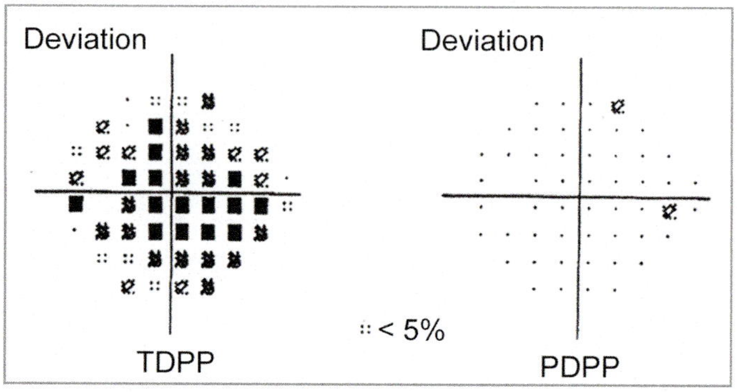

Uniform generalized depression
Foveal sensitivity 30 dB
7th best deviation point of TDNP -4 dB
MD -5.45 dB P < 0.5%
PSD 1.44 dB

Left eye SFA printout also shows uniform generalized field defect. Since there is no localized scotoma in the generalized depression, the pattern deviation plots are normal. So, the visual field is not suggestive of glaucoma.

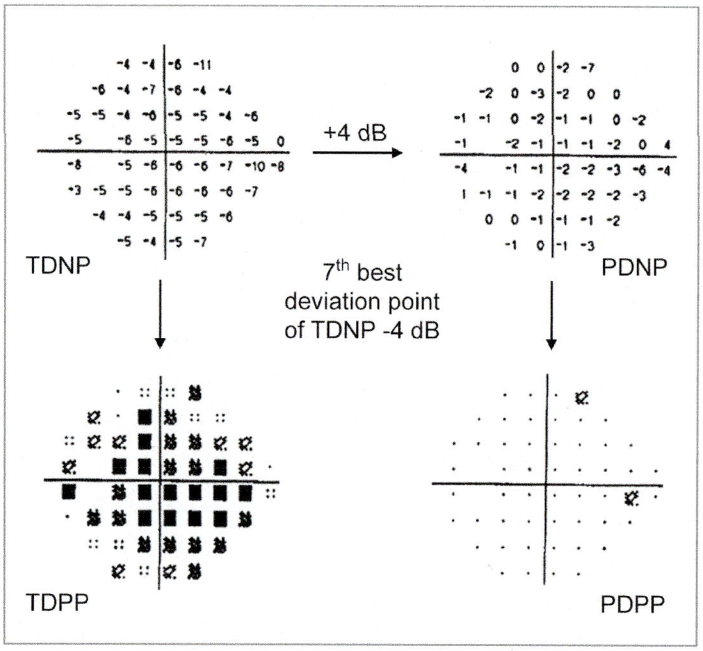

By elevating each point's sensitivity by 4 dB, the 7th best deviation point of total deviation numerical plot became normal (0 deviation) and the first six best deviation points of TDNP became points without significant P values in the PDNP. The deviation values in PDNP are varying mostly from 2 dB deviation to -3 dB deviation. So the sensitivity of most of the points of PDNP are in the normal range and hence are not represented by any significant P value symbol and thus a normal pattern deviation probability plot.

Case 27 LE Glaucoma suspect on the basis of cup/disc disparity between both the eyes in a case of cataract

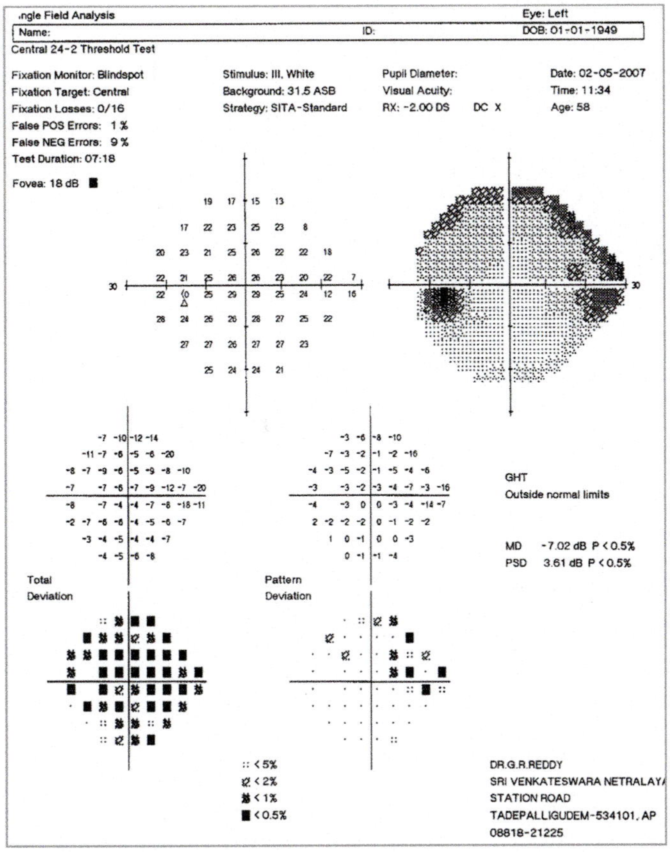

24-2, SITA Standard, FL 0/16; FP 1%; FN 9%

MD -7.02 dB P < 0.5%

PSD 3.61 dB P < 0.5%

Fovea 18

7th best deviation point of TDNP is -4 dB

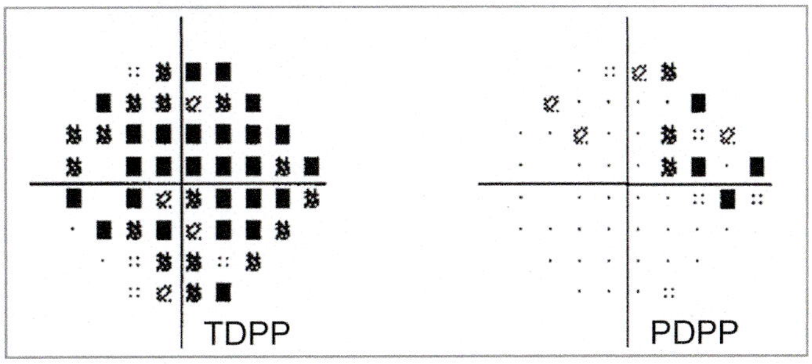

In this irregular generalized depression, TDPP is showing generalized depression and localized scotoma in generalized depression is highlighted in PDPP field. The other features of irregular generalized depression are different shades in grey scale, localized field defect in PDPP, PSD with P value and the 7th best deviation point's dB value and MD index are different values.

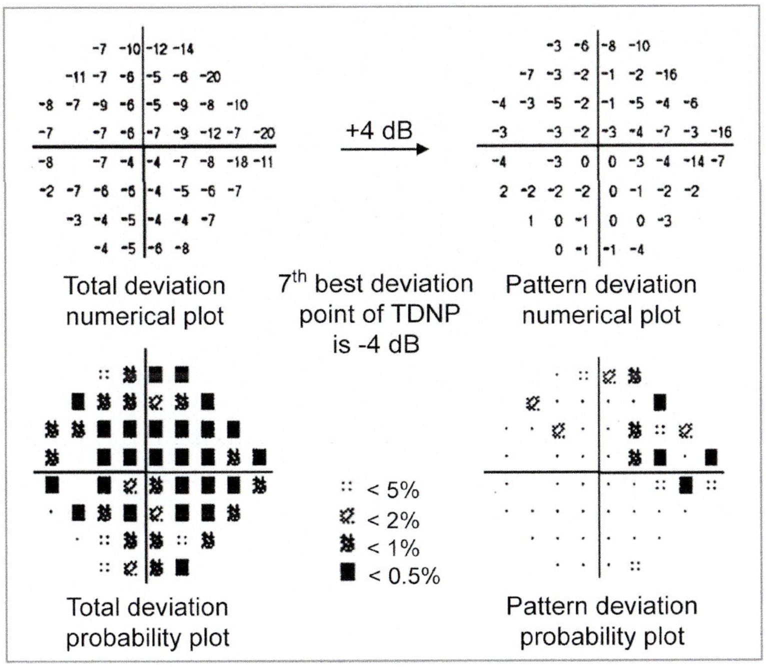

By elevating each point's sensitivity of TDNP by 4 dB, most of the deviation values of PDNP came to normal range except the points of the upper nasal quadrant which retained their P value. So, concentrate on the pattern deviation plots to estimate the location, extent and depth of the field defect caused by glaucoma. The field defect in the pattern deviation probability plot is fulfilling the Anderson's criteria to label the field defect as glaucomatous field defect.

Case 28 LE Glaucoma suspect on the basis of notch and RNFL defect in a case of cataract

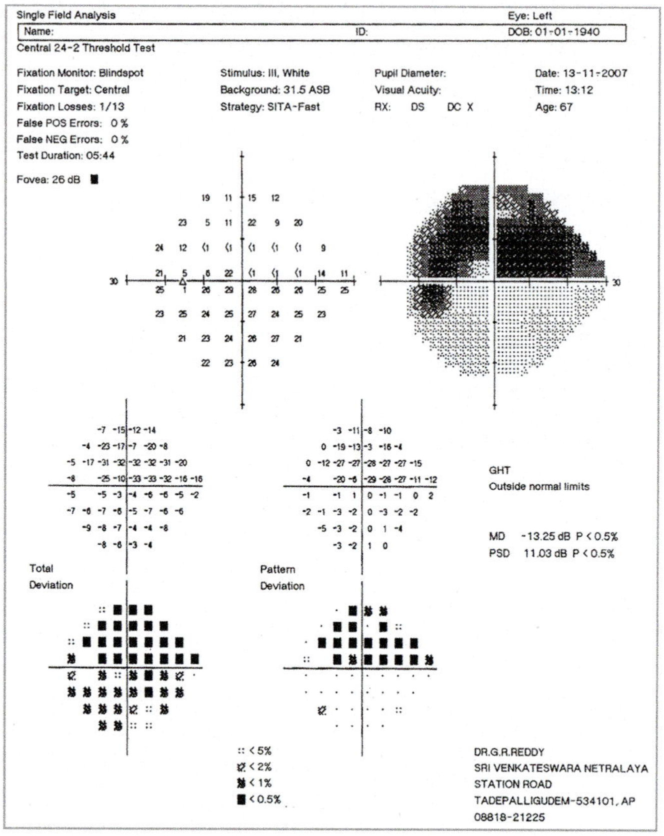

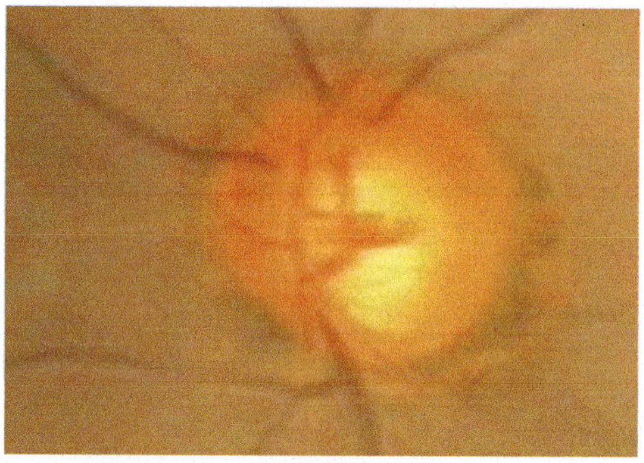

24-2, SITA Fast, FL 1/13; FP 0%; FN 0%
MD -13.25 dB P < 0.5%
Foveal sensitivity 26 dB
7th best deviation point of TDNP (-4 dB)

By elevating each point's sensitivity of TDNP by 4 dB, loss of sensitivity of the points in the lower half PDNP came to normal range except the points of the upper half of the field which retained their P values. So, concentrate on the pattern deviation plots to estimate the location, extent and depth of the field defect caused by glaucoma.

Loss of sensitivity of the points in the upper half of the field points is due to cataract and glaucoma. The loss due to cataract is around 6 dB and the remaining loss of sensitivity is due to glaucoma.

Loss of sensitivity of the points in the upper half of the field points is due to glaucoma and is highlighted in pattern deviation plots after removing the generalized depression caused by cataract.

Loss of sensitivity at all points is around 6 dB due to cataract.

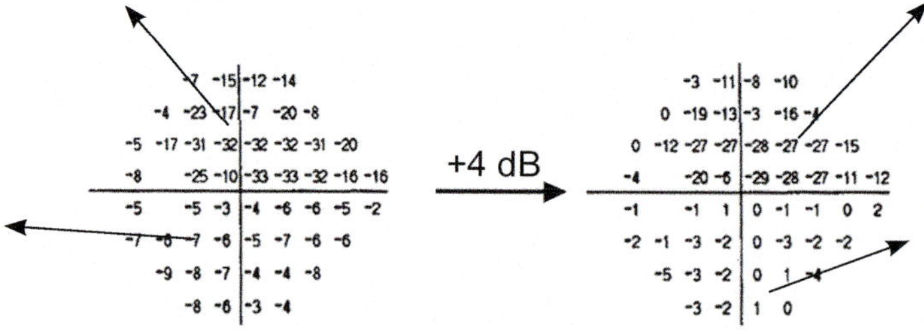

Total deviation numerical plot

Pattern deviation numerical plot

The points in the lower half of the field became normal after removing the generalized depression caused by cataract.

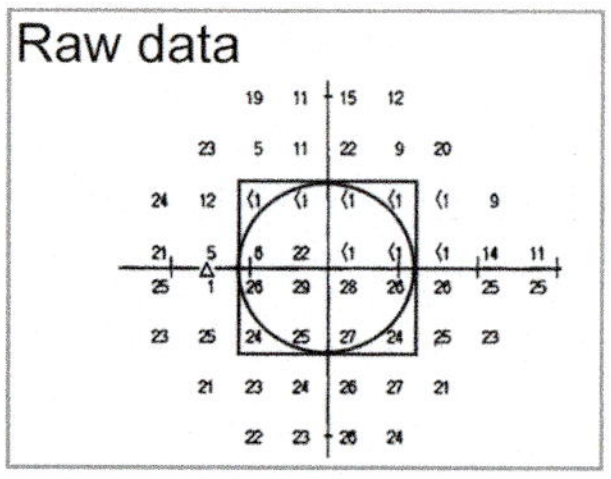

(<1) in the raw data indicates to replace the projecting bulb.

The loss of sensitivity due to glaucoma is very severe and most of the points became absolute scotomas. Though MD -13.25 dB P < 0.5%, in truth the mean deviation of the field defect due to glaucoma will be around 20 dB (Average of 26 points). The field defect extended to 30 points in the upper half of the field. It effected the foveal sensitivity also. The sensitivity at fovea is >10 dB which includes the loss due to cataract which is around 5 dB. The test should be repeated with 10-2 point pattern to know foveal status.

Case 29 RE

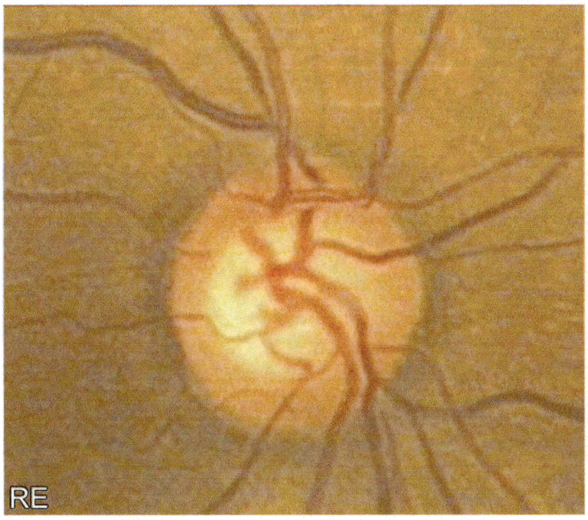

Case 29 LE

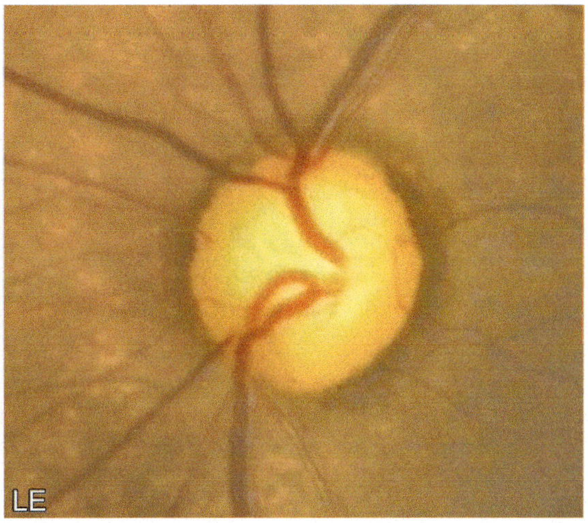

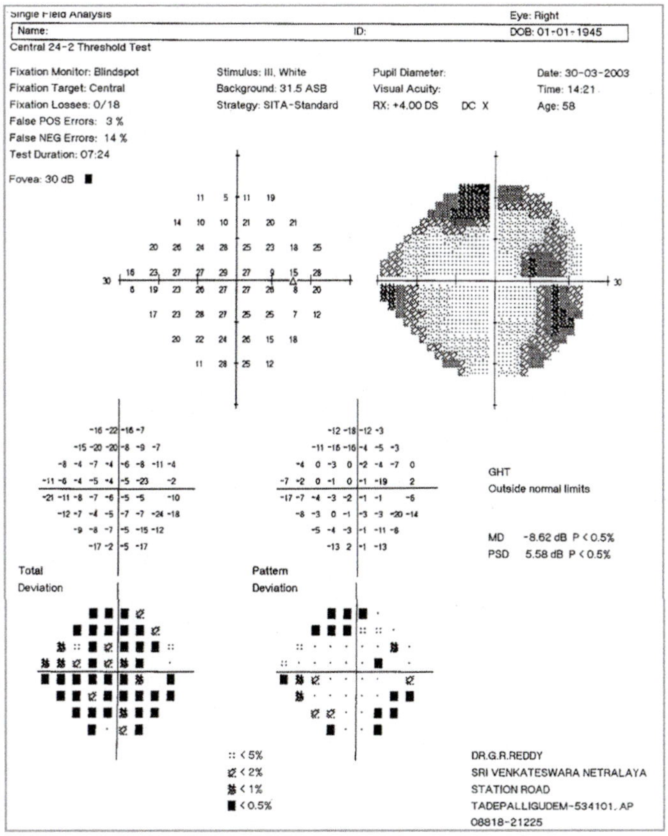

24-2, SITA Standard
FL 0/18; FP 3%; FN 14%
MD -8.62 dB P < 0.5%
PSD 5.58 dB P < 0.5%
Foveal sensitivity 30 dB
7th best deviation point of TDNP is -4 dB

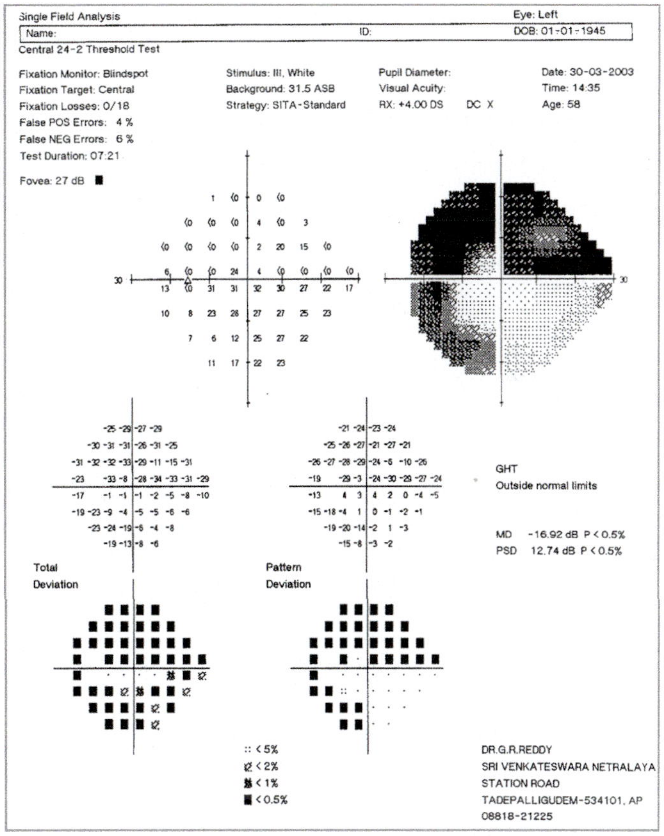

24-2, SITA Standard
FL 0/18; FP 4%; FN 6%
MD -16.92 dB P < 0.5%
PSD 12.74 dB P < 0.5%
Foveal sensitivity 27 dB
7th best deviation point of TDNP is -5 dB

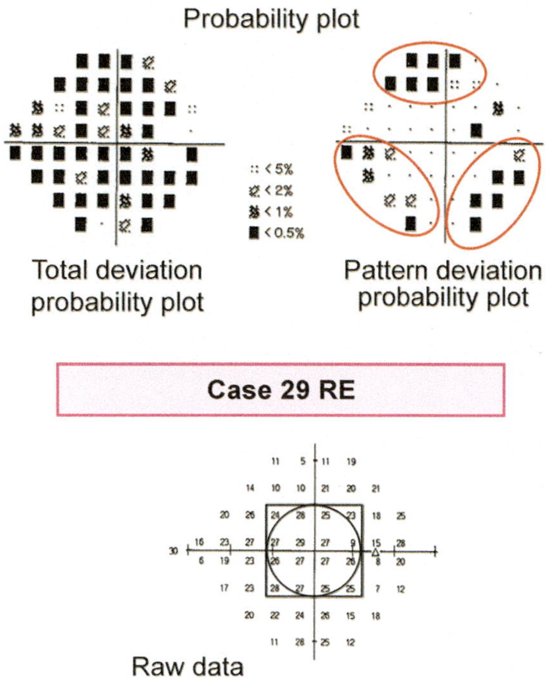

Case 29 RE

By elevating each point's sensitivity of TDNP by 4 dB, three localized field defects in the generalized field defect retained their P values in the PDPP.

This is Type 1 glaucoma associated with cataract.

7th best deviation point of TDNP is -4 dB.
Foveal sensitivity 30 dB.
MD -8.62 dB P < 0.5%.

Existing sensitivity: The measured sensitivity is around 25 dB at most of the points. In this case right eye's, the nerve damage is not severe when compared to the left eye. So there is no need to keep the target IOP at very low level. In this case, the left eye is an established case of glaucoma and the right eye shows a very early field defect.

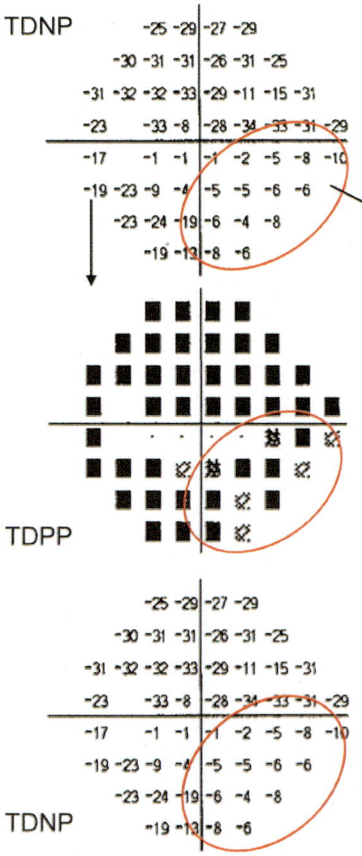

7th best deviation point
of TDNP is -5 dB
+5 dB

Loss of sensitivity at all points due to cataract is around 5 dB. This area is unaffected by glaucoma. In the remaining three quadrants loss of sensitivity is due to cataract and glaucoma. The loss of sensitivity at all points in PDNP is due to glaucoma.

Loss of sensitivity due to cataract is eliminated by elevating each point's sensitivity by 5 dB. The loss of sensitivity is very severe. Some of the points became absolute scotomas. There are absolute scotomas in the 10° area. We should repeat the test with 10-2 point pattern to know foveal status.

We should aim at low target IOP

Case 29 LE

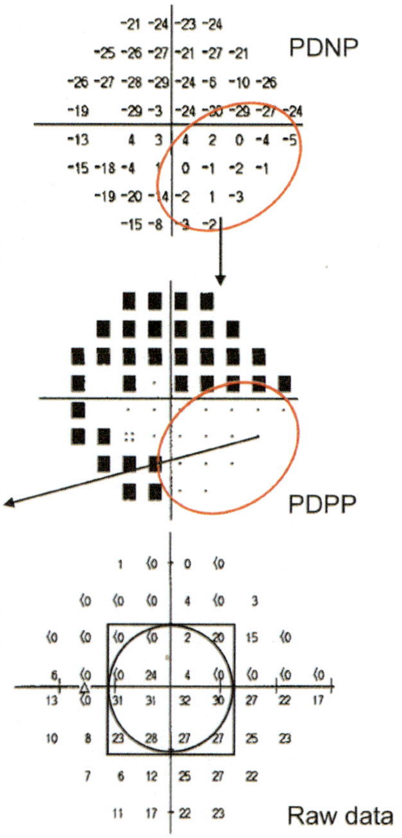

In this case, glaucoma is suspected on the basis of retinal nerve fiber layer (RNFL) defect in both the eyes and the visual fields were recorded. It is known that cataract will produce uniform generalized field defect and when it is associated with glaucoma, it will produce irregular generalized field defect.

Case 30 RE

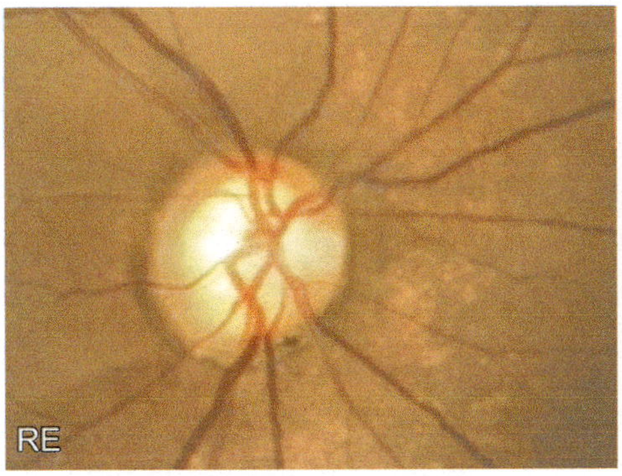

24-2, SITA Standard
FL 2/16; FP 4%; FN 0%
MD -19.01 dB P < 0.5%;
PSD 12.70 dB P < 0.5%
Foveal sensitivity 29 dB
7th best deviation point of TDNP is -5 dB

Case 30 LE

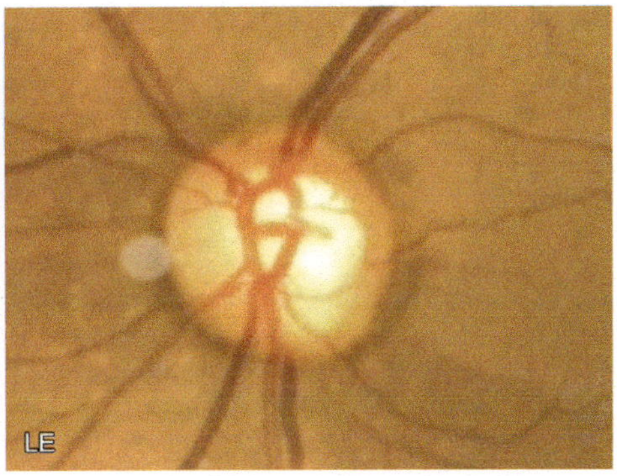

24-2, SITA Standard
FL 2/16; FP 5%; FN 5%
MD -9.03 dB P < 0.5%
PSD 6.36 db P < 0.5%
Foveal sensitivity 30 dB
7th best deviation point of TDNP is -5 dB

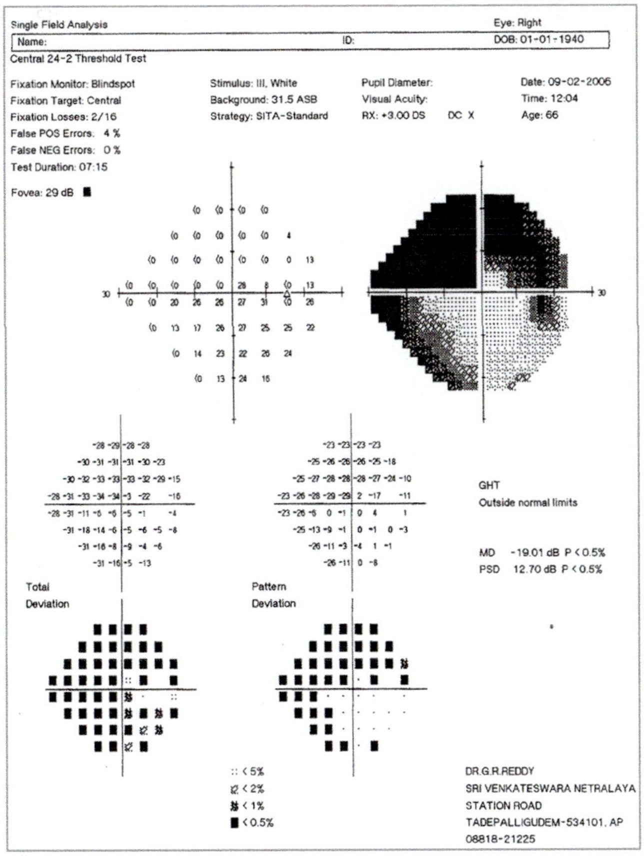

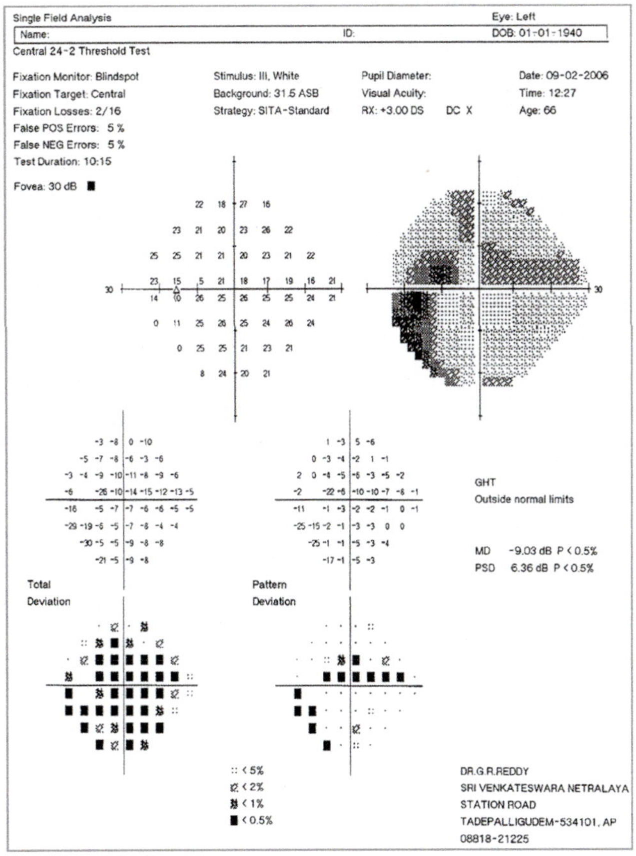

Case 30 RE

Cataract causes generalized depression so loss of sensitivity occurs in all quadrants due to cataract. The further loss of sensitivity is seen due to glaucoma in all quadrants except lower temporal quadrants.

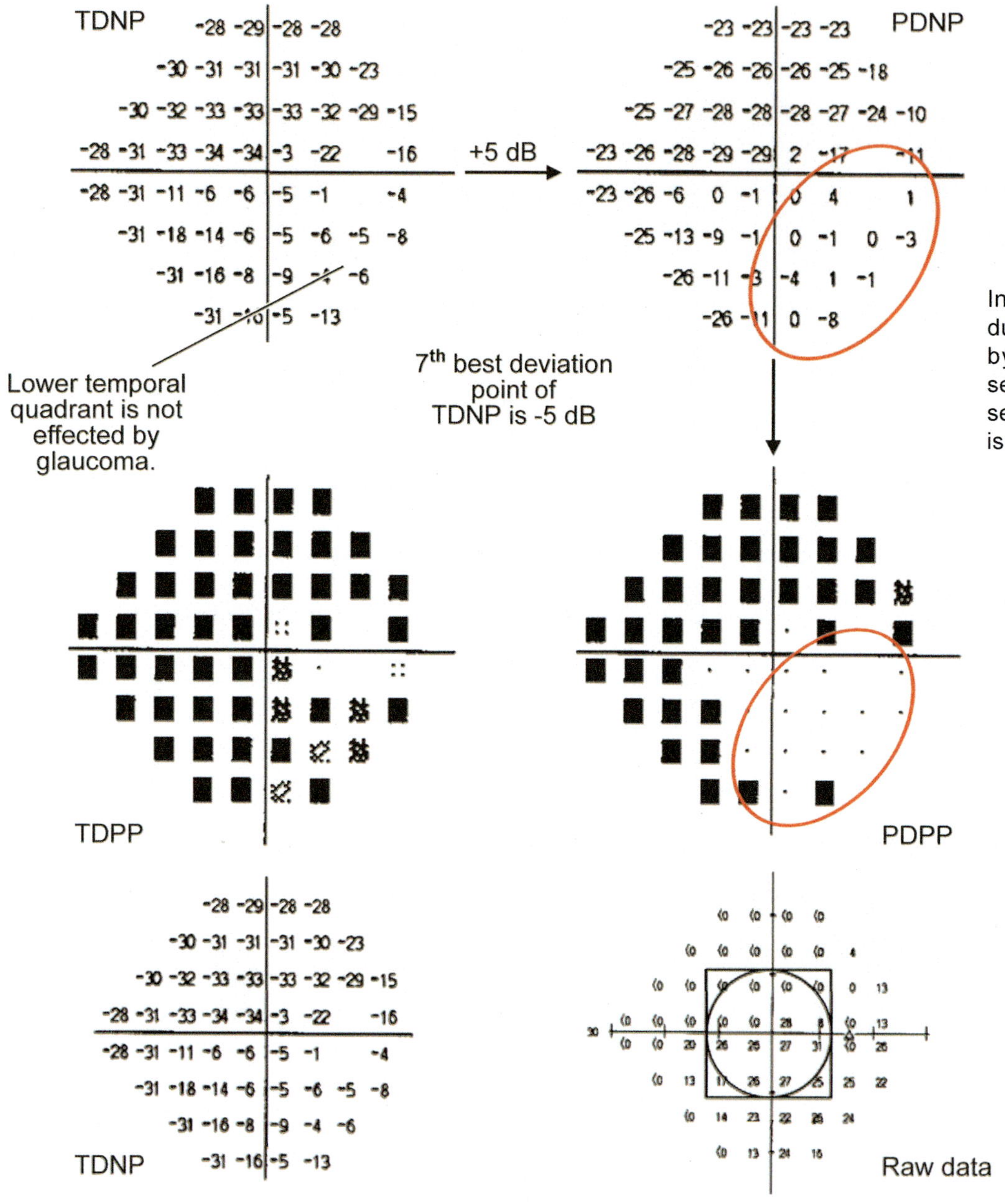

FOVEAL SENSITIVITY 29 DB

In PDNP—Loss of sensitivity due to cataract is eliminated by elevating each point's sensitivity by 5 dB. So loss of sensitivity at all points in PDNP is due to glaucoma.

MD -19.01 dB P < 0.5%
PSD 12.70 dB P < 0.5%
Foveal sensitivity 29 dB

The loss of sensitivity is very severe and some points became absolute scotomas. There are absolute scotomas in the 10° area so we should repeat the test with 10-2 point pattern to know foveal status.

In this case we should aim for low target IOP.

Case 30 LE

***Case*: In this case, glaucoma is suspected in a cataract patient on the basis of RNFL defect in both the eyes. Cataract produces uniform generalized field defect and when it is associated with glaucoma, it will produce irregular generalized field defect.**

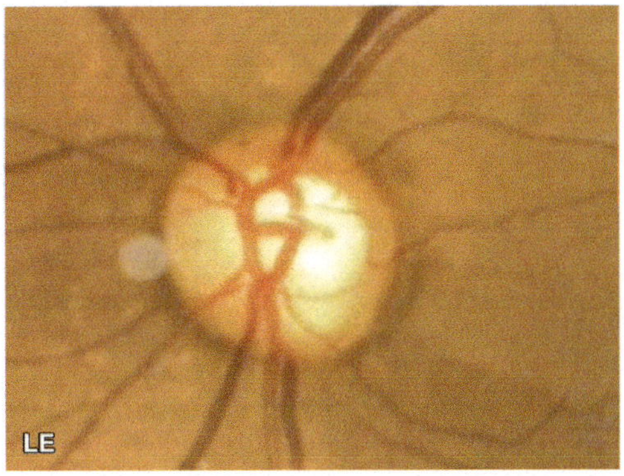

24-2, SITA Standard
FL 2/16; FP 5%; FN 5%
MD -9.03 dB P < 0.5%
PSD 6.36 db P < 0.5%
Foveal sensitivity 30 dB
7th best deviation point of TDNP is -5 dB

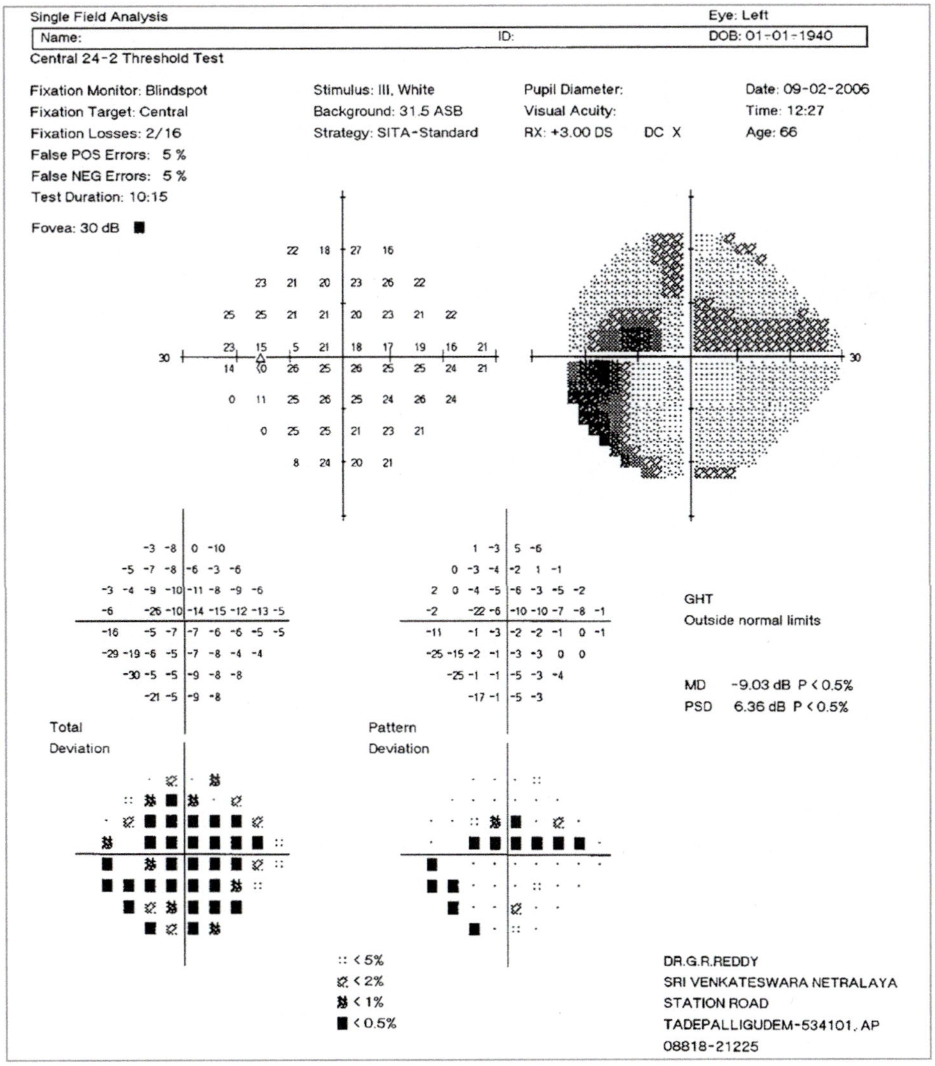

Case 30 LE

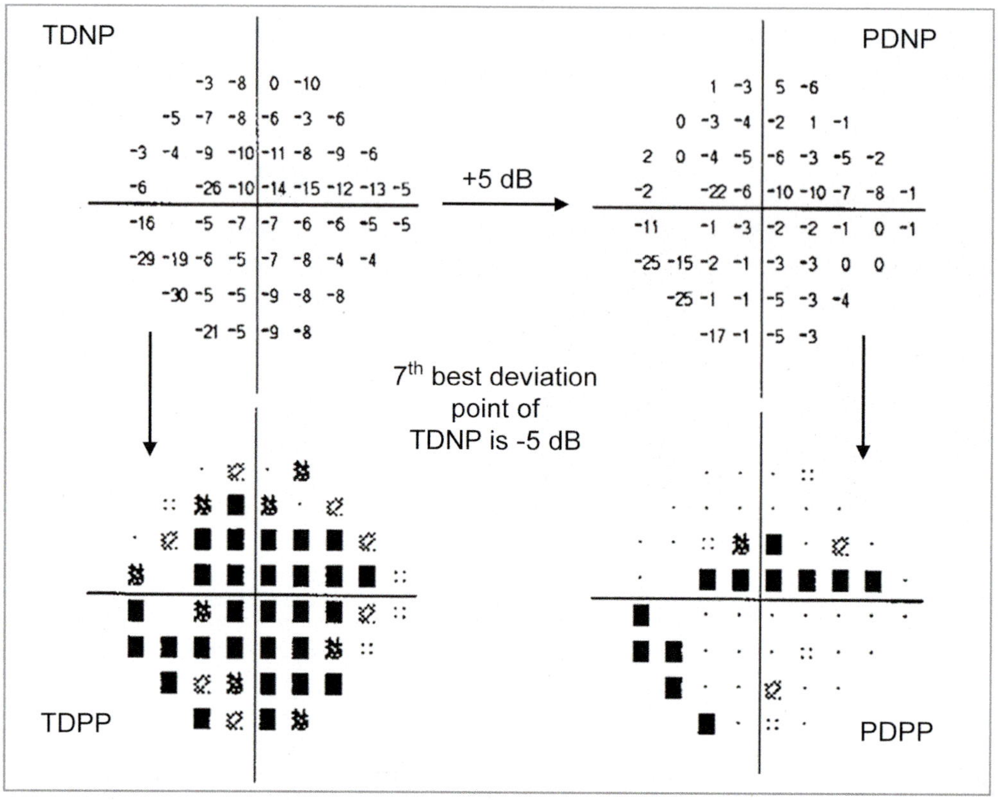

In this irregular generalized depression, TDPP is showing generalized depression and two localized field defects in generalized depression are highlighted in PDPP. One localized field defect is within 10° circle area and the second field defect is in the lower temporal quadrant. This case belongs to type 3 glaucoma. (Field defect dominant in and outside 10° circle area).

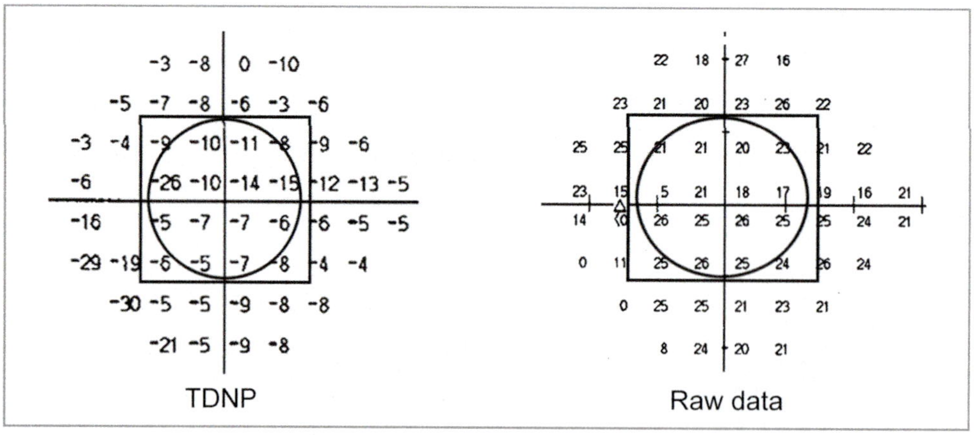

In type 3 glaucoma. (Field defect dominant in and outside 10° circle area.) We should repeat the test with 10-2 point pattern and should aim for low target IOP.

In this example, I will be showing how the SFA printouts look in a case of glaucoma suspect with cataract and after cataract surgery.

Case 31 RE

Fundus—the media is hazy due to cataract

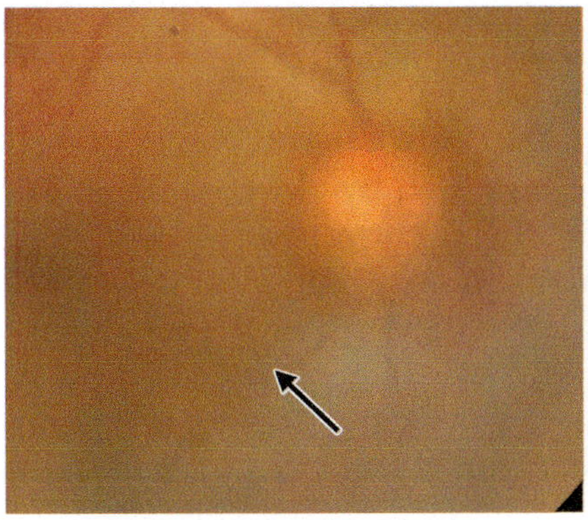

?RNFL defect seen at 6 to 8 clock position.

Fundus—the media is clear after cataract surgery

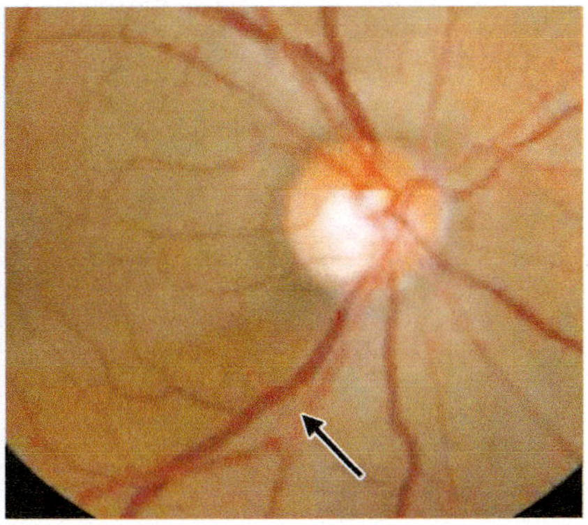

RNFL defect is well appreciated at 6 to 8 clock position after cataract surgery

Case 31 RE

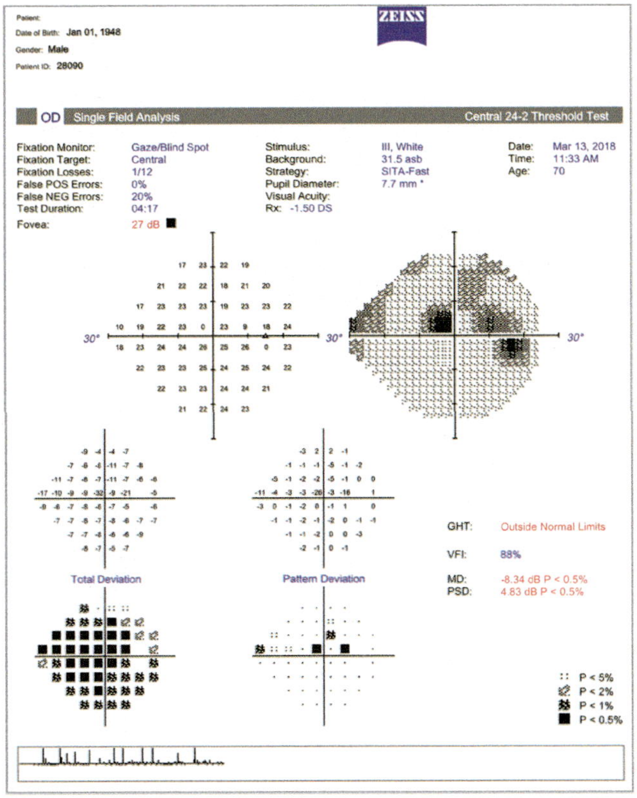

Global indices cataract + glaucoma
MD -8.34 dB P < 0.5%
PSD 4.83 dB P < 0.5%

Case 31 LE

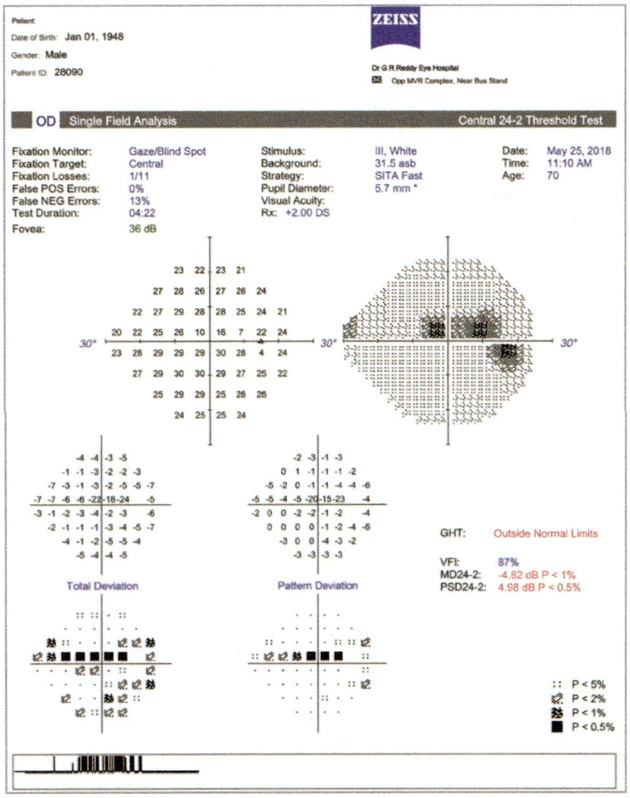

Global indices with glaucoma and after cataract removal
MD -4.62 dB P < 0.5%
PSD 4.98 dB P < 0.5%

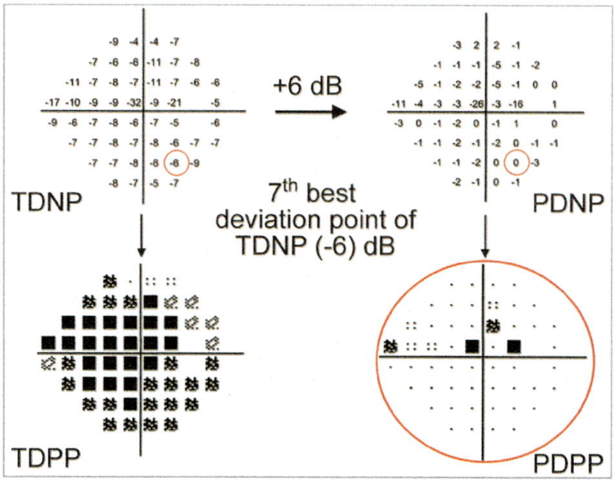

SFA in a glaucoma suspect in a cataract patient

- Uniform generalized field defect → Cataract not associated with glaucoma
- Irregular generalized field defect → Cataract associated with glaucoma

In TDNP, the generalized depression due to cataract is eliminated by elevating each point's sensitivity by 6 dB during conversion of TDNP to PDNP. So the loss of sensitivity at all points in PDNP is due to glaucoma. The PDPP is highlighting the localized scotomas, masked in the TDPP by generalized depression due to cataract and the field defect in PDPP is corresponding to the RNFL defect. The diagnosis of glaucoma is confirmed.

The important role of visual fields is to set target IOP which depends on location, depth, direction of progression and extent of the field defect due to glaucoma.

In this case glaucoma is starting within 10° and there is absolute scotoma in the field defect. We have to repeat the test with 10-2 point pattern to know the foveal status. And accordingly, we should plan the target IOP.

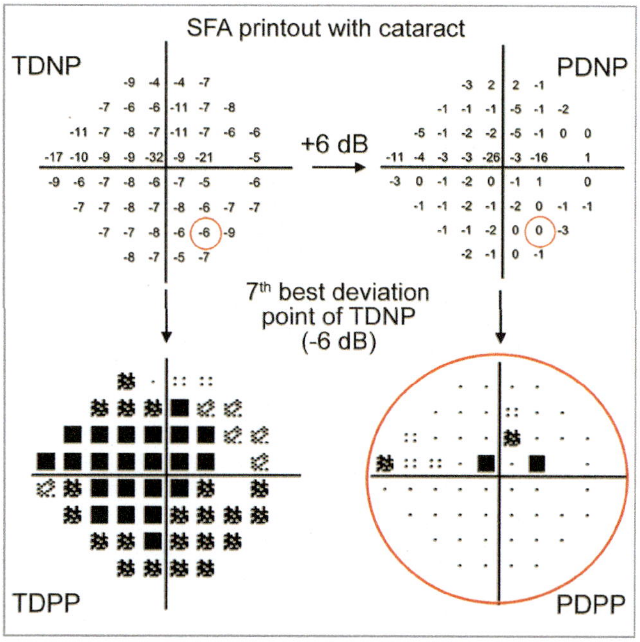

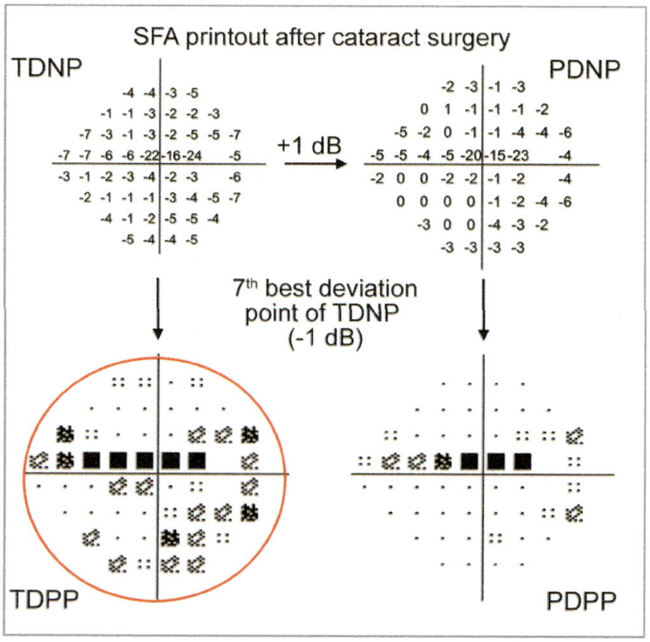

SFA printout of the same patient after clear corneal phaco with foldable intraocular lens (IOL) implantation. Because the cataract is removed there will not be generalized depression in the TDPP produced due to cataract. So the localized scotoma is highlighted in the TDPP itself in SFA printout after cataract surgery. The TDPP in the SFA after cataract removal and PDPP in the SFA with cataract will be almost similar.

Fundus—Media is hazy before cataract surgery in a Fundus—Media is clear after cataract surgery in a case of cataract with glaucoma suspect.

Case 32 RE

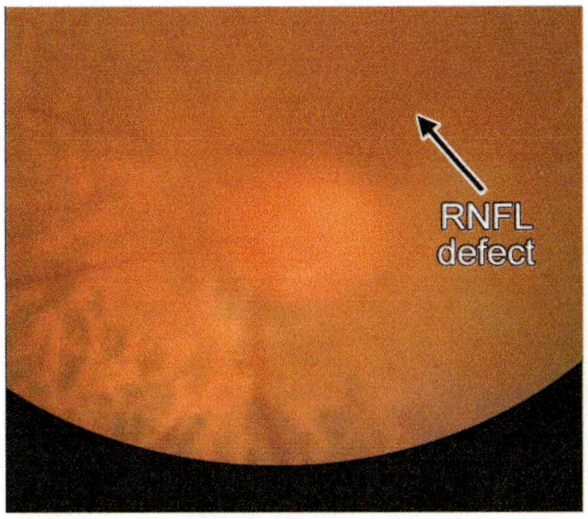

Fundus—The media is hazy due to cataract RNFL defect seen at 12 to 1 clock position.

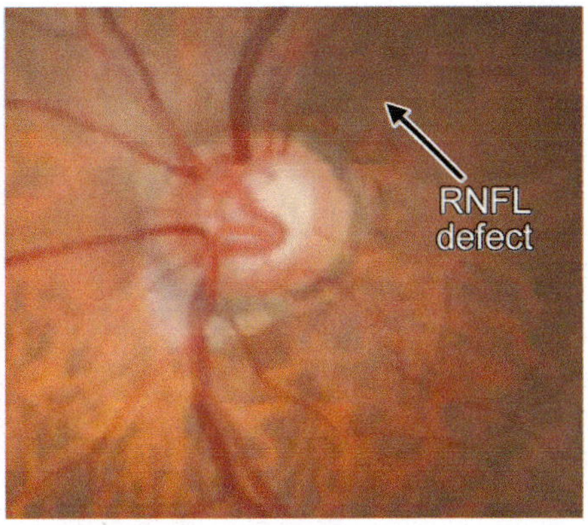

Fundus—The media is clear and RNFL defect is well appreciated at 12 to 1 clock position after cataract surgery.

SFA printout before cataract surgery in a case of cataract with glaucoma suspect

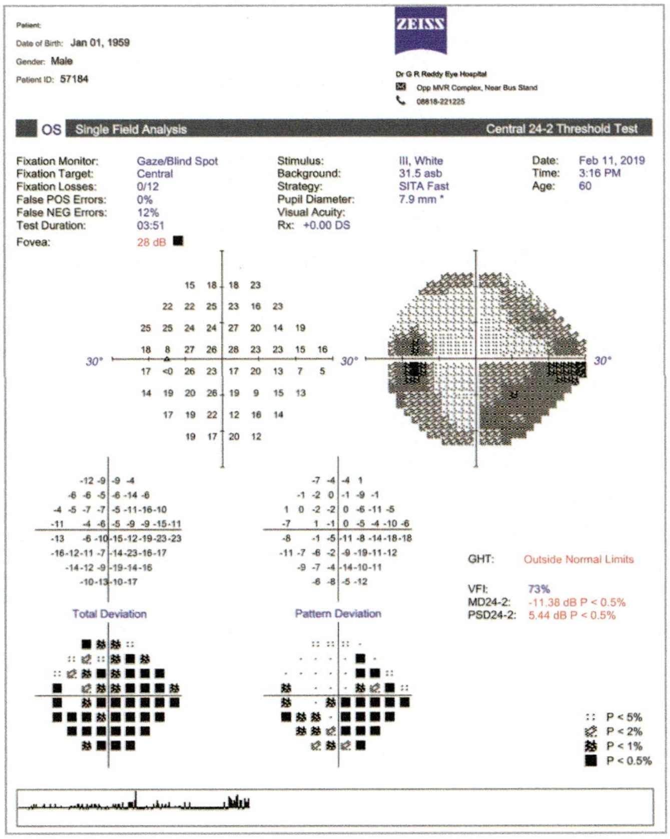

GHT-ONL; VFI 73%

MD -11.38 dB P < 0.5%; PSD 5.44 dB P < 0.5%

SFA printout after cataract surgery in a case of glaucoma suspect

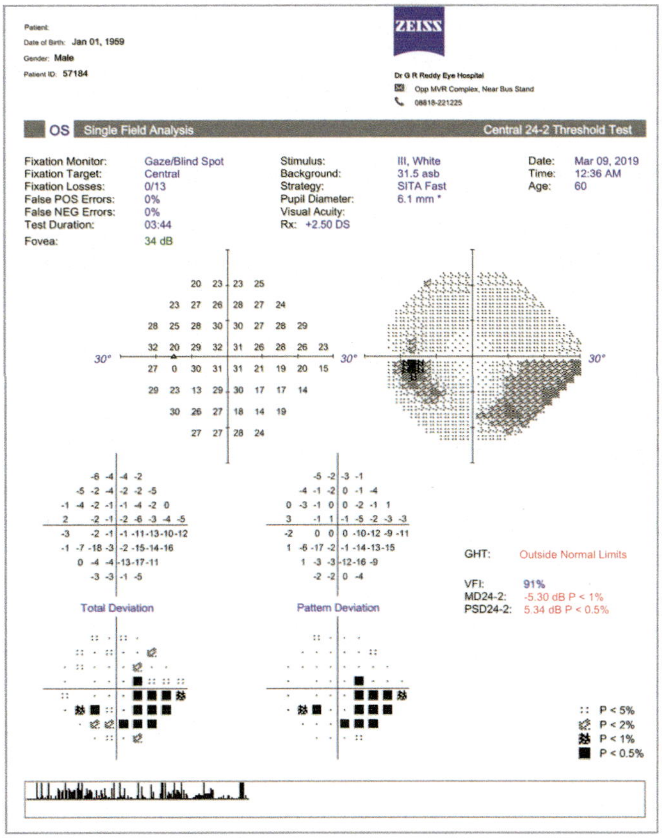

GHT-ONL; VFI 91%

MD -5.30 dB P< 1%; PSD 5.34 dB P < 0.5%

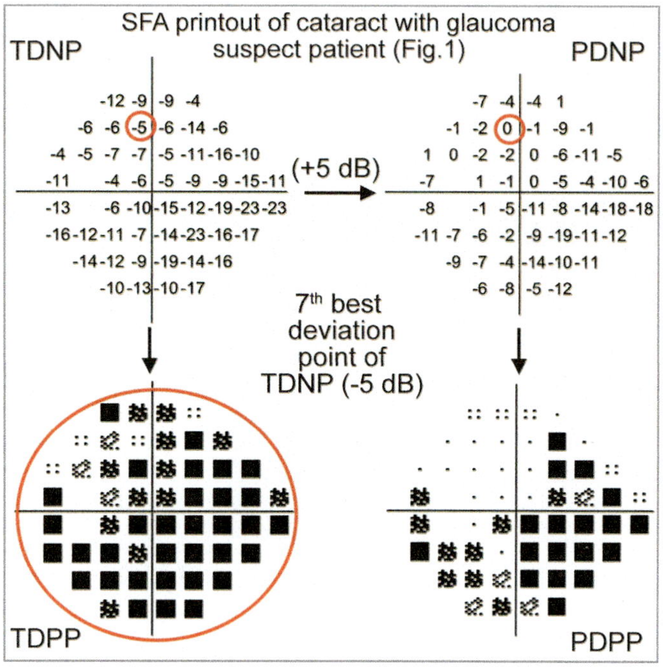

Case 32 RE

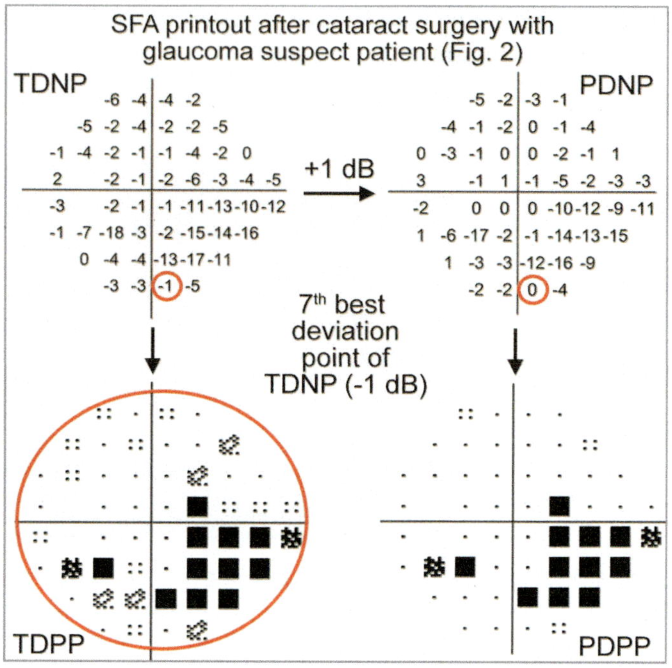

Case 32 LE

SFA printout of cataract with glaucoma suspect patient (Fig. 1).

Probability plots: Irregular generalized depression—The generalized depression in TDNP is due to cataract. By elevating each point's sensitivity by 5 dB during conversion of TDNP to PDNP, generalized depression is eliminated and the localized field defect in generalized depression was highlighted in PDPP.

SFA printout after cataract surgery with glaucoma suspect patient (Fig. 2).

Probability plots: Localized field defect in TDPP.

The generalized depression in TDPP due to cataract (Fig. 1) is eliminated by surgical removal of the cataract and localized field defect in generalized depression was highlighted in TDPP itself (Fig. 2). In a localized field defect TDPP and PDPP look similar.

When we suspect glaucoma associated with cataract, always consider pattern deviation plots for diagnosis and to set target IOP. Note that GHT and VFI are derived from PDNP. In Figure 1, TDNP is converted to PDNP by elevating each point's sensitivity of TDNP by (+5 dB) the dB value that converts the 7th best deviation point to 0 dB deviation. The fields were repeated in the same patient after cataracts removal. Due to cataract removal the generalized depression caused by cataract was removed from the TDNP.

The generalized depression caused by cataract and the dB value that converts the 7th best deviation point to 0 dB will be almost same.

> Note there is no change in PSD. Because generalized depression was removed by cataract extraction there will not be change in the contour of hill of vision and hence it will not affect the PSD value.

Global indices cataract + glaucoma		Global indices after cataract removal
Foveal sensitivity 28 dB	→	Foveal sensitivity 34 dB
MD -11.35 dB P < 0.5%	→	MD -5.39 dB P < 0.5%
PSD 5.44 dB P < 0.5%	→	PSD 5.34 dB P < 0.5%

CHAPTER

10

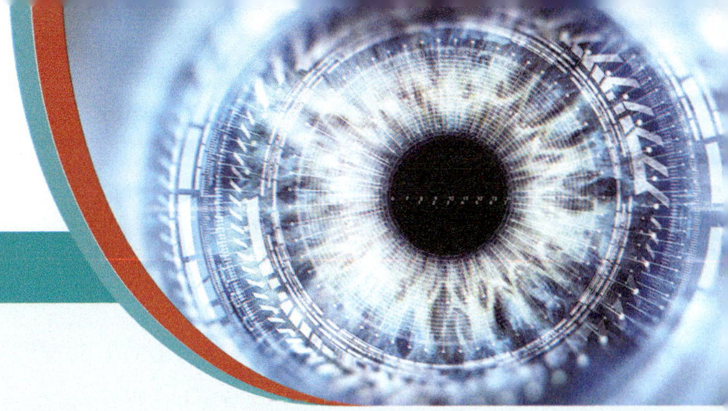

Assessing Glaucoma Progression

The most important aim in the management of glaucoma is to set target intraocular pressure (IOP) to prevent progression of the existing field defect and to prevent the onset of new field defects early and reliably. Uncontrolled IOP is the most important clinical clue to suspect glaucoma progression. Disc evaluation in the follow-up visits is very important to detect progression. Gold standard method is yet to be developed to detect progression early and reliably. Basically the ganglion cell loss can be assessed by either functional tests (visual fields) or structural tests (OCT and HRT). Progression analysis on the basis of structural analysis is still not well established. We will concentrate on the role of visual fields to detect progression of glaucoma.

For the analysis of glaucoma progression the most important prerequisite is to have a baseline field and follow-up field. Baseline field—as you know there are three types of glaucomas.

Type 1: Ganglion cell damage dominant outside 10° circle.

Type 2: Ganglion cell damage dominant inside 10° circle.

Type 3: Ganglion cell damage dominant inside and outside 10° circle.

Once glaucoma is suspected, we should perform the field test either with 24-2 or 30-2 point patterns. From this single field analysis (SFA) printout we know the type of glaucoma and accordingly we will repeat the test with 10-2 point pattern.

Follow-up field—depending on the baseline field the follow-up SFA printout will be performed.

Now we have a baseline field and follow-up field. Then MD index and visual field index (VFI) are the two indices are required for the assessment of glaucoma progression.

The glaucoma progression includes enlargement of the existing field defect (Horizontal progression), deepening of existing defect (Vertical progression) and onset of new field defect.

Baseline field MD index and VFI → Follow-up field MD index and VFI

↓

Increase in MD index or decrease in VFI in the follow-up field

↓

Progression (+)

↓

Deepening of existing defect, enlargement of the existing field defect and onset of new field defect

Most important point to be noted is VFI is not present in 10-2 printouts. So we cannot assess glaucoma progression analysis in type 2 and type 3 glaucomas based on VFI index. So for these types of glaucomas, progression analysis will depend on change in MD index between the baseline field and the follow-up field. The most important positive point is VFI index. Its value is independent of cataract because the VFI is derived from pattern deviation numerical plot (PDNP). But development of cataract will have affect on the value of MD index. We should carefully evaluate the value of MD index keeping in mind reliability indices, refractive error correction and influence of cataract on foveal sensitivity.

The most important point to be noted is VFI is not present in 10-2 SFA printout so glaucoma progression can not be assessed on VFI-based progression analysis in Type 2 and Type 3 glaucomas.

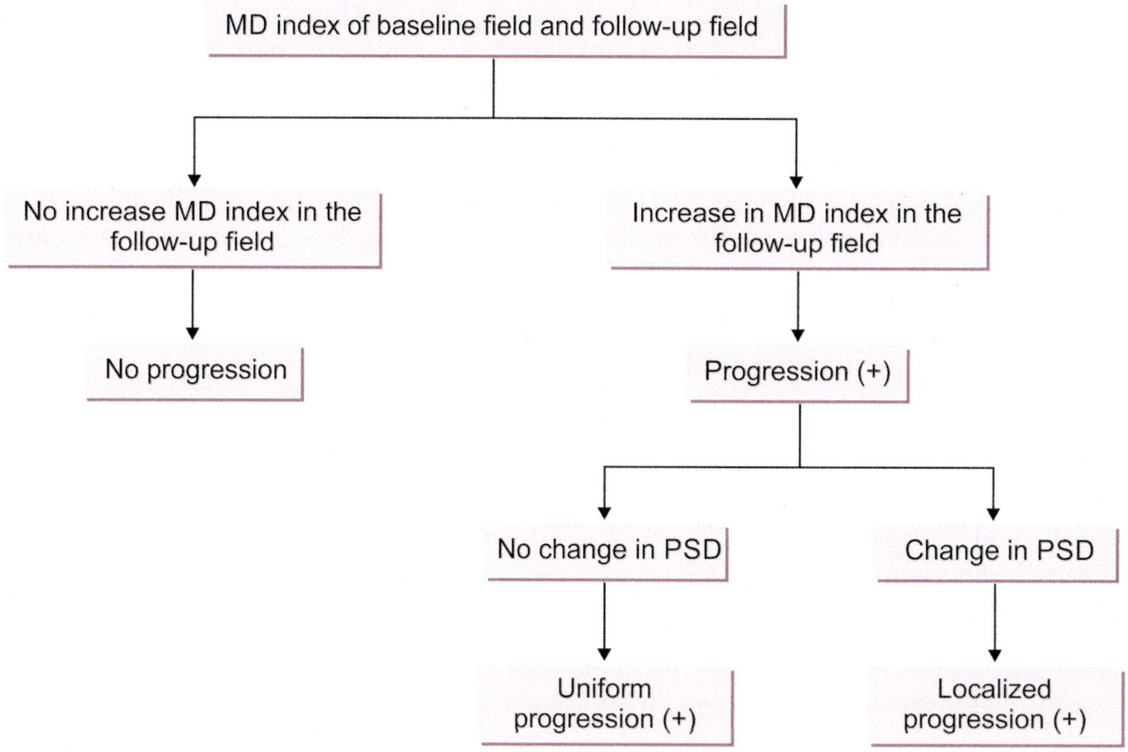

It is always better to keep the same parameters of the baseline printout to the follow-up field. Better to have the same point pattern (we cannot compare the MD index of 24-2 with 10-2 MD index), same strategy and refractive error correction for near should be given properly. Reliability indices, size of the pupil should be taken into consideration before comparing the MD index of both the tests.

The STATPAC ANALYSIS of the measured retinal sensitivity will be given in two formats

Single field analysis printout

Overview printout

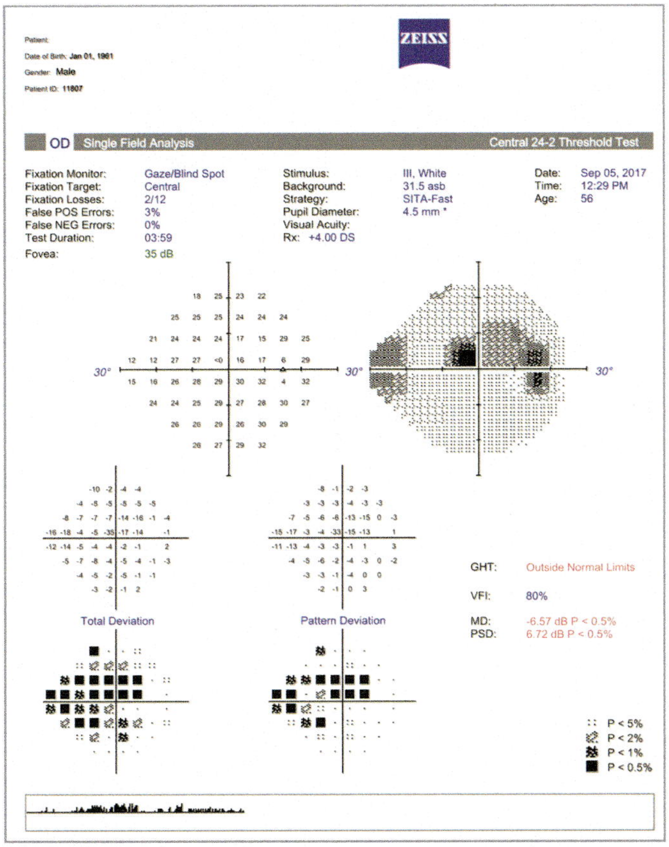

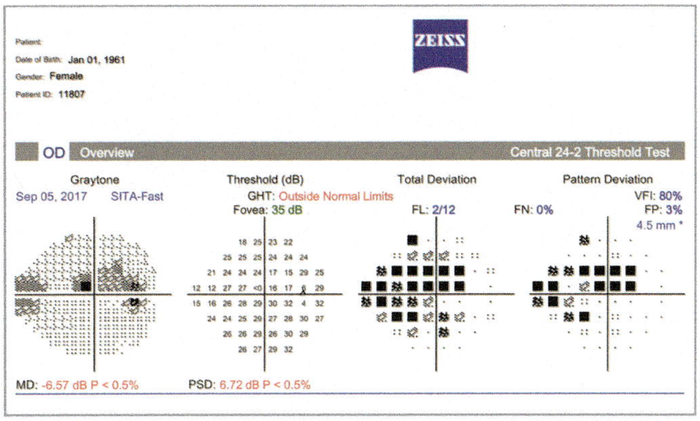

ZONE 8	PDPP
ZONE 9	Global indices
ZONE 10	GHT
ZONE 11	Gaze tracking

ZONE 5	TDNP (Not displayed in overview printout)
ZONE 7	PDNP (Not displayed in overview printout)

Zone 1	Patient data and test
Zone 2	Reliability data and foveal sensitivity
Zone 3	Raw data
Zone 4	Grey scale
Zone 5	TDNP
ZONE 6	TDPP
ZONE 7	PDNP

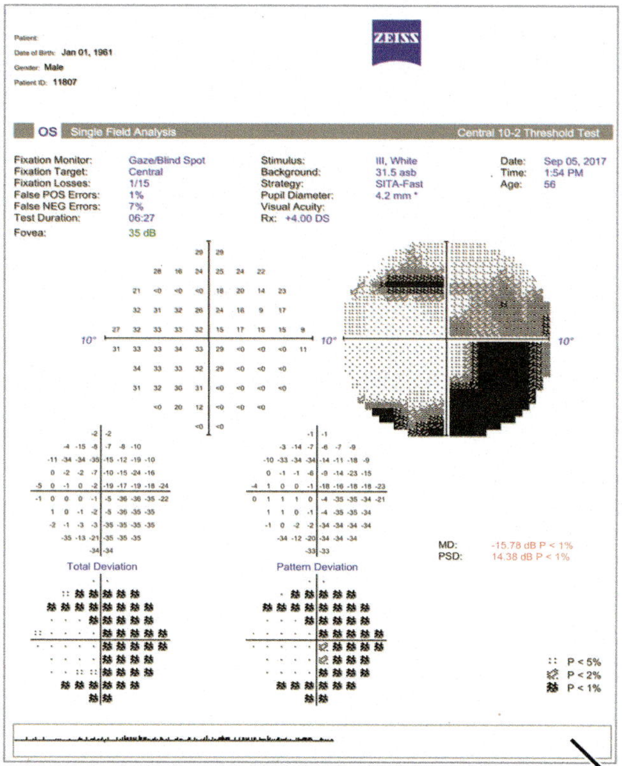

Single analysis printout September 2017

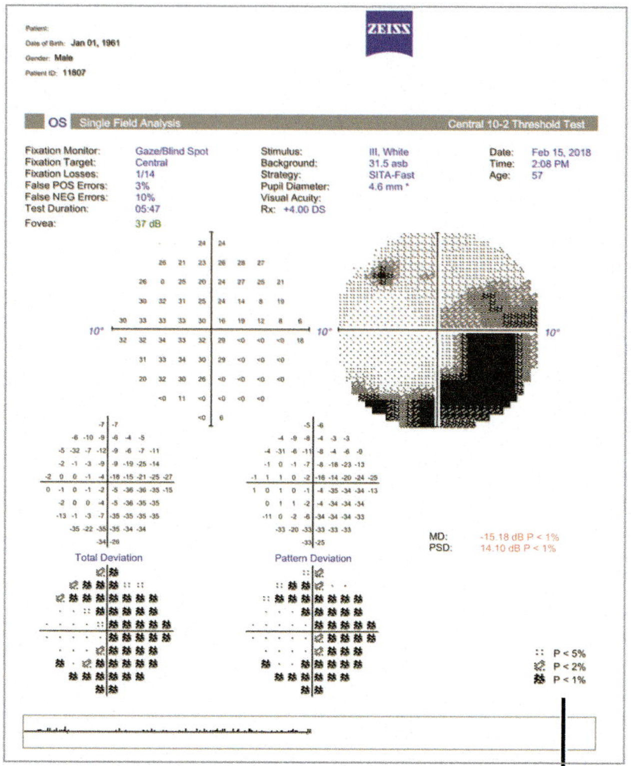

Single analysis printout April 2018

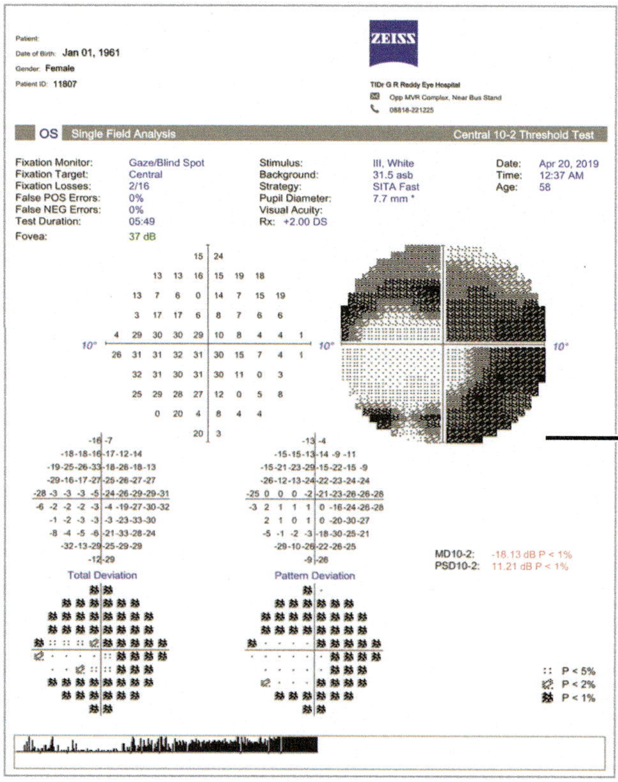

Single analysis printout April 2019

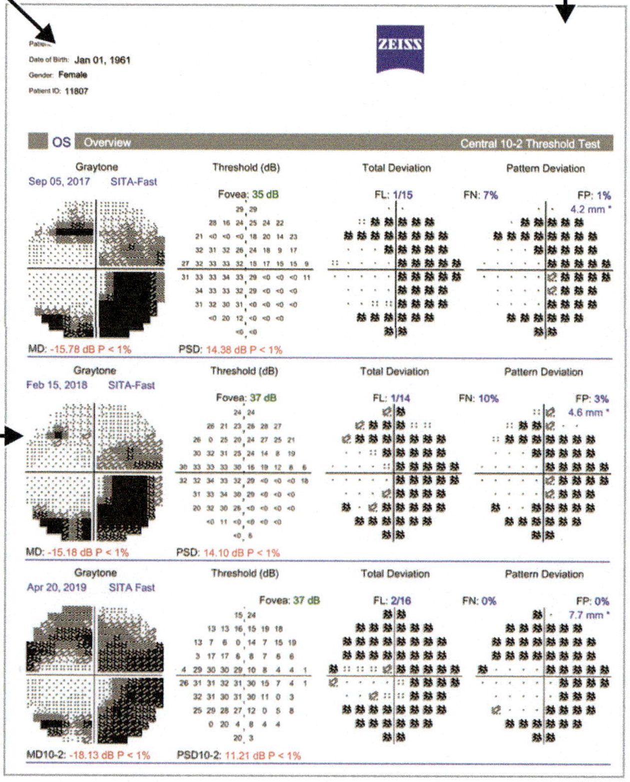

Overview printout of all the three tests on a single sheet

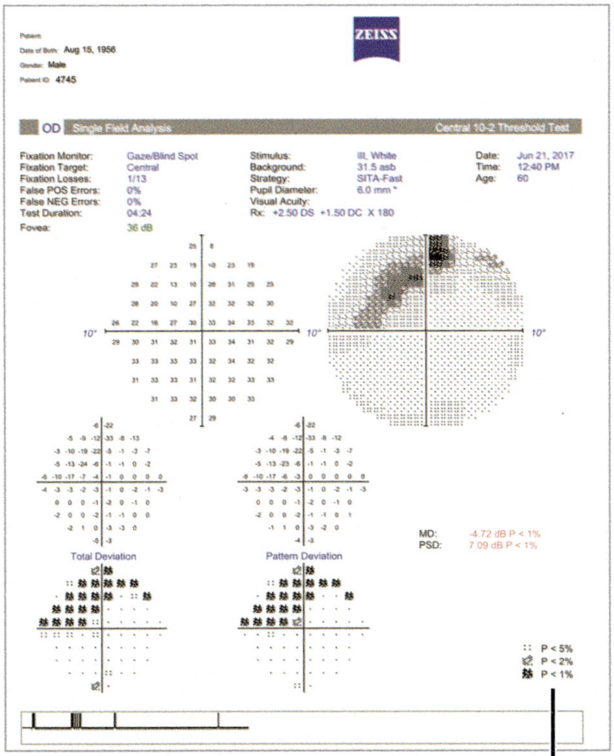

Single analysis printout September 2017

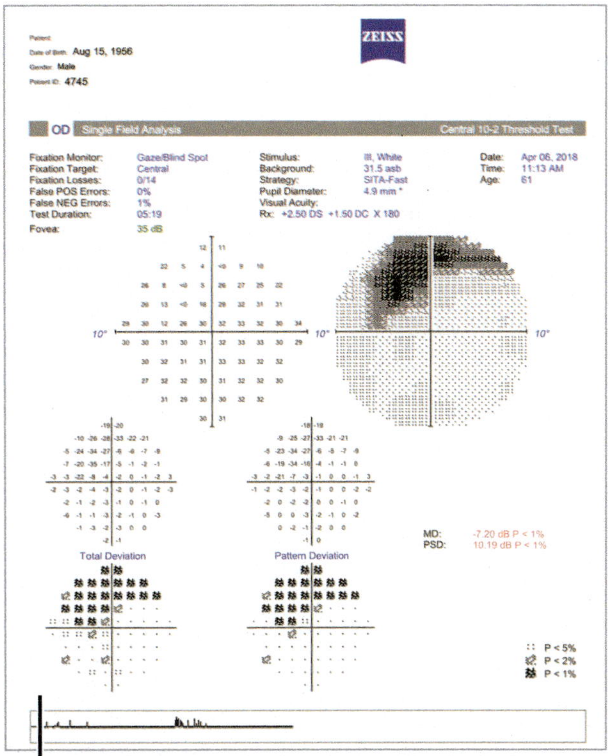

Single analysis printout April 2018

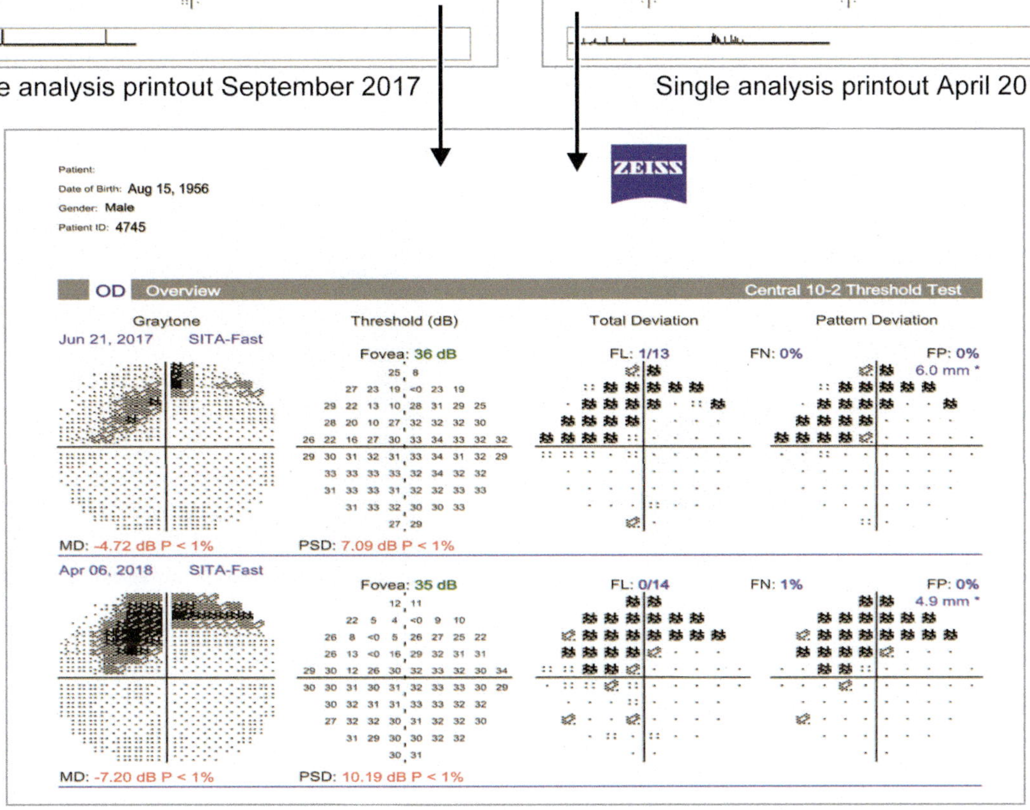

FL 1/13; FP 0%; FN 0%
Fovea 36 dB
MD -4.72 dB P < 1%
PSD 7.09 dB P < 1%

FL 0/14; FP 0%; FN 1%
Fovea 35 dB
MD -7.20 dB P < 1%
PSD 10.19 dB P < 1%

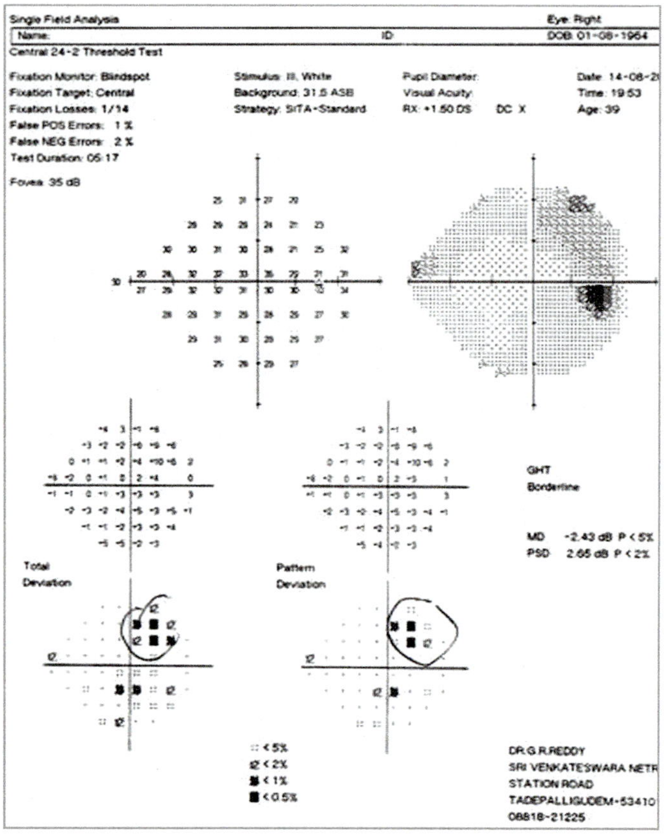

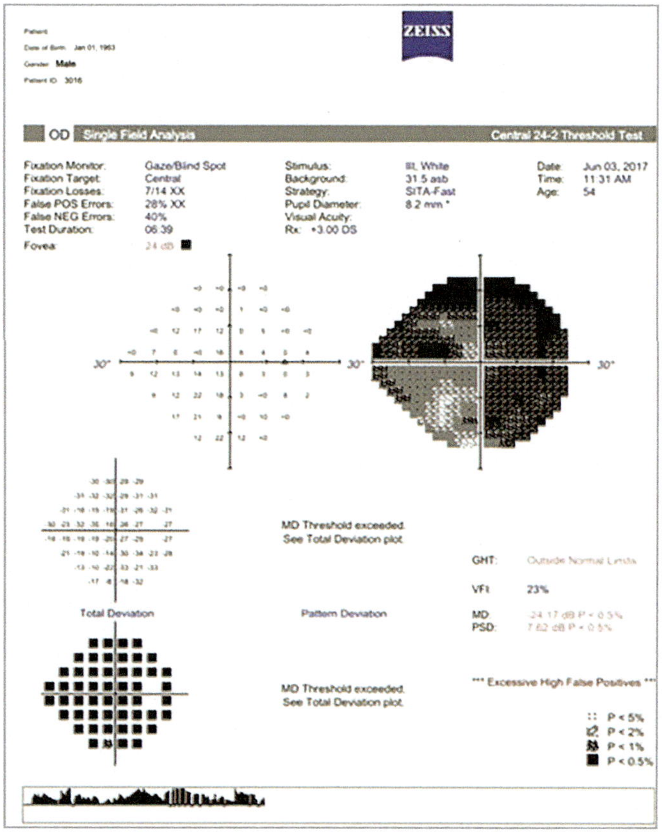

Case 33 RE (2003)

FL 1/14; FP 1%; FN 2%
Fovea 35 dB
2003 MD -2.43 dB P < 5%

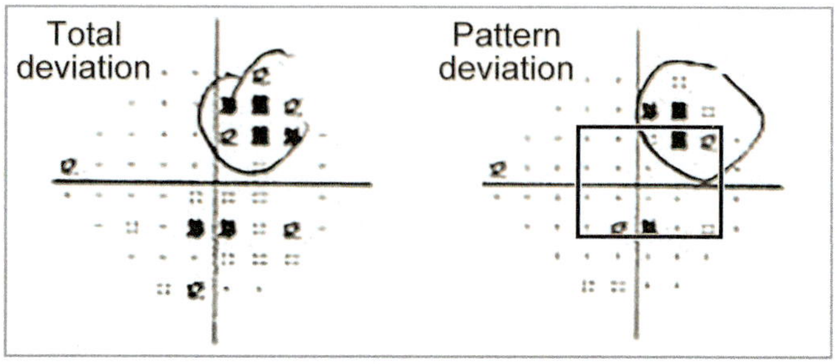

Case 33 RE After 15 years (2018)

This case was seen in 2003 Fundus picture was not taken due to lack of facility. In this eye, glaucoma started almost within 10° circle. I lost the follow-up of this case 33 RE (I saw this case as an advanced case of glaucoma in 2018).

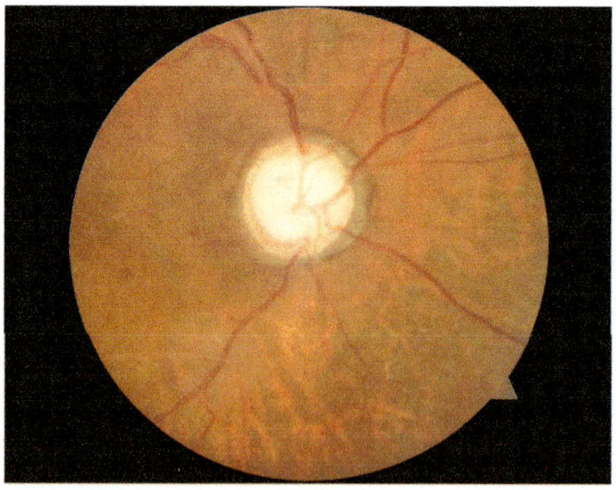

FL 7/14; FP 28%; FN 40%
Fovea 24 dB; VFI 23%
MD -24.17 dB P < 0.5%

This case stands for an example for glaucomas starting within 10° circle.

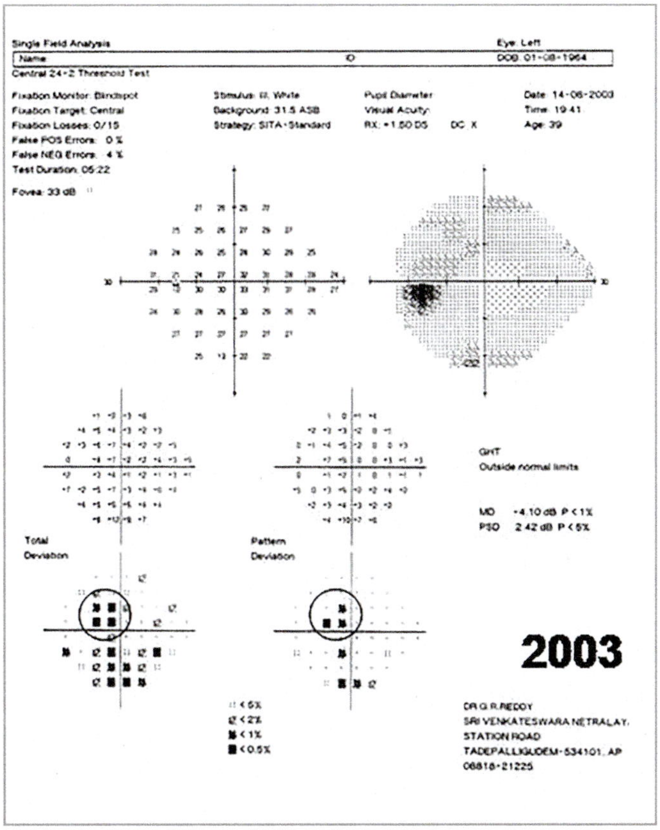

Case 33 LE (2003)

FL 0/15; FP 0%; FN 4%
Fovea 33 dB
2003 MD -4.10 dB P < 1%

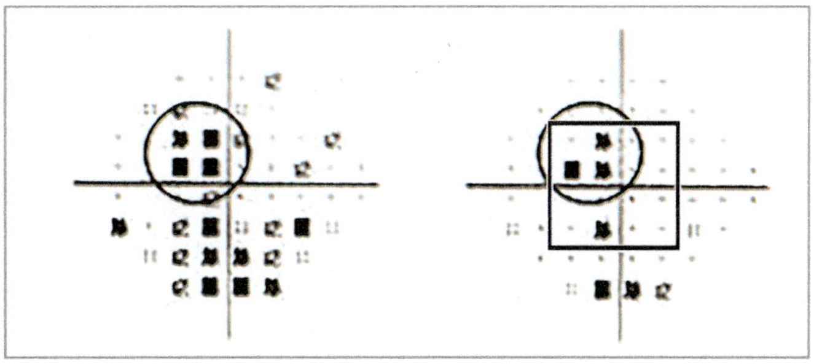

CASE 33 LE after 15 years (2018)

This case was seen in 2003, fundus picture was not taken due to lack of facility. In the left eye also glaucoma almost started within 10° circle. I lost the follow-up case 33 LE (I saw the case in 2018 as an advanced case of glaucoma).

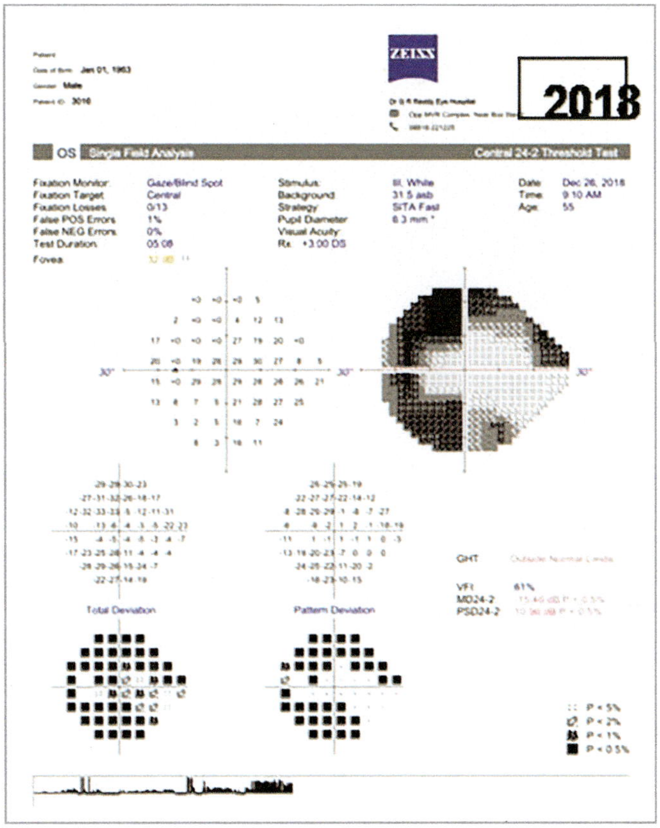

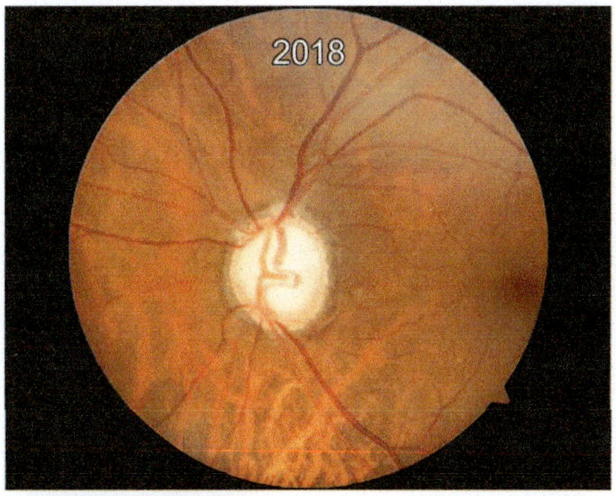

FL 0/13; FP 1%; FN 0%
Fovea 32 dB; VFI 61%
MD -15.47 dB P < 0.5%

The most important take home message in this case is direction of progression. Though the glaucomatous damage started within 10° circle, the direction of progression is not towards fixation. This is the reason why I always give importance to the direction of progression.

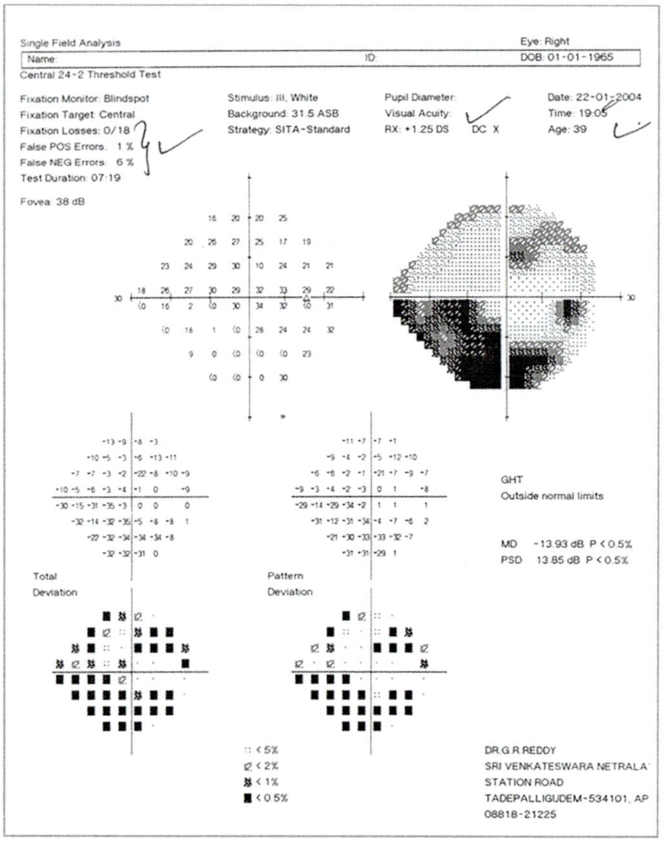

Case 34 RE

FL 0/18; FP 1%; FN 6%
Fovea 38 dB
MD -13.93 dB P < 0.5%

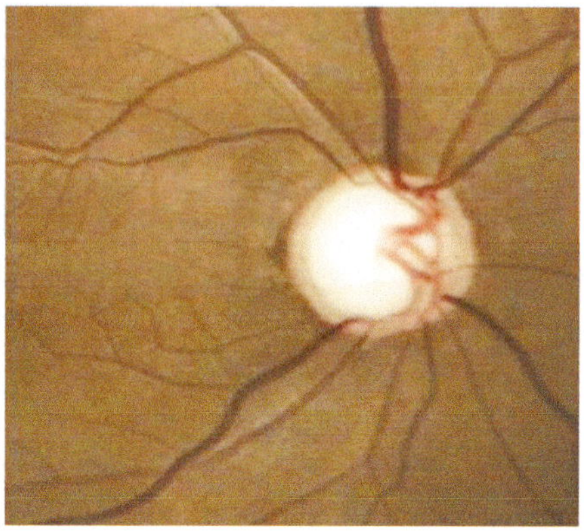

This case was seen in 2004

Since then IOP was under control.

Case 34 RE after 13 years (2017)

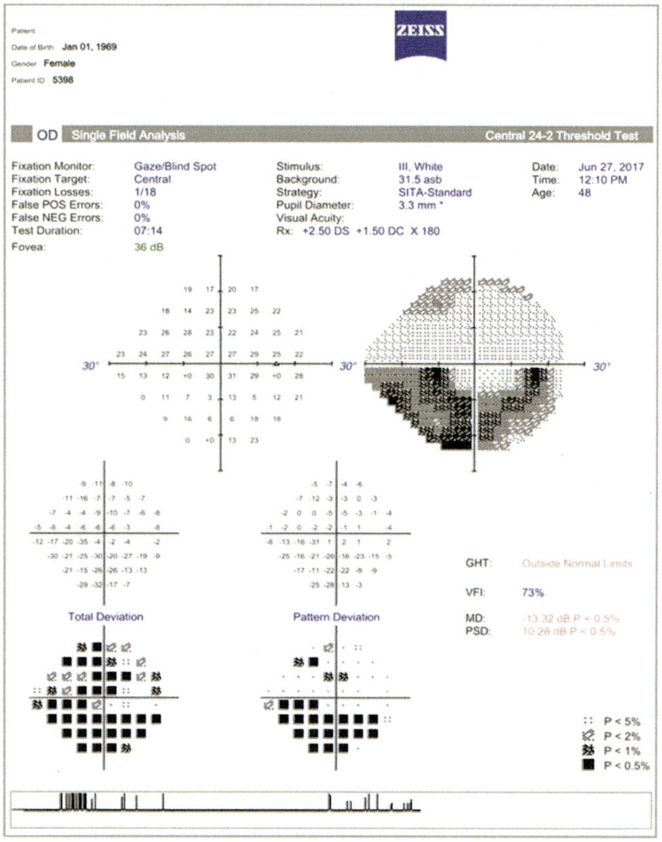

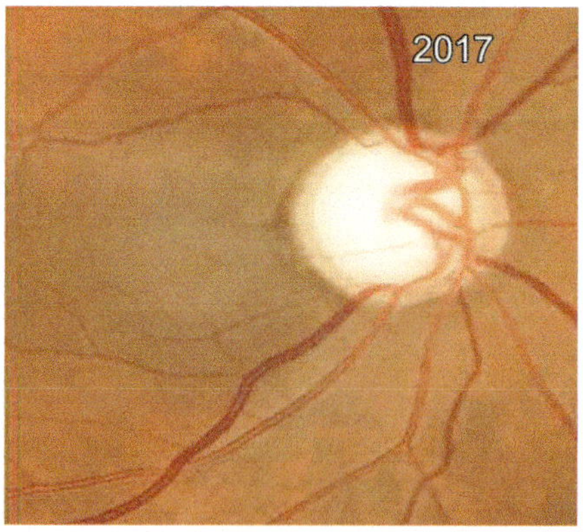

FL 1/18; FP 0%; FN 0%
Fovea 36 dB
VFI 73%
MD -13.32 dB P < 0.5%

There is no change in MD index

This indicates that glaucoma is stable.

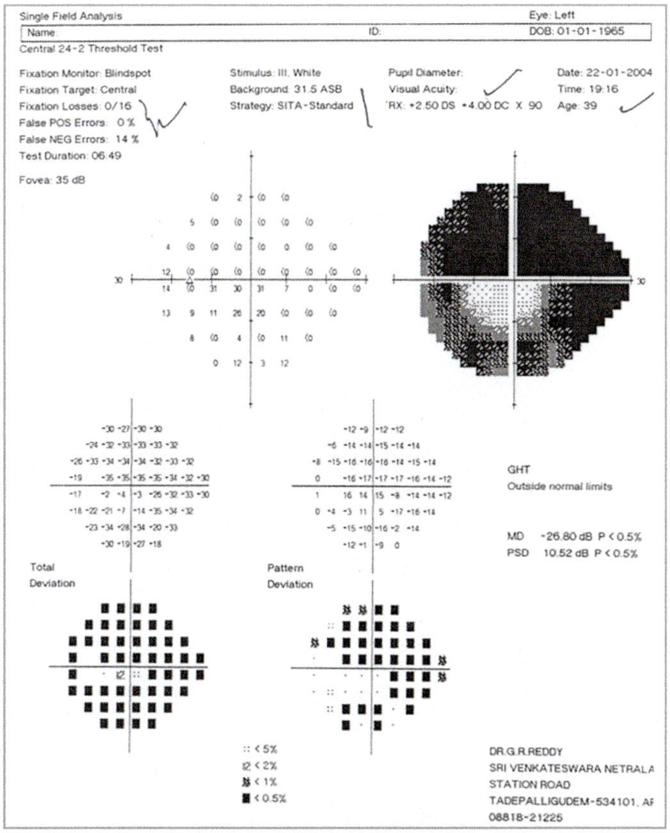

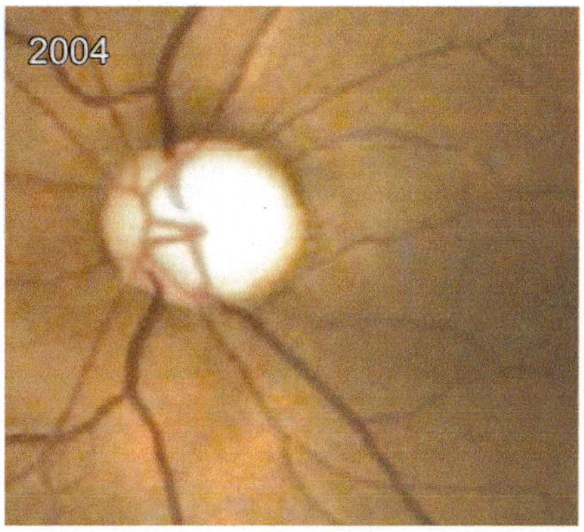

Case 34 LE

FL 0/16; FP 0%; FN 14%
Fovea 35 dB
MD -26.80 dB   P < 0.5%

Case 34 LE after 13 years (2017)

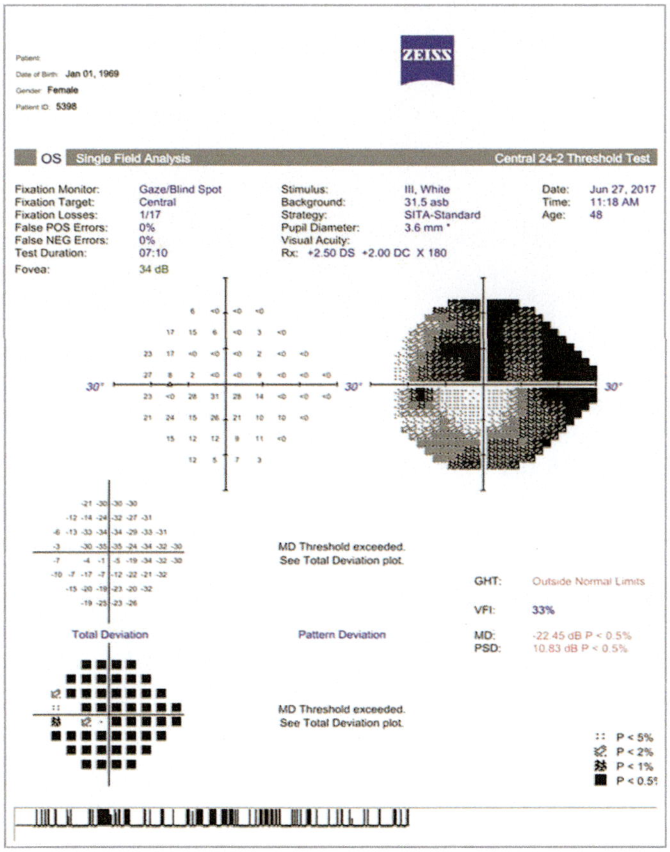

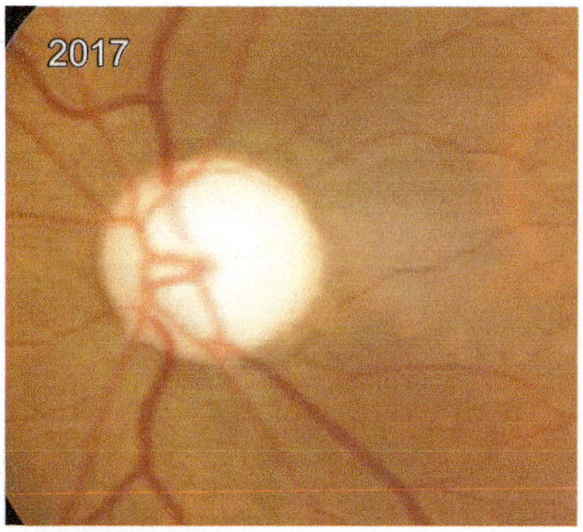

FL 1/17; FP 0%; FN 0%
Fovea 34 dB
VFI 33%
MD -22.45 dB   P < 0.5%

Glaucoma is stable since 2004

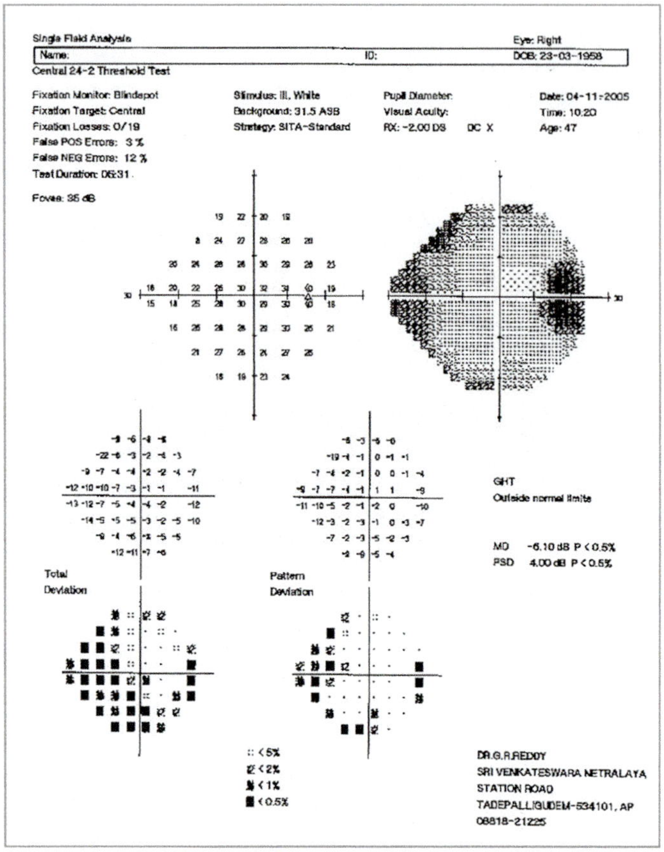

Case 35 RE (2006)

FL 0/19; FP 3%; FN 12%;
Fovea 36 dB
MD -6.10 dB P < 0.5%

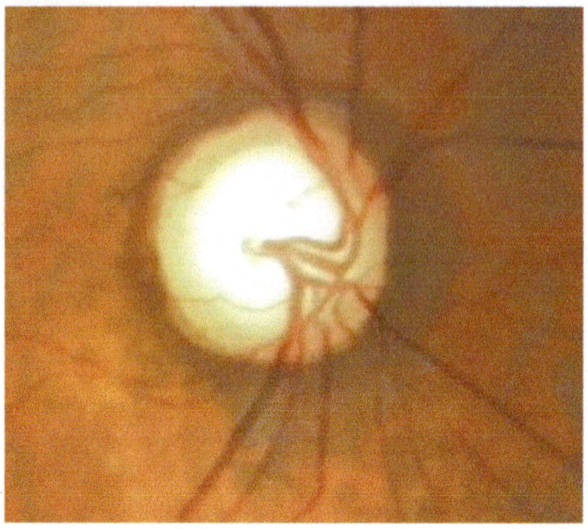

Case 35 RE after 10 years (2016)

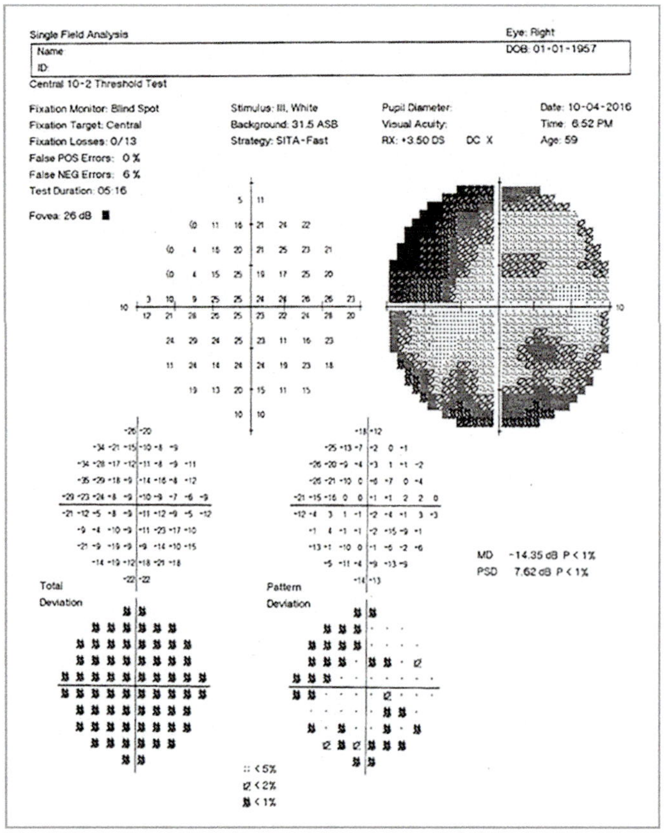

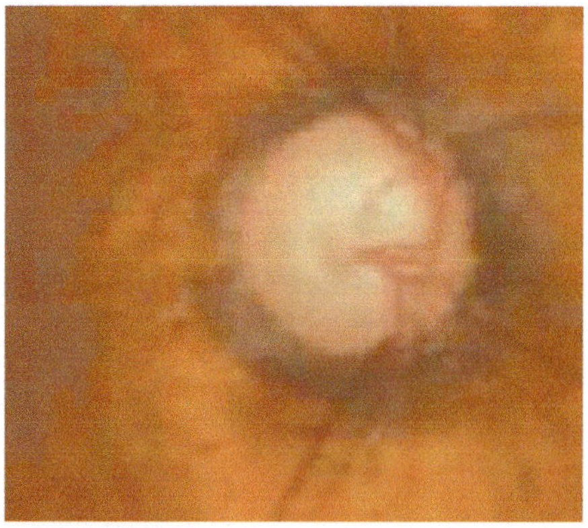

FL 0/13; FP 0%; FN 6%
Fovea 26 dB
MD -14.35 dB P < 1%

This case was seen in 2006. There is no clue in the fundus to say it is a case of glaucoma. This glaucoma belongs to Type 1 group with field defects outside 10° circle. Lost the follow-up and again I saw the case in 2016 as an advanced case of glaucoma.

Case 35 LE (2006)

FL 0/19; FP 6%; FN 7%
Fovea 34 dB
MD -10.15 dB P < 0.5%

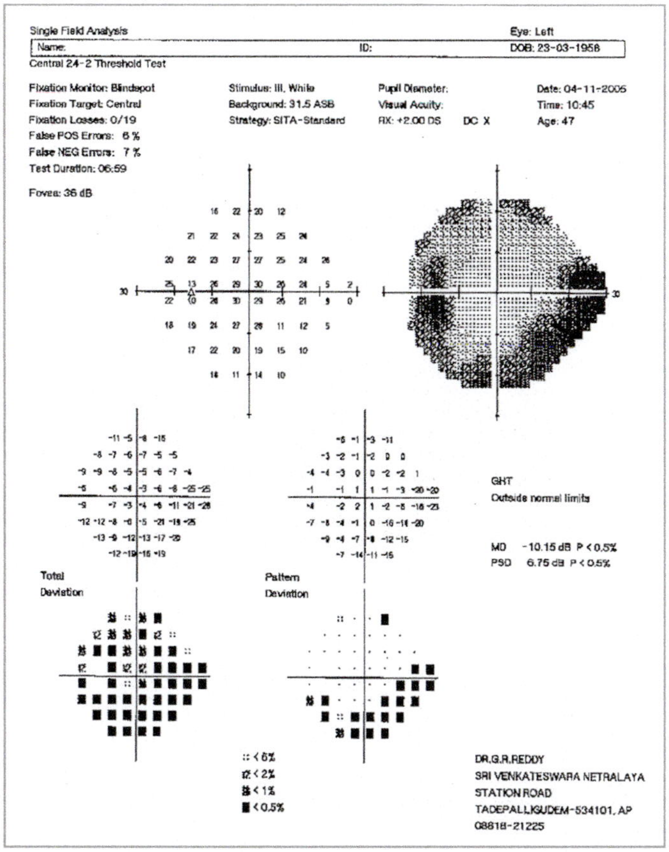

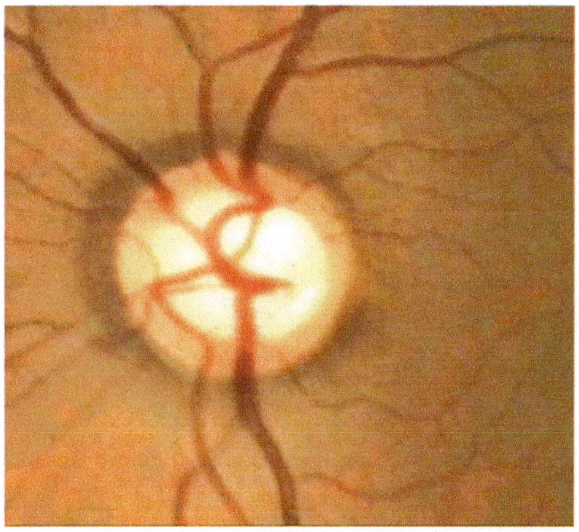

Case 35 LE after 10 years (2016)

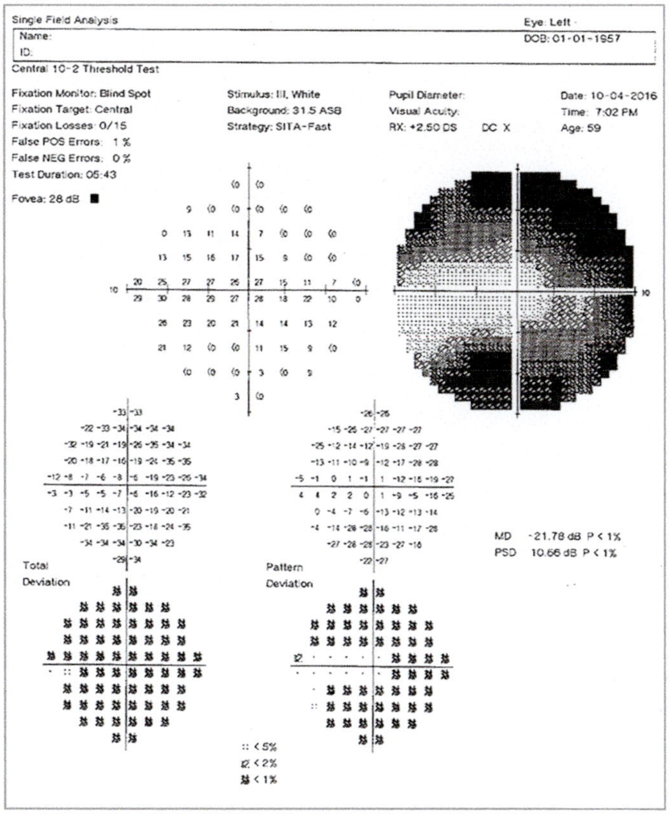

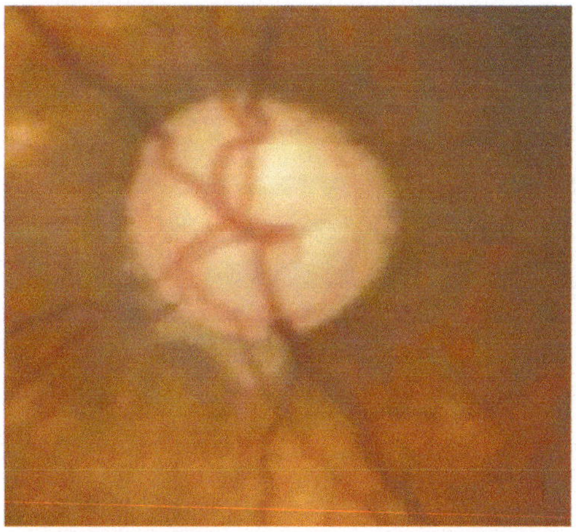

Case 34 LE
FL 0/15; FP 1%; FN 0%
Fovea 28 dB
MD -21.78 dB P < 1%

This case was seen in 2006. There is no clue in the fundus to say it is a case of glaucoma. This glaucoma belongs to Type 1 group with field defects outside 10° circle. Lost the follow-up and again I saw the case in 2016 as an advanced case of glaucoma.

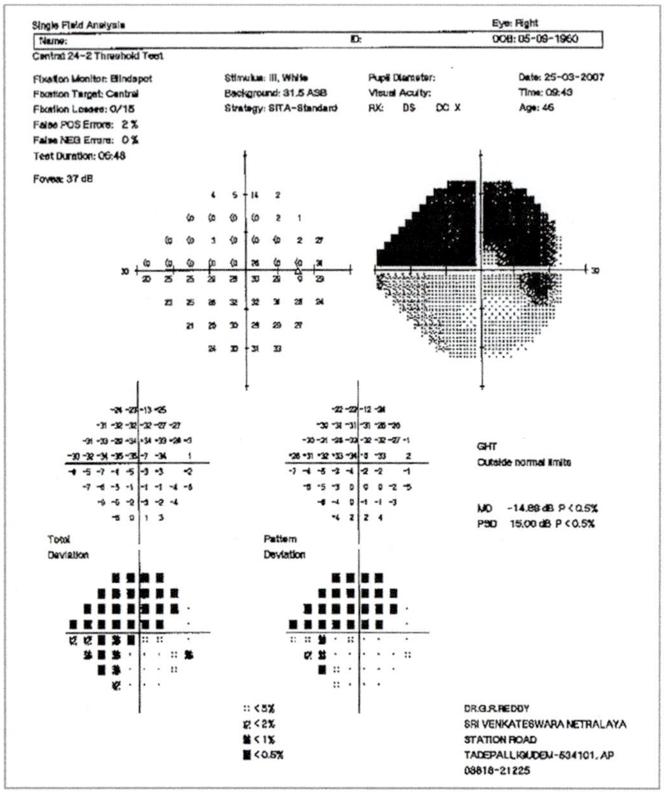

Case 36 RE (2007)

Fovea 37 dB
MD -14.88 dB P < 0.5%

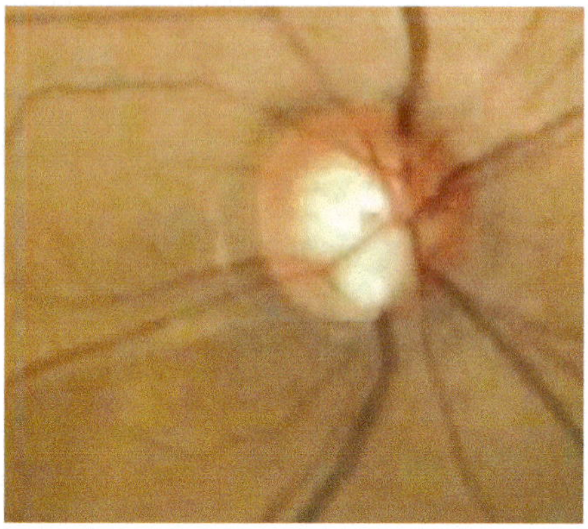

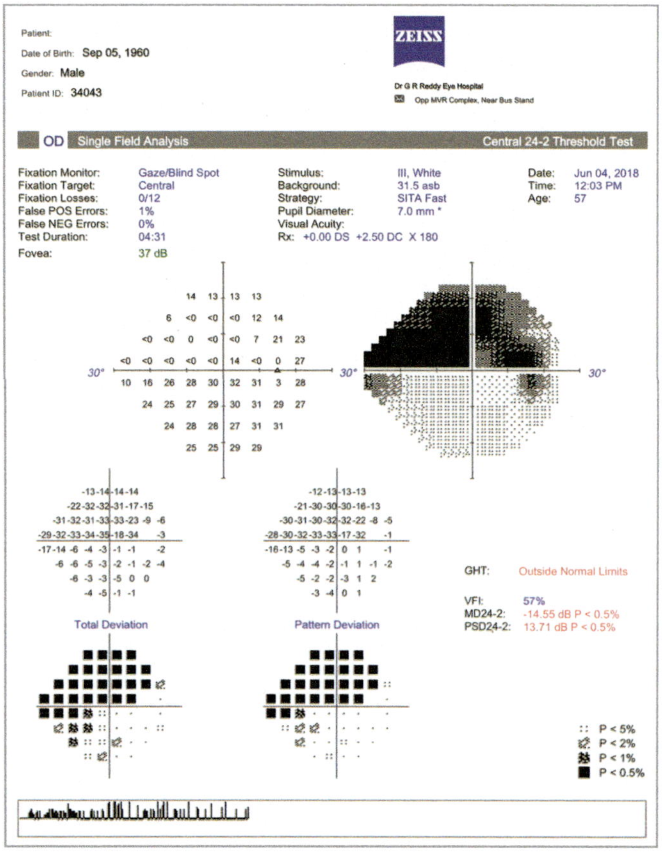

Case 36 RE after 11 years (2018)

FL 0/12; FP 1%; FN 0%
Fovea 37 dB

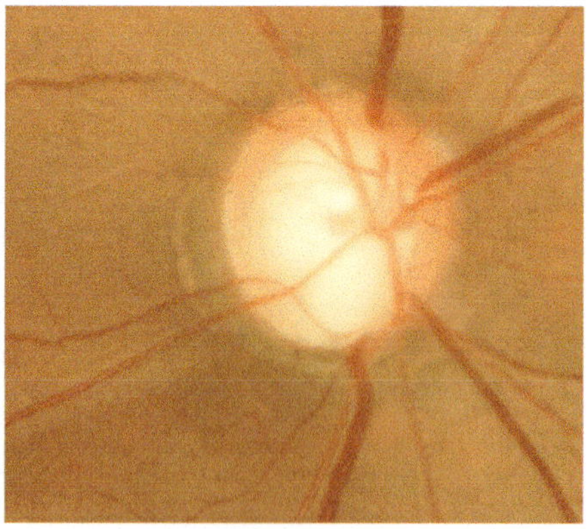

VFI 57%
MD -14.55 dB P < 0.5%

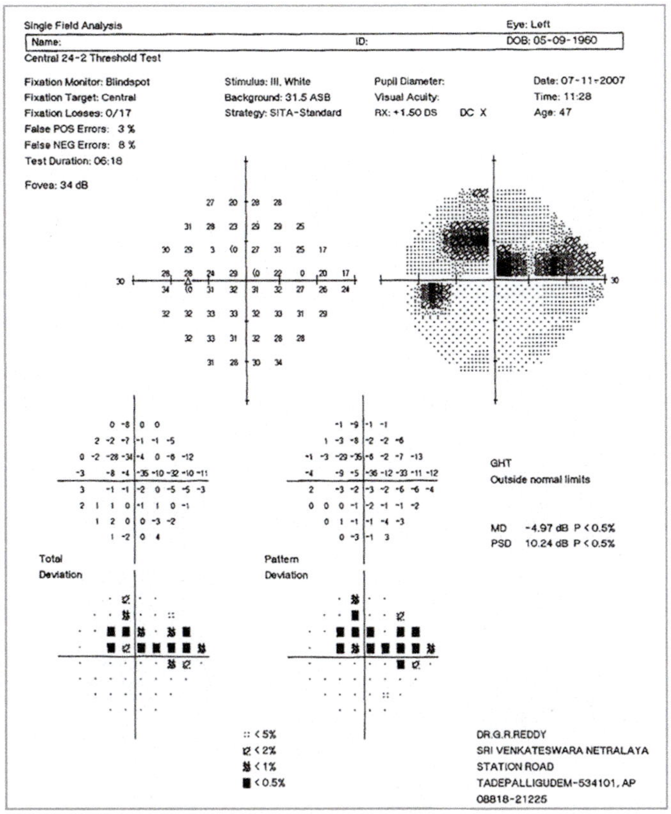

Case 36 LE (2007)

MD -4.97 dB P < 0.5%

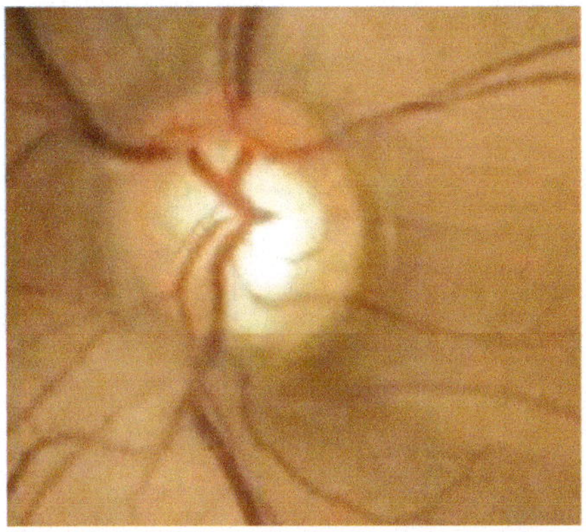

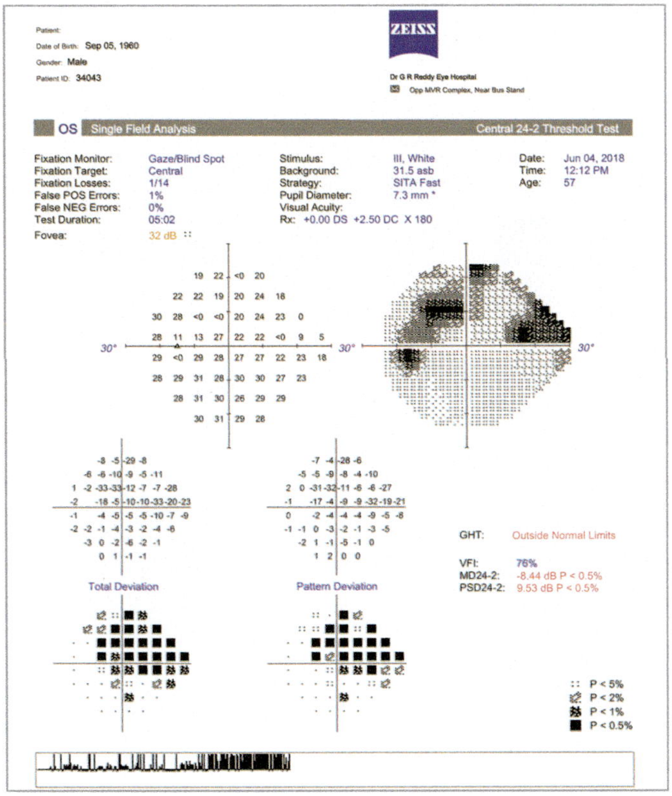

Case 36 LE after 11 years (2018)

This case belongs to type 3 glaucoma. Isolated field defects in and outside 10° circle are appreciated in the grey scale and probability plots. In 2007, I did not know how to evaluate 10° circle area to know the indications to repeat the test with 10-2 point pattern. In this case glaucoma is stable in 24-2 print-out. We cannot comment on progression in 10-2 printouts since. As we did not do 10-2 fields at that time.

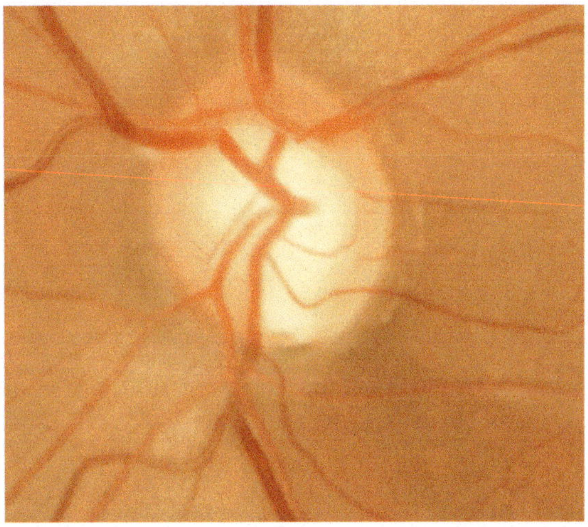

VFI 76%
MD -8.44 dB P < 0.5%

Case 37 RE

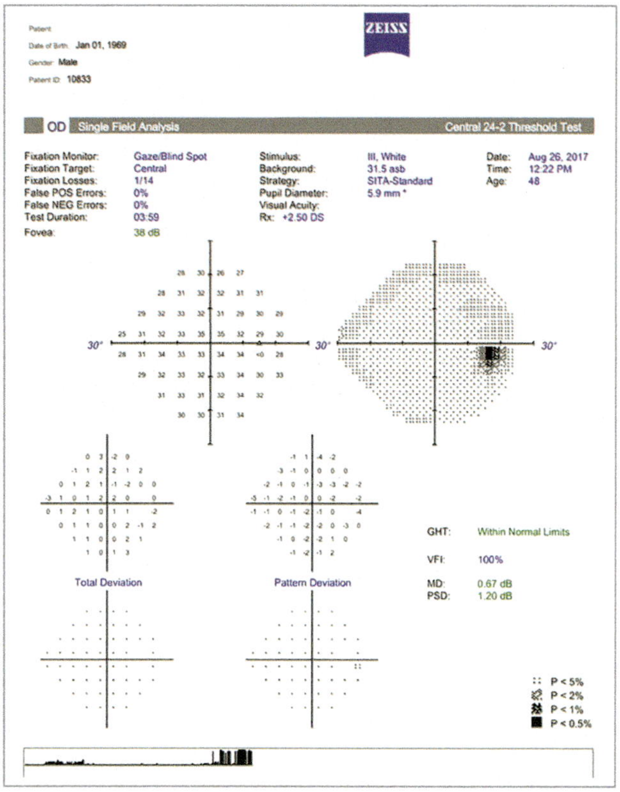

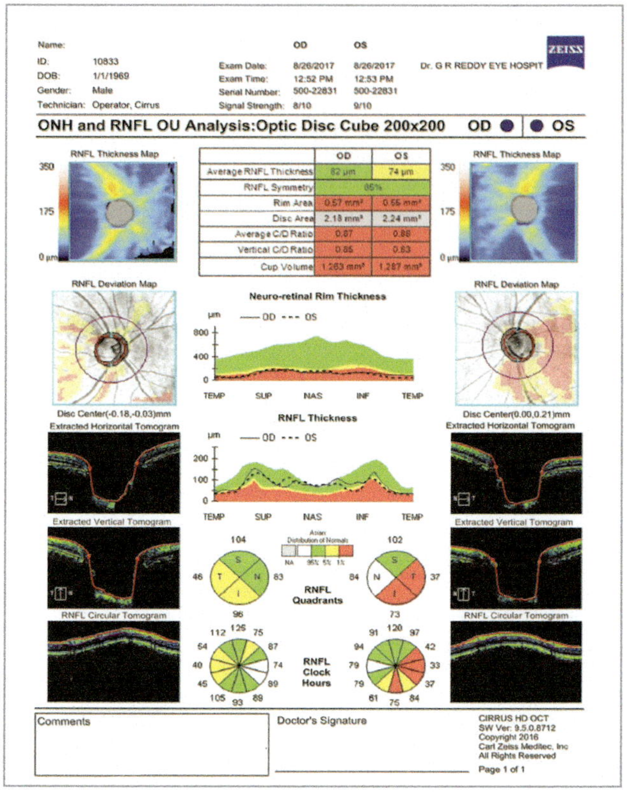

Case 36 RE

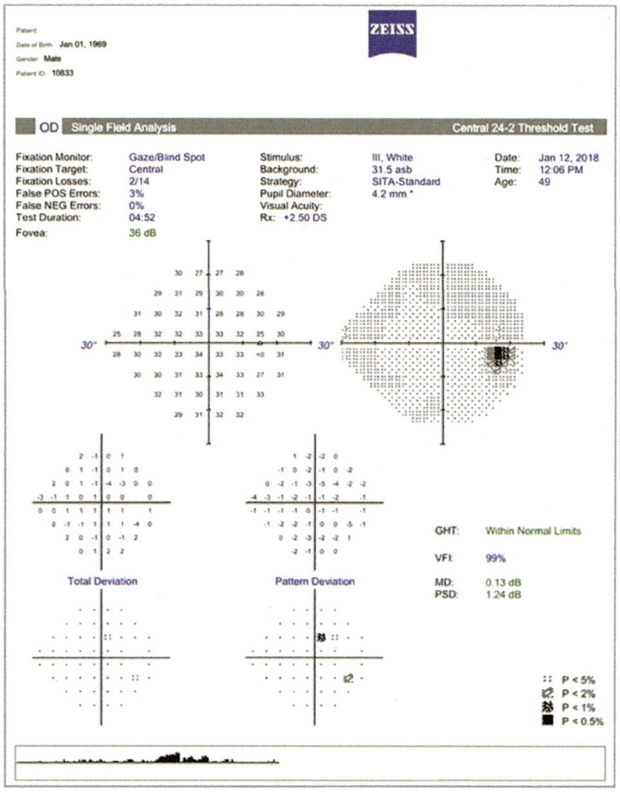

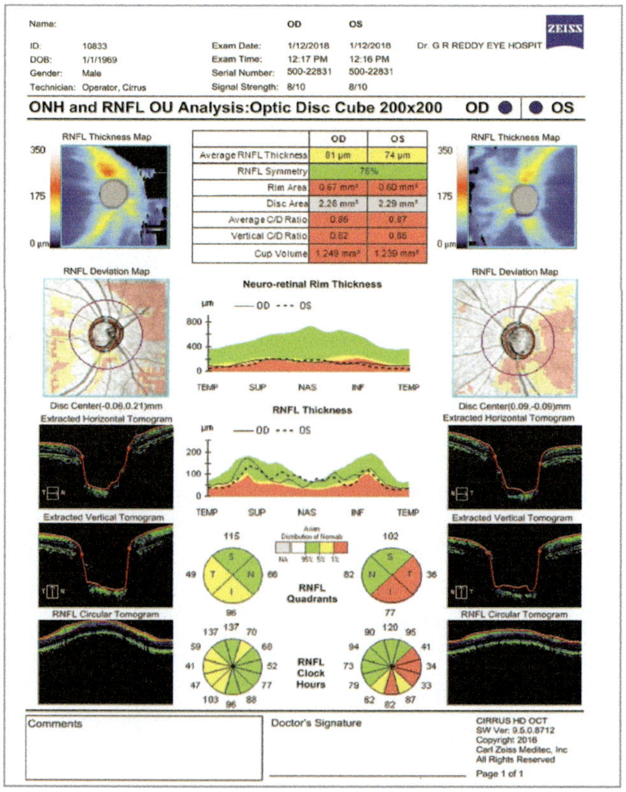

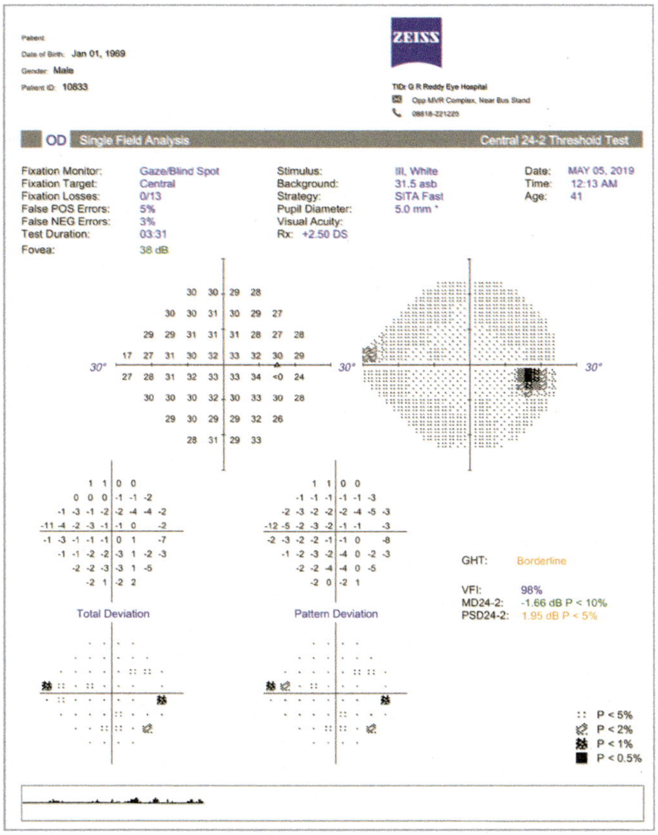

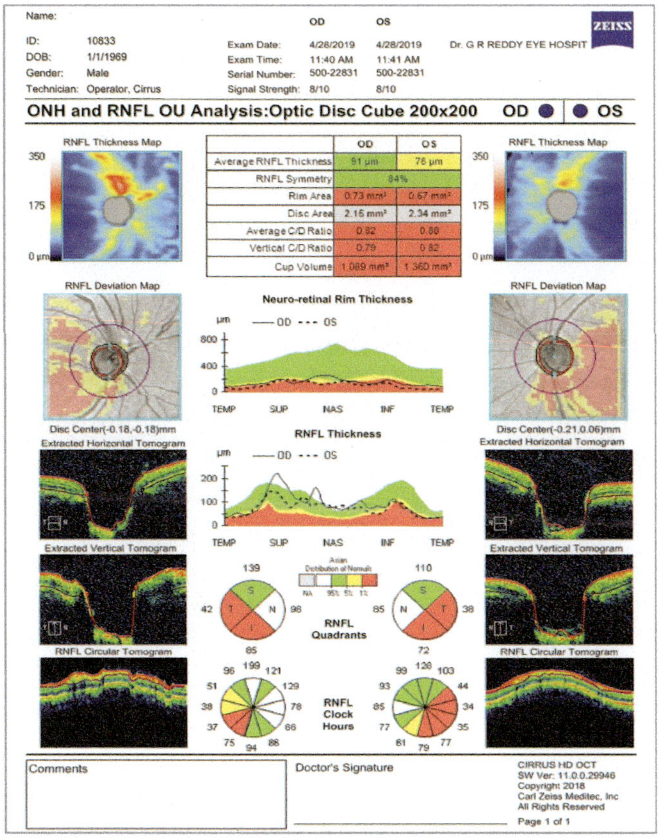

Case 37 RE

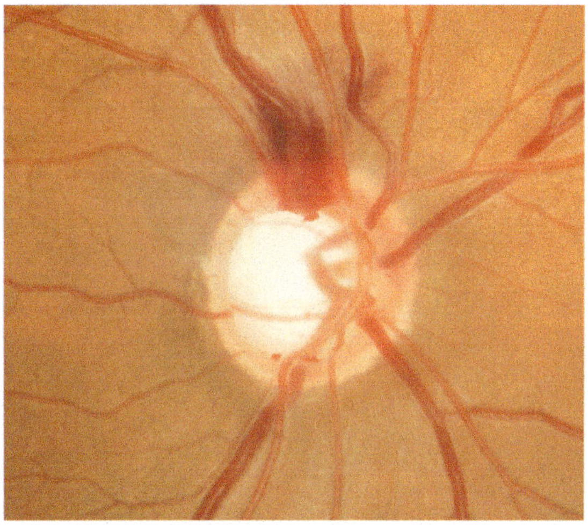

The main aim of presenting this case is to say that the concept of picking up glaucoma very early by OCT when compared to visual fields may not be always be true.

LE is an established case of glaucoma since 2017. The patient is on IOP lowering agents since 2017 for both the eyes.

2017—RE visual fields and OCT are normal

2018—RE visual fields and OCT are normal

2019—RE developed disc hemorrhage.

Visual fields and OCT are showing the changes in 2019 printout.

I always tell we should look at visual fields and OCT as complimentary to each other.

In this case, OCT did not pickup ganglion cell defect earlier to visual fields. Both picked up the RNFL loss at the same time.

Case 38 RE

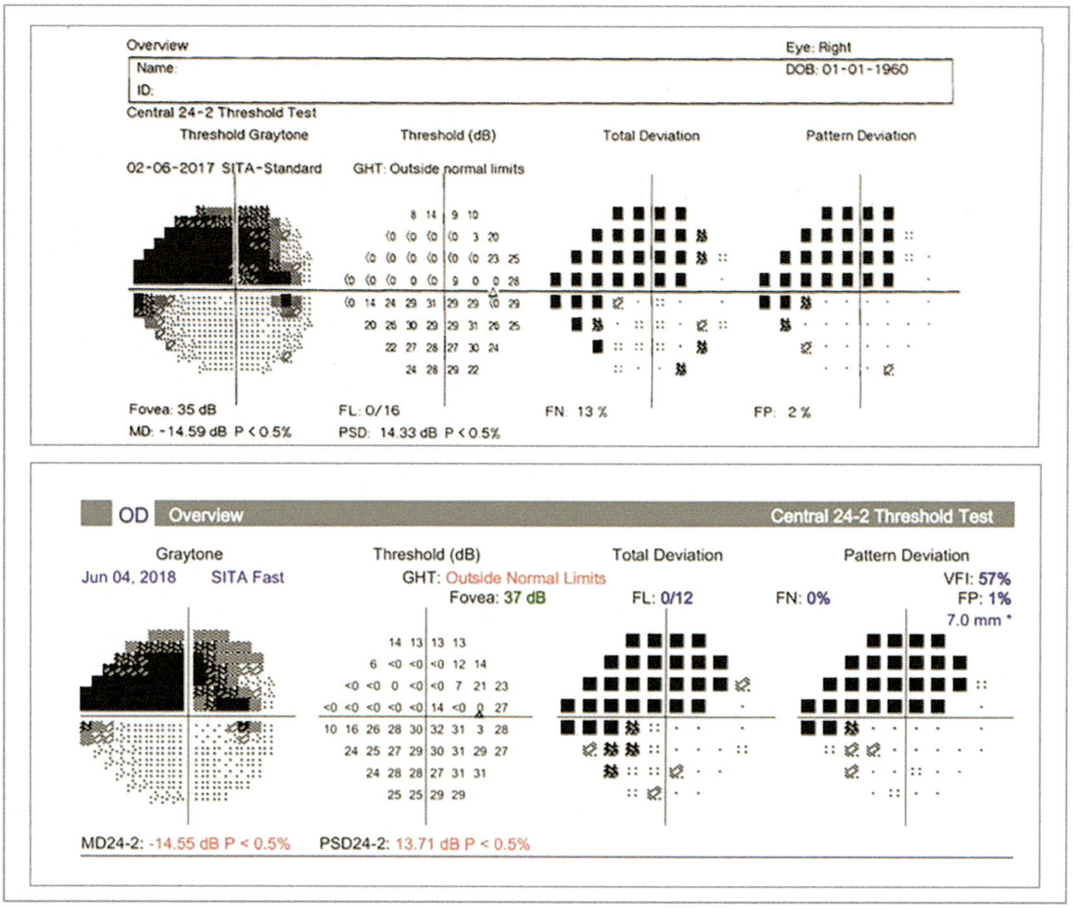

Date	*Point pattern strategy*	*Reliability indices*	*Fovea*	*VFI*	*MD index*
2-6-2017	24-2 SITA Standard	FL 0/16; FP 2%; FN 13%	35 dB		-14.59 dB P < 0.5%
4-6-2018	24-2 SITA Fast	FL 0/12; FP 1%; FN 0%	37 dB	57%	-14.55 dB P < 0.5%

The grey scales and probability plots give rough idea regarding progression. In this overview print-out there is no significant change either in grey scale or in the probability plots between 2017 and 2018 tests. Finally we should see whether there is increase in MD index or not. In this case, there is no change in MD index between 2017 and 2018 tests. So, glaucoma is stable.

Case 38 RE 10-2

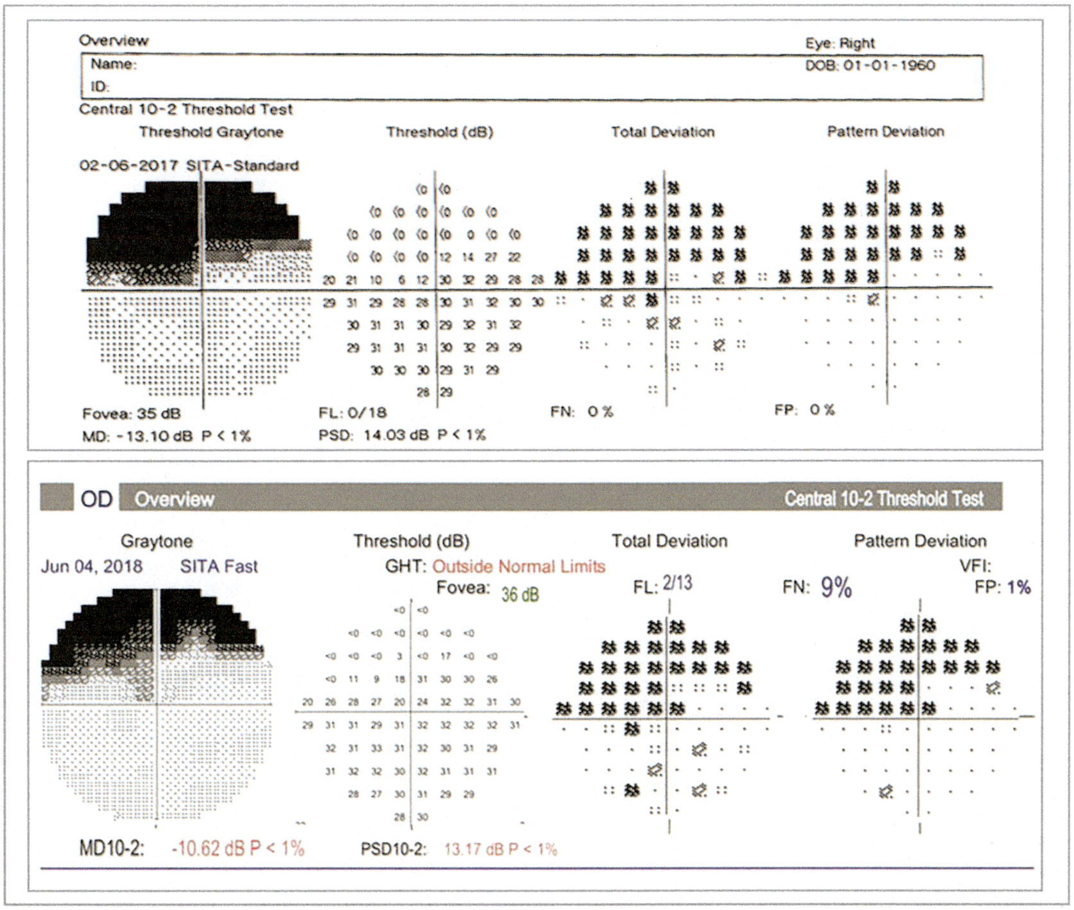

Date	Point pattern strategy	Reliability indices	Fovea	VFI	MD index
2-6-2017	10-2 SITA Standard	FL 0/18; FP 0%; FN 0%	35 dB		-13.10 dB P < 1%
4-6-2018	10-2 SITA Fast	FL 2/13; FP 1%; FN 9%	36 dB		-10.62 dB P < 1%

In this overview printout the probability plots are looking similar. From the probability plots, it is clearly evident that there is no horizontal progression. Since already all the points in the localized field defect are already represented by P < 1%, further vertical progression will not be appreciated in the probability plots. 2018 grey scale is looking better than the 2017 grey scale. Finally, we should see whether there is increase in MD index or not. In this case, MD index is improved by 2.48 dB. This may be due to high FL so glaucoma is stable.

Case 38 LE

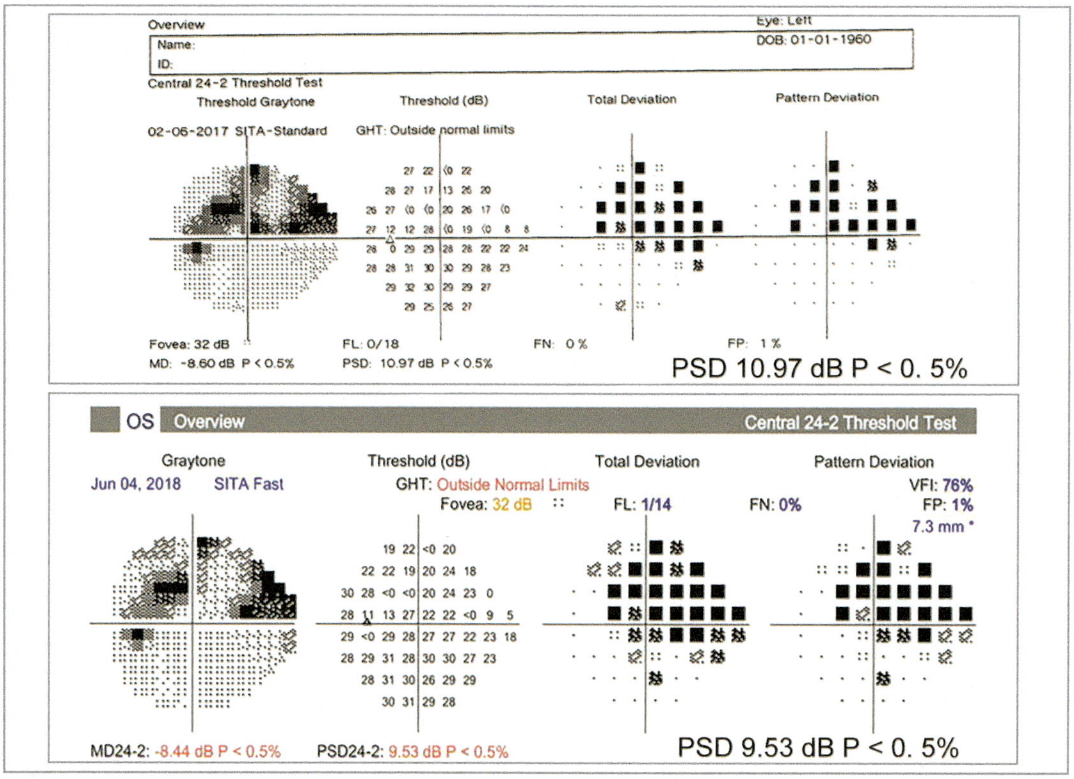

Date	Point pattern strategy	Reliability indices	Fovea	VFI	MD index
2-6-2017	24-2 SITA Standard	FL 0/18; FP 1%; FN 0%	32 dB		-8.60 dB P < 0.5%
4-6-2018	24-2 SITA Fast	FL 1/14; FP 1%; FN 0%	32 dB	76%	-8.44 dB P < 0.5%

Both grey scale and probability plots of 2018 are looking better than the 2017 grey scale and probability plots of 2017. Finally, we should see whether there is increase in MD index or not. 2017 MD index -8.60 dB P < 0.5% 2018—MD index -8.44 dB P < 0.5%. Since there is no increase in the MD glaucoma is stable.

Case 38 LE 10-2

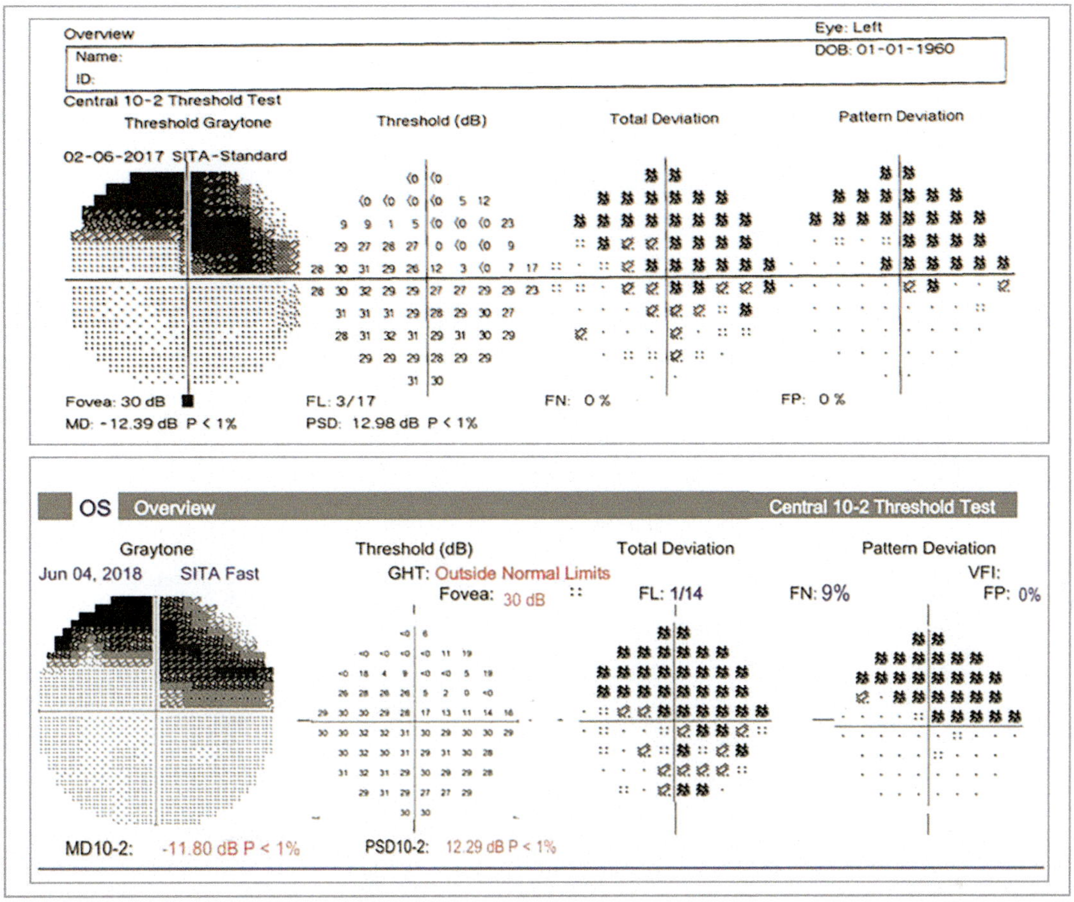

Date	Point pattern strategy	Reliability indices	Fovea	VFI	MD index
2-6-2017	10-2 SITA Standard	FL 3/17; FP 0%; FN 0%	30 dB		-12.39 dB P < 1%
4-6-2018	10-2 SITA Fast	FL 1/14; FP 0%; FN 9%	30 dB		-11.80 dB P < 1%

Grey scales and probability plots give rough idea regarding progression. In this overview printout there is no significant change either in grey scale or in the probability plots between 2017 and 2018 tests. The 2018 MD index is -11.80 dB and 2017 MD index is -12.39 dB. The high value of 2017 MD index is due to high fixation losses (3/17).

Case 39 RE

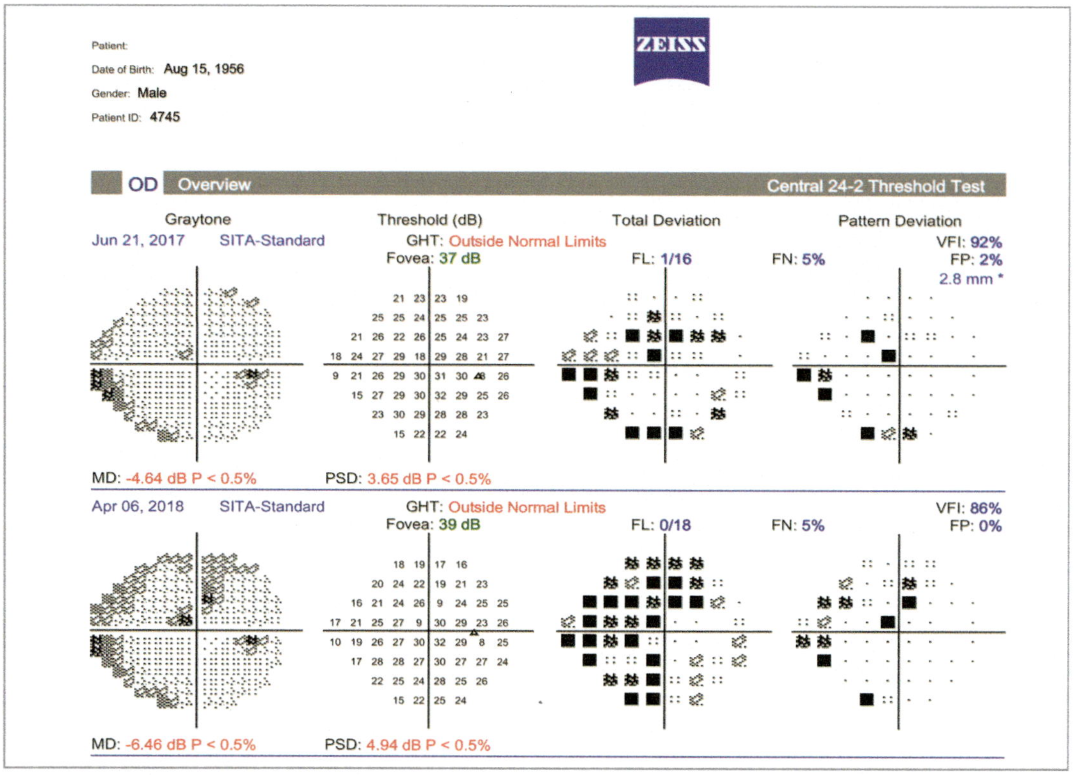

Date	Point pattern strategy	Reliability indices	Fovea	VFI	MD index
21-6-2017	24-2 SITA Standard	FL 1/16; FP 2%; FN 5%	37 dB	92%	-4.64 dB P < 0.5%
6-4-2018	24-2 SITA Standard	FL 0/18; FP 0%; FN 5%	39 dB	86%	-6.46 dB P < 0.5%

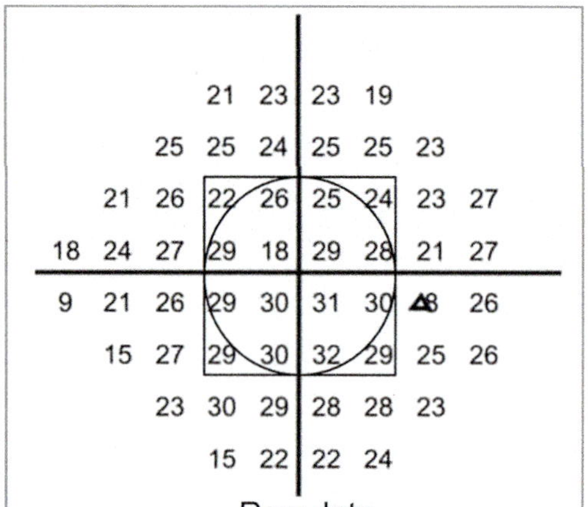

Raw data

There is increase in MD index by -1.12 dB which is significant in a localized scotoma. VFI fell from 92% to 86%. From the grey scale and raw data, the progression is significant in the 10° circle area. Both the vertical and horizontal expansion is well appreciated in the grey scale. Horizontal expansion is well appreciated in the probability plots. Though the sensitivity in the 10° circle area is good, grey scale and probability plots are giving indications to repeat the test with 10-2 point pattern.

Case 39 LE 10-2

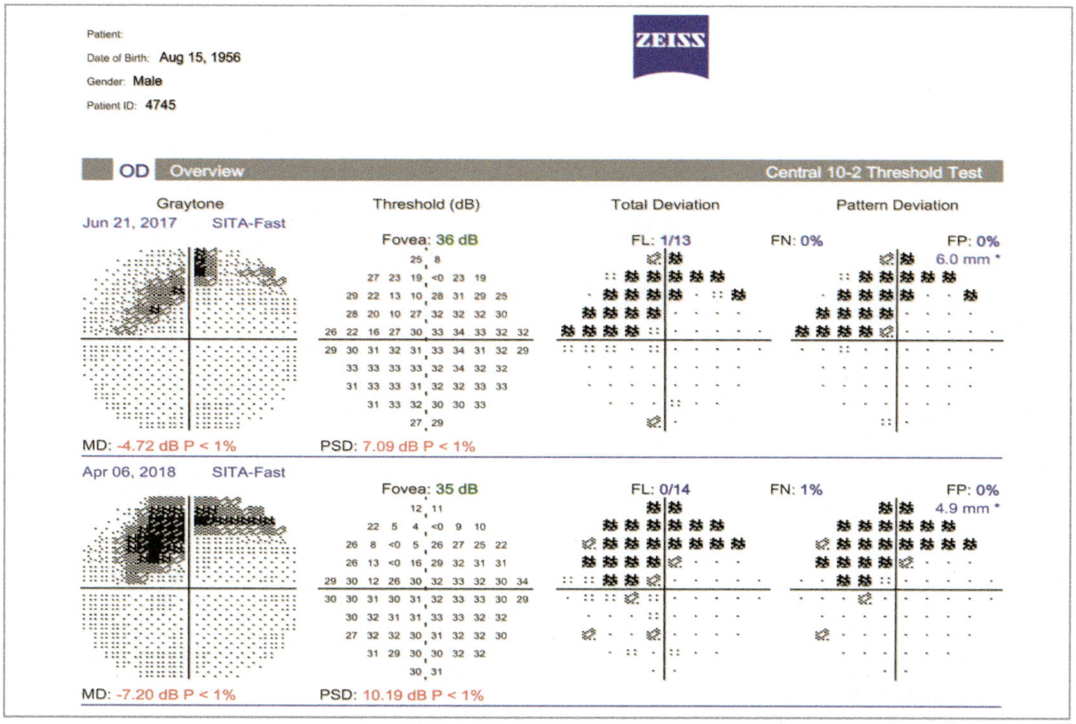

Date	Point pattern strategy	Reliability indices	Fovea	VFI	MD index
21-6-2017	10-2 SITA-Fast	FL 1/13; FP 0%; FN 0%	36 dB		-4.72 dB P < 1%
6-4-2018	10-2 SITA-Fast	FL 0/14; FP 0%; FN 1%	35 dB		-7.20 dB P < 1%

There is increase in MD index by -2.48 dB which is very significant in a localized scotoma. VFI is not calculated in 10-2 printouts. So progression in 10-2 printouts can not be analyzed by VFI based progression analysis. We have to depend on change in MD. The horizontal and vertical progression is well appreciated in the grey scale and raw data, the progression is significant in the 10° circle area. Both the vertical and horizontal expansion is well appreciated in the grey scale. Horizontal expansion is well appreciated in the probability plots. The vertical progression can not be appreciated at these points as they are already represented by P <1%. In this case the progression is more significant in 10° circle area than out side 10° circle. So the most important in progression analysis is proper base line printouts. In this case we require both 24-2 printouts and 10-2 printouts for progression analysis.

Case 39 LE

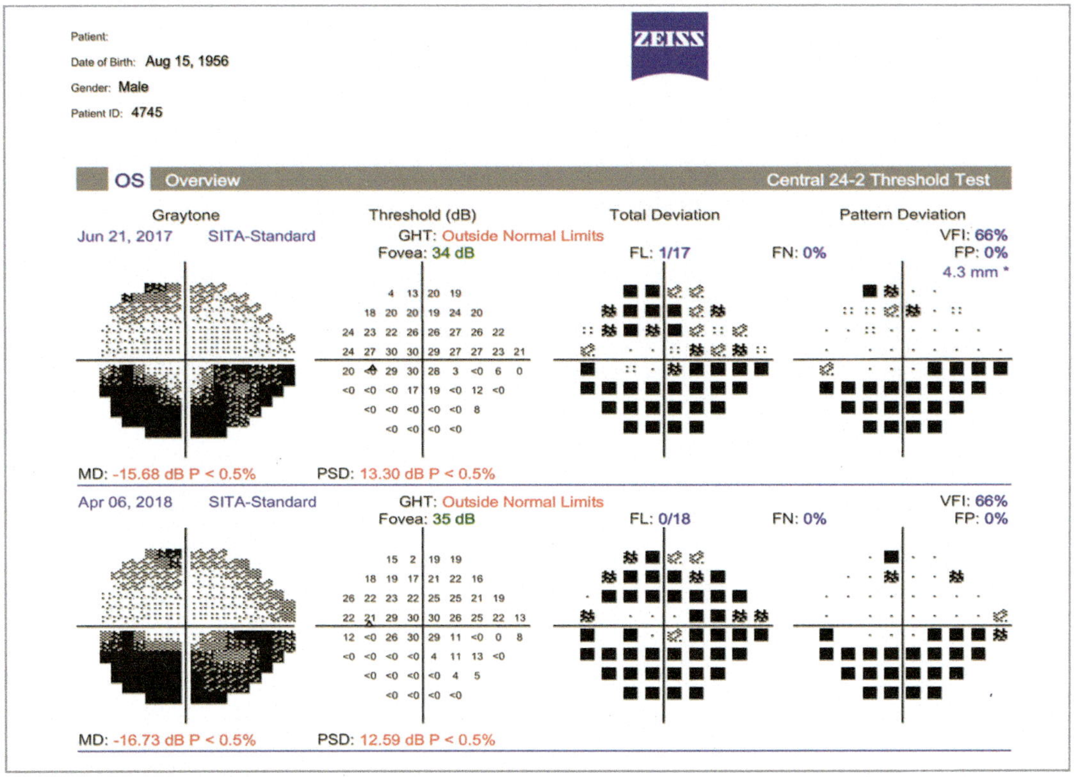

Date	Point pattern strategy	Reliability indices	Fovea	VFI	MD index
21-6-2017	24-2 SITA Standard	FL 1/17; FP 0%; FN 0%	34 dB	66%	-15.68 dB P < 0.5%
6-4-2018	24-2 SITA Standard	FL 0/18; FP 0%; FN 0%	35 dB	66%	-16.73 dB P < 0.5%

The loss of sensitivity points in the probability plots are already represented by P < 0.5%. So vertical progression will not be appreciated in the probability plots, if loss occurs at the same location. Horizontal expansion will be appreciated in the pattern deviation probability plot when TDPP shows generalized depression. The increase in MD index by -1.05 dB.

There is no significant change in the MD index. So glaucoma is stable.

CASE 39 LE 10-2

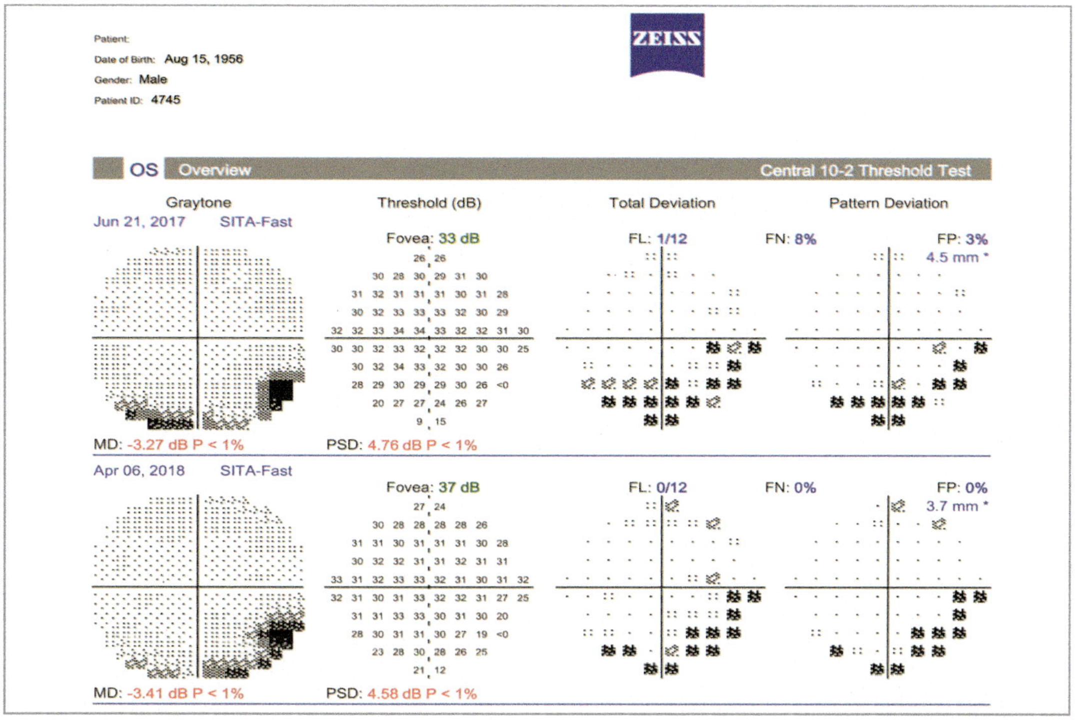

Date	*Point pattern strategy*	*Reliability indices*	*Fovea*	*VFI*	*MD index*
21-6-2017	10-2 SITA Fast	FL 1/12; FP 3%; FN 8%	33 dB		-3.27 dB P < 1%
6-4-2018	10-2 SITA Fast	FL 0/12; FP 0%; FN 0%	37 dB		-3.41 dB P < 1%

There is no significant change in the MD index, VFI index is absent in 10-2 printouts. Glaucoma is stable.

Case 40 RE

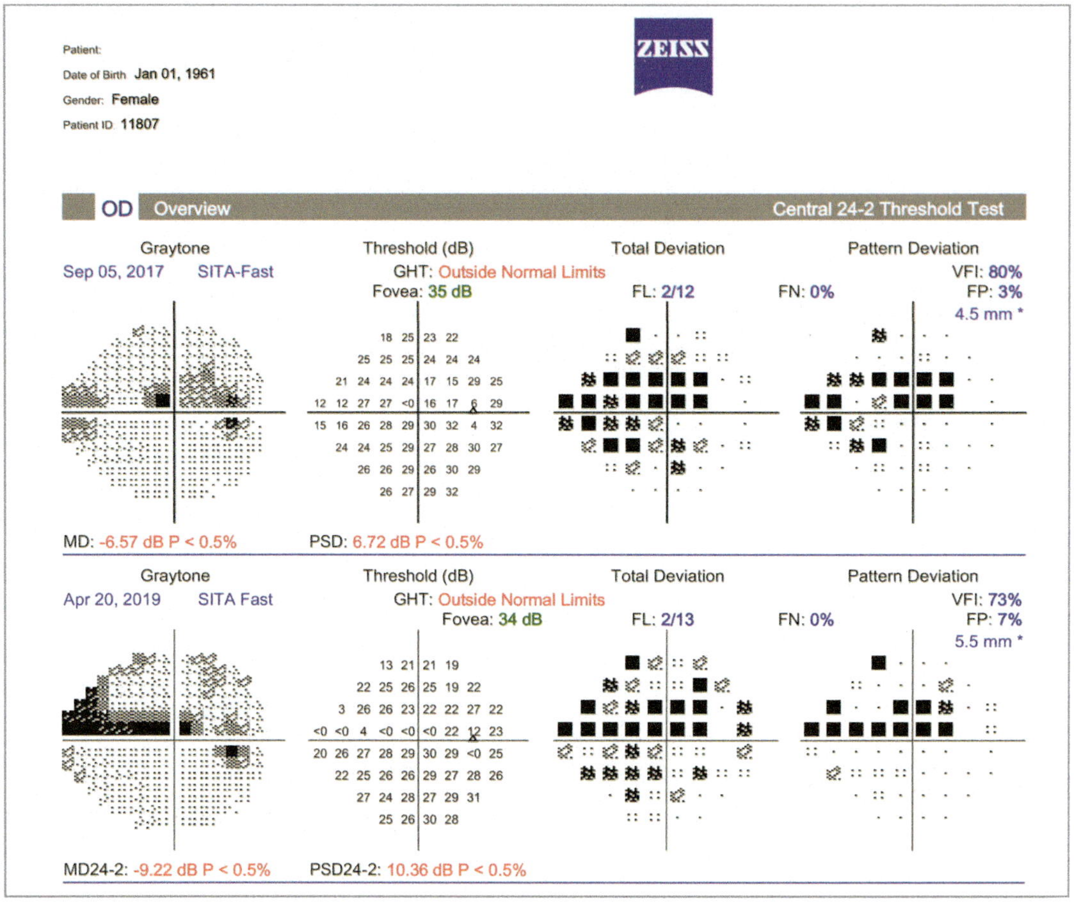

Date	Point pattern strategy	Reliability indices	Fovea	VFI	MD index
5-9-2017	24-2 SITA Fast	FL 2/12; FP 3%; FN 0%	35 dB	80%	-6.57 dB P < 0.5%
20-4-2019	24-2 SITA Fast	FL 2/13; FP 7%; FN 0%	34 dB	73%	-9.22 dB P < 0.5%

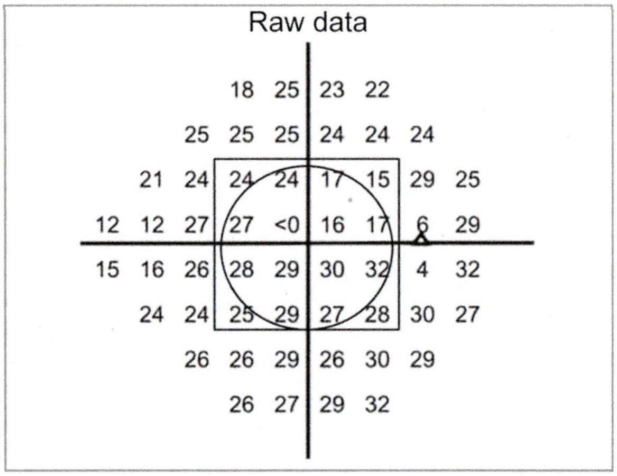

There is increase in MD index by -2.65 dB which is significant in a localized scotoma. VFI fell from 80% to 73%. From the grey scale, the progression is significant in the 10° circle area. Both the vertical and horizontal expansion is well appreciated in the grey scale. The progression is not appreciated in the probability plots. There is an absolute scotoma in the 10° circle area and it is an indication to repeat the test with 10-2 point pattern.

Case 40 RE 10-2

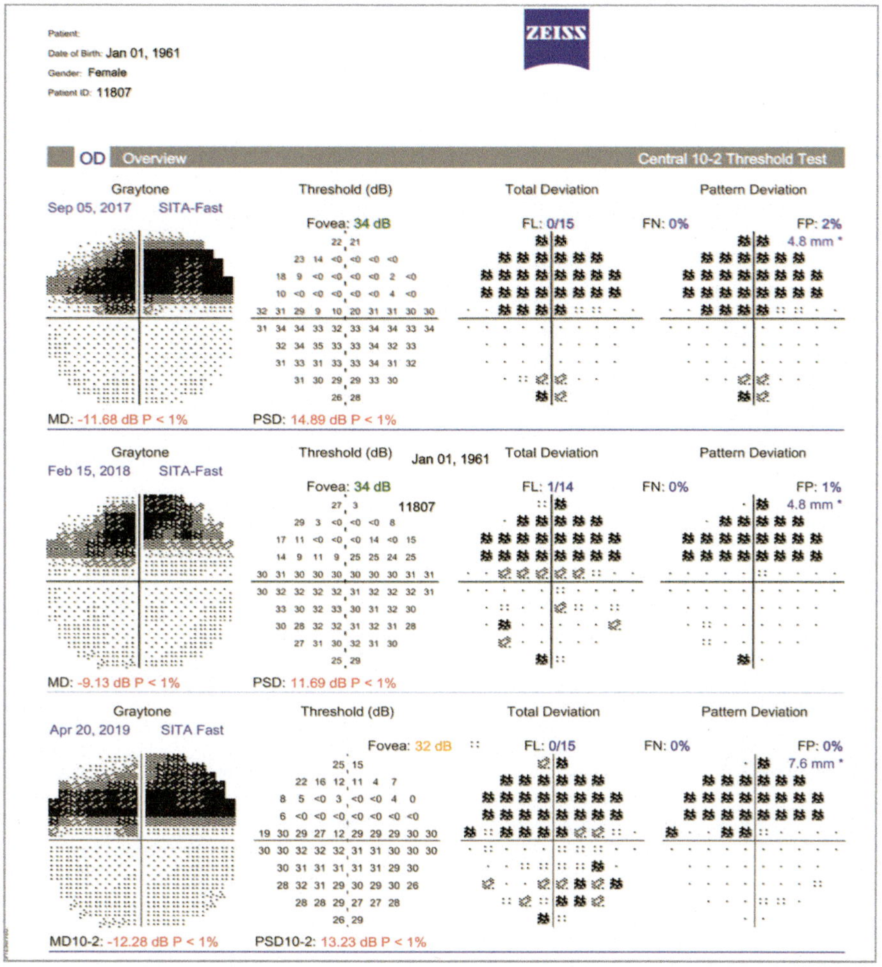

Date	Point pattern strategy	Reliability indices	Fovea	VFI	MD index
5-9-2017	10-2 SITA Fast	FL 0/15; FP 2%; FN 0%	34 dB		-11.68 dB P < 1%
15-2-2018	10-2 SITA Fast	FL 1/14; FP 1%; FN 0%	34 dB		-9.13 dB P < 1%
20-4-2019	10-2 SITA Fast	FL 0/15; FP 0%; FN 0%	32 dB		-12.28 dB P < 1%

There is increase in MD index by 0.60 dB which is not significant. Glaucoma is stable. The grey scale and probability plots are looking similar in all follow-up tests:

2017—24-2 MD -6.57 dB P < 0.5% and 2019—10-2 MD index -11.68 dB P <1%

2019—24-2 MD -9.22 dB P < 0.5% and 2019—10-2 MD index -12.28 dB P <1%

This case belongs to type-3 glaucoma in which we have to keep the target IOP very low. The field defect within 10° circle area is stable and the field defect outside 10° circle area is progressing.

Case 40 LE

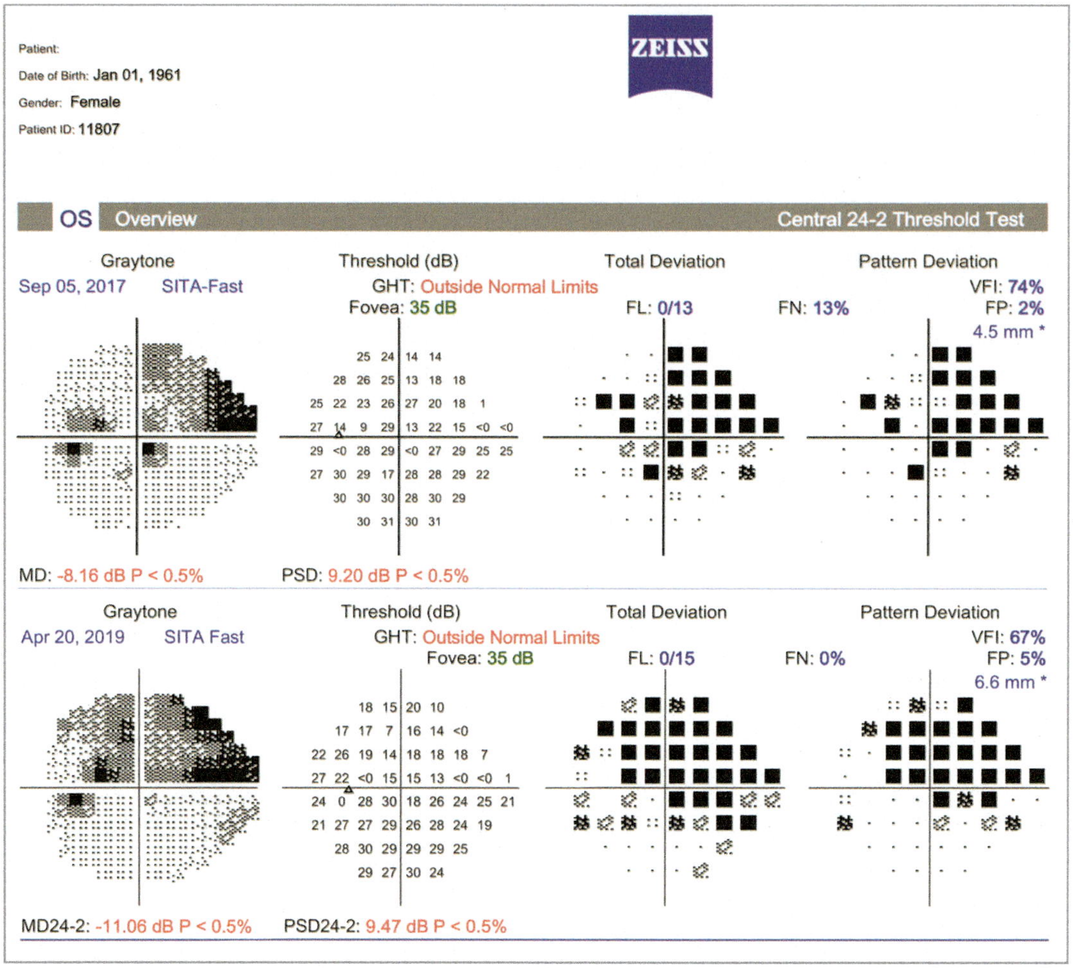

Date	Point pattern strategy	Reliability indices	Fovea	VFI	MD index
5-9-2017	24-2 SITA Fast	FL 0/13; FP 2%; FN 13%	35 dB	74%	8.16 dB P < 0.5%
20-4-2019	24-2 SITA Fast	FL 0/15; FP 5%; FN 0%	35 dB	67%	-11.06 dB P < 0.5%

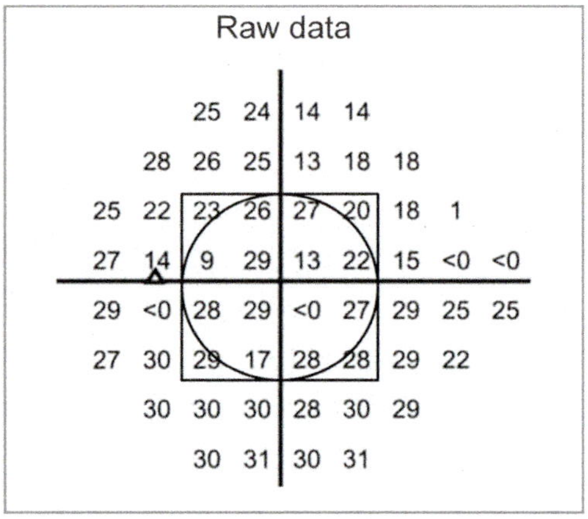

The increase in MD index by -2.90 dB in a localized field defect is very significant and the VFI came down from 74% to 67%. Glaucoma is not stable. The progression of glaucoma is mainly horizontal progression. Which is appreciated in both grey scale and probability plots. Further loss of sensitivity at the points which are already represented by P < 0.5% (black squares) in the probability plots (vertical progression) will not be appreciated in the probability plots. Horizontal expansion will be appreciated in the pattern deviation probability plot when TDPP shows generalized depression.

Case 40 LE 10-2

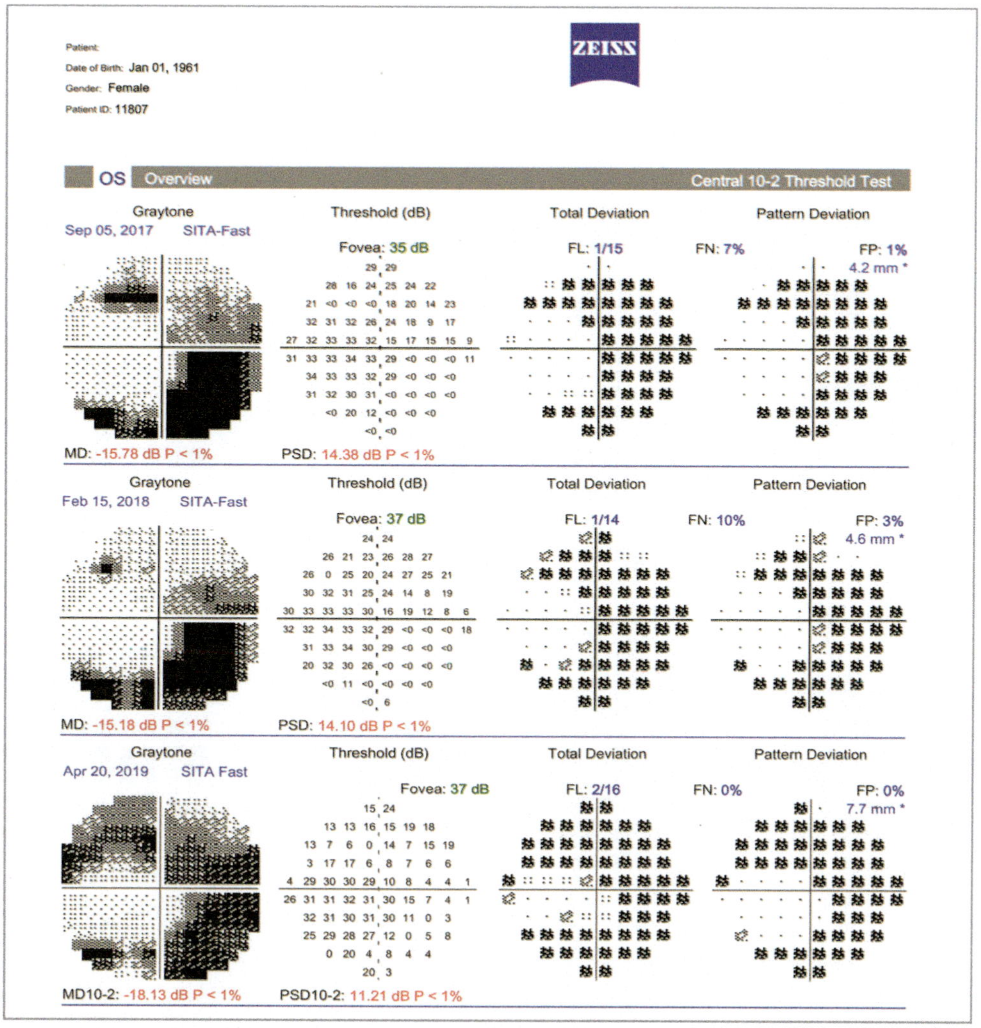

Date	Point pattern strategy	Reliability indices	Fovea	VFI	MD index
5-9-2017	10-2 SITA Fast	FL 1/15; FP 1%; FN 7%	35 dB		-15.78 dB P < 1%
15-2-2018	10-2 SITA Fast	FL 1/14; FP 3%; FN 10%	37 dB		-15.18 dB P < 1%
20-4-2019	10-2 SITA Fast	FL 2/16; FP 0%; FN 0%	37 dB		-18.13 dB P < 1%

There is increase in MD index by-2.35 from 2017 to 2019 dB which is significant in a localized scotoma. VFI is not calculated in 10-2 printouts. In the grey scale the vertical and horizontal progression is well appreciated. In this case we require both 24-2 and 10-2 printouts for progression analysis. Progression is occurring in both 24-2 and 10-2 point patterns. Since progression is taking place in 10° circle area, we should aim for low target IOP or, early filtering surgery is indicated.

Case 41 RE

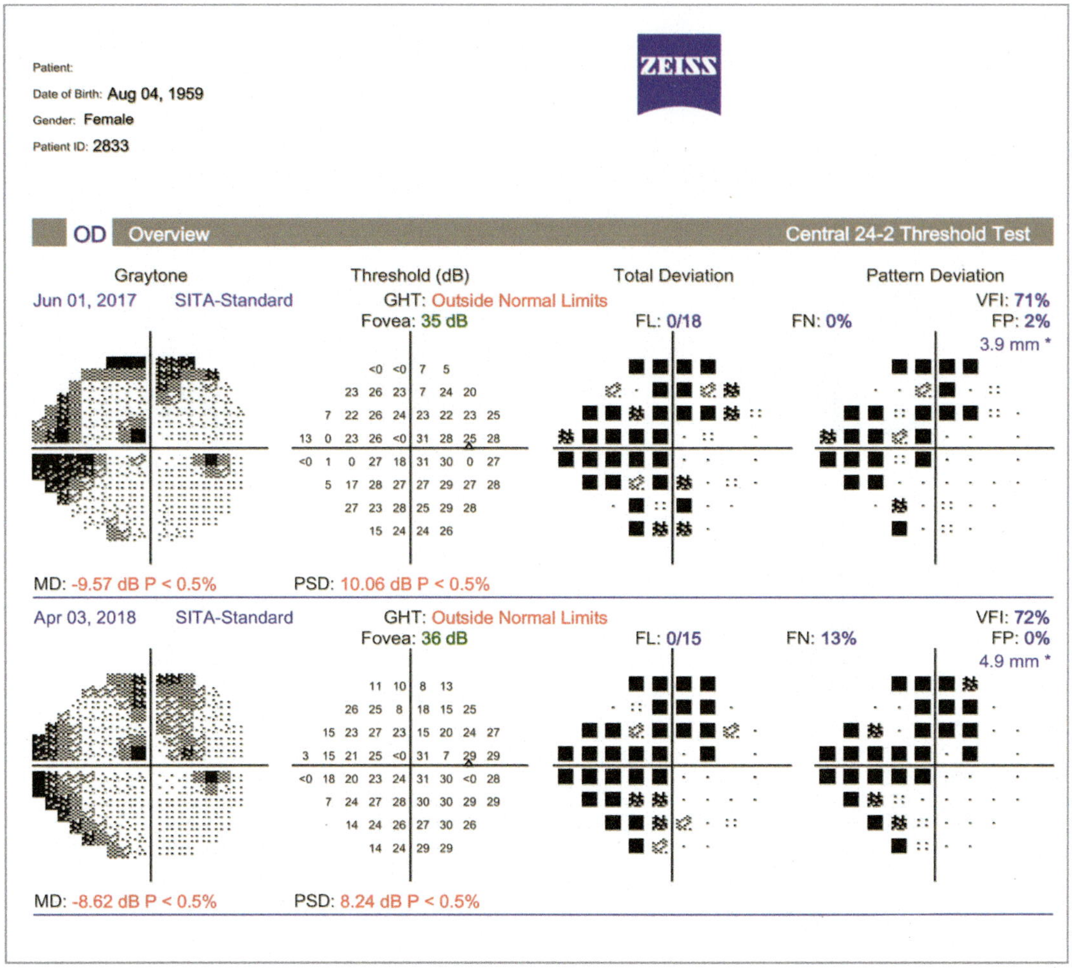

Date	Point pattern strategy	Reliability indices	Fovea	VFI	MD index
1-6-2017	24-2 SITA Standard	FL 0/18; FP 2%; FN 0%	35 dB	71%	-9.57 dB P < 0.5%
3-4-2018	24-2 SITA Standard	FL 0/15; FP 0%; FN 13%	36 dB	72%	-8.62 dB P < 0.5%

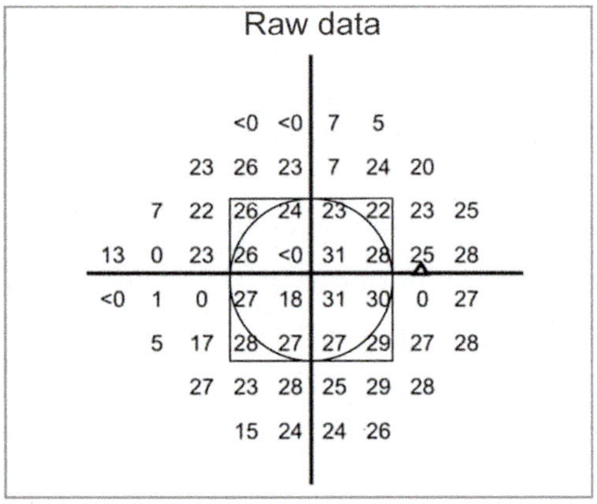

2017—24-2 MD -9.57 dB P < 0.5%

2018—24-2 MD -8.62 dB P < 0.5%

The MD index became better in 2018 and VFI is stable.

Grey scale, probability plots and raw data are giving indications to repeat the test with 10-2 point pattern.

Case 41 RE 10-2

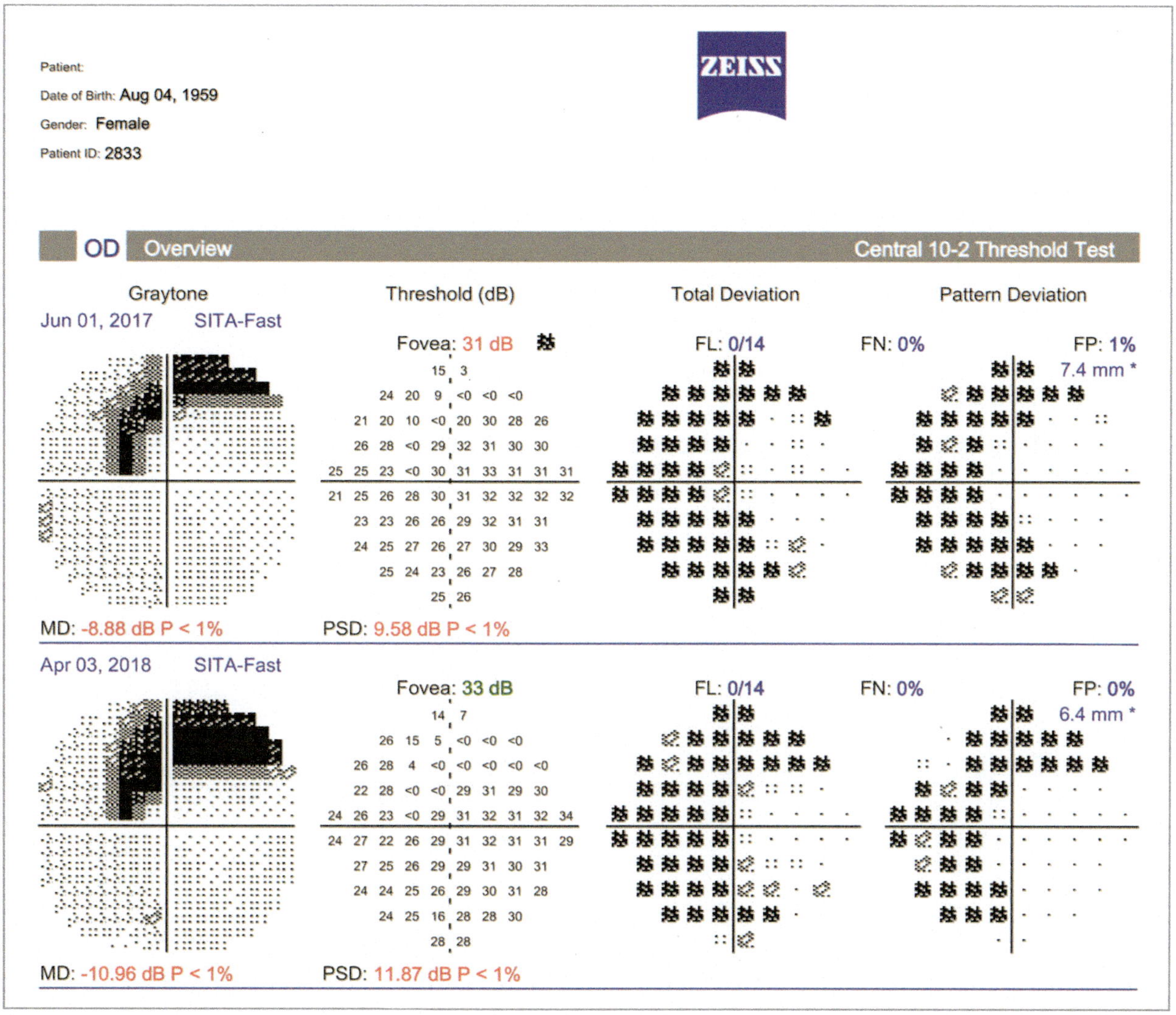

Date	Point pattern strategy	Reliability indices	Fovea	VFI	MD index
1-6-2017	10-2 SITA Fast	FL 0/14; FP 1%; FN 0%	31 dB		-8.88 dB P < 1%
3-4-2018	10-2 SITA Fast	FL 0/14; FP 0%; FN 0%	33 dB		-10.96 dB P < 1%

2017—10-2 MD index -8.88 dB P < 1%

2018—10-2 MD index -10.96 dB P < 1%

There is increase in MD index by 2.08 dB which is significant in a localized scotoma. VFI is absent in 10-2 printouts. In this case field defect outside 10° circle area is very stable and the field defect in 10° circle area is progressing. We should keep target IOP very low.

Case 41 LE

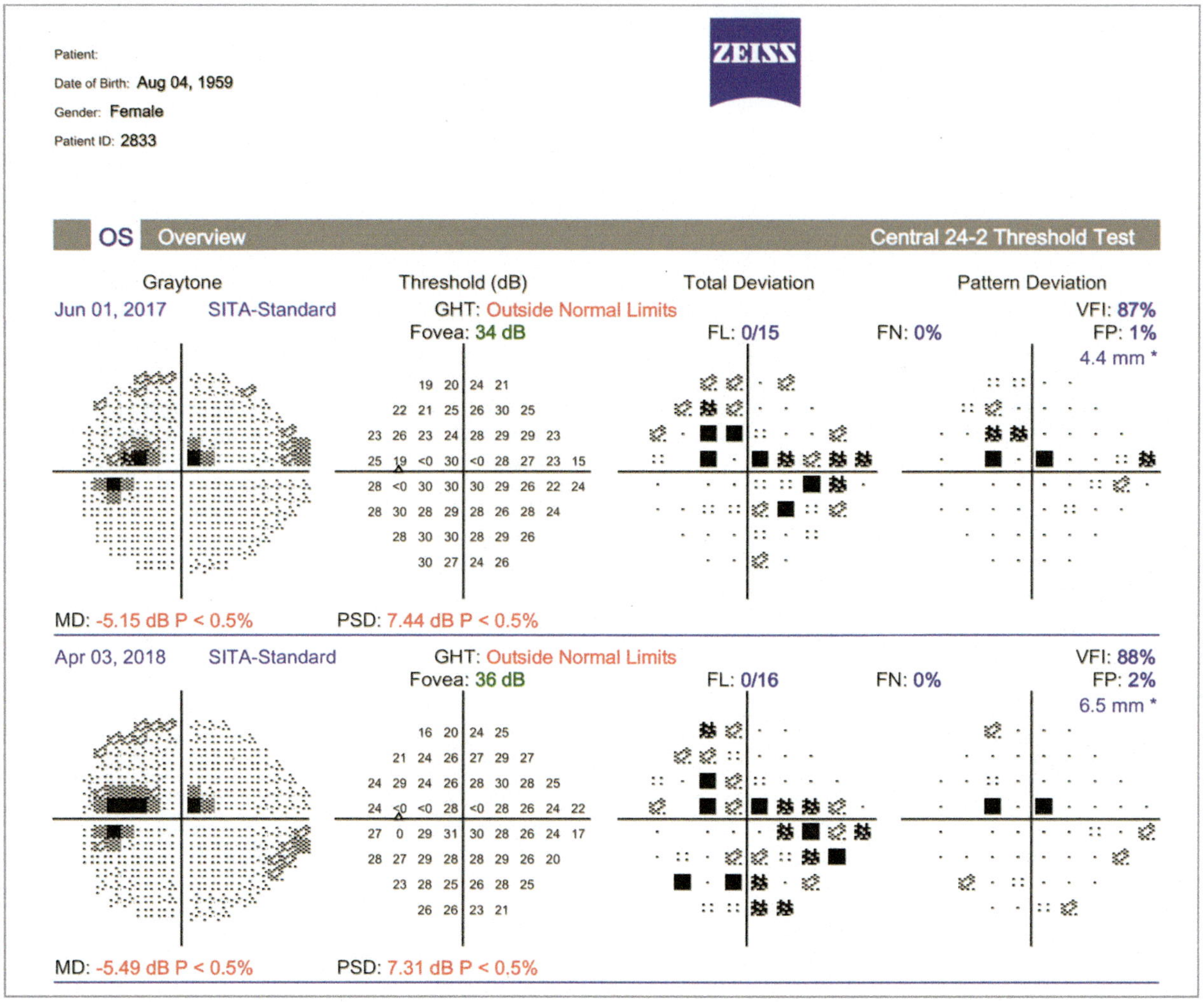

Date	Point pattern strategy	Reliability indices	Fovea	VFI	MD index
1-6-2017	24-2 SITA Standard	FL 0/15; FP 1%; FN 0%	34 dB	87%	-5.15 dB P < 0.5%
3-4-2018	24-2 SITA Standard	FL 0/16; FP 2%; FN 0%	36 dB	88%	-5.49 dB P < 0.5%

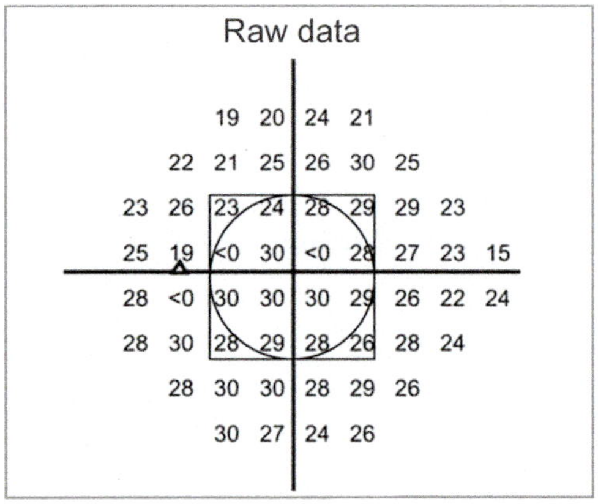

2017—24-2 MD -5.15 dB P < 0.5%

2018—24-2 MD -5.49 dB P < 0.5%

No change in VFI.

Almost there is no progression.

Grey scale, probability plots and raw data are giving indications to repeat the test with 10-2 point pattern.

Case 41 LE 10-2

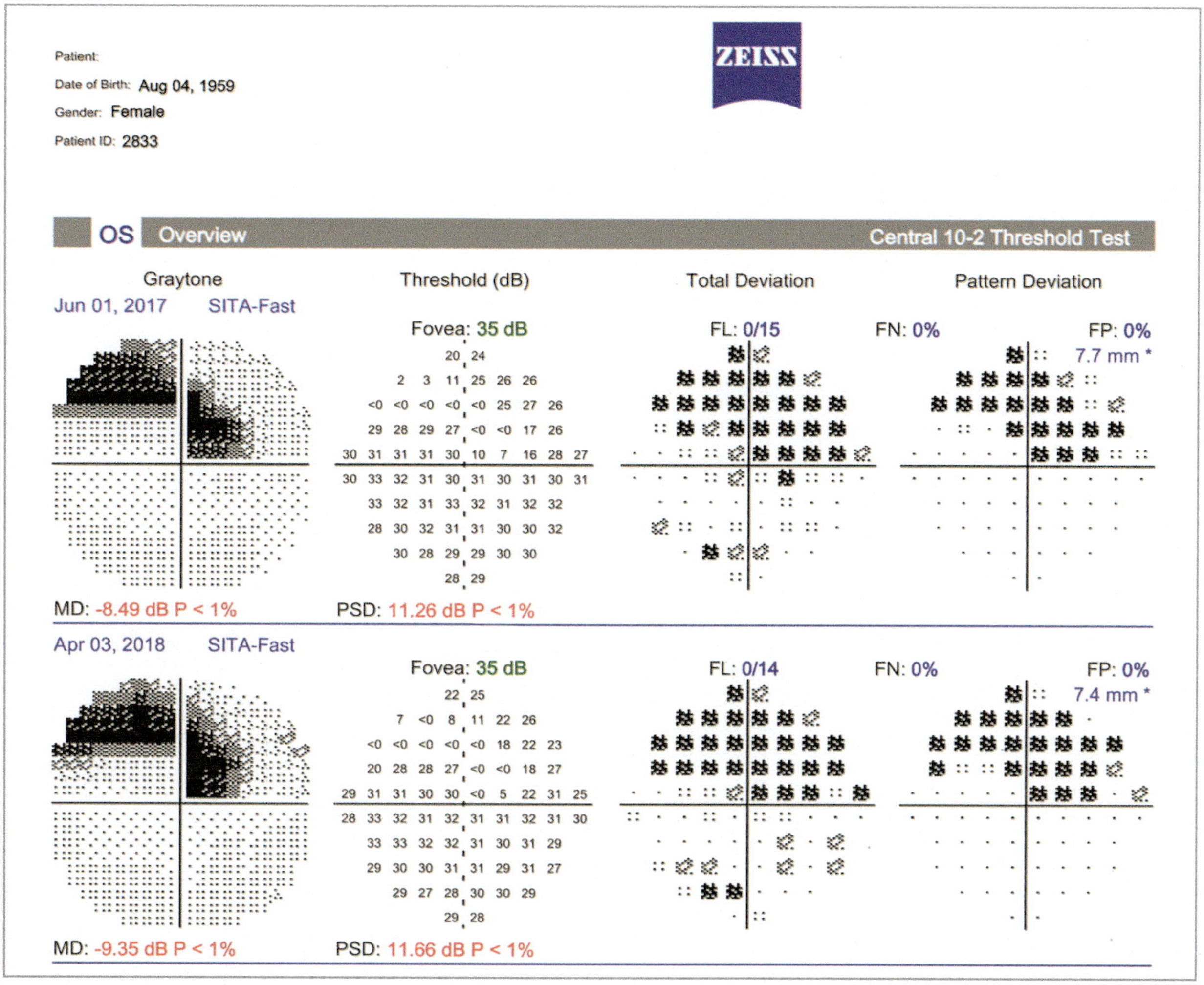

Date	Point pattern strategy	Reliability indices	Fovea	VFI	MD index
1-6-2017	10-2 SITA Fast	FL 0/15; FP 0%; FN 0%	35 dB		-8.49 dB P < 1%
3-4-2018	10-2 SITA Fast	FL 0/14; FP 0%; FN 0%	35 dB		-9.35 dB P < 1%

2017—10-2 MD index -8.49 dB P < 1%

2018—10-2 MD index -9.35 dB P < 1%

Increase in MD index is 0.86 dB which is a significant number in a localized scotoma.

In this case field defect outside 10° circle area is very stable and the field defect in 10° circle area is progressing. We should keep target IOP very low.

Case 42 RE

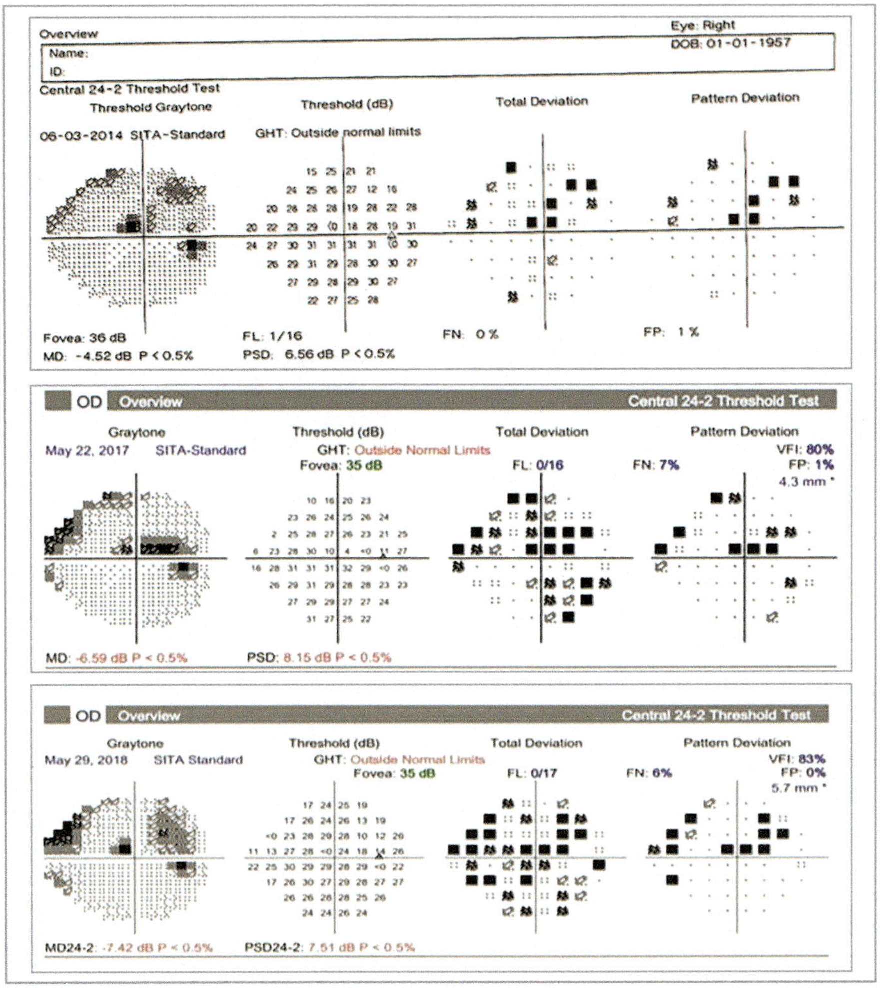

Date	Point pattern strategy	Reliability indices	Fovea	VFI	MD index
2014	24-2 SITA Standard	FL 1/16; FP 1%; FN 0%	36 dB		-4.52 dB P < 0.5%
22-5-2017	24-2 SITA Standard	FL 0/16; FP 1%; FN 7%	35 dB	80%	-6.59 dB P < 0.5%
29-5-2018	24-2 SITA Standard	FL 0/17; FP 0%; FN 6%	35 dB	83%	-7.42 dB P < 0.5%

2014—24-2 MD index -4.52 dB P < 0.5%

2018—24-2 MD index -7.42 dB P < 0.5%. Increase in MD index by -2.90 dB which is a significant number in a localized scotoma.

Grey scale, probability plots and raw data are giving indications that there is a definite progression in macular area and giving indications to repeat the test with 10-2 point pattern.

Case 42 RE 10-2

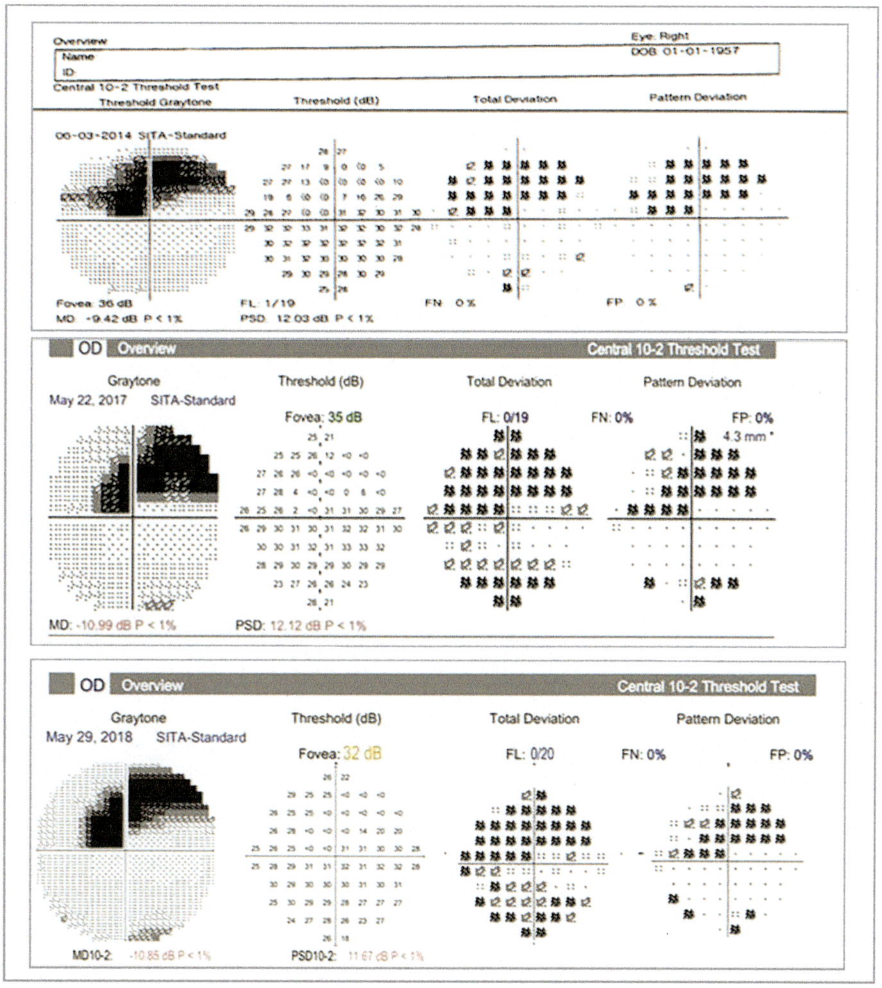

Date	Point pattern strategy	Reliability indices	Fovea	VFI	MD index
2014	10-2 SITA Standard	FL 1/19; FP 0%; FN 0%	36 dB		-9.42 dB P < 1%
22-5-2017	10-2 SITA Standard	FL 0/19; FP 0%; FN 0%	35 dB		-10.99 dB P < 1%
29-5-2018	10-2 SITA Standard	FL 0/20; FP 0%; FN 0%	32 dB		-10.85 dB P < 1%

2014—10-2 MD index -9.42 dB P < 1%

2018—10-2 MD index -10-85 dB P < 1%

There is increase in MD index by -1.43 dB. VFI is absent in 10-2 printouts. In this case the progression of the field is appreciated in the grey scale and to some extent in the probability plots. In this case the location of the field defect is very important. The field defect started very close to fixation. The progression is more in the macular area. We should aim for low target IOP to arrest progression. In this case we require both 24-2 and 10-2 printouts as baseline fields.

Case 42 LE

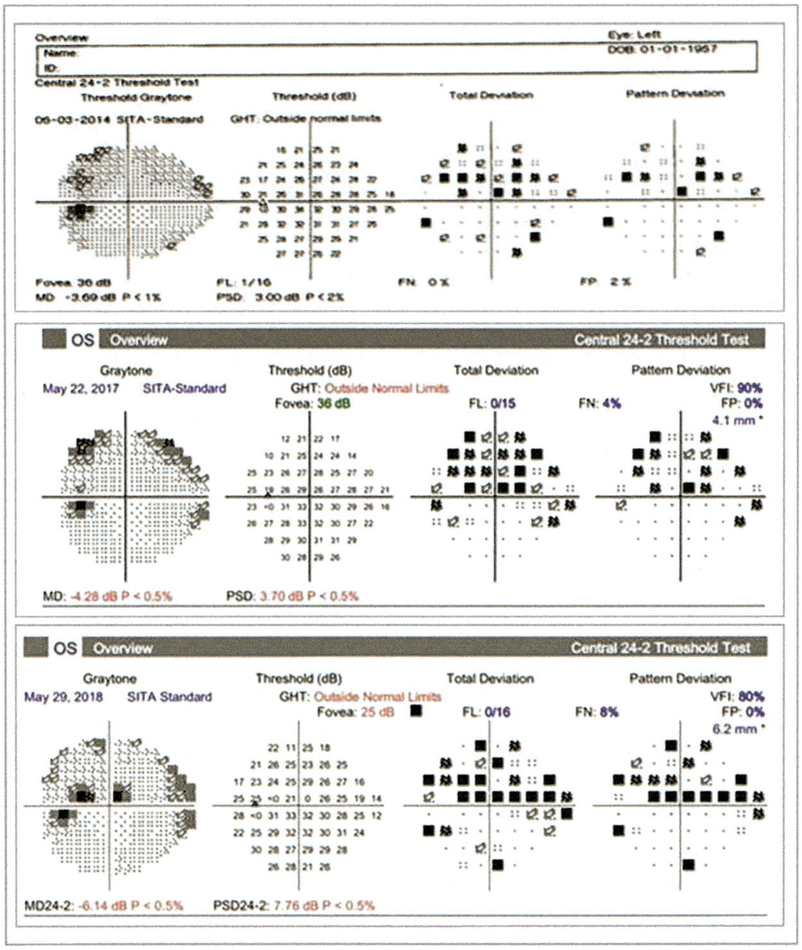

Date	Point pattern strategy	Reliability indices	Fovea	VFI	MD index
May 2014	24-2 SITA Standard	FL 1/18; FP 2%; FN 0%	36 dB		-3.69 dB P < 1%
22-5-2017	24-2 SITA Standard	FL 0/15; FP 4%; FN 0%	36 dB	90%	-4.26 dB P < 0.5%
29-5-2018	24-2 SITA Standard	FL 0/16; FP 0%; FN 8%	25 dB	80%	-6.14 dB P < 0.5%

2014—24-2 MD -3.69 dB P < 1%

2018—24-2 MD 6.14 dB P < 0.5%. Increase in MD index by -2.45 dB which is a significant number in a localized scotoma.

Grey scale, probability plots and raw data are giving indications that there is a definite progression in macular area and giving indications to repeat the test with 10-2 point pattern.

Case 42 LE 10-2

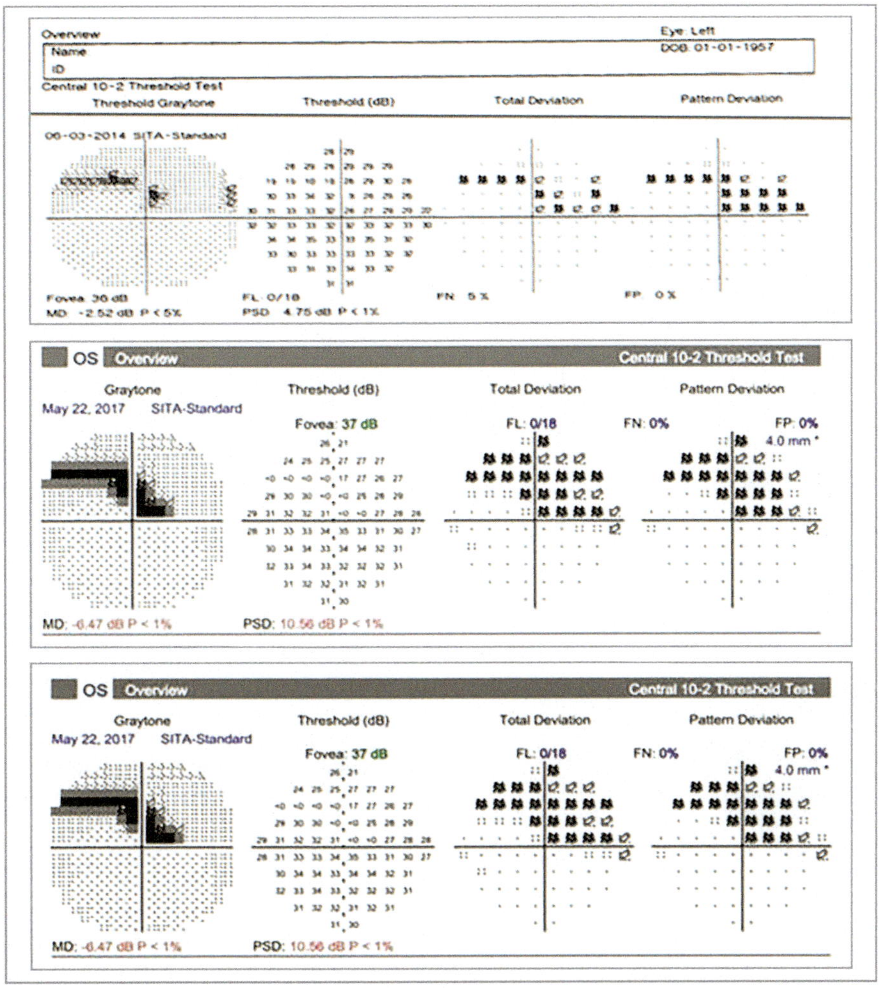

Date	Point pattern strategy	Reliability indices	Fovea	VFI	MD index
2014	10-2 SITA Standard	FL 0/18; FP 0%; FN 5%	36 dB		-2.52 dB P < 5%
22-5-2017	10-2 SITA Standard	FL 0/18; FP 0%; FN 0%	37 dB		-6.47 dB P < 1%
29-5-2018	10-2 SITA Standard	FL 0/19; FP 0%; FN 0%	32 dB		-6.74 dB P < 1%

2017—10-2 MD index -2.52 dB P < 1%

2018—10-2 MD index -6.74 dB P < 1%

There is increase in MD index by -4.22 dB which is significant in a localized scotoma. VFI is absent in 10-2 printouts. In this case the progression of the field is appreciated in the grey scale and to some extent in the probability plots. In this case the progression is more in the macular area. In this case we require both 24-2 and 10-2 printouts as baseline fields.

Case 43 LE

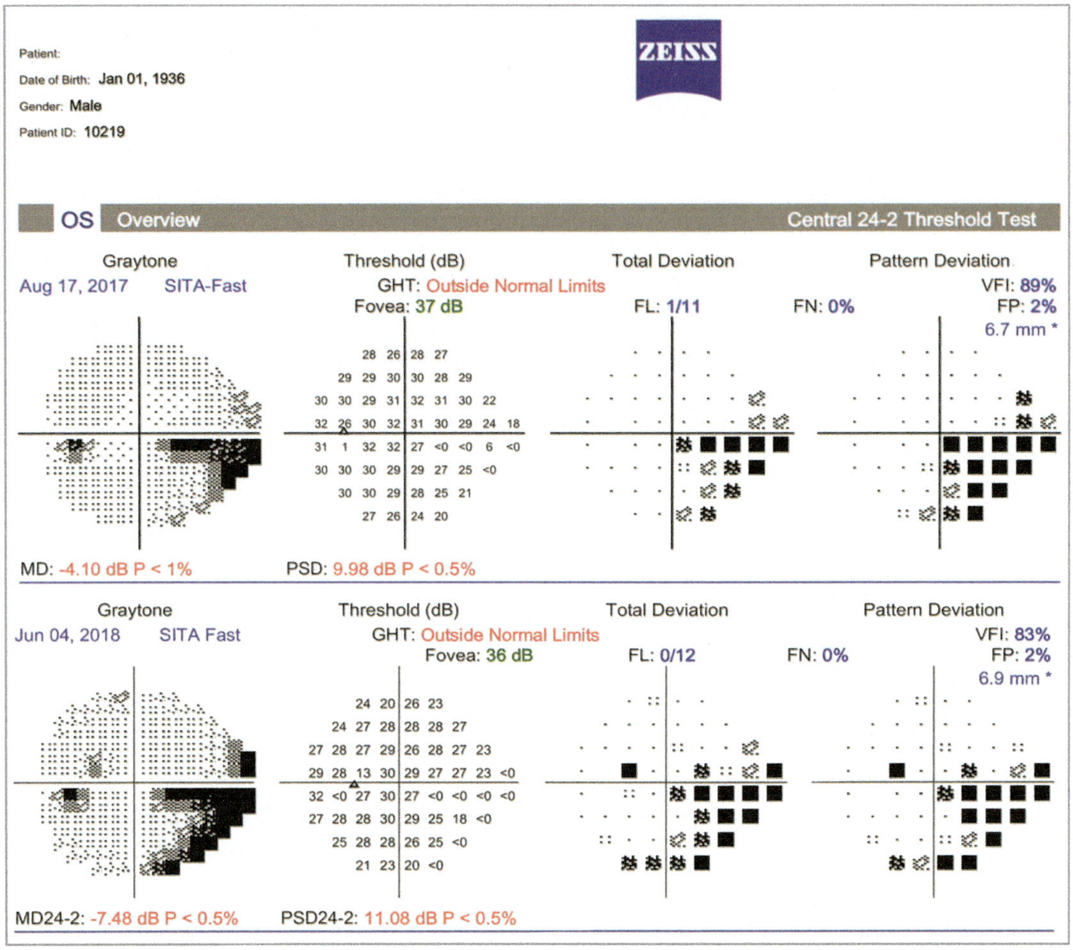

Date	*Point pattern strategy*	*Reliability indices*	*Fovea*	*VFI*	*MD index*
17-8-2017	24-2 SITA Fast	FL 1/11; FP 2%; FN 0%	37 dB	89%	-4.10 dB P < 1%
4-6-2018	24-2 SITA Fast	FL 0/12; FP 2%; FN 0%	36 dB	83%	-7.48 dB P < 0.5%

Aug 2017—24-2 MD -4.10 dB P < 1%

June 2018—24-2 MD -7.48 dB P < 0.5% increase in MD index by -3.38 dB which is a significant number in a localized scotoma.

Grey scale is giving indications that there is a definite horizontal progression. The probability plots are almost similar. No clue from the probability plots regarding progression. The most important decision in this case is asking for the repetition of the test with 10-2 point pattern. If the loss of sensitivity is severe even at one point among the 16 points in the 10° circle area, we should repeat the test with 10-2 point pattern. In 24-2, there is huge bare area between 3° and 9° circle points in the 10° circle area.

Case 43 LE 10-2

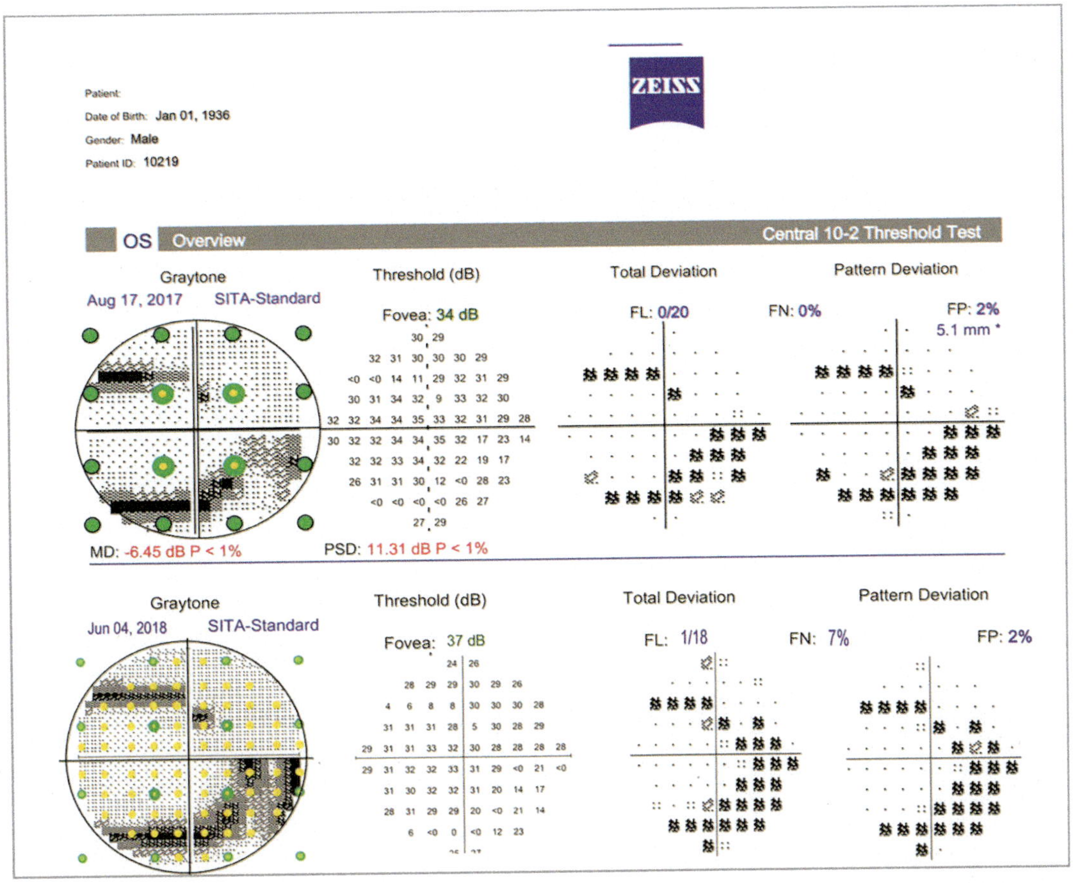

Date	Point pattern strategy	Reliability indices	Fovea	VFI	MD index
17-8-2017	10-2 SITA Standard	FL 0/20; FP 2%; FN 0%	34 dB		-6.45 dB P < 1%
4-6-2018	10-2 SITA Standard	FL 1/18; FP 2%; FN 7%	37 dB		-8.63 dB P < 1%

Aug. 2017—10-2 MD -6.45 dB P < 1%; June 2018—10-2 MD -8.63 dB P < 1%. Increase in MD index by -2.18 dB which is a significant number in a localized scotoma. Biarcuate scotoma in 10° circle & close to fixation requires low target IOP to arrest progression.

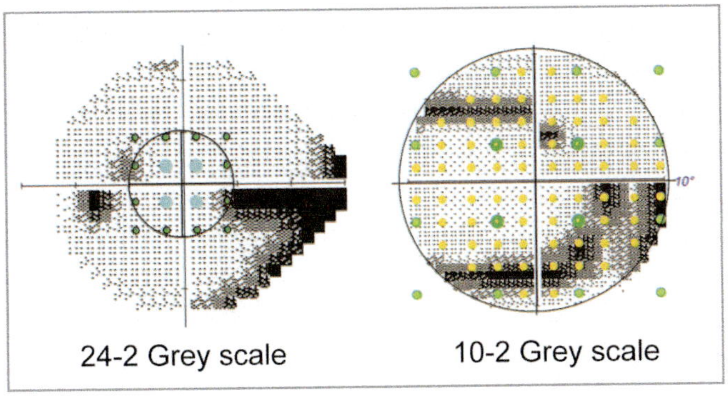

In this case a new scotoma started between 3° and 9° circle points and progressed between these points. Since there are no points in between 3° and 9° points in 24-2 point pattern, the scotoma is not appreciated in the grey scale and probability plots of 24 -2 point pattern. Since the new scotoma is also progressing, we have to keep the target IOP more low or we have to go for filtering surgery.

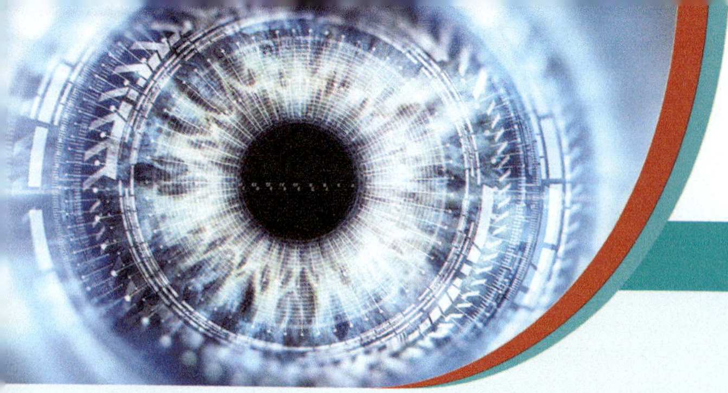

CHAPTER

11

Single Field Analysis Printouts of Clinically Important Cases

In this chapter I am presenting six cases of visual field defects of clinical importance.

Case 44	A case of AION
Case 45	A case of optic neuritis
Case 46	A case of neuroretinitis
Case 47	Head injury with optic nerve and brain tissue damage
Case 48	A case of papilledema
Case 49	Coloboma of optic nerve head and retina
Case 50	Occlusion of upper branch of central retinal artery
Case 51	A case of right posterior cerebral artery occlusion
Case 52	Bitemporal hemianopia.

Case 44 AION (Right Eye)

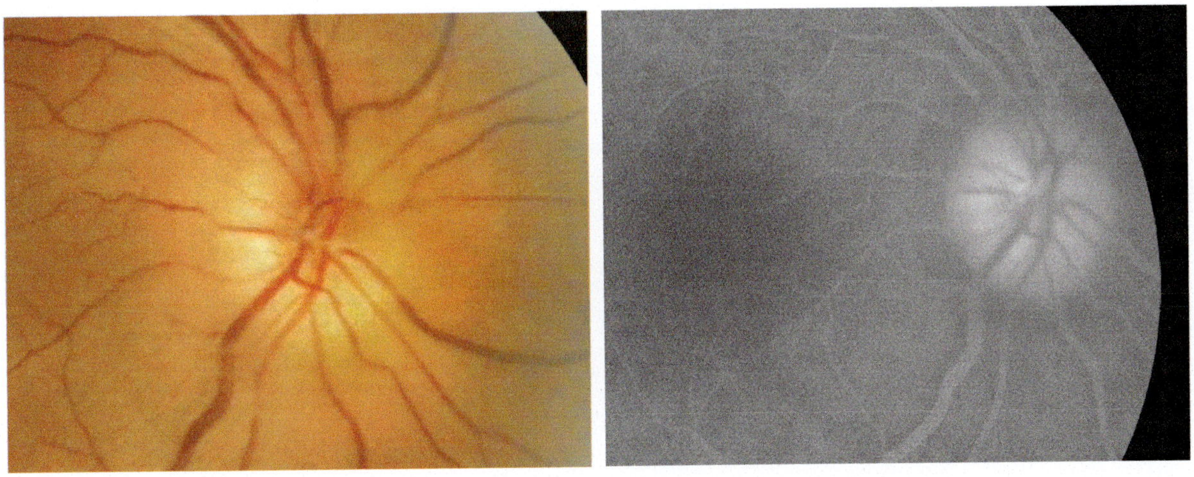

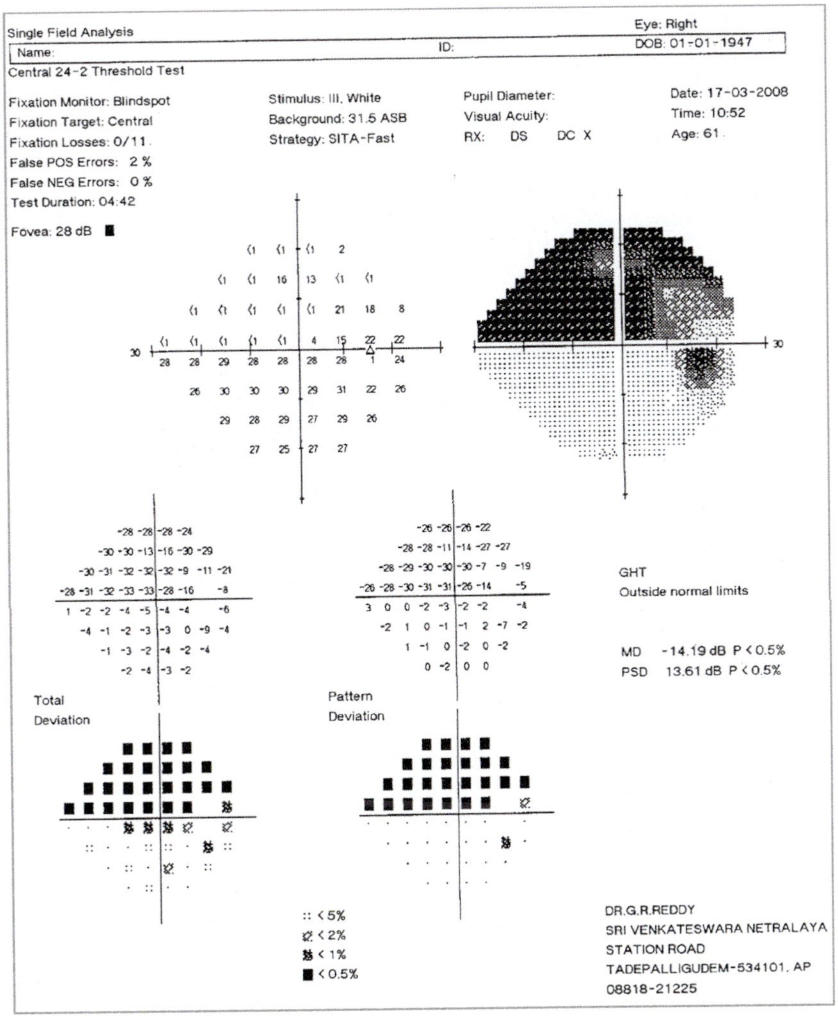

Single Field Analysis
Eye: Right
Name:
ID:
DOB: 01-01-1947
Central 24-2 Threshold Test

Fixation Monitor: Blindspot
Fixation Target: Central
Fixation Losses: 0/11
False POS Errors: 2 %
False NEG Errors: 0 %
Test Duration: 04:42

Stimulus: III, White
Background: 31.5 ASB
Strategy: SITA-Fast

Pupil Diameter:
Visual Acuity:
RX: DS DC X

Date: 17-03-2008
Time: 10:52
Age: 61

Fovea: 28 dB

<1 <1 <1 2
<1 <1 16 13 <1 <1
<1 <1 <1 <1 <1 21 18 8
<1 <1 <1 <1 <1 4 15 22 22
30 28 28 29 28 28 28 28 1 24
26 30 30 30 29 31 22 26
29 28 29 27 29 26
27 25 27 27

-28 -28 -28 -24
-30 -30 -13 -16 -30 -29
-30 -31 -32 -32 -32 -9 -11 -21
-28 -31 -32 -33 -33 -28 -16 -8
1 -2 -2 -4 -5 -4 -4 -6
-4 -1 -2 -3 -3 0 -9 -4
-1 -3 -2 -4 -2 -4
-2 -4 -3 -2

Total
Deviation

-26 -26 -26 -22
-28 -28 -11 -14 -27 -27
-28 -29 -30 -30 -30 -7 -9 -19
-26 -28 -30 -31 -31 -26 -14 -5
3 0 0 -2 -3 -2 -2 -4
-2 1 0 -1 -1 2 -7 -2
1 -1 0 -2 0 -2
0 -2 0 0

Pattern
Deviation

GHT
Outside normal limits

MD -14.19 dB P < 0.5%
PSD 13.61 dB P < 0.5%

:: < 5%
< 2%
< 1%
■ < 0.5%

DR.G.R.REDDY
SRI VENKATESWARA NETRALAYA
STATION ROAD
TADEPALLIGUDEM-534101, AP
08818-21225

Pale disk edema and altitudinal field defects are suggestive of anterior ischemic optic neuropathy (AION). Later the diagnosis was confirmed by angiogram.

Case 45 Optic neuritis

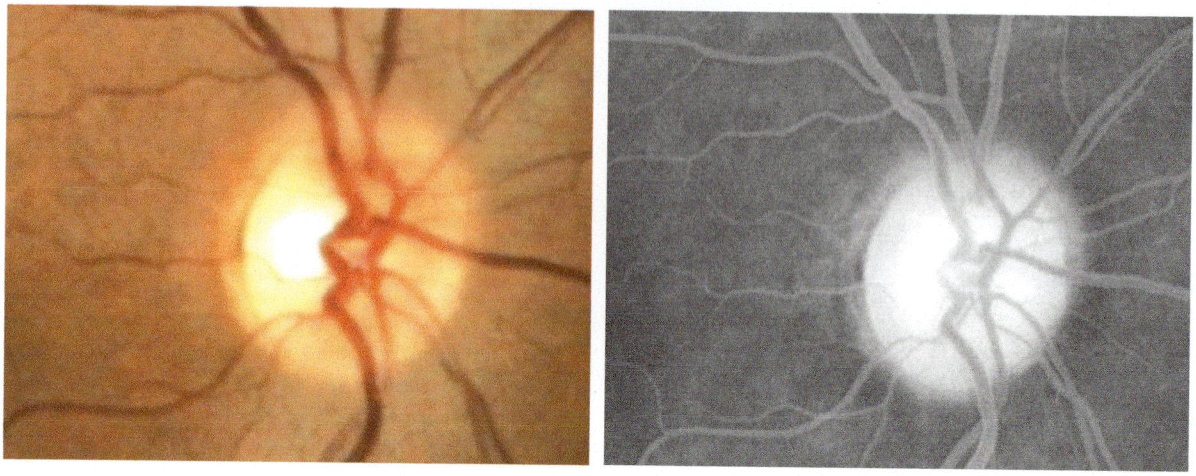

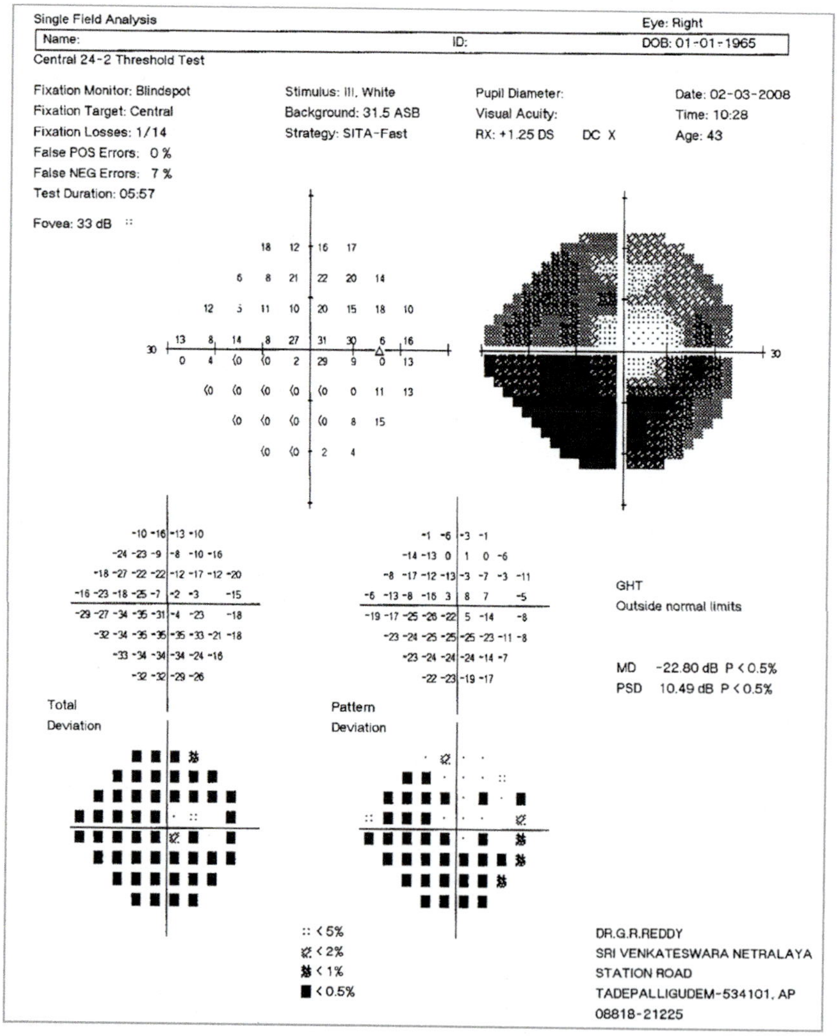

Optic neuritis presenting with irregular generalized depression with MD index -22.80 dB.

Case 46 Neuroretinitis

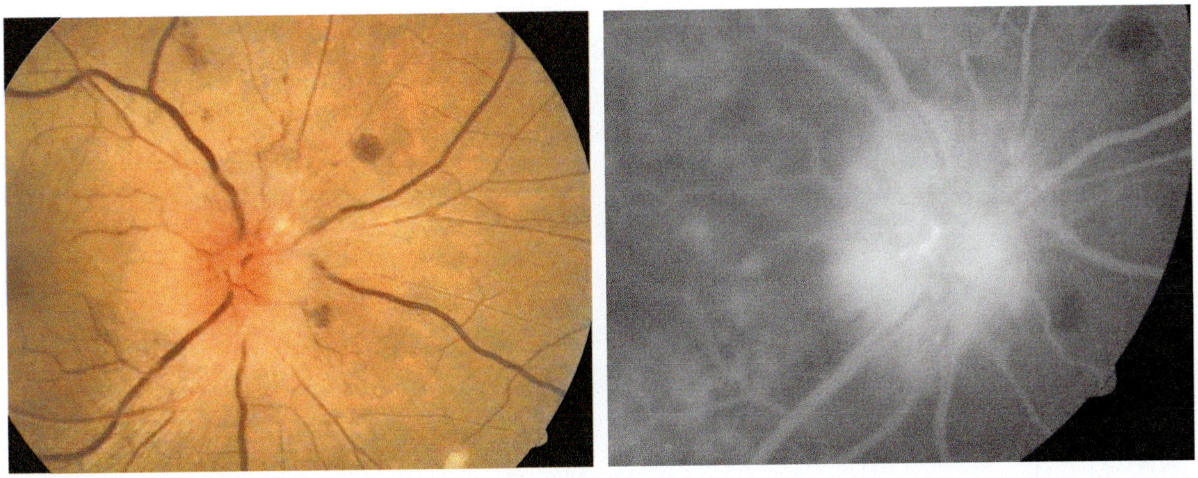

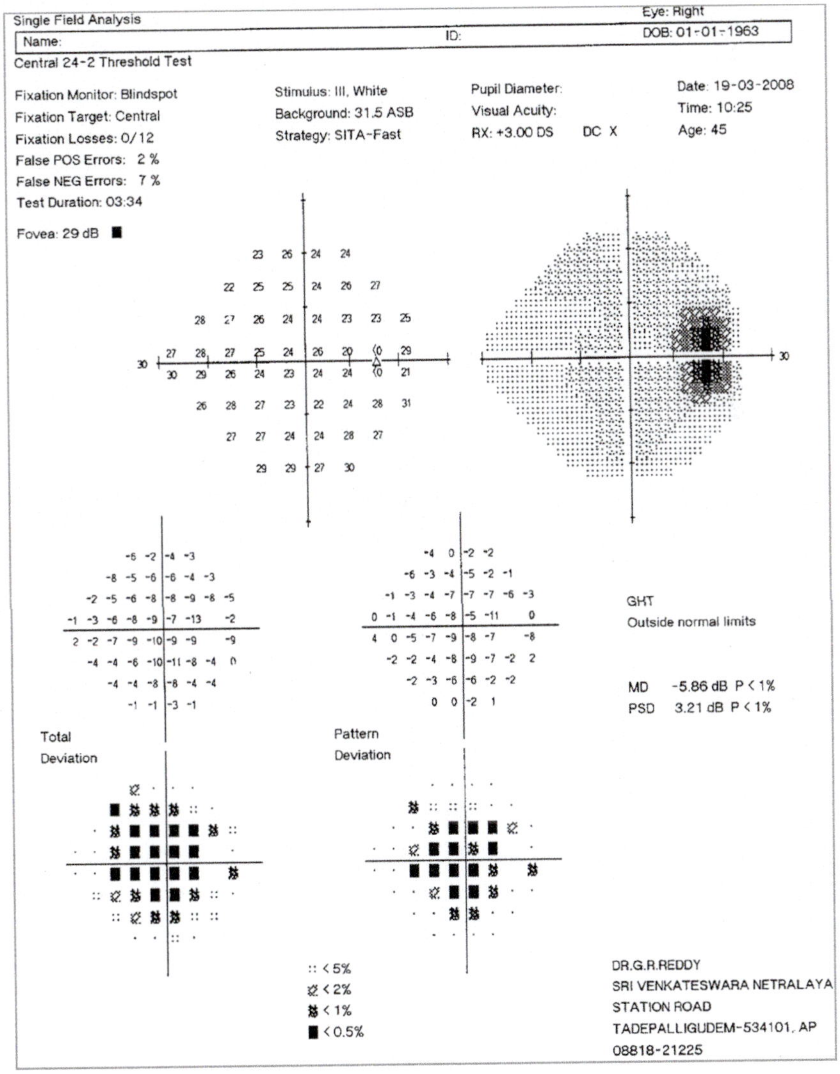

Central relative scotoma in a case of neuroretinitis.

In this case of neuroretinitis, we are seeing the involvement of central macular fibers. Note that it is a relative scotoma.

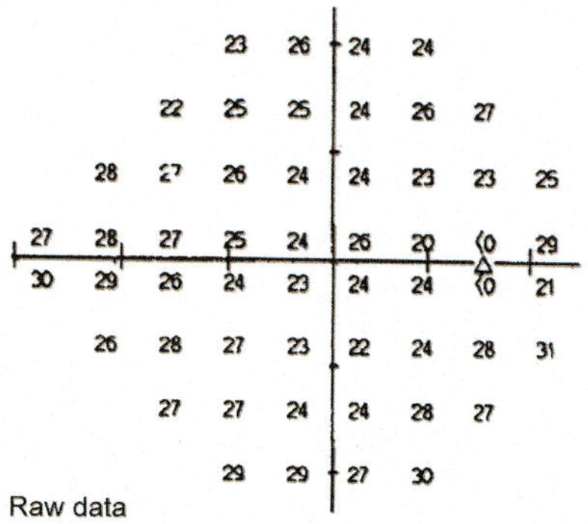

Raw data

In the raw data, the sensitivity is around 25 dB and there is no absolute scotoma in the raw data.

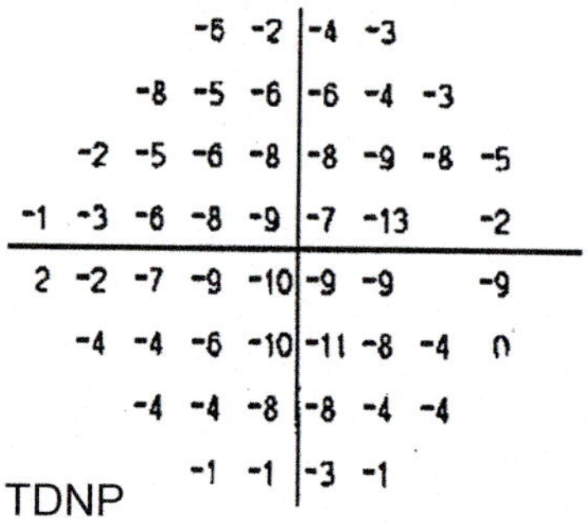

TDNP

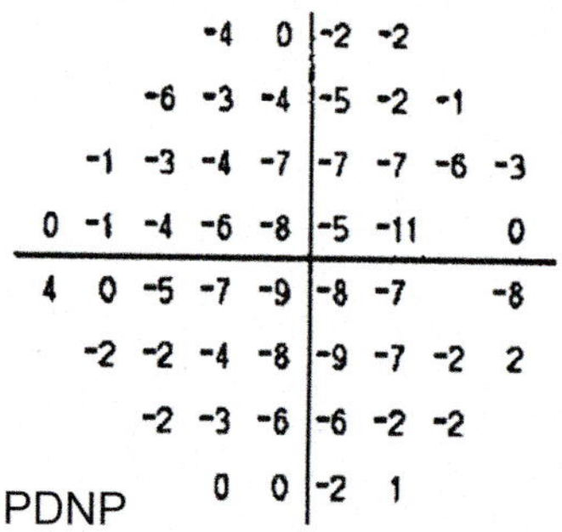

PDNP

The total deviation numerical plot is showing loss at almost all points. Note that the worst sensitivity point is -11 dB and the 7th best sensitivity point is -2 dB.

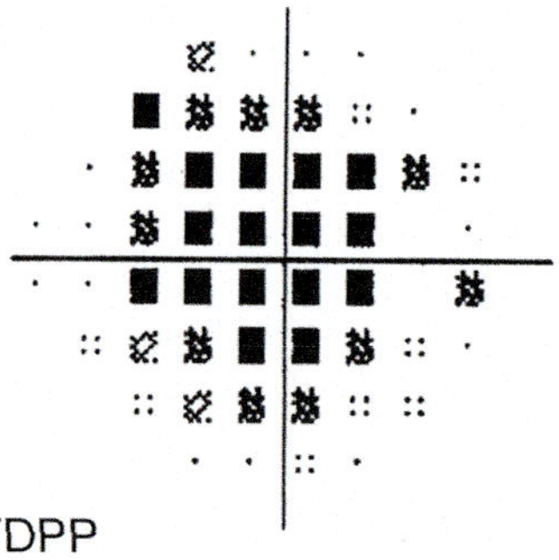

TDPP

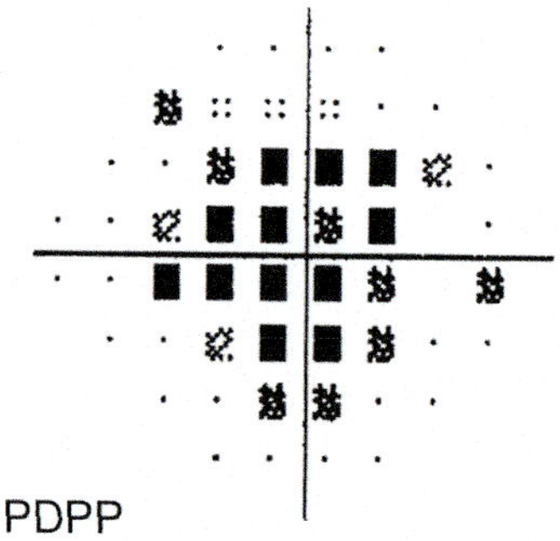

PDPP

The probability plots are giving an impression that the central scotoma is a deep scotoma. But if we see the total deviation numerical plot, we know that, the worst sensitivity point is -11 dB in this scotoma.

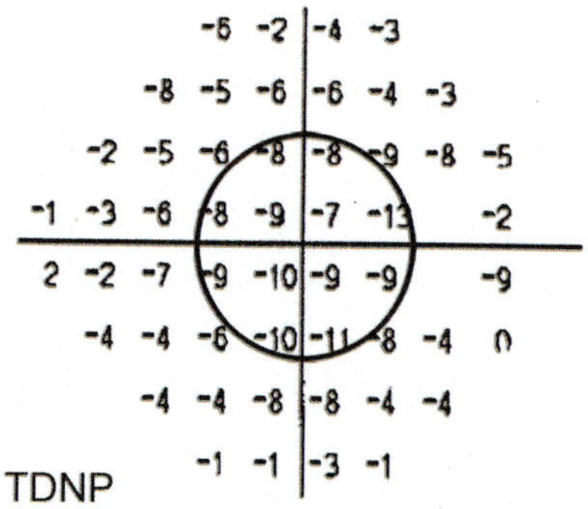

TDNP

Please note that if the loss of sensitivity is more than 5 dB to 8 dB within 10° circle and if the loss of sensitivity is more than 6 dB to 10 dB outside 10° circle, they will be represented by black squares. This is the reason why we see black squares in this fields defect though the the loss of sensitivity is less than 11 dB at any point.

Case 47

Here I am presenting a case of bilateral optic atrophy R > L with a history of head injury one year back CT scan. **Showed compression injuries to brain tissue proper fundus-optic atrophy R > L**

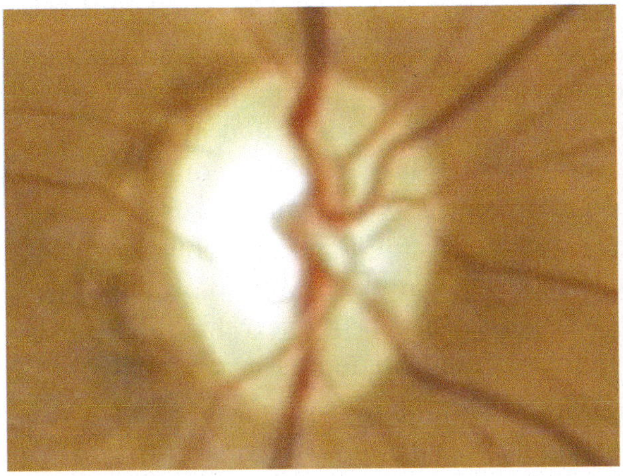

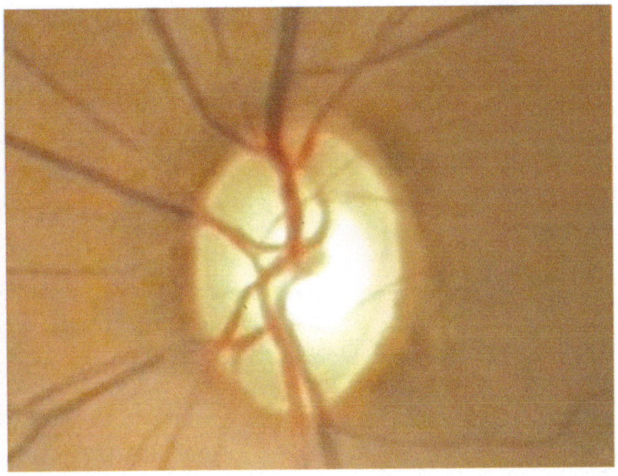

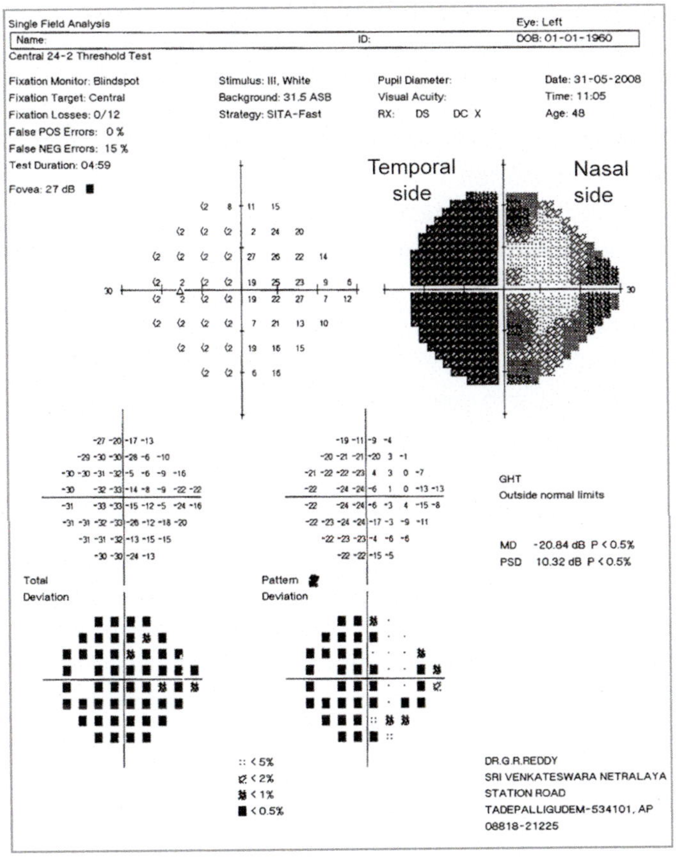

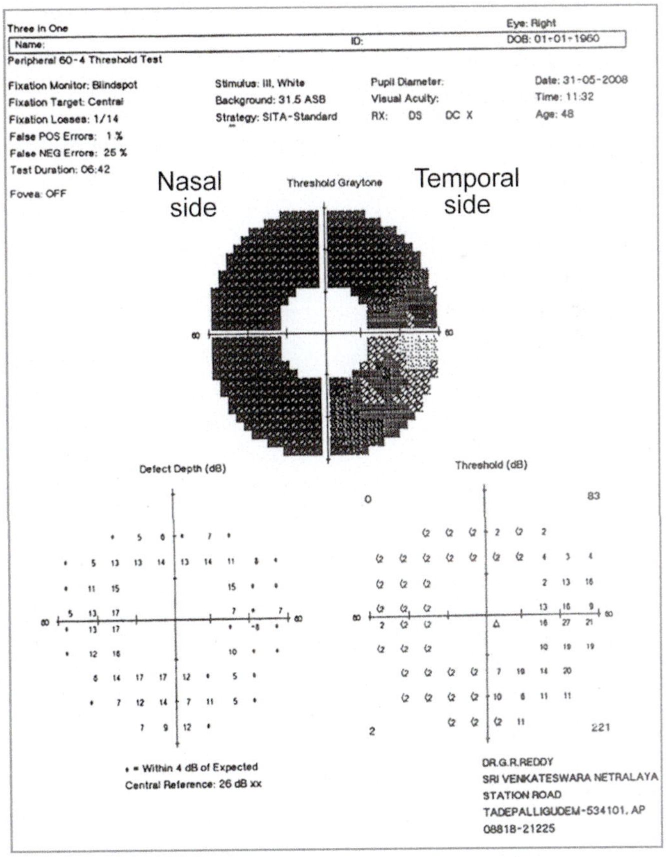

Left homonymous hemianopia due to occipital lobe injury and generalized depression due to B/L optic atrophy.

This case is the best example to tell the importance of pattern deviation plot to identify the localized field defect caused by occipital lobe injury in a case of generalized field defect due to optic atrophy.

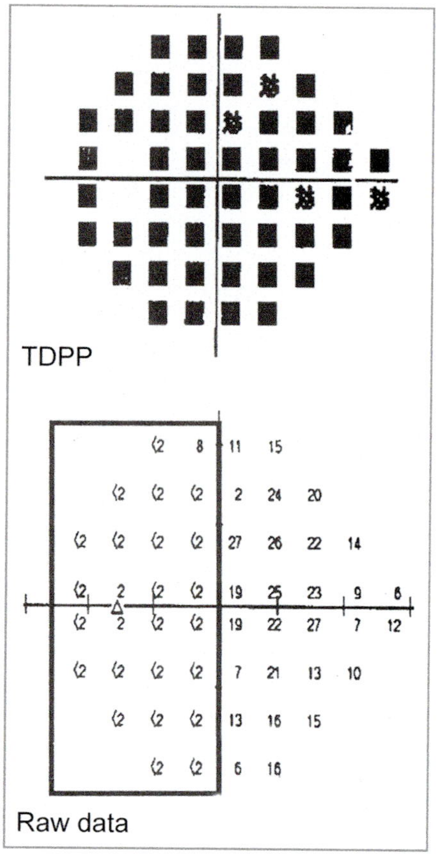

Total deviation probability plot shows generalized depression due to optic atrophy with almost all the points representing P < 0.5% (black squares). A case of optic atrophy will produce uniform generalized depression. This case is also associated with **occipital lobe injury**. So the localized field defect cannot be identified in this total deviation probability plot as already all points are represented by black squares. In this situation, the pattern deviation plot will help us to pickup localized field defects which are masked by the generalized field defect in the total deviation probability plot. The pattern deviation probability plot helps us to diagnose many neurological conditions by highlighting the pattern of deep scotomas in the generalized depression.

This is raw data of the patient with B/L optic atrophy in a case of head injury. There is a generalized depression of sensitivity and the most important point is that the entire temporal half of the field is absolute scotoma. There is a definite vertical line of demarcation between the absolute scotoma and the relative scotoma.

Absolute scotoma involving the entire temporal half of the field in the generalized depression of the left eye. The generalized depression is due to optic atrophy and the super added localized field defect involving the entire temporal field of the left eye is due to right occipital lobe injury. It is well appreciated in the pattern deviation probability plot.

Pattern deviation probability plot shows a deep scotoma mainly involving the entire temporal field (all the points in the temporal field are represented by P < 0.5%). The lower nasal and upper nasal quadrants are also involved with different P values.

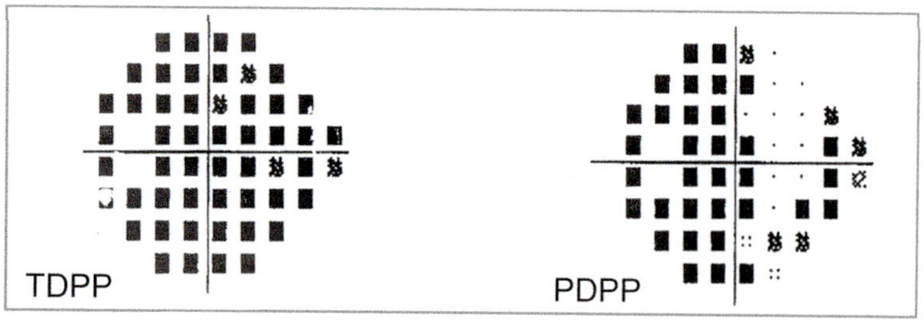

Suppose a person with cataract gets occipital lobe infarct, we know that occipital lobe infarct will produce homonymous hemianopia. But the vertical half of the absolute scotoma will be masked by generalized depression due to cataract in the total deviation probability plot. The absolute scotomas in the generalized depression will be brought out in the pattern deviation probability plot. So the homonymous hemianopia pattern of field defect will be appreciated in the pattern deviation probability plots in a case of cataract or in any clinical condition which causes generalized depression.

Case 48 Papilledema

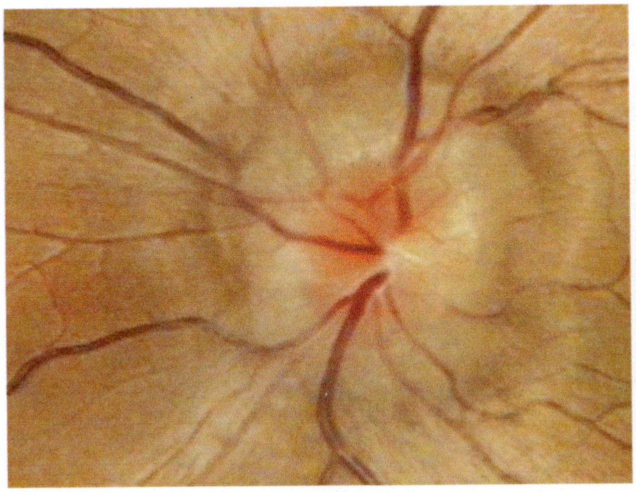

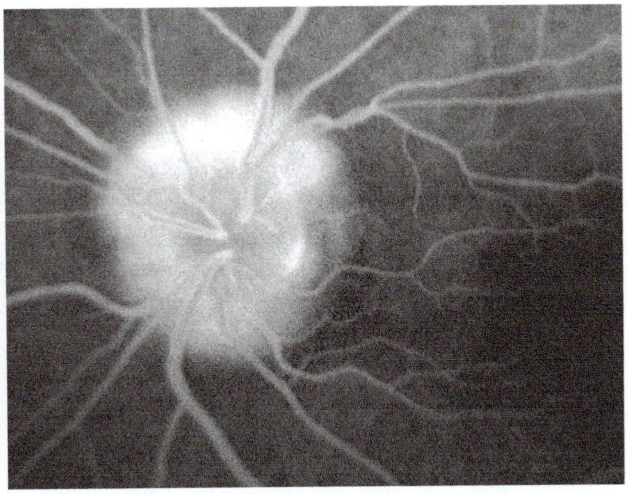

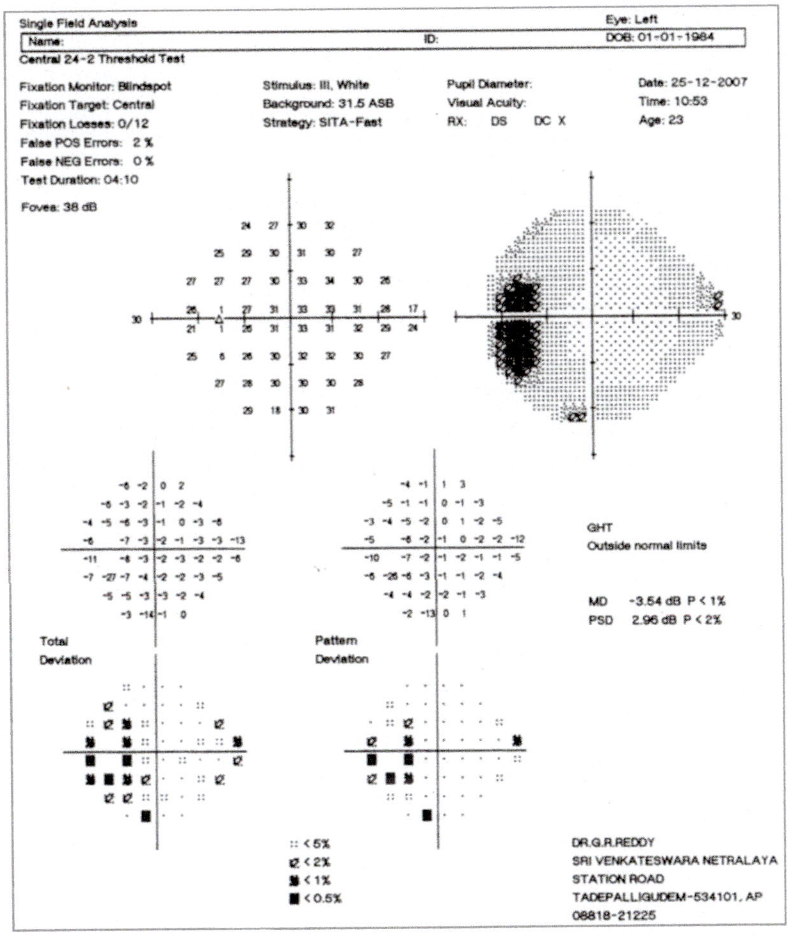

Note the enlargement of blind spot in a case of papilledema. The enlargement of blind spot is better appreciated in the grey scale. Please note that we do not see generalized depression in a case of papilledema.

SINGLE FIELD ANALYSIS PRINTOUT OF COLOBOMA OF LOWER HALF OF THE DISK AND RETINA

Case 49

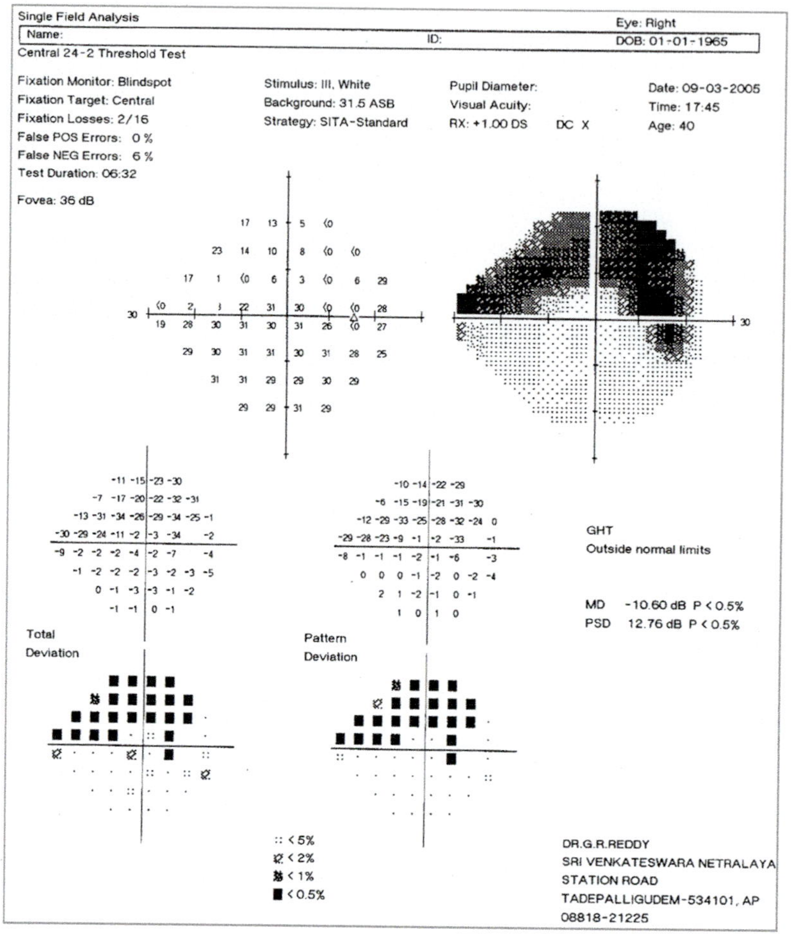

SINGLE FIELD ANALYSIS PRINTOUT OF OCCLUSION OF UPPER BRANCH OF CENTRAL RETINAL ARTERY

Case 50

Selection of the test	:	24-2 SITA Standard
Probability plots	:	Lower horizontal field defect
Mean deviation index	:	-18.19 dB P value < 0.5%
Interpretation	:	Occlusion of upper branch of CRA (Field defects are corresponding to the fundus changes)

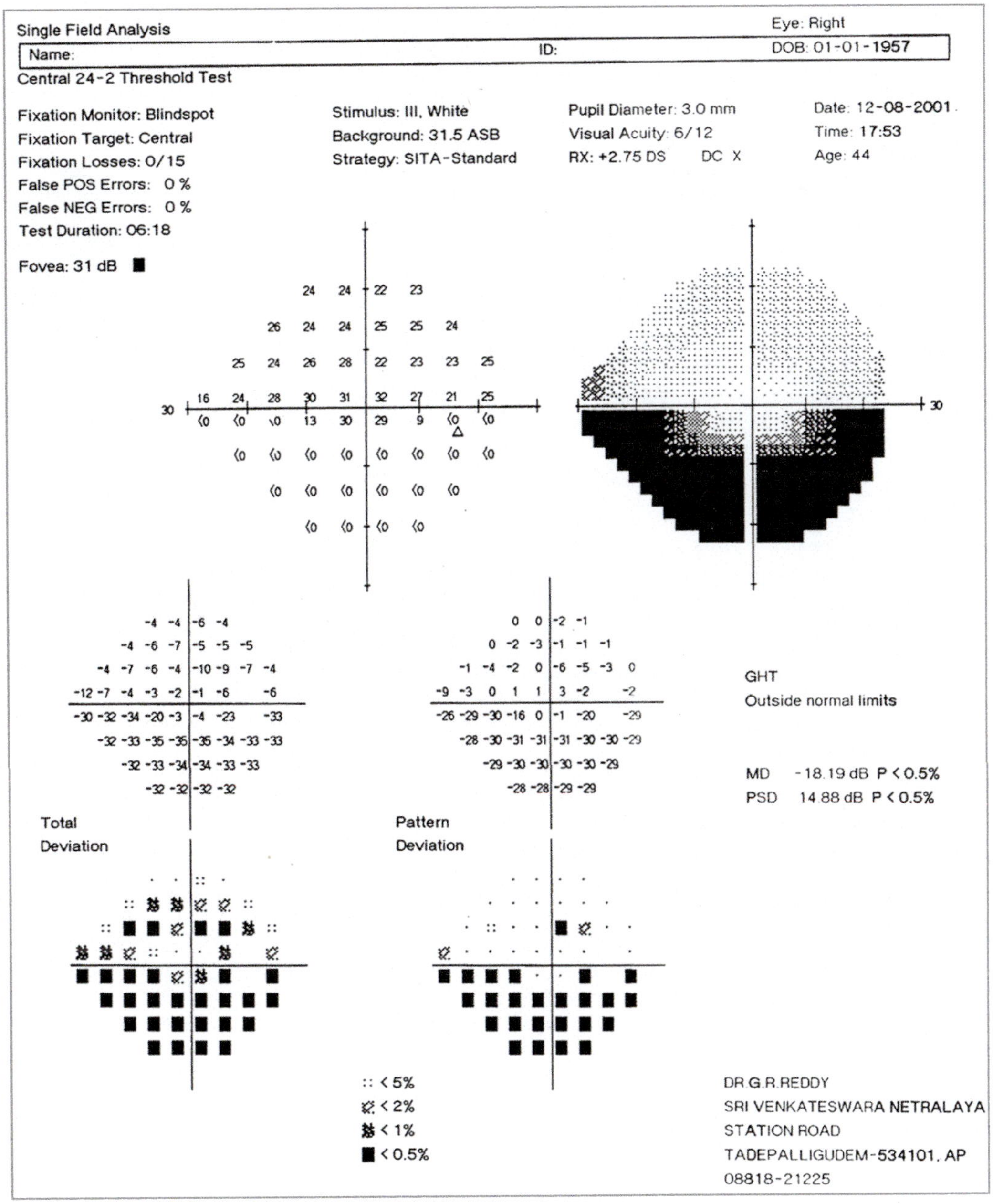

SINGLE FIELD ANALYSIS PRINTOUT OF RIGHT POSTERIOR CEREBRAL ARTERY OCCLUSION

Case 51 Homonymous hemianopia

Left Homonymous Hemianopia

Complaint ataxic gait: Fundus—within normal limits. Field—field showed left homonymous hemianopia.

Diagnosis: Right posterior cerebral artery occlusion. Later the diagnosis was confirmed by CT scan brain, which showed right occipital lobe infarct.

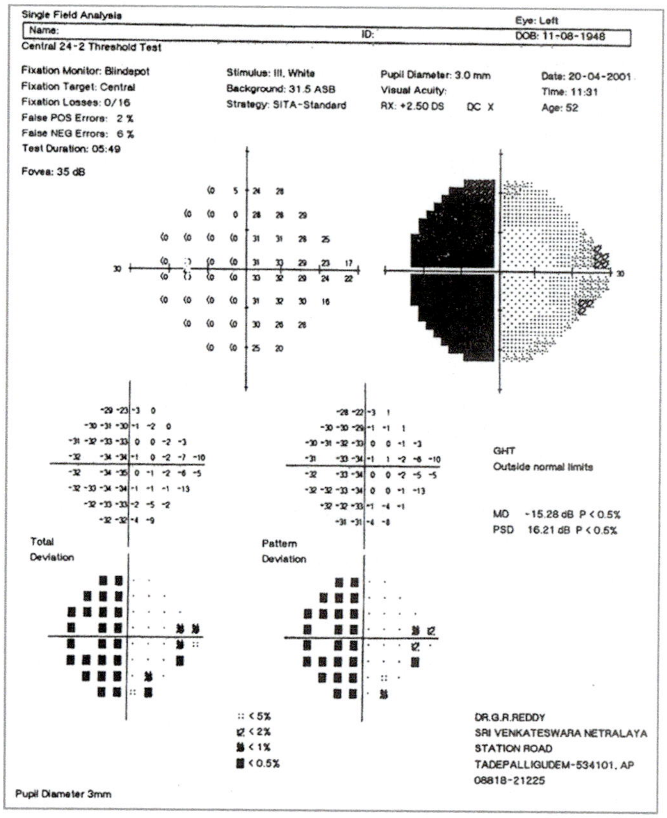

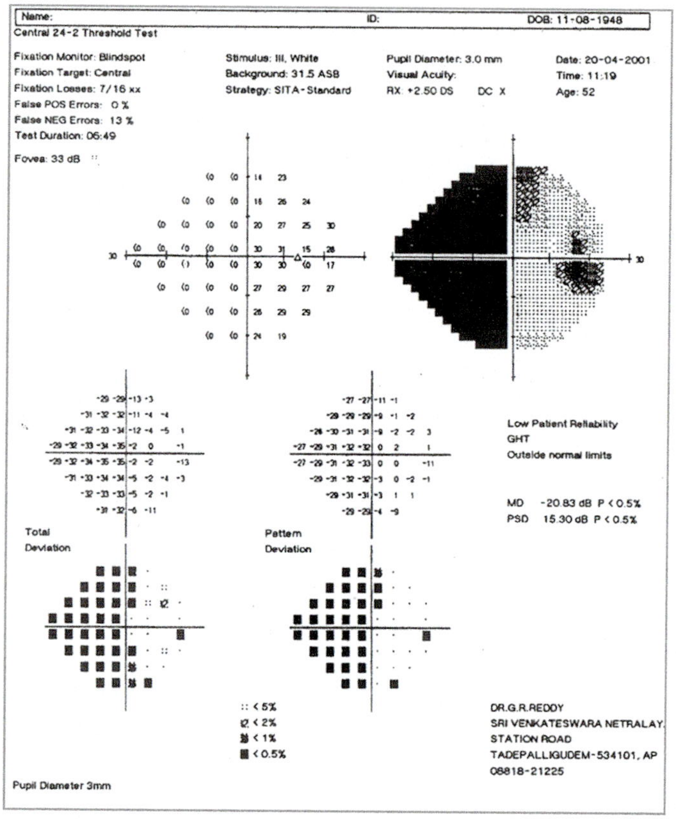

STEP 1: When we interpret the single field analysis (SFA) of both the eyes at the same time, we should hold the right eye's field with right hand and left eye's field with left hand.

STEP 2: Identification of temporal and nasal halves of the field. The blind spot will be present in the temporal half of the field. In this case right eye is showing nasal half of the field and left eye is showing temporal half of the field. (If we cannot locate blind spot in the grey scale, we can locate it in probability plots).

Case 52 Field chart of bitemporal hemianopia

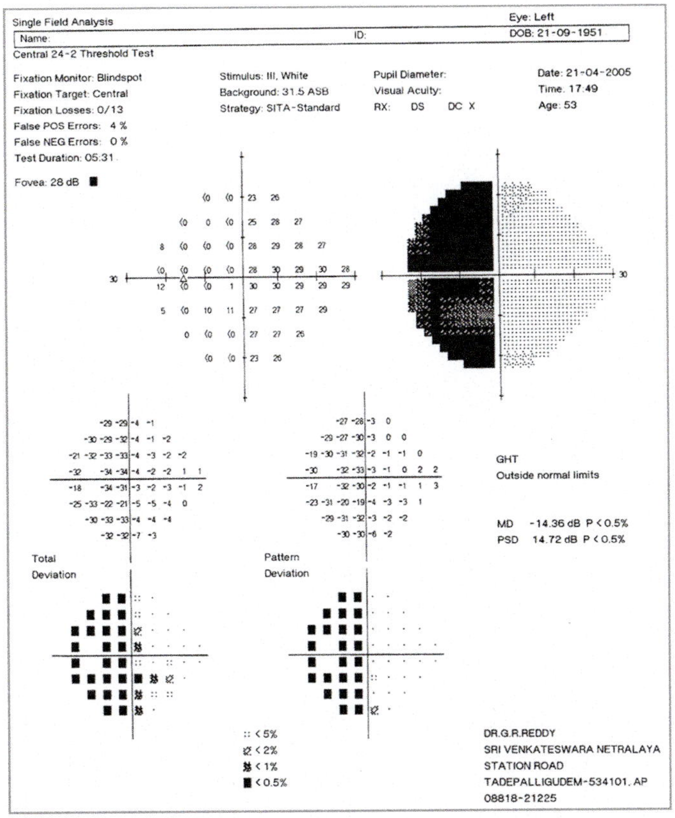

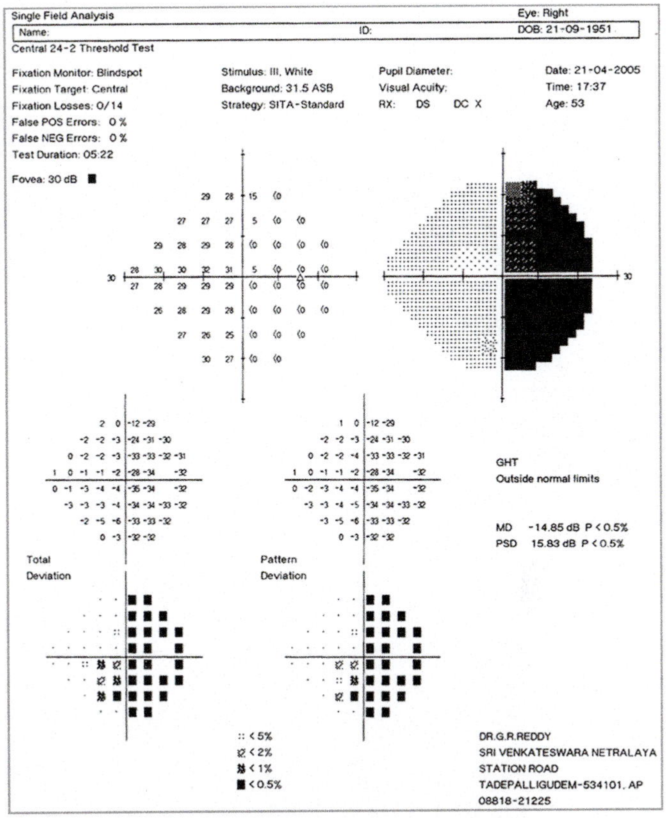

This is a case of bitemporal hemianopia. The CT scan showed a large aneurysm pressing the central fibers of optic chiasma. Some other important causes of bitemporal hemianopia are pituitary tumors, craniopharyngioma, meningiomas, anterior communicating artery aneurysms, etc.

CHAPTER

12

New Point Pattern 24-2 C Sita Faster

24-2 C POINT PATTERN

New point pattern 24-2 C is introduced to reduce the extent of the bare area present between the **3° circle points and 9° circle points.**

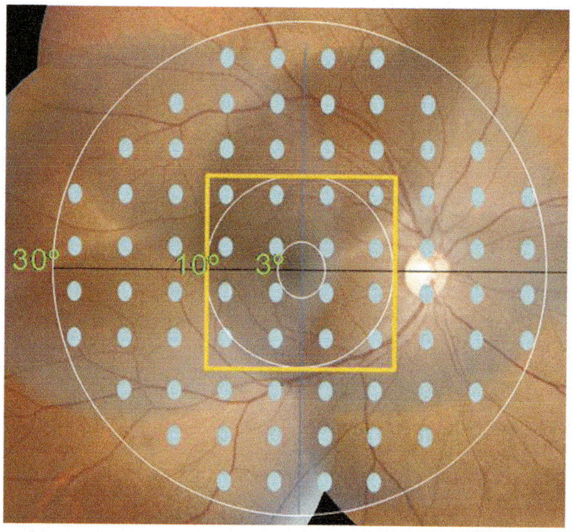

30-2 point pattern

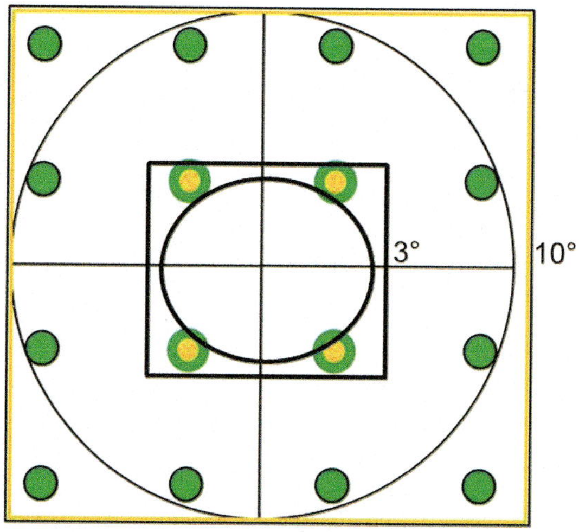

10° circle area of either 30-2 or 24-2 point pattern

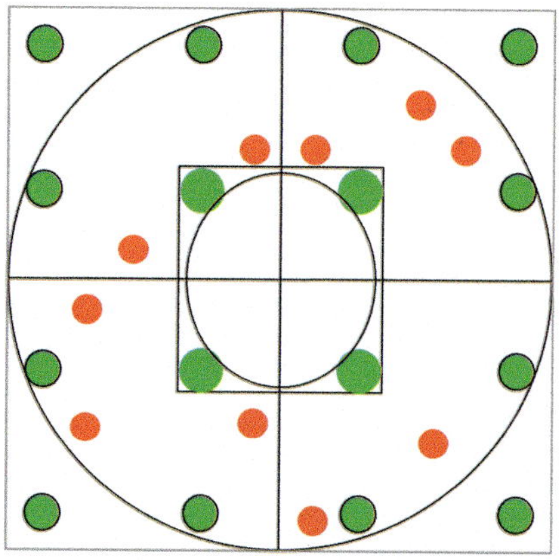

24-2 C point pattern

The bare area present between 3° circle points and 9° circle points is filled with 10 points

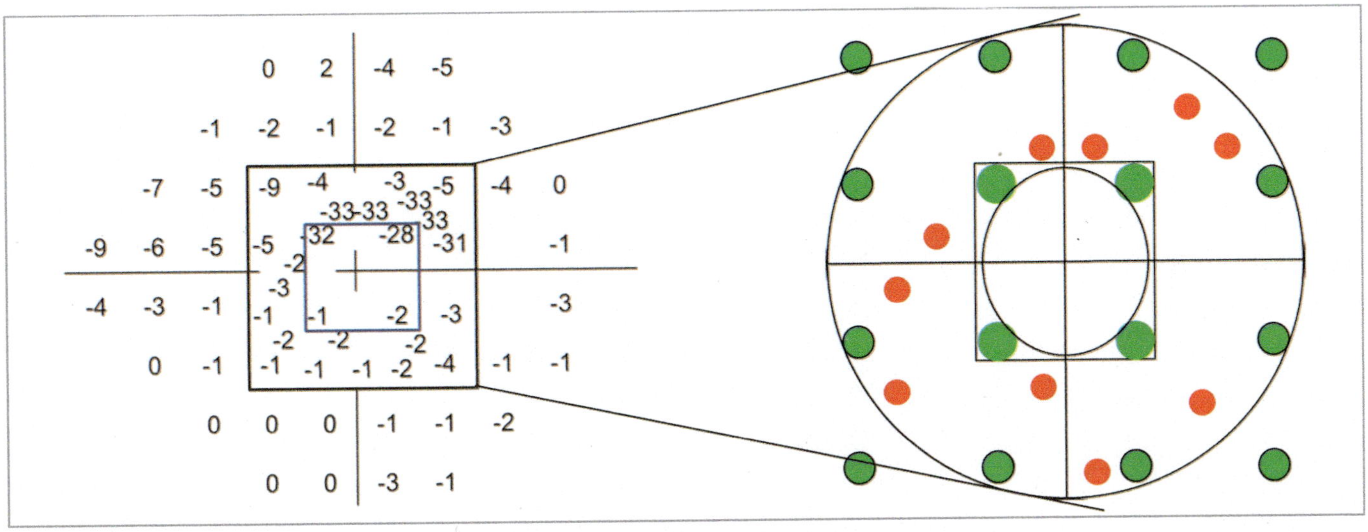

2 points in the upper nasal quadrant.
3 points in the upper temporal quadrant.
2 points in the lower temporal quadrant.
3 points in the lower nasal quadrant.

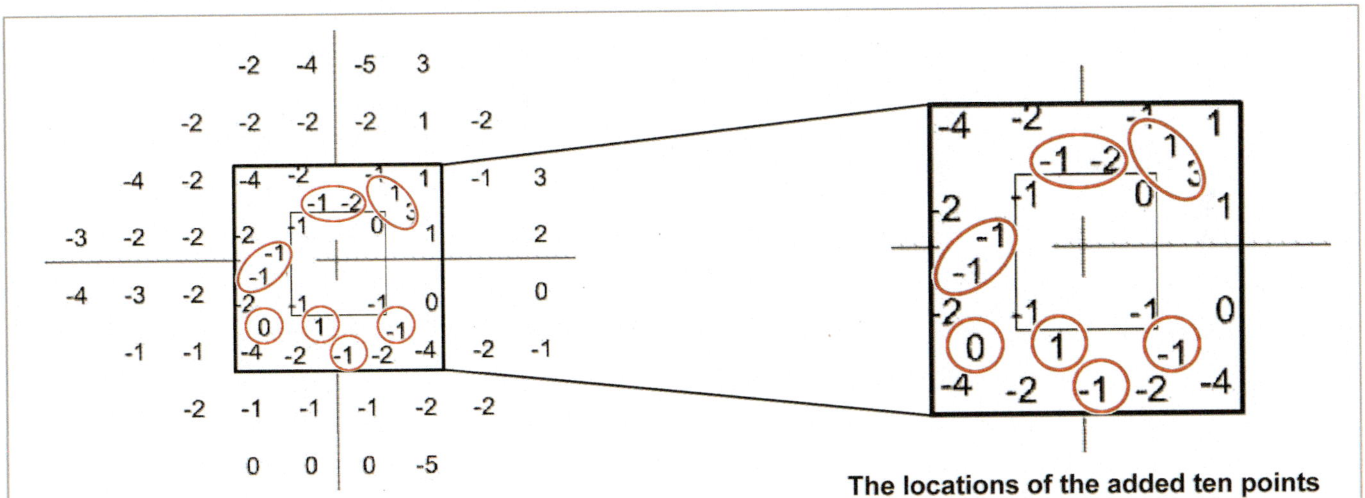

24-2 C point pattern

The locations of the added ten points in 10° circle area of 24-2 C

The main advantage of the new 24-2 C is the extent of the field defects in 10° circle area will be better appreciated compared to 24-2 point pattern. We see more number of significant P value symbols in 24-2 C point pattern than in 24-2 point pattern. So we do not miss to ask the test to be repeated with 10-2 point pattern.

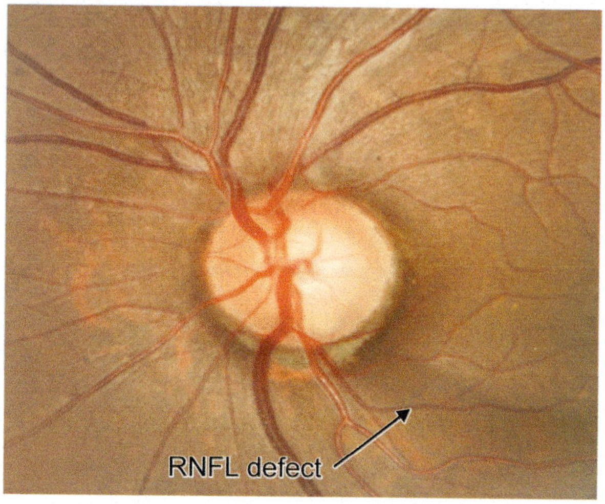

The patient is tested on both 24-2 and 24-2 C. Now, we study the difference between 24-2 SFA printout and 24-2 C SFA printout. These printouts are correlated with 10-2 printout.

Example 1

Direction of the RNFL defect is giving clue to repeat the test with 10-2 point pattern.

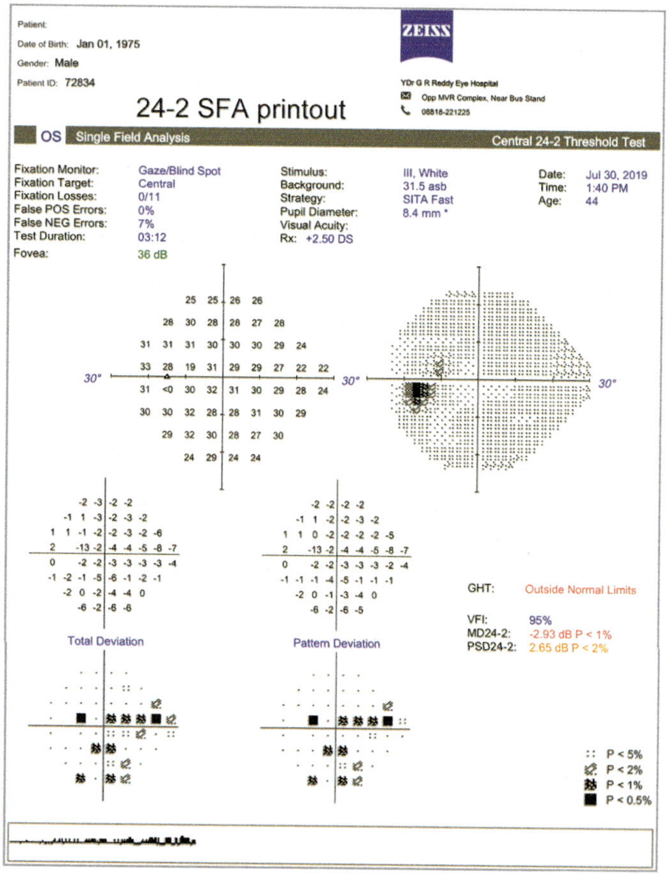

FL 0/11; FP 0%; FN 7%
Fovea 36 dB; VFI 95%
MD -2.93 dB P < 1%

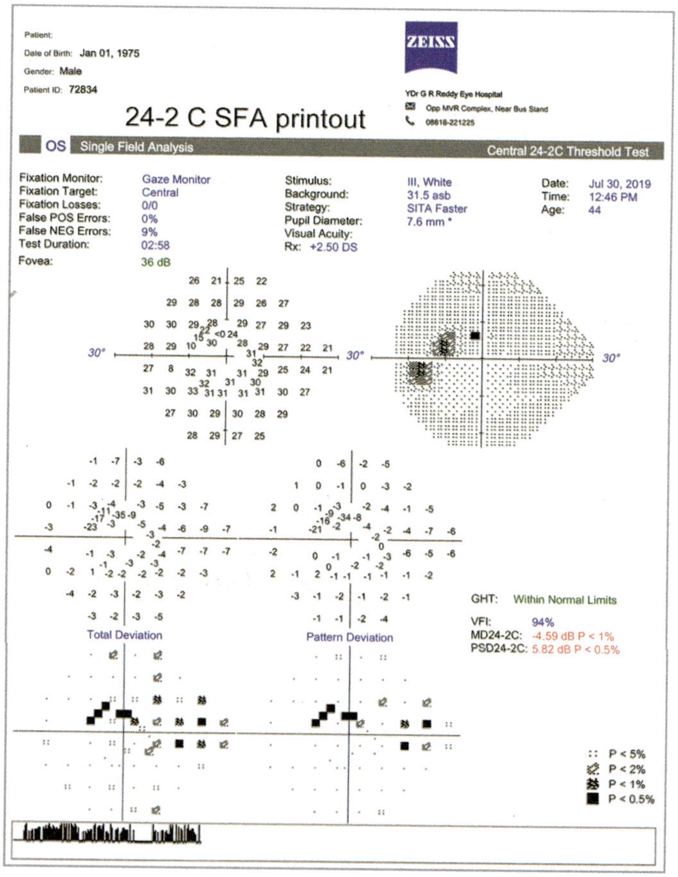

FL 0/0; FP 0%; FN 9%
Fovea 36 dB; VFI 94%
MD -4.59 dB P < 1%

24-2 SFA printout

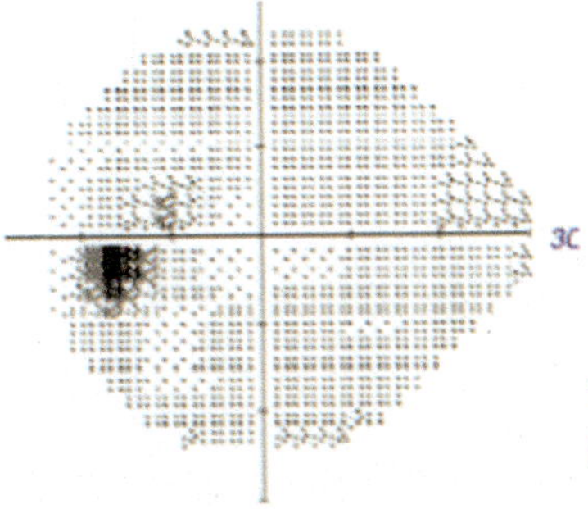

24-2 grey scale

Grey scale is looking normal

VFI 95%
MD -2.93 dB

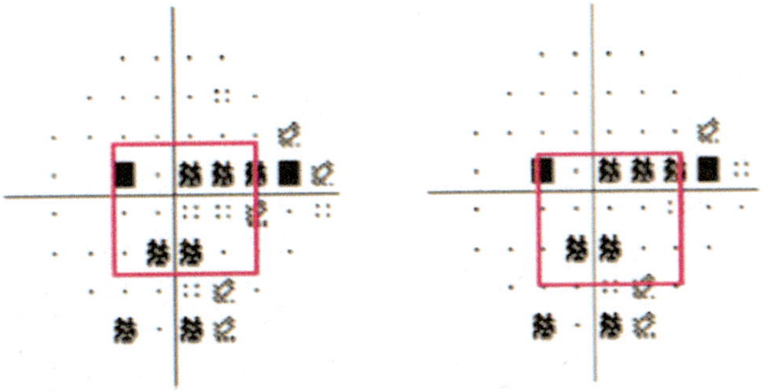

24-2 probability plots

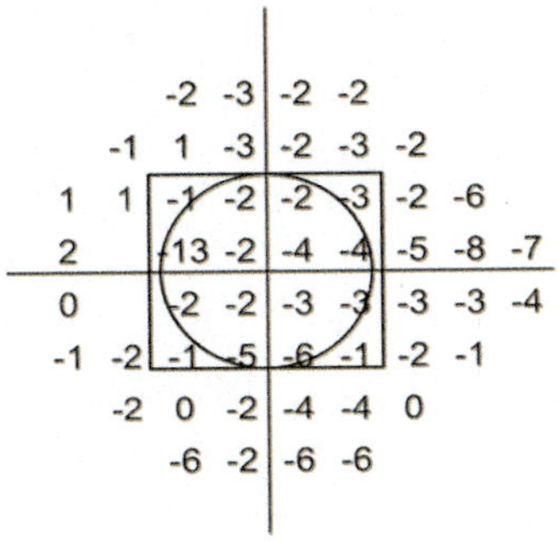

24-2 TDNP

Black square in the probability plot and 13 dB loss of sensitivity point in the 10° circle area of 24-2 are the indications to repeat the test with 10-2 point pattern.

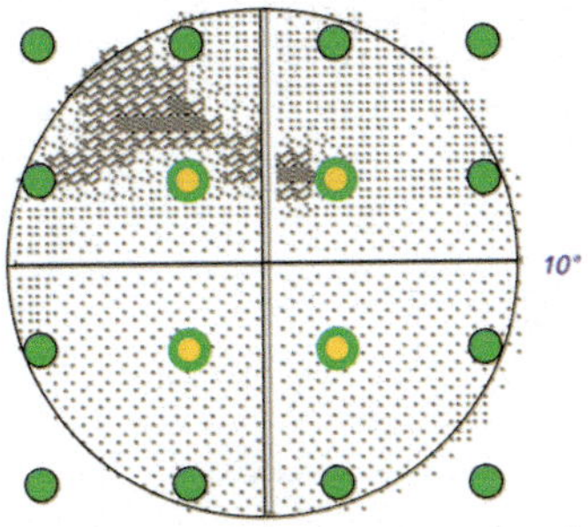

10-2 grey scale

24-2C SFA printout

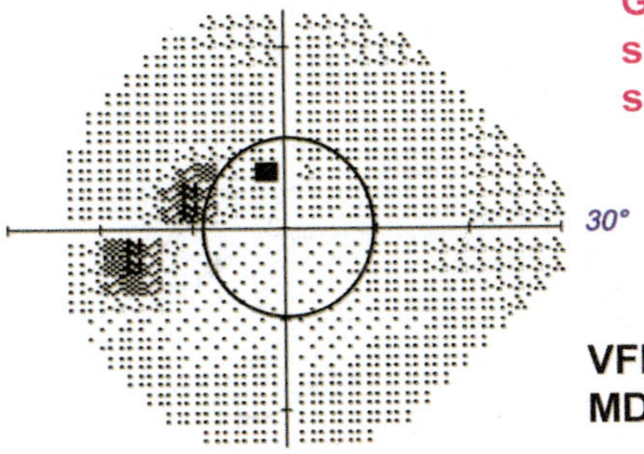

24-2 C gray scale

Grey scale is showing the shade

VFI 94%
MD -4.59 dB

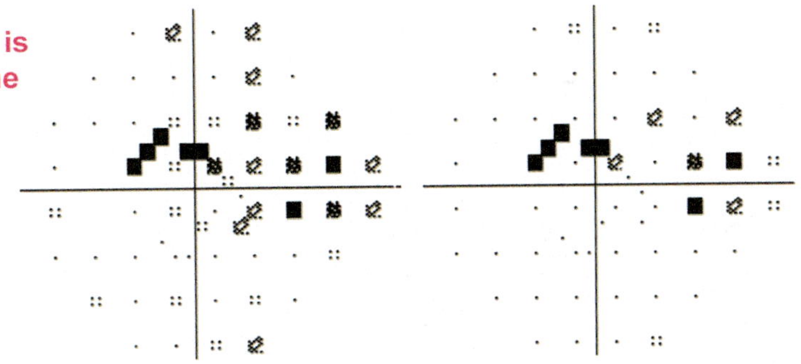

24-2 C probability plots

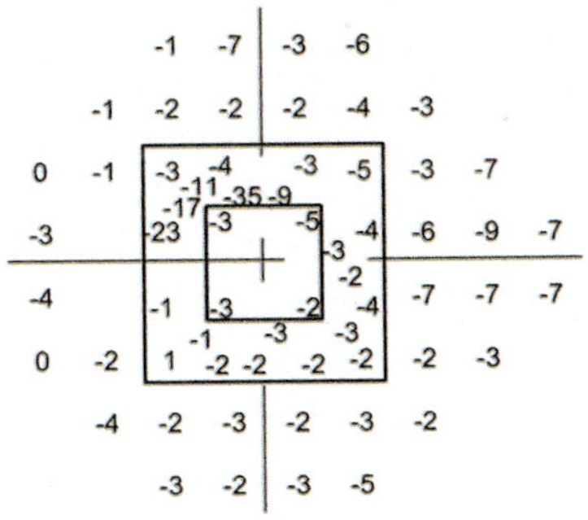

24-2 C TDNP

24-2 C grey scale probability plots and raw data or TDNP are giving indications to repeat the test with 10-2 point pattern.

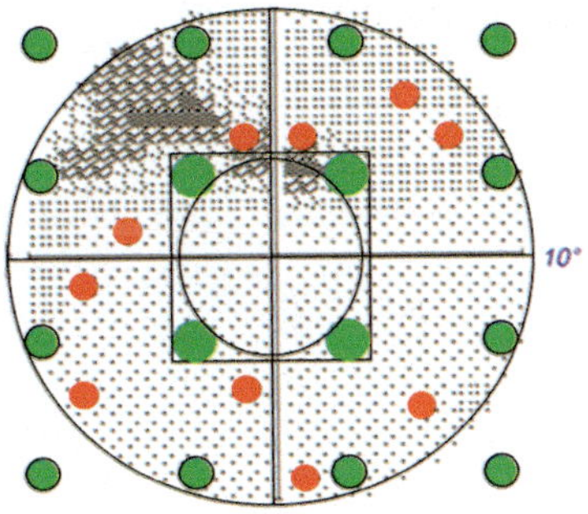

10-2 grey scale

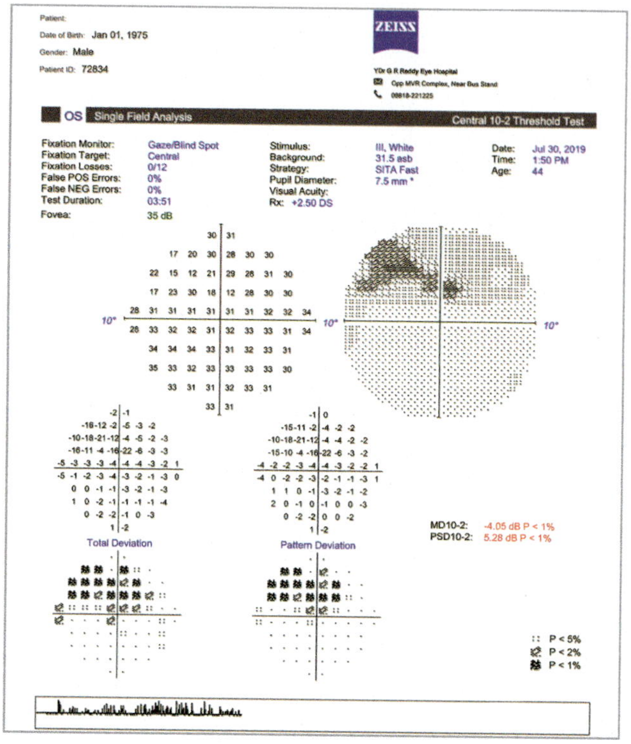

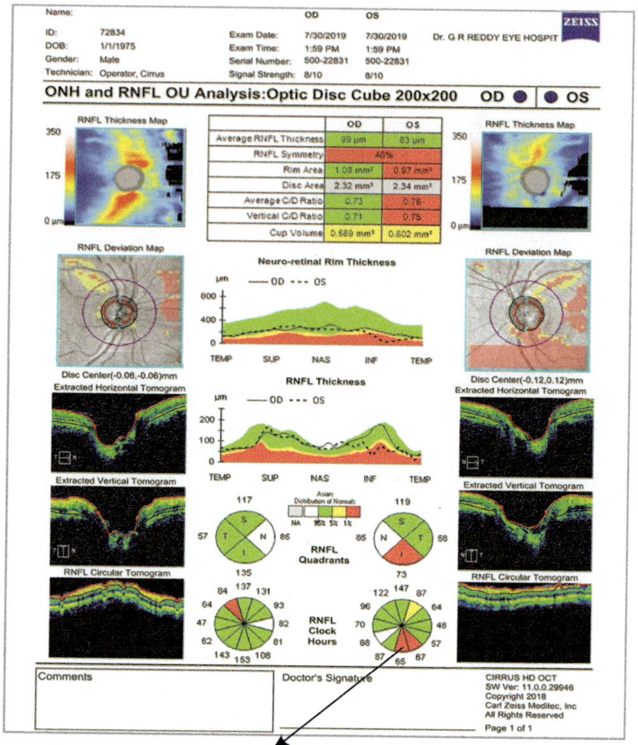

In OCT, thinning of RNFL between 5 and 6 clock hours is an indication (left eye) to repeat the test with 10-2 point pattern

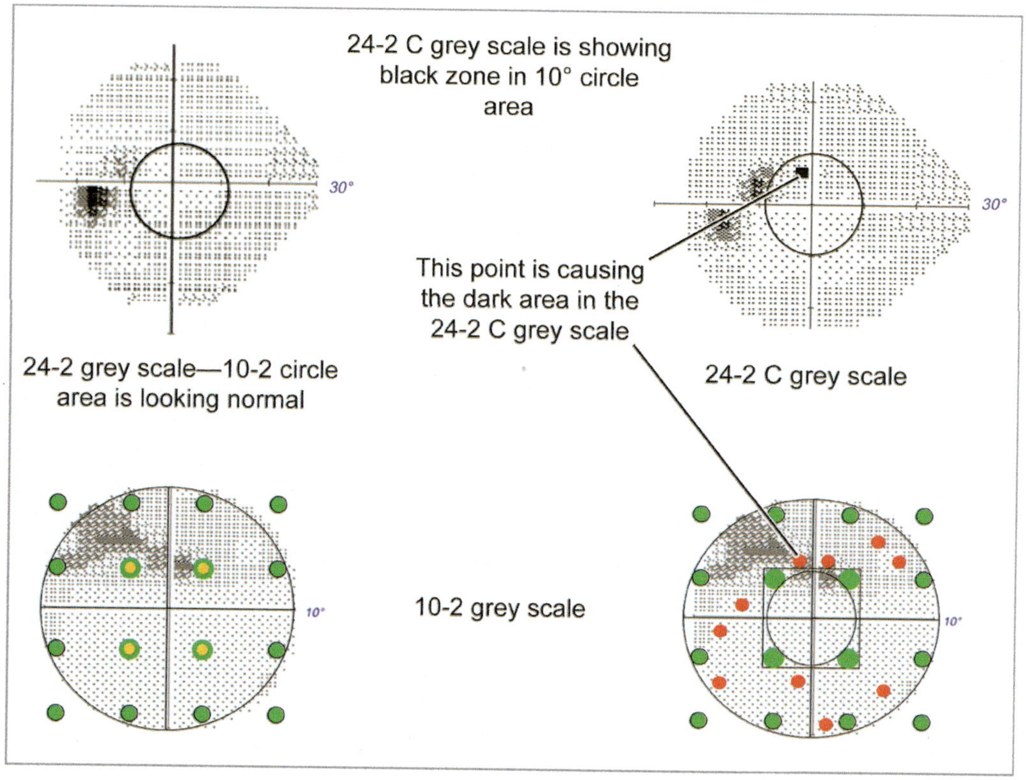

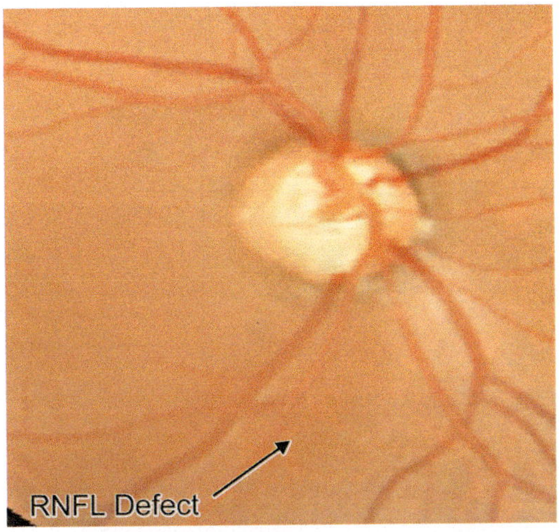

Example 2

Direction of the RNFL defect is giving clue to repeat the test with 10-2 point pattern.

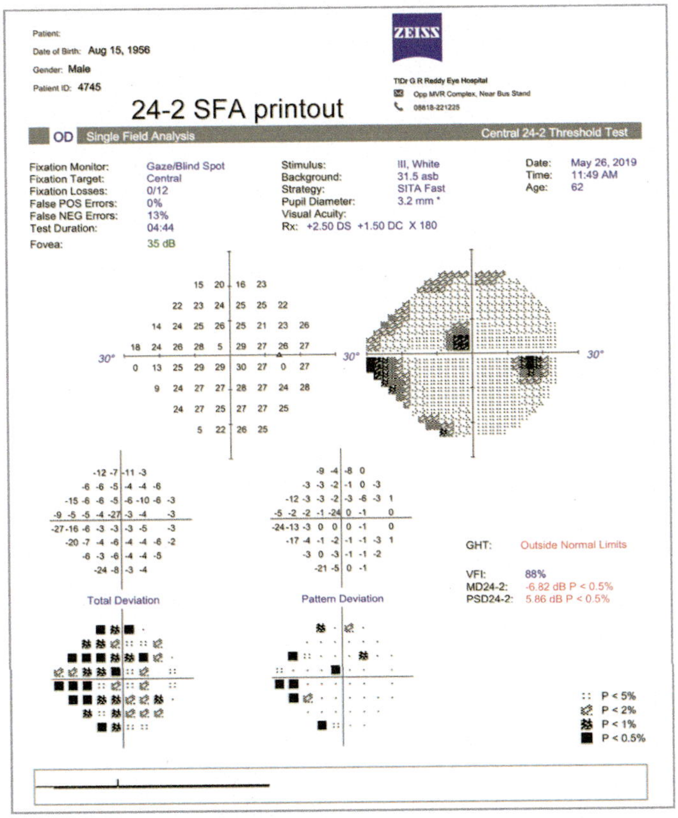

FL 0/12; FP 0%; FN 13%
Fovea 35 dB; VFI 88%
MD -6.82 dB P < 1%

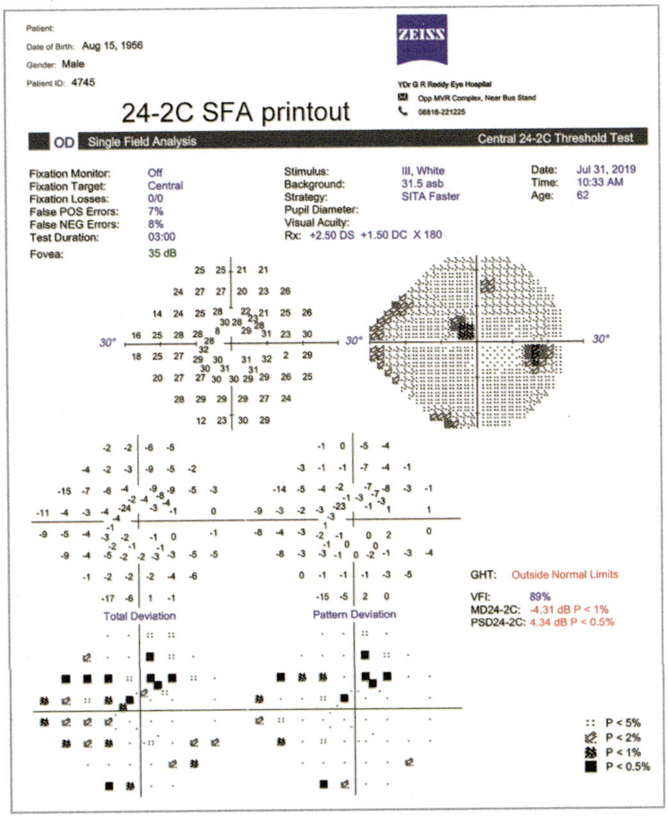

FL 0/0; FP 7%; FN 6%;
Fovea 35 dB; VFI 89%
MD -4.31 dB P < 1%

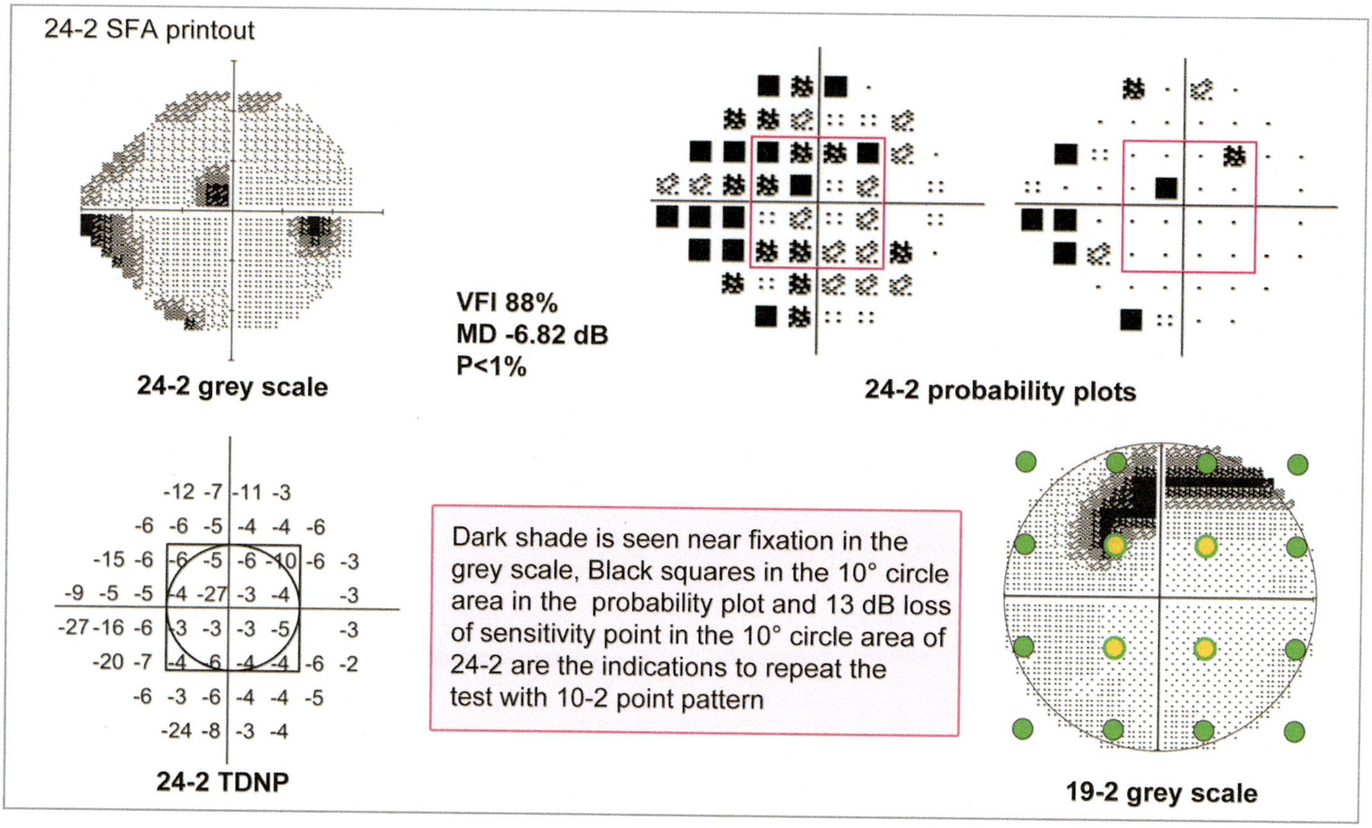
24-2 SFA printout
24-2 grey scale
VFI 88%
MD -6.82 dB
P<1%
24-2 probability plots
-12 -7 -11 -3
-6 -6 -5 -4 -4 -6
-15 -6 -6 -5 -6 -10 -6 -3
-9 -5 -5 -4 -27 -3 -4 -3
-27 -16 -6 -3 -3 -3 -5 -3
-20 -7 -4 -6 -4 -4 -6 -2
-6 -3 -6 -4 -4 -5
-24 -8 -3 -4
24-2 TDNP
Dark shade is seen near fixation in the grey scale, Black squares in the 10° circle area in the probability plot and 13 dB loss of sensitivity point in the 10° circle area of 24-2 are the indications to repeat the test with 10-2 point pattern
19-2 grey scale

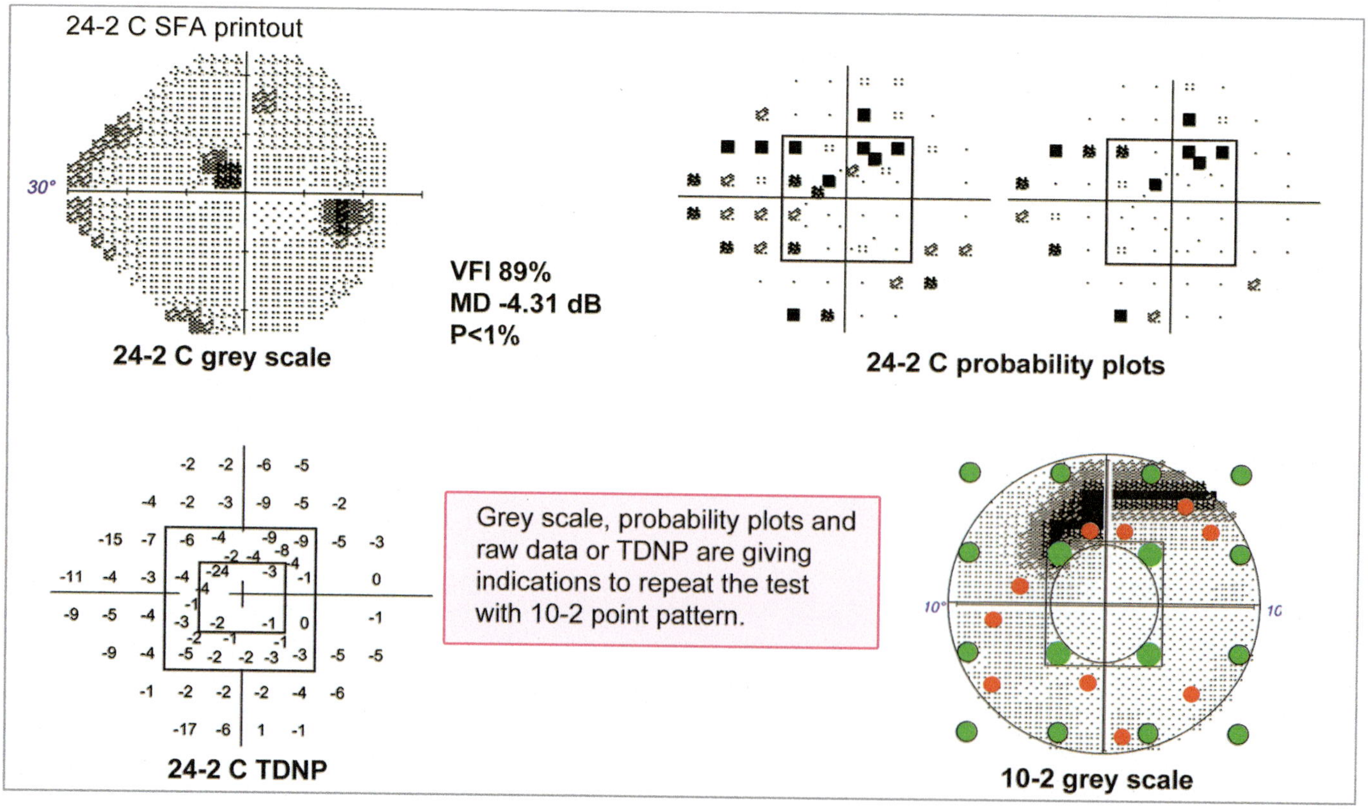
24-2 C SFA printout
30°
24-2 C grey scale
VFI 89%
MD -4.31 dB
P<1%
24-2 C probability plots
24-2 C TDNP
Grey scale, probability plots and raw data or TDNP are giving indications to repeat the test with 10-2 point pattern.
10°
10-2 grey scale

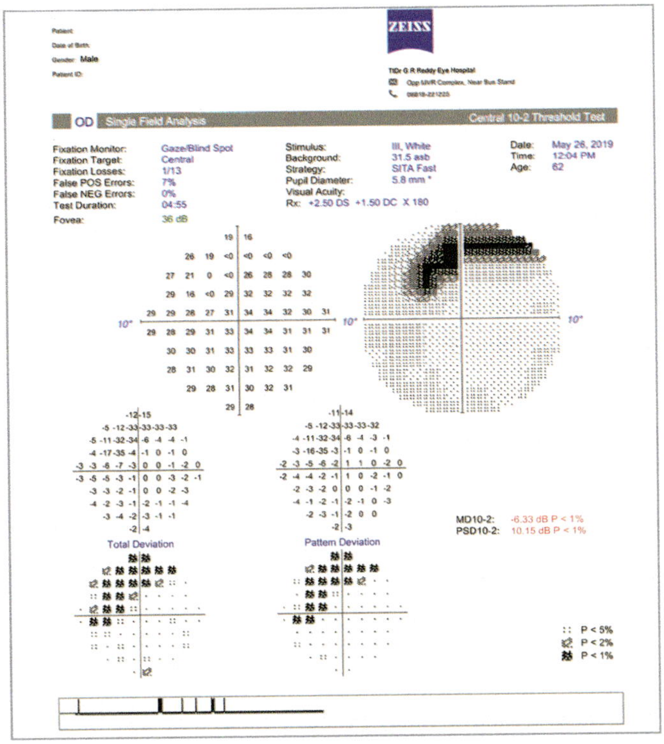

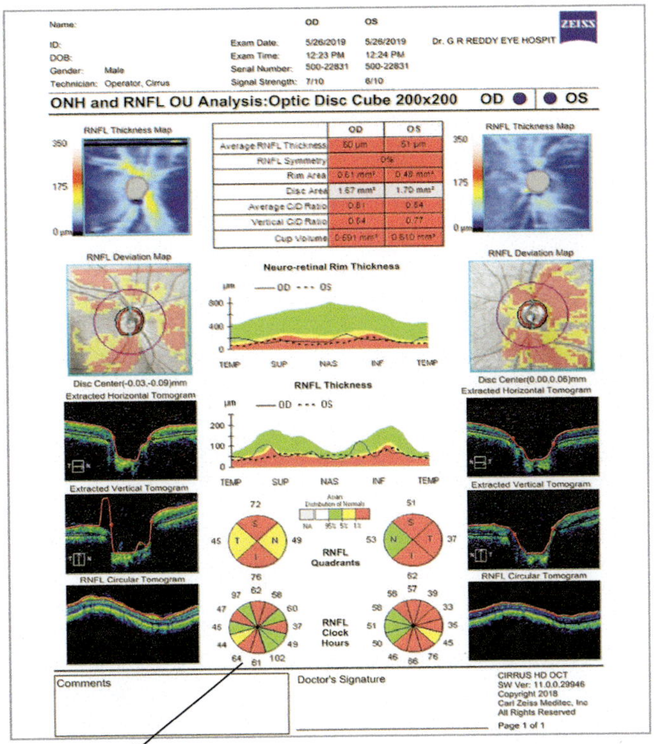

In OCT, thinning of RNFL between 6 and 7 clock hours (right eye) is an indication to repeat the test with 10-2 point pattern

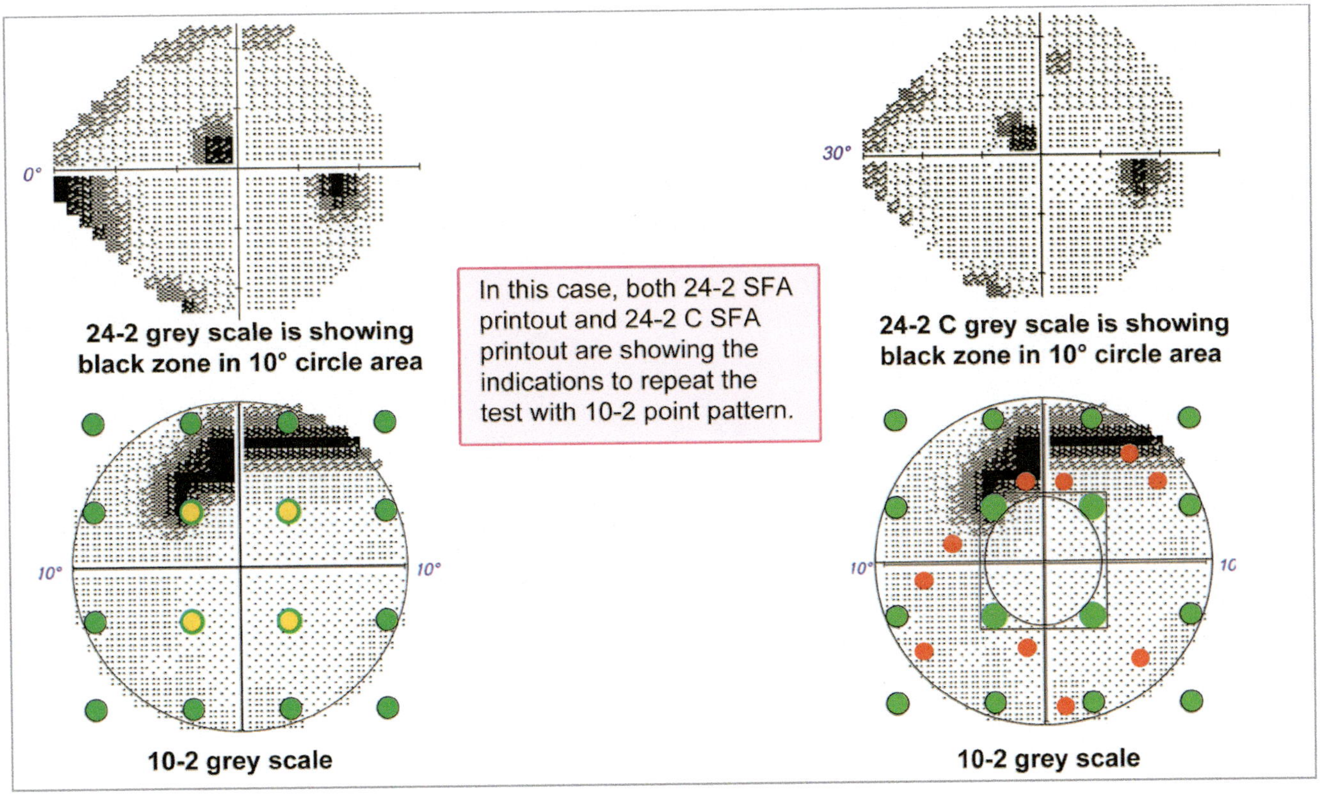

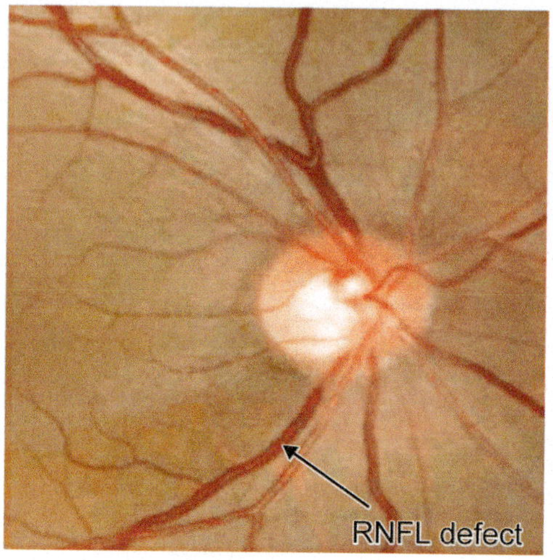

Example 3

Direction of the RNFL defect is giving clue to repeat the test with 10-2 point pattern.

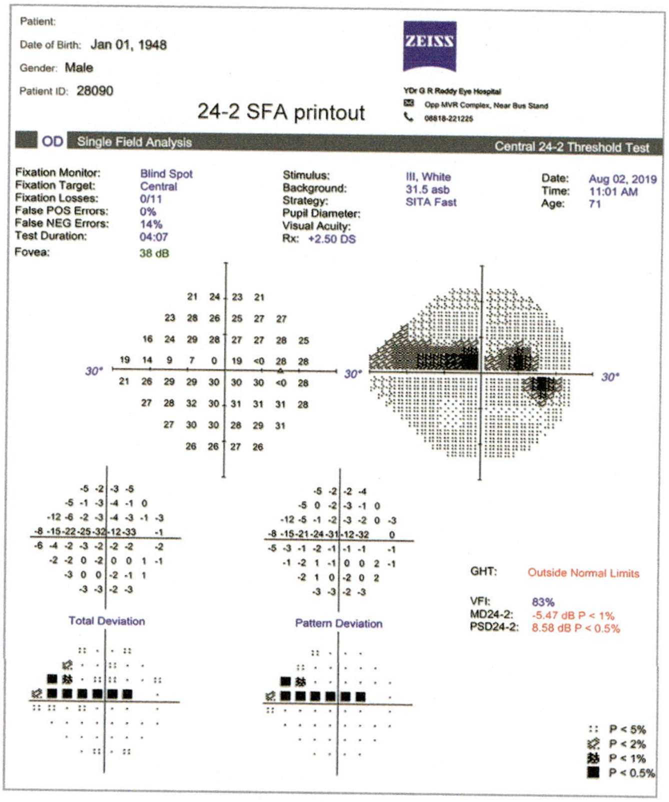

FL 0/11; FP 0%; FN 14%
Fovea 38 dB; VFI 83%
MD -5.47 dB P < 1%

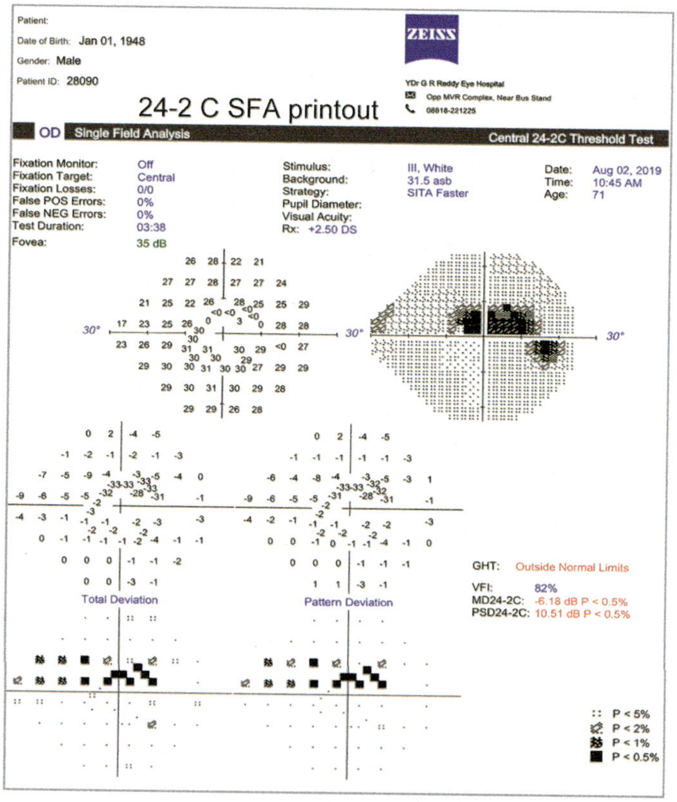

FL 0/0; FP 0%; FN 0%
Fovea 35 dB; VFI 82%
MD -6.18 dB P < 0.5%

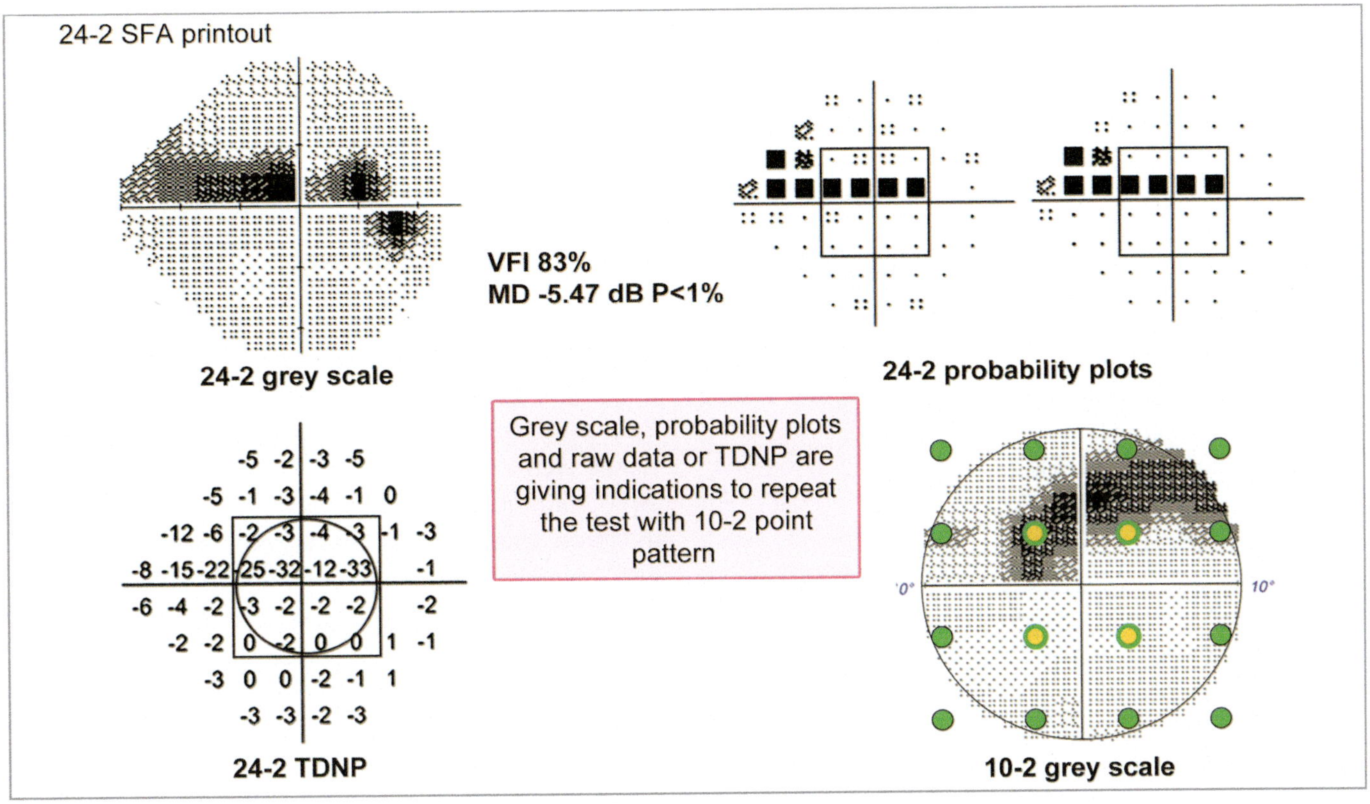
24-2 SFA printout
24-2 grey scale
VFI 83%
MD -5.47 dB P<1%
24-2 probability plots
-5 -2 -3 -5
-5 -1 -3 -4 -1 0
-12 -6 -2 -3 -4 -3 -1 -3
-8 -15 -22 -25 -32 -12 -33 -1
-6 -4 -2 -3 -2 -2 -2 -2
-2 -2 0 -2 0 0 1 -1
-3 0 0 -2 -1 1
-3 -3 -2 -3
24-2 TDNP
Grey scale, probability plots and raw data or TDNP are giving indications to repeat the test with 10-2 point pattern
10°
10°
10-2 grey scale

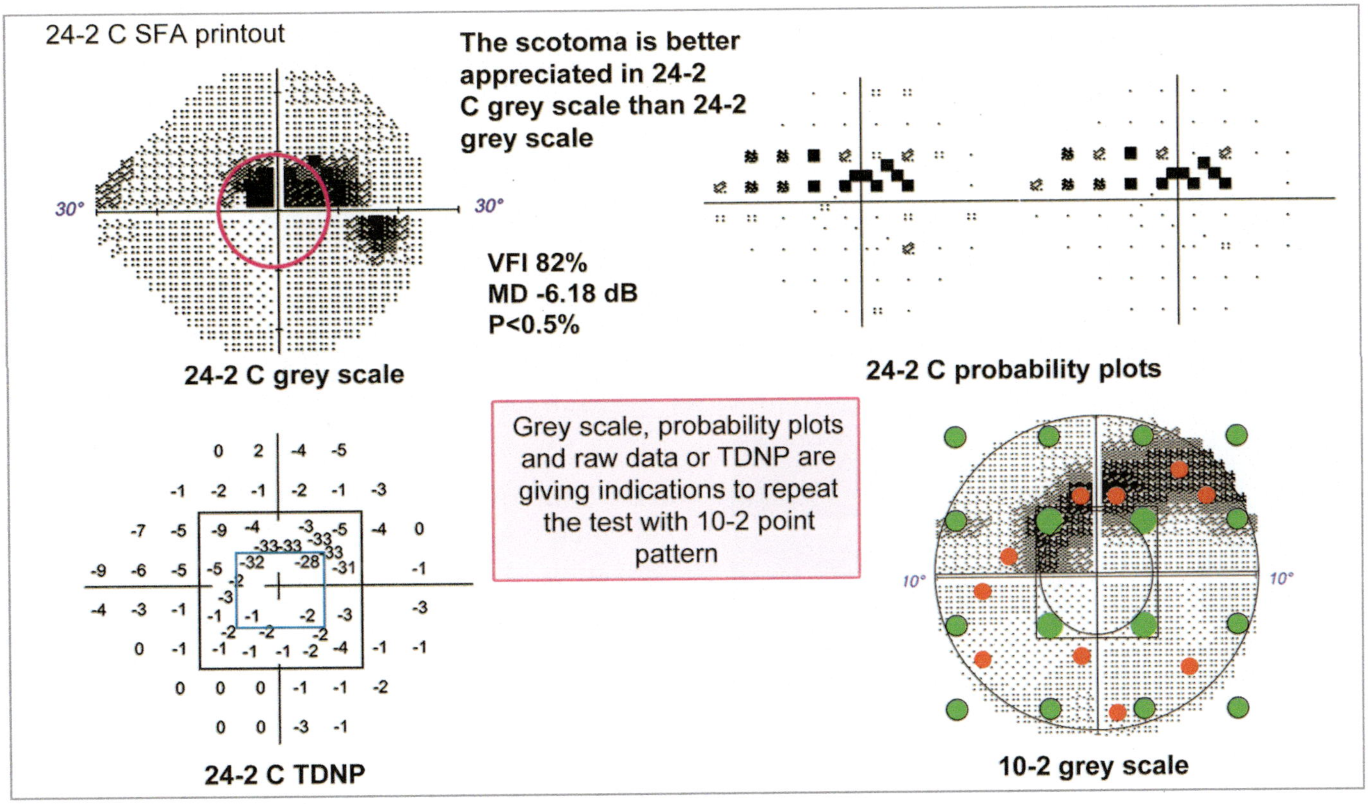
24-2 C SFA printout
The scotoma is better appreciated in 24-2 C grey scale than 24-2 grey scale
30°
30°
24-2 C grey scale
VFI 82%
MD -6.18 dB
P<0.5%
24-2 C probability plots
24-2 C TDNP
Grey scale, probability plots and raw data or TDNP are giving indications to repeat the test with 10-2 point pattern
10°
10°
10-2 grey scale

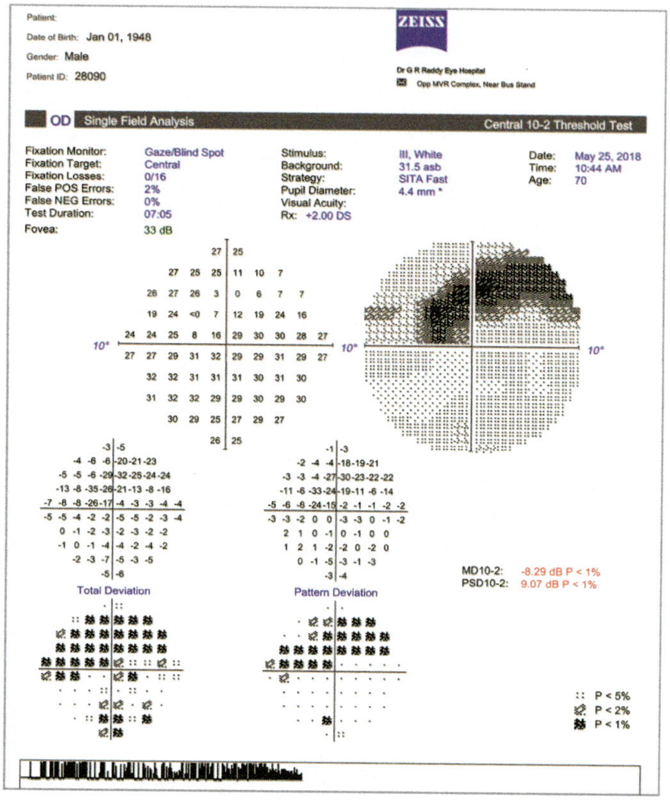

FL 0/16
FP 2%
FN 0%
Fovea 33 dB
MD Index -8.18 dB P < 1%

In type 2 and type 3, the plan of treatment depends on the 10-2 printouts. In type 2 and type 3 glaucomas, 24-2 SFA helps in giving indications to repeat the test with 10-2 point pattern. I selected the three known patients of type 2 glaucoma who were already having 24-2 and 10-2 SFA printouts. These patients were tested with 24-2C SITA Faster. Now older 24-2 and 24-2C printouts are compared with each other. In all the three cases I did not see any additional advantage with the newer 24-2 C SITA Faster over the older 24-2 SFA printout in giving additional information to repeat the test with 10-2 point pattern.

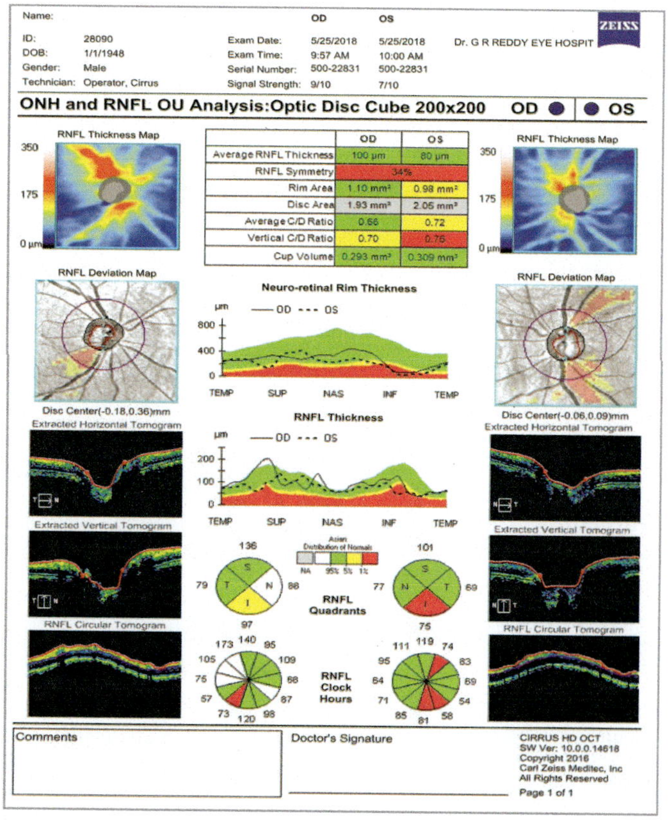

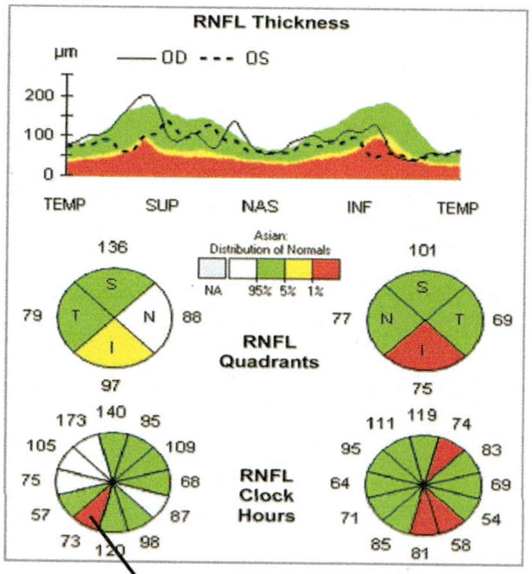

In OCT, thinning of RNFL between 7-8 clock hours (right eye) is an indication to repeat the test with 10-2 point pattern

Glossary

Box plot: The decibel deviations of a total deviation numerical plot of the single field analysis printout are divided into three groups according to their degree of decibel deviations. And these 3 groups constitute the box plot. The best 15% sensitive points are represented by upper tail, the next 70% best points are represented by box proper and the least 15% sensitive points are represented by lower tail.

Catch trial: This entire category includes fixation losses, false positive errors and false negative errors. They are called catch trials. Because they monitor patient reliability and attentiveness. If any one of these parameters falls outside the established norms, an 'xx' will be printed alongside the associated fraction numbers to indicate a statistically significant error rate.

Central reference level (CRL): Hypothetical threshold sensitivity at the center of the field, ignoring foveal peak. It may be a value projected on the basis of the normal slope of the "hill of vision" and empirically determined thresholds at 4 to 5 locations or an assigned value (by age, or as a minimal value). It is used to determine expected threshold values throughout the field to guide testing or to calculate defect depth.

Change analysis: A printout that displays statistical summaries of a series of field tests in the form of box plots and a summary of 4 global indices. The indices are the same four presented in the single field analysis, but this time they are plotted overtime to indicate changes in the patient' visual field.

Corrected pattern standard deviation: It is one of the four global indices. It is the corrected form of pattern standard deviation by removing the effect of short-term fluctuation from the PSD, we get the CPSD. So, CPSD depends on the both PSD and SF (CPSD-PSD-SF).

0 decibel: The maximum intensity of light that is projected by any perimeter is designated as 0 decibel.

Decibel: In the context of perimetry, the intensity of light is expressed as 0.1 log unit attenuation of the maximum available stimulus (10000 asb for the current Humphrey perimeters).

Defect depth: It is the difference of threshold at a location between the measured threshold value, and the calculated CRL or the assigned threshold value (by age or as a minimal value).

False negative rate (FN): The frequency at which the patient fails to respond to stimuli that are expected to be visible. The basis of the calculation and the interpretation of the result is not identical to SITA and non-SITA strategies.

False positive rate (FP): The frequency with which the patient responds to the stimuli, that actually could not have been seen. The manner of determining the rate differs in the SITA and non-SITA strategies, but the interpretation is the same.

FASTPAC: Threshold algorithm in which stimuli are presented in 3 dB steps, and the threshold value is assigned based on the first cross-over form seeing to non-seeing or vice versa.

Fixation losses rate (FL): With the blind spot method of Heijl-Krakou, the number of times the patient responds per catch trial in which a stimulus is presented in the expected position of the physiological blind spot.

Glaucoma change probability printout: Comparison of threshold data in a follow-up field to baseline, in which points are highlighted if they change by amounts that are larger than the typically seen in stable glaucoma patients. Similarly, MD values changing by more than typical values are also figured.

Glaucoma Hemifield test (GHT): Plain language analysis of a single threshold 30-2 or 24-2 test analysis is based on normative database and a pathological model for glaucoma field loss.

Global indices: Single numerical values which each characterize certain aspects of visual fields. For Humphrey parameters, MD, PSD, SF and CPSD are the global indices.

Grey scale: Threshold sensitivity values displayed as shades of grey, smoothed with interpolated values between actual test locations.

Long-term fluctuations: True changes in threshold sensitivity overtime, after removal of variability due to single measurement error.

Macular test: A pattern for threshold testing that includes the foveal point and 16 locations, 2 degree apart in a 4 × 4 grid centering on the point of fixation. In the HFA-1, each point is tested in triplicate and the HFA-1 non-SITA strategies, each point is tested twice.

Mean deviation (MD): The weighted average of the total deviation values in a visual field tests. Deviations near the center of the field are counted more heavily than those at the edge.

Overview printout: Summary printout in which the whole series of test results are shown chronologically. Grey scale, threshold value map, total deviation probability map and pattern deviation probability plot for each field are displayed in a horizontal plot along with reliability parameters, global indices and foveal threshold.

Pattern deviation decibel and probability plots: Display of localized loss of each test points after removal of effects of any generalized loss. Pattern deviation dB values are the total deviation dB values minus the general height. The pattern deviation probability map highlights locations where deviation exceeds those found in fewer than 5%, 2%, 1% or 0.5% of normal sensitivity.

Pattern standard deviation (PSD): The global indices that represents the standard deviation around the mean of total deviation. It is the index of localized field loss.

Short-term fluctuation: The test–re-test (the intra-test) variability of the threshold sensitivity values obtained on repeat testing within the same testing session, representing measurement error, SF is expressed as the standard deviation of distribution of repeat values obtained on replicate testing at a location of visual field.

Short wavelength automated perimetry (SWAP): Test that isolates the blue-sensitive portion of the visual system for testing, also known as blue-yellow perimetry.

Single field analysis: Basic STATPAC display of the results of a single field examination, showing threshold sensitivity values, reliability parameters, global indices and the statistical calculations to compare the results with the range of values expected from the eyes with no ocular disease.

STATPAC: Trademark for Humphrey software that performs a series of statistical calculations on the visual field results, with displays that include single field analysis, change analysis, glaucoma change probability and overview printouts.

Swedish interactive thresholding algorithm (SITA): Recently available strategy to measure the threshold sensitivity and reliability parameters efficiently, to achieve optimal measurements with minimal time.

Total deviation value and probability maps: The total deviation decibel values are the difference between the measured threshold sensitivity and age-corrected normal sensitivity at each location. The total deviation probability map highlights locations where deviation exceeds those found in fewer than 5%, 2%, 1% or 0.5% of normal.

Index

E

F

G

T

U

V

Y

Z